Workbook to Accompany
Mosby's

PARAMEDIC TEXTBOOK

Third Edition

About the Authors

Kim D. McKenna, RN, BSN, CEN, EMT-P is the Director of Education for the St. Charles County Ambulance District, located in the metropolitan St. Louis, Missouri area. For 6 years Kim served as the Chief Medical Officer for the Florissant Valley Fire Protection District in Florissant, Missouri. Kim has been involved in prehospital education since 1985. She has served the EMS community through active participation on the board, ad hoc committees, and as chair of the Publications Committee of the National Association of EMS Educators.

Mick J. Sanders, MSA, EMT-P received his paramedic training in 1978 from St. Louis University Hospitals. He earned a Bachelor of Science degree in 1982 and a Master of Science degree in 1983 from Lindenwood College in St. Charles, Missouri. He has worked in various health care systems as a field paramedic, emergency department paramedic, and EMS instructor. For 12 years, Mr. Sanders served as Training Specialist with the Bureau of Emergency Medical Services, Missouri Department of Health, where he oversaw EMT and paramedic training and licensure in St. Louis City and the surrounding metropolitan area.

Workbook to Accompany
Mosby's

PARAMEDIC TEXTBOOK

Third Edition

Kim D. McKenna, RN, BSN, CEN, EMT-P

Director of Education
St. Charles County Ambulance District
St. Peters, Missouri

Mick J. Sanders, MSA, EMT-P

EMS Training Specialist
St. Charles, Missouri

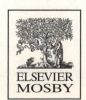

ELSEVIER
MOSBY

ELSEVIER
MOSBY

11830 Westline Industrial Drive
St. Louis, Missouri 63146

Notice

Knowledge and best practice in this field are constantly changing. As new research and experience broaden our knowledge, changes in practice, treatment and drug therapy may become necessary or appropriate. Readers are advised to check the most current information provided (i) on procedures featured or (ii) by the manufacturer of each product to be administered, to verify the recommended dose or formula, the method and duration of administration, and contraindications. It is the responsibility of the practitioner, relying on their own experience and knowledge of the patient, to make diagnoses, to determine dosages and the best treatment for each individual patient, and to take all appropriate safety precautions. To the fullest extent of the law, neither the Publisher nor the authors assumes any liability for any injury and/or damage to persons or property arising out or related to any use of the material contained in this book.

Acquisitions Editor: Linda Honeycutt
Development Editor: Laura Bayless
Publishing Services Manager: Julie Eddy
Project Manager: Rich Barber

Printed in the United States

Last digit is the print number: 9 8 7 6 5 4 3 2 1

To my children—Ginny, Becky, Maggie, Grant—and to my husband, Don.

Thanks for helping me remember to enjoy life.

KDM

Preface

The *Workbook to Accompany Mosby's Paramedic Textbook,* third edition, has been written to enhance the paramedic student's understanding and retention of the material presented in the textbook. This has been accomplished using a variety of questions designed to encourage the various levels of learning necessary in this field, from recall and memorization to application of concepts. Some of the features of this workbook include the following:

- A special section on studying and test-taking skills (see p. viii) so that good habits can begin early in the program
- A format that follows *Mosby's Paramedic Textbook,* third edition, chapter by chapter, with answers referenced to the appropriate objective
- Summaries from the textbook chapters to refresh key information
- An entirely new *Wrap It Up* section in each chapter that offers an additional opportunity to use learning in context
- Matching questions that reinforce key terms or content within the chapters
- Extensive use of case study–based questions to help visualize the real-life application of information
- Self-assessment sections that offer the opportunity to review material using multiple-choice questions, a testing format often used by instructors for examinations
- Complete rationale for all answers that ensures understanding of material
- A programmed review of basic math skills that precedes the drug dose calculation section
- Illustrations for student identification of anatomy, patient management techniques, and special equipment
- Paramedic career opportunities section (see p. xi) that introduces some of the choices in the paramedic profession

Electrocardiogram and drug flashcards at the end of the book can be removed for easy reference and study purposes. Flashcards are completed by the students and are keyed to questions in the workbook. The electrocardiogram flashcards show actual patient rhythms, and the drug flashcards are based on patient care scenarios. Three blank drug flashcards will allow students to create cards for regional drugs.

Before completing each chapter of the workbook, you should read the accompanying chapter in *Mosby's Paramedic Textbook,* third edition, and review the learning objectives. When you encounter areas of difficulty while completing the questions, reread the text and attempt the questions again. We hope that this workbook, when used effectively, will facilitate mastery of the complex knowledge necessary to become a paramedic. Enjoy!

Acknowledgments

This workbook, of course, would never have been possible without the terrific manuscript of *Mosby's Paramedic Textbook,* third edition, written by Mick J. Sanders. His commitment to excellence is reflected throughout the text, and his encouragement and suggestions made the completion of the workbook possible.

Many thanks to Catherine Parvensky, who wrote the studying and test-taking tips and the paramedic career opportunities sections of the workbook.

For the original patient electrocardiogram strips, I am indebted to the staff of the intensive care unit and especially to my former colleagues in the emergency department at St. John's Mercy Medical Center. A debt of gratitude goes to Gary Denton of Acute Coronary Syndrome Consultants, Inc., and to Wolff Medical Publishing, Inc. for the 12-lead electrocardiogram tracings included in this edition of the text.

To all of my paramedic students, past and present, I sincerely appreciate all that you have taught me and your suggestions for the content of this workbook.

And to the fellow paramedics and EMTs with whom I work in the field, thanks for showing me where the textbook ends and reality begins.

I am also grateful to the reviewers of this and past editons: Bob Nixon, BA, EMT-P; Monroe Yancie, NREMT-P; Jeff DeGraffenreid, Johnson County Medical Action Emergency Medical Services, Olathe, Kansas; and Janet Fitts, RN, EMT-P for their suggestions and fresh ideas.

Thanks to the staff at Elsevier, especially Laura Bayless, who worked so diligently to make this project happen; to Rich Barber whose attention to detail is evident throughout the text; and to Joy Knobel in Marketing who cheered us all on. We are forever grateful.

Kim D. McKenna
Mick J. Sanders

Study Tips

For all the emphasis placed on furthering education, little guidance is given for how to be a good student. Learning the following studying and test-taking tips can help you get the most out of your paramedic course and other classes in the future.

STUDY SESSIONS

The way that an individual studies may determine the likelihood of successful completion of a training program. You need to develop a routine pattern for studying and stick to it. The following are methods to increase the effectiveness of study sessions:

- Set a regular time for studying each day.
- Pace yourself by scheduling a specific amount of time for each subject or chapter.
- Take periodic breaks to prevent burnout.
- Read lesson information before each session and review notes immediately after the class.
- Do not wait until the last minute and expect to cram information and do well. Instead, pace yourself throughout the course.
  - Be aware of distractions, internal and external.
  - Internal distractions include hunger, tension, fatigue, illness, glucose levels, and daydreaming and getting sidetracked.
  - External distractions include room temperature (hot or cold), noise levels, and lighting.
- Make a game of it; drill the information by using the following:
  - Flash cards for memorizing facts
  - Jeopardy cards
  - Trivial Pursuit cards
- When frustration sets in, do the following:
  - Take a break.
  - Have a snack. (Sugar helps.)
  - Take a walk. (Increased cardiovascular activity increases blood flow to the brain.)
  - Take a few deep breaths and relax.

WHERE AND WHEN DO YOU STUDY BEST?

Everyone has a particular time and place in which they are most productive. For some it is late at night, and for others it is early in the morning. Determine when you are at your peak and study daily at that time.

- Where do you do the best work?
  - At a desk or table?
  - In front of the television? (Some people need background noise to focus.)
- Decide whether you work better studying alone or in work groups. Sometimes, work sessions are a great motivation for studying.

- Decide what form of studying works best for you:
  - Writing notes from the book
  - Highlighting information in the book
  - Taking copious notes
  - Listening to the instructor and asking questions

INCREASING RETENTION

There are many ways to increase retention of material, including association, mnemonics, imagery, and recitation. Try them all and see what works best for you:

Association—Relate information to something you understand. Build new information on what is already known.

Mnemonics—Use letters or words to remember facts. For example, use "AVPU" to determine a patient's level of consciousness: *A*lert, *V*erbal, *P*ainful stimuli, or *U*nconscious.

Imagery—Visualize a picture of the information. Memorize a chart or picture of the body and associated organs, and then remember that picture for questions on anatomy.

Recitation—Read notes out loud or discuss the information with peers. Hearing information repeatedly helps retention.

TEST-TAKING TIPS

Test taking is a skill that can be learned. Most state examinations are multiple-choice questions and are graded solely on the number of correct answers. There is no penalty for guessing, so do not leave any questions unanswered because they will be marked incorrect.

Multiple-choice questions are made up of two parts: the stem (question) and possible answers. These types of questions can be factual or situational:

Factual: During one-person cardiopulmonary resuscitation, the ratio of compressions to ventilations is
a. 15 to 2
b. 5 to 1
c. 10 per minute
d. 20 per minute

Situational: A 55-year-old man was shoveling his driveway when he developed shortness of breath and pain in the middle of his chest. He is most likely suffering from which of the following?
a. Myocardial infarction
b. Congestive heart failure
c. Emphysema
d. Angina pectoris

When answering a question, thoroughly analyze it. To accomplish this, do the following:
- Read the stem without looking at the answers. Evaluate the question, looking for key words such as *not, except, first,* or *final.*
- Identify key content words such as *one rescuer, adult victim, radiating pain, slurred speech,* or *conscious victim.*
- Think of a correct answer and then look at all the choices to see whether your answer is there. If not, find the next *best answer.*
- Do not read into the question.
- Eliminate obviously wrong answers and select from those remaining.
- Do not change answers. Your first hunch is usually correct.

PREPARING FOR TESTS

You can take some simple steps to prepare yourself for a test:
- Get a good night's sleep before the examination.
- Avoid milk products because they tend to induce sleep.
- Eat a good meal but not too much before the examination. (Blood flow is forced to the digestive tract the first hour after eating a large meal, which tends to induce sleep.)

- Exercise moderately to increase blood supply to the brain.
- Layer clothes so that you can add or remove layers as necessary to be comfortable during the examination.
- Use a wristwatch to pace yourself.
- Sit away from friends or other distractions.
- Be prepared and be positive. If you have studied properly, you know the material and will do well on the examination.

STRATEGIES FOR INCREASING TESTING PERFORMANCE

If you use the following strategies, you are sure to improve your performance during tests:
- Pace yourself to make certain that you have enough time to answer all questions.
- Use scrap paper to work through questions.
- At the end, make certain you have answered *all* questions. Do not change answers unless you initially misread the question.
- Make sure that you complete the answer sheet correctly. Fill in circles completely, and do not leave stray marks. Make certain that you check the number on the answer sheet against the number on the test every 10 questions to avoid the unnecessary stress of finding yourself on the wrong line.

Paramedic Career Opportunities

Since its inception in 1967, emergency medical services (EMS) has developed into a sophisticated profession with various levels of care that result in improved care of the sick and injured. With the evolution of EMS have come career opportunities for emergency medical technicians, paramedics, nurses, and physicians. Although specific job opportunities depend on geographical locations, in general, opportunities for prehospital emergency responders have emerged from volunteer to paid career positions. For a certified EMT-Paramedic, many options are available.

OTHER AREAS OF INTEREST

Aside from traditional prehospital roles, some paramedics have taken on expanded duties. Although much controversy has surrounded the use of paramedics within the emergency department, some hospitals in the United States employ paramedics to use their full skills and knowledge. Others may hire them as orderlies, pathology assistants, intravenous team members, phlebotomists, suture technicians, and respiratory therapists.

Some hospitals also have extended emergency departments in which paramedics have an expanded function. These facilities offer treatment for minor illnesses or injuries, physical examinations, and health screenings. They often are located within industrial settings, universities, or stand-alone buildings not part of hospitals.

Finally, paramedics who pursue advanced education can find additional opportunities. Many universities offer credit hours toward a bachelor's degree for any individual with a paramedic certification. For a field paramedic with experience, other advanced opportunities may include training as a nurse or physician's assistant.

POSITION

A *field paramedic* requires current certification as an EMT-Paramedic. Some states and organizations also require National Registry certification.

A *paramedic supervisor* usually requires substantial experience as a field provider and supervisory experience.

A *flight paramedic* usually requires substantial experience as a field provider and the ability to work under pressure. Additional certifications or training may be required by the individual service.

An *interhospital transport medic* usually requires certification/licensure as a paramedic. Additional specialized training may be required or provided by the employer.

An *EMS administrator,* in addition to paramedic certification/licensure, often requires advanced degrees in EMS, business, or health care administration.

An *EMS educator* usually requires paramedic certification and experience as an instructor.

Specialized training in education to meet the minimum requirements set forth by each state usually is needed. Advanced-degree certification often is desired for high-level training programs.

DESCRIPTION

Many paramedics enjoy the day-to-day operations of a field provider, administering emergency care to the sick and injured. Roles and responsibilities of paramedics undoubtedly will grow as the emergency department extends into the community through advanced life support personnel.

An advanced life support supervisor is usually an experienced paramedic with administrative or management skills. Responsibilities for this position generally include recruitment, scheduling, discipline, and supervision of emergency care personnel.

Flight paramedics use their knowledge and skills to care for victims who require air medical evacuation and rapid transport to hospitals. A flight crew usually is composed of a pilot, a flight medic, and a flight nurse. Some organizations hire paramedics to assist with the interhospital, intercontinental, or international transfer of patients requiring monitored transportation. Responsibilities for this position generally include monitoring of patients during transport and initiation of emergency care when necessary. Additional training for specialty skills often is necessary in this role to meet the needs of high-risk infants, children, or other patients who are critically ill or injured.

Experienced paramedics with backgrounds in management can act in administrative capacities within various organizations. Although advanced training often is necessary, administrative positions in hospitals, government emergency services organizations, and independent companies are possibilities.

Many colleges and universities offer programs in EMS, including paramedic certification programs, associate's degrees, bachelor's degrees, and even master's degrees. Paramedics with experience in education can obtain positions as instructors for such programs.

Contents

PART ONE

IN THIS PART

EMS Systems: Roles and Responsibilities

READING ASSIGNMENT

Chapter 1, pages 1-21, in *Mosby's Paramedic Textbook,* ed. 3

OBJECTIVES

Upon completion of this chapter, the paramedic student will be able to do the following:

1. Outline key historical events that influenced the development of emergency medical services (EMS) systems.
2. Identify the key elements necessary for effective EMS systems operations.
3. Differentiate among training and roles and responsibilities of the four nationally recognized levels of EMS licensure/certification: first responder (Emergency Medical Responder), EMT-Basic (Emergency Medical Technician), EMT-Intermediate (Advanced Emergency Medical Technician), and EMT-Paramedic (Paramedic).
4. List the benefits of membership in professional EMS organizations.
5. Describe the benefits of continuing education.
6. Differentiate among professionalism and professional licensure, certification, and registration.
7. Describe the paramedic's role in patient care situations as defined by the U.S. Department of Transportation.
8. Describe the benefits of each component of off-line (indirect) and online (direct) medical direction.
9. Outline the role and components of an effective, continuous quality improvement program.
10. Identify the key components of prehospital research and its benefits to the EMS system.

SUMMARY

- The roots of prehospital emergency care may date back to the military.
- In the early twentieth century through the mid-1960s, prehospital care in the United States was provided in a few ways. Care was provided mostly by urban hospital-based systems. These systems later developed into municipal services. Care also was provided by funeral directors and volunteers who were not trained in these services.
- The operations of an effective EMS system include citizen activation, dispatch, prehospital care, hospital care, and rehabilitation.
- The various levels of providers have their own distinct roles and duties. These roles include telecommunicators (dispatchers), first responders (Emergency Medical Responders [EMR]), EMT-Basics (Emergency Medical Technicians [EMT]), EMT-Intermediates (Advanced Emergency Medical Technicians [AEMT]), and EMT- (Paramedics). These levels combine to make an effective prehospital EMS system.
- Many professional groups and organizations help to set the standards of EMS. These groups exist at the national, state, regional, and local levels. The groups take part in development, education, and implementation. Being active in such a group helps to promote the status of the paramedic.

- Continuing education is crucial. It provides a way for all health care providers to maintain basic technical and professional skills.
- Professionalism refers to the way in which a person conducts himself or herself. Professionalism also refers to how one follows the standards of conduct and performance established by the profession.
- The roles and duties of the paramedic can be divided into two categories. These groups are *primary* and *additional* duties.
- The two types of medical direction are online (direct) and off-line (indirect) medical direction. Both are equally important. They help to ensure that the components of quality medical care are in place in an EMS system.
- A CQI program identifies and attempts to resolve problems in areas such as medical direction, financing, training, communication, prehospital management and transportation, interfacility transfer, receiving facilities, specialty care units, dispatch, public information and education, audit and quality assurance, disaster planning, and mutual aid.
- Quality EMS research helps shed light on the efficacy, effects, and cost-effectiveness of EMS interventions. The research is based on experimental data. Such research can lead to changes in professional standards and training. The research also can lead to changes in equipment and procedures.
- When planning research, the researcher should consider involving an institutional review board.

REVIEW QUESTIONS

1. While working late, a 56-year-old man develops chest pain. The man is alone in his office when the chest pain increases, and he falls to the floor, suffering a cardiac arrest.

    Identify the missing components of the EMS system in Fig. 1-1 that are necessary to effectively resuscitate this victim and return him to a productive role in society.

    a. _Dispatch_

    b. _Advanced Life Support_

    c. _Hospital Delivery_

    d. _Rehabilitation and Education_

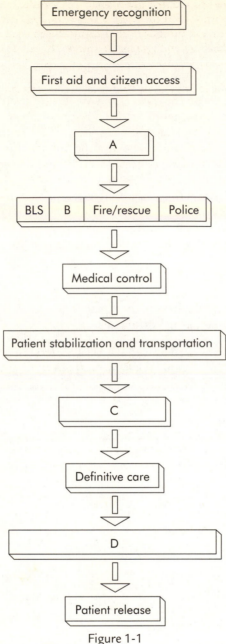

Figure 1-1

Questions 2 and 3 pertain to the following case study:

After attending a continuing education lecture on advances in trauma care, you report to work for your 12-hour shift. You carefully check out your vehicle for equipment and mechanical readiness for a call and then head to the company fitness room to exercise. Just as you finish your workout, the tones sound. You are dispatched to a nursing home for a person with "difficulty breathing." The street alarm is activated, and as you pull out, you carefully glance to ensure that traffic has come to a stop before proceeding onto the busy roadway in front of your station. Upon arrival at the nursing home, you obtain a rapid history from the nursing home staff and begin your assessment of the 87-year-old patient. She is in obvious respiratory distress, and you recognize the need for rapid interventions to prevent further deterioration of her condition. Your partner administers oxygen and prepares to insert an intravenous (IV) line as you contact on-line medical direction. You briefly describe your patient's condition and request orders for nitroglycerin and furosemide. The physician advisor agrees with your treatment plan. As soon as your partner secures the IV line, you administer the drugs, carefully checking for allergies and appropriate dosing before giving them. A repeat assessment of the patient in 5 minutes shows some improvement. You continue plans to transfer her into the ambulance. The nursing home staff tells you she should be transported to the city hospital. This is consistent with your medical protocols, so you agree. As you depart, another evaluation demonstrates even more improvement. On arrival at the hospital, you give a report and transfer care of the patient to the nursing staff and then complete your patient report. You ask the physician about another drug that you had considered requesting, but she agrees that in this patient's circumstance, the treatment plan you had chosen was appropriate. Back at base, you restock the vehicle with the drugs and equipment used on the call. Then you head down to the classroom to help teach the 8 pm community cardiopulmonary resuscitation (CPR) class.

2. List 10 primary responsibilities of the paramedic that were demonstrated in this simulated call.

a. Physical preparedness for the Job

b. Having appropriate supplies

c. Responding in a safe manner

d. Performing quick pt assessment

e. Contacting med control for opinion on care plan

f. Handling emergency appropriately

g. Stabilizing pt in the field

h. Transporting to appropriate facility.

i. Giving pt report

j. Replacing equipment and debriefing the call

3. List two additional responsibilities of the paramedic that were demonstrated in this scenario.

a.

b.

Match the historical role in EMS in column I with the appropriate person or event in column II. Use each answer only once.

Column I	Column II
4. __c__ First use of helicopter for medical evacuation during an armed conflict.	**a.** American Red Cross
5. __f__ Demonstrated the value of mouth-to-mouth ventilation.	**b.** Belfast, 1966
6. __g__ Twentieth century battlefield ambulance corps developed.	**c.** Korean conflict
7. __B__ Dr. Eugene Nagel trains firefighters as paramedics.	**d.** Miami, 1967
8. ___ Earliest documented mobile coronary unit performs prehospital defibrillation.	**e.** Napoleonic Wars
9. __A__ Clara Barton performs battlefield emergency medical care and brings this organization to the United States.	**f.** Peter Safar, MD, 1958
10. __e__ Jean Larry transports wounded in covered cart.	**g.** World War I
11. __h__ Fixed-wing medical transports were developed in this conflict.	**h.** World War II
	i. Vietnam conflict

Match the description in column I with the appropriate licensure and certification level in column II. Use each answer only once.

Column I	Column II
12. __A__ Trained in basic life support, including defibrillation	**a.** EMT-B (EMT)
13. __C__ Trained in all aspects of basic and advanced life support	**b.** EMT-I (AEMT)
14. __B__ Trained in all aspects of basic life support and IV therapy	**c.** EMT-P (Paramedic)
	d. First responder (Emergency Medical Responder)

Match the activity in column I with the appropriate term in column II. You may use each term *more* than once.

Column I

15. _____ Education and training of EMS personnel
16. _____ Personnel selection for employment
17. _c_ Appropriate equipment choice selection
18. _c_ Clinical protocol guidance and direction
19. _____ Clinical problem resolution
20. _____ Interface among EMS systems
21. _____ Advocacy within medical community
22. _c_ On-line communication with physicians and EMS
23. _b_ Patient care report reviews
24. _____ Establish standards of care
25. _____ Serve as resource experts
26. _A_ Introduction of new information

Column II

a. Continuing education
b. Continuous quality improvement
c. Medical direction
d. Professional associations

Questions 27 to 35 pertain to the following research abstract, which was published in *Prehospital Emergency Care,* 2(3), 1998. Read the abstract carefully and then answer each question.

Efficacy of Midazolam for Facilitated Intubation by Paramedics

Authors: Edward T. Dickinson, MD, NREMT-P
Jason E. Cohen, BA, EMT-P
C. Crawford Mechem, MD

Affiliation: Department of Emergency Medicine, University of Pennsylvania School of Medicine, Philadelphia, Pennsylvania

Objective: The use of pharmacological agents by paramedics to facilitate endotracheal intubation (ETI) is becoming increasingly common. This study was done to determine the efficacy of intravenous midazolam, a short-acting benzodiazepine, as a drug to facilitate ETI in patients resistant to conventional ETI.

Methods: The study was conducted in a suburban municipal EMS system over a 22-month period. All paramedics were trained in the use of midazolam for facilitated intubation prior to allowing the use of midazolam in the system. All calls in which midazolam was used were reviewed on a monthly basis by investigators via retrospective review of the prehospital care reports.

Results: During the study period, 13,212 emergency responses occurred, resulting in 154 ETIs by paramedics. Midazolam was used to facilitate 20 (13%) of these ETIs. "Clenched teeth" and failed intubation attempt were the most commonly cited indications for facilitated intubation. Eleven patients had medical complaints, and nine were trauma patients. Successful ETI with midazolam was achieved in 17 of 20 (85%) cases. In 88% (15 of 17) of these cases, a single dose of midazolam was sufficient for ETI; mean dose 3.6 mg (standard deviation [SD] 1.1 mg). The three patients with failed ETI received multiple doses of midazolam; mean dose 5 mg (SD 2 mg).

Conclusion: The prehospital use of single-dose IV midazolam is generally effective in accomplishing facilitated ETI in patients resistant to conventional (nonpharmacological) endotracheal intubation.

27. What was the purpose of this study (i.e., what problem or question are the authors trying to solve)?

_____

_____

28. Is the hypothesis stated in this abstract? _____ If you answered yes, what is it? If you answered no, what do you think it is?

_____

29. What is the study population?

_____

30. What are the sample and sample size for this research?

_____

31. Was a random sampling procedure used? Yes/No Explain your answer.

_____

32. Did this study use a qualitative or quantitative approach?

_____

33. The study indicates a standard deviation for the mean dose of 1.1 mg. What does that mean?

_____

34. What are some weaknesses or unanswered questions related to this research?

_____

35. Are the findings of this study important to the EMS community?

_____

STUDENT SELF-ASSESSMENT

36. Which federal law enabled creation of the U.S. Department of Transportation and the National Highway Traffic Safety Administration and provided funding for EMS?
   a. Accidental Death and Disability Act
   b. Consolidated Omnibus Reconciliation Act
   c. Emergency Medical Services Systems Act
   d. Highway Safety Act

37. Which of the following is _not_ a component of the EMS system?
   a. Disaster planning   **c.** Intensive care units
   b. Insurance providers   **d.** Paramedic training

38. How has health care reform affected emergency medical services?
   a. It results in larger reimbursement amounts for each call.
   b. It may increase the distance for transport based on insurance restrictions for hospitals.
   c. It has caused a decrease in emergency ambulance transports.
   d. It will restrict the scope of practice for the EMS provider.

39. Which of the following describes the manner in which a paramedic follows the practice, guidelines, and ethical considerations of prehospital emergency care?
   a. Certification   **c.** Professionalism
   b. Licensure   **d.** Registration

40. Which of the following is _not_ a role of the paramedic as defined by the U.S. Department of Transportation?
   a. Assessing and providing emergency patient care
   b. Coordinating collection of outstanding patient bills
   c. Documenting and communicating patient care
   d. Making sure the ambulance is adequately stocked

41. The EMS physician medical director is responsible for which of the following:
   a. Ensuring maintenance of ambulances and equipment
   b. Monitoring the quality of EMS care
   c. Negotiating staff salary and benefit disputes
   d. Providing patient care in the field on advanced life-support units

42. A man who claims to be an emergency department physician is attempting to direct care in an inappropriate manner on a cardiac arrest call. You should do which of the following:
   a. Contact on-line medical direction for instructions
   b. Follow his orders because he has appropriate credentials

   c. Ignore him and carry on as you see appropriate

   d. Immediately ask the police to arrest him

43. Which of the following demonstrates a prospective method of a continuous quality improvement model?

   a. Continuing education programs

   b. Listening to audio tapes of EMS reports

   c. Observation of prehospital care by the medical director

   d. Reviewing prehospital patient care records

44. You are conducting research for a drug to treat cardiac arrest. Only you and your partner have been trained to gather the data, so the drug will be used only on days that you work. This type of subject selection is called which of the following:

   a. Alternative time sampling   **c.** Statistical table sampling

   b. Convenience sampling   **d.** Systemic sampling

45. You are doing a study on the variability of scene response times according to time of day. Here are the data you collected (in minutes) for one group: 1, 2, 3, 4, 4, 4, 4, 4, 5, 5, 5, 5, 6, 6, 6, 7, 7, 8, 9. What is the mode for this set of data?

   a. 4

   b. 5

   c. 6

   d. 7

46. Before your research is approved by an institutional review board, what must you prove?

   a. Consent will be obtained.

   b. The hypothesis is true.

   c. No risks will be incurred.

   d. Your sample is large enough.

WRAP IT UP

Your rural EMS service responds to a call for a vehicle accident with possible rescue. Your ambulance arrives on the scene first, and you provide the scene size-up on the radio for the incoming units: "4017 on the scene, two vehicles involved, major damage, investigating." A bystander shouts to you that he called 9-1-1 on his cell phone and that there is a guy "hurt real bad" in one of the cars. You and your EMT partner split up, going to separate cars to triage the injured. Major damage to the car prevents access through the doors, so you break a window to gain access. The driver, an unrestrained teenage boy, has trauma to the head. He is taking agonal gasps and has a rapid radial pulse. You shout to your partner that you have a critical patient and immediately call dispatch to send a helicopter and a second ambulance. As you begin to manage the patient's airway and to ventilate him, the rescue pumper arrives. Your partner tells you that there are two patients in the second car: a woman with minor lacerations and her 9-year-old daughter, who has significant cervical spine tenderness and is hysterical. The second ambulance crew arrives, and you tell them that extrication is needed. You direct the paramedic on the rescue pumper to manage the two patients in the second car while you and your partner care for your critically injured patient as extrication efforts proceed. Your patient has apparent head, chest, and abdominal injuries. Dispatch notifies you that the helicopter has a 2-minute estimated time of arrival (ETA). Police have blocked the highway for safety and are assisting with the landing zone. Moments before the helicopter lands, rescue crews remove the car door, and you perform rapid extrication. You carefully move the patient to the spine board, secure him, and move him to your ambulance. With your partner's assistance, you intubate the patient using in-line spinal immobilization. Then, as your partner ventilates the patient, you initiate an IV line while firefighters assist with monitoring and assessment of vital signs. The air medical crew arrives. You give them a rapid, thorough report and direct them to take the patient to the closest level I trauma center. The rescue pumper paramedic reports that the two patients from the second vehicle are being transported by ground past the local hospital to the trauma center. You quickly clean your rig and return in service to the station to write your patient care report.

1. What role did citizens play in this call?

_____

2. What steps did dispatch take to coordinate the activities in this call?

_____

3. What role, if any, did medical direction play in this call?

_____

4. Why was the use of the helicopter indicated in this situation when the other two patients were taken by ground to the same facility?
   a. The male patient needed intubation.
   b. The ETA of the second ambulance was delayed.
   c. Prolonged extrication was needed.
   d. Multiple trauma patients were involved.
5. Why were the patients taken to the trauma center rather than a closer hospital?
   a. Definitive care is rapidly available for the trauma patient at a trauma center.
   b. Mileage charges are greater to a more distant hospital.
   c. Helicopters transport only to trauma centers.
   d. Local hospitals have poorer quality of care.
6. Why were you performing the advanced skills on this call rather than your partner?
   a. The attending paramedic always performs the skills.
   b. The first person reaching the patient performs invasive skills.
   c. Your partner is an EMT, and these skills exceed his license in many states.
   d. The most experienced crew member is designated to perform skills.
7. Rank the attributes of the professional paramedic that you think would be most important on this call from 1 to 11, with 1 the most important and 11 the least important.
   _____ Integrity   _____ Empathy
   _____ Self-motivation   _____ Appearance and personal hygiene
   _____ Self-confidence   _____ Communication
   _____ Time management   _____ Teamwork and diplomacy
   _____ Respect   _____ Patient advocacy
   _____ Careful delivery of service
8. Would your rankings from the question above change for the following situations? If you answer yes, indicate how they would change.
   a. A 75-year-old patient who is despondent over the loss of his wife is threatening to kill himself. Yes/No

_____

_____

   b. A 27-year-old woman has just miscarried a 20-week pregnancy; this is her sixth miscarriage in 2 years. Yes/No

_____

_____

   c. A 54-year-old patient in the mayor's chambers has chest pain, and electrocardiogram (ECG) readings suggest a heart attack. He does not want to be transported to the hospital. Yes/No

_____

_____

9. Place a ✔ beside the roles/responsibilities of the paramedic used on this call.
   _____ Preparation   _____ Response
   _____ Scene assessment   _____ Patient assessment
   _____ Recognition of injury or illness _____ Patient management
   _____ Appropriate patient disposition   _____ Patient transfer
   _____ Documentation   _____ Returning to service

CHAPTER 1 ANSWERS

REVIEW QUESTIONS

1. a. Dispatcher; b. Advanced life support; c. Hospital delivery; d. Patient rehabilitation and education
   (Objective 2)

2. a. Physical preparation for the job (exercise program)
   b. Having appropriate equipment and supplies
   c. Responding to the scene in a safe manner
   d. Performing a quick patient assessment to determine priorities for care
   e. Contacting medical direction for assistance with the care plan
   f. Managing the emergency in the appropriate manner
   g. Stabilizing the patient in the field
   h. Providing transport by the appropriate means to the correct facility
   i. Reporting to the staff regarding the patient's condition on arrival
   j. Replacing equipment and debriefing the call
   (Objective 7)

3. a. Advocating citizens' role in the EMS system by teaching community programs such as CPR.
   b. Continuing personal professional development by attending continuing education programs
   (Objective 7)

4. c
5. f
6. g
7. d
8. b
9. a
10. e
11. h
    (Questions 4-11: Objective 1)

12. a or d
13. c
14. b
    (Questions 12-14: Objective 3)

15. a, b, c, d
16. c
17. a, b, c
18. b, c, d
19. a, b, c, d
20. c, d
21. c, d
22. b, c
23. b, c
24. b, c, d
25. c, d
26. a, c, d
    (Questions 15-26: Objectives 4, 5, 8, 9)

27. To determine the efficacy of IV midazolam to aid in prehospital intubations that failed conventional methods
28. No. No hypothesis is stated. The hypothesis could have been that the use of midazolam will facilitate intubation in patients who could not be intubated by conventional means.

29. The study population is the 154 ETIs that occurred within the study period.
30. The sample is the patients who could not be intubated by conventional means (sample size is 20 patients).
31. No. Random sampling was not done. All patients who met the criterion (failed intubation) were included.
32. Descriptive statistics were used to report the findings in this quantitative paper.
33. This means that about 65% of the patients received 3.6 mg ± 1.1 mg of midazolam in the successful ETI group.
34. Many other things could be considered. For example, did the age of the patients affect the success? Were the missed patients trauma or medical patients, and did that influence success rates? Is 20 a large enough sample size to make a broad generalization to all EMS patients? What was the experience level of the paramedics in the "success" group versus the "fail" group?
35. The use of any drug is associated with potential risks and complications. Objective data on the effectiveness of drugs, especially in the unique prehospital environment, support the standards and practice of paramedic care. (Questions 27-35: Objective 10)

STUDENT SELF-ASSESSMENT

36. d. This act, passed in 1966, required states to develop effective EMS programs or lose federal construction funds. It enabled large amounts of money to be spent for development of EMS and advanced life support (ALS) pilot programs. Accidental Death and Disability: the Neglected Disease of Modern Society (the "white" paper) was not an act but a report published by the National Academy of Sciences–National Research Council through its Committee on Trauma and Shock. The committee's recommendations paved the way for the Highway Safety Act of 1966. The EMSS act of 1973 developed regional EMS organizations. It identified 15 required components of the EMS system. The Consolidated Omnibus Reconciliation Act (COBRA) eliminated federal funds for EMS and redistributed them under state block grants.
(Objective 1)

37. b. Although insurance reimbursement is necessary for many EMS systems to operate, the insurance providers are not considered a part of the system.
(Objective 2)

38. b. Patients' health plans now often restrict their choice of hospitals. Except in life-threatening emergencies, patients must seek care from their preferred provider or lose reimbursement. In some places this has resulted in expanded transport areas if EMS agencies are to meet the needs of the health care consumers they serve. Generally, the health care changes have resulted in decreases rather than increases in reimbursement.
(Objective 2)

39. c. Certification authorizes a person who has met specific qualifications to participate in an activity. Licensure grants a license to practice a profession. Registration is the act of enrolling a person's name in a book of record.
(Objective 6)

40. b. Although this role may fall to the paramedic in some systems, it is not defined by the government as an integral role.
(Objective 3)

41. b. Other personnel should assume patient care and administrative and maintenance duties. The primary role of the EMS physician medical director is to ensure quality patient care.
(Objective 8)

42. a. On-line medical direction should be contacted to attempt to arbitrate the situation. If this is impossible, police intervention may be recommended. Written policies addressing this issue should be prepared by the medical director so that actions to be taken in this situation are clearly defined.
(Objective 8)

43. a. The continuing education program can be offered to introduce new material, concepts, or skills so that appropriate patient care is delivered when that knowledge or skill is needed. This is done to ensure quality before a problem occurs. Direct observation of care is a concurrent method of CQI, and review of records and tapes is done after the actual care is delivered (retrospectively).
(Objective 9)

44. b. Alternative time sampling selects participants based on a predetermined time interval (e.g., day of the week, month). Sampling using a statistical table involves selection of patients based on a table that predetermines which patient will be following a selected protocol. Systemic sampling enrolls patients in the order in which they are encountered. For example, it may be established that every other patient encountered gets the test intervention.
(Objective 10)

45. a. The number 4 occurs most frequently. The *mean,* or average of the sum of the times, is 5, as is the *median,* or middle of the group.
(Objective 10)

46. a. Although traditional informed consent is not always possible, an acceptable alternative must be demonstrated to the IRB before your project is approved. The purpose of the research is to prove or disprove the hypothesis; this can be determined only after the study is completed. If risks are associated with the research, you must demonstrate that the potential benefit of the study warrants the risk. The primary responsibility of the IRB is to consider ethical, not procedural, issues with the research.
(Objective 11)

WRAP IT UP

1. Citizens recognized the emergency, called 9-1-1, and provided information to responding EMS units.
(Objective 2)

2. Dispatch identified the nature of the emergency, dispatched the proper apparatus to the correct location, dispatched the helicopter and an additional ambulance when directed, and updated the scene crew on the status of the helicopter.
(Objective 2)

3. Although no on-line medical direction was identified on this call, undoubtedly the crews notified on-line medical direction of their status. In addition, on-line medical direction should have had a role in determining the treatment protocols used, the protocol for using air medical services, and the protocol determining use of the trauma center. Medical direction also should be involved in a review of the call at a later time to monitor quality of care.
(Objective 8)

4. c. Most systems provide for dispatch of air medical crews when prolonged extrication is likely and the patient's condition warrants it. In other situations, even when the patient's condition is critical, the time to the appropriate hospital and other factors would be considered and should be established by protocol in collaboration with medical direction.
(Objective 2)

5. a. Protocols should define when patients are taken to a trauma center. Typically these are based on the mechanism of injury, the anatomical injuries involved, and the patient's physiological status. Definitive care (surgery) for the trauma can be most effectively delivered at a trauma center, where appropriate resources (personnel and equipment) are readily available.
(Objective 2)

6. c. In many states, advanced invasive skills such as intubation and vascular access are not within the scope of practice of an EMT.
(Objective 3)

7. Responses will vary by individual opinion; however, careful delivery of service, time management, self-confidence, and communication likely would rank very high on this type of call.
(Objective 6)

8. All attributes are critical for the paramedic; however, responses will vary by individual opinion. The following attributes are more likely to be ranked higher.
   a. Yes. Communication, respect, empathy, and patient advocacy
   b. Yes. Empathy, respect, and careful delivery of service
   c. Yes. Careful delivery of service, communication, teamwork and diplomacy, and appearance and personal hygiene.
   (Objective 6)

9. All of these roles and responsibilities are used on this call.
(Objective 7)

The Well-Being of the Paramedic

READING ASSIGNMENT
Chapter 2, pages 22-41, in *Mosby's Paramedic Textbook,* ed. 3

OBJECTIVES
Upon completion of this chapter, the paramedic student will be able to do the following:
1. Describe the components of wellness and associated benefits.
2. Discuss the paramedic's role in promoting wellness.
3. Outline the benefits of specific lifestyle choices that promote wellness, including proper nutrition, weight control, exercise, sleep, and smoking cessation.
4. Identify risk factors and warning signs of cancer and cardiovascular disease.
5. Identify preventive measures to minimize the risk of work-related illness or injury associated with exposure, lifting and moving patients, hostile environments, vehicle operations, and rescue situations.
6. List signs and symptoms of addiction and addictive behavior.
7. Distinguish between normal and abnormal anxiety and stress reactions.
8. Give examples of stress-reduction techniques.
9. Outline the 10 components of critical incident stress management.
10. Given a scenario involving death or dying, identify therapeutic actions you may take based on your knowledge of the dynamics of this process.
11. List measures to take to reduce the risk of infectious disease exposure.
12. Outline actions to be taken following a significant exposure to a patient's blood or other body fluids.

SUMMARY
- Wellness has two main aspects: physical well-being and mental and emotional health.
- As health care professionals, paramedics have a responsibility to serve as role models in disease prevention.
- Physical fitness can be described as a condition that helps individuals look, feel, and do their best.
- Sleep helps to rejuvenate a tired body.
- Steps to reduce cardiovascular disease include the following: improving cardiovascular endurance, eliminating cigarette smoking, controlling high blood pressure, maintaining a normal body-fat composition, maintaining good total cholesterol/high-density lipoprotein ratio, monitoring triglyceride levels, controlling diabetes, avoiding excessive alcohol, eating healthy foods, reducing stress, and making a periodic risk assessment.
- Most common cancers are linked to one of three environmental risk factors: smoking, sunlight, and diet.

- Injuries on the job can be minimized. Knowledge of body mechanics during lifting and moving is helpful. Also, being alert for hostile settings is key. Prioritization of personal safety during rescue situations is wise. In addition, paramedics must practice safe vehicle operations. They must use safety equipment and supplies as well.
- The misuse and abuse of drugs and other substances may lead to chemical dependency (addiction). This may have a wide range of effects on physical and mental health.
- "Good" stress is eustress. Eustress is a positive response to stimuli and is considered protective. "Bad" stress is distress. Distress is a negative response to environmental stimuli and is the source of anxiety and stress-related disorders.
- Adaptation is a process where persons learn effective ways to deal with stressful situations. This dynamic process usually begins with using defense mechanisms. Next, one develops coping skills, followed by problem solving, and culminating in mastery.
- Critical incident stress management is designed to help emergency personnel understand their reactions. The process reassures them that what they are experiencing is normal and may be common to others involved in the incident.
- Often news of a sudden death must be given to a family. The paramedic's initial contact can influence the grief process greatly.
- The paramedic's duty is to be familiar with laws, regulations, and national standards that address issues of infectious disease. The paramedic also must take personal protective measures to guard against exposure.
- Actions to take after a significant exposure include disinfection, documentation, incident investigation, screening, immunization, and medical follow-up.

REVIEW QUESTIONS

Complete the following table to describe your wellness behaviors, analyze risks or benefits associated with those behaviors, and identify opportunities to improve them.

Behavior	Current practice	Risk/benefit of this behavior	Improvement plan
Diet (fats, vitamins, carbohydrates)			
Weight			
Cardiovascular endurance			
Strength/flexibility			
Sleep (hours/day)			

Continued

Behavior	Current practice	Risk/benefit of this behavior	Improvement plan
Cardiovascular disease risk factors			
Cancer risk factors			
Injury prevention			
Substance abuse			
Smoking			

Match the defense mechanism in column II with the appropriate example in column I. Use each defense mechanism only once.

Column I

1. **h** A rape victim who cannot recall anything from the time she was abducted until the police find her
2. **e** A paramedic who, when passed over for a promotion, states that the boss always plays favorites
3. **i** A paramedic who is upset by a violent death and washes all the vehicles in the garage
4. **B** A victim of an automobile accident who refuses to acknowledge that he cannot move his legs
5. **D** An EMT who gave poor care, yet complains about the patient's hospital treatment
6. **g** A 10-year-old who begins to suck his thumb en route to the hospital after sustaining a fracture from a fall

Column II

a. Compensation
b. Denial
c. Isolation
d. Projection
e. Rationalization
f. Reaction formation
g. Regression
h. Repression
i. Substitution

Questions 7 to 11 pertain to the following case study:

You respond to a call for an assault. Police on the scene tell you that an 18-year-old man has been stabbed. You find the patient, who turns out to be your nephew, at a party on the fourth floor of an apartment complex that has no working elevators. The patient is alert and crying and has a briskly bleeding puncture wound in the midaxillary line. He complains of having severe difficulty breathing and abdominal pain, and he has a rapid radial pulse. Oxygen is administered, and as you prepare for rapid transport and treatment, some party goers begin to get belligerent.

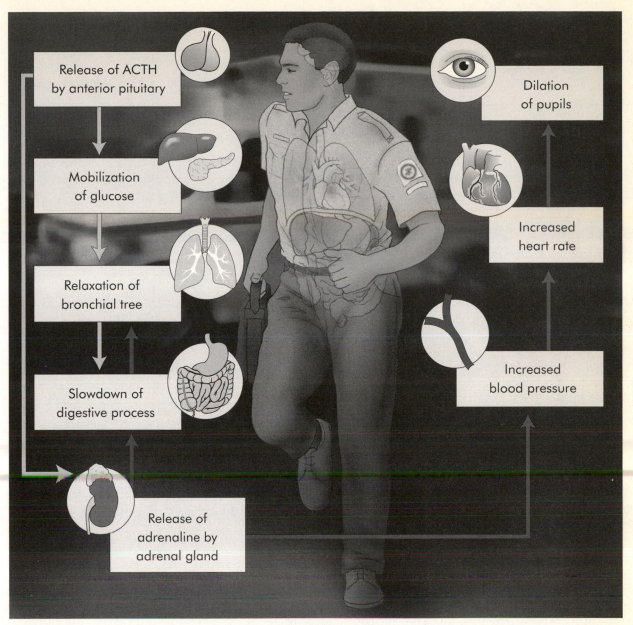

Release of ACTH
by anterior pituitary

Mobilization
of glucose

Relaxation of
bronchial tree

Slowdown of
digestive process

Release of
adrenaline by
adrenal gland

Dilation
of pupils

Increased
heart rate

Increased
blood pressure

Figure 2-1

7. Describe three measures that you should take to reduce the risk of work-related illness and injury on this type of call in each of the following areas:

a. Infectious disease

PROPER BSI PRECAUTIONS, Gloves, etc.

b. Lifting and moving

Proper lifting technique

   c. Hostile environments

_____

   d. Vehicle operation

_____

8. Briefly explain how each area of the body labeled in Fig. 2-1 responds to stress during the alarm reaction in this type of situation.

   a. _____

   b. _____

   c. _____

   d. _____

   e. _____

   f. _____

   g. _____

   h. _____

9. Describe two daily wellness practices that may benefit you as a paramedic when you respond to this type of situation.

   a.

   b.

10. List two reasons you, your crew, or both might use the services of the critical incident stress debriefing team after this call.

_____

_____

11. Which of the services that can be provided by a critical incident stress debriefing team may be of benefit after this call?

_____

_____

12. List five causes of stress that are job related and five that are not job related.

   a. Job-related stressors:

_____

   b. Non–job-related stressors:

_____

13. List three potential symptoms of decompensation from the effects of long-term stress.

a.

b.

c.

14. Name five effective stress-management techniques that can minimize the effects of EMS job-related stress. (After you complete this, survey paramedics you know to see what strategies they use.)

a.

b.

c.

d.

e.

Questions 15 to 17 pertain to the following case study:

You arrive at a family gathering where you find a 46-year-old man in full cardiopulmonary arrest. His mother is crying and begging, "Please, Lord, don't take him, take me." His wife is distraught, pacing and saying, "It's going to be OK; it's not as bad as it seems." The brother yells at you as you enter, "What took you so long? Hurry up! What are you waiting for?"

15. Identify which of the stages of grief described by Dr. Kubler-Ross each family member is exhibiting in this situation.

a. Mother:

b. Wife:

c. Brother:

16. How should you care for these family members to promote normal grieving?

_____

_____

_____

17. How can you deal with the pent-up emotions you must suppress while caring for dying patients and their families on calls like this?

_____

_____

18. Identify which of the following situations represents an exposure to blood or body fluids. If exposure is involved, describe a measure that could have prevented it.

a. After using a lancet to obtain a blood sample from your patient for dextrose measurement, you puncture your hand with the lancet. Exposure? Yes/No
Preventive measure:

_____

b. Blood sprays from a patient's endotracheal tube, hitting you in the face. You aren't sure if any got in your eyes or mouth. Exposure? Yes/No

Preventive measure:

_____

c. Your bare forearm brushes against a bloody sheet. You have no open wounds on your arm. Exposure? Yes/No

Preventive measure:

_____

d. You put the IV bag in your mouth to hold it up as you move the patient, and your partner points out that blood is splattered over the bag. Exposure? Yes/No

Preventive measure:

_____

19. At the scene of a motor vehicle collision, glass punctures your glove and cuts your finger. The patient's blood penetrates the glove and comes in contact with your cut. List at least four actions you should take after this exposure.

a.

b.

c.

d.

STUDENT SELF-ASSESSMENT

20. Which of the following is true regarding a healthy diet?
   a. Amino acids are produced by the body in the liver.
   b. Fats should be completely eliminated from the diet.
   c. Vitamin supplements are necessary for normal health.
   d. Water is one of the most important nutrients.

21. Which of the following is true regarding a routine physical fitness program?
   a. A decrease in muscle mass and metabolism will occur.
   b. A decrease in resting blood pressure may occur.
   c. A decrease in resistance to injury will occur.
   d. It should not be done if you have any preexisting illness.

22. Which of the following is a lifestyle modification associated with a decreased risk of heart disease?
   a. Reducing cigarette smoking
   b. Maintaining blood pressure at 120/80 mm Hg
   c. Reducing the very-low-density lipoprotein (VLDL) triglyceride level to 400 mg/dL
   d. Maintaining the low-density lipoprotein (LDL) cholesterol level at 190 mg/dL

23. Which of the following signs or symptoms is commonly listed as a warning sign of cancer?
   a. Indigestion or change in bowel habits
   b. Irregular heart beats or palpitations
   c. Lifelong presence of warts or moles
   d. Persistent nasal congestion

24. Actions that may prevent you from becoming infected with a communicable disease while practicing as a paramedic include which of the following?
   a. Annual skin testing for tuberculosis
   b. Frequent hand washing during all patient care activities
   c. Recapping of needles after patient use
   d. Use of body substance isolation for high-risk patients

25. How can you minimize your risk of injury while lifting or moving patients?
    a. Bend at the hips and knees
    b. Hold the load 18 inches from your body
    c. Lift with your back, not your legs
    d. Move backward rather than forward

26. Which of the following may indicate the potential for addiction or addictive behavior?
    a. Your partner asks you to drive him home from a bar because he feels he has had too much to drink.
    b. Your partner tells her husband she only had six beers instead of the 12 she actually drank.
    c. Your partner mentions that he is going out to have a few beers with some friends after work.
    d. Your partner says she can't handle booze the way she used to and now prefers beer to hard liquor.

27. You are called to a scene to assume care from a rescue unit. You immediately recognize the paramedic caring for the patient as an individual with whom you consistently disagree over patient care issues. What type of stress is this call likely to produce?
    a. Environmental   c. Personality
    b. Managerial   d. Psychosocial

28. Generalized feelings of apprehension are known as:
    a. Anxiety   c. Reaction formation
    b. Phobias   d. Stress

29. A paramedic student has just failed his practical examination station because of improper airway management technique. He states, "Well, I would have done it, but we never practiced it in class this way." This is an example of which defense mechanism?
    a. Projection   c. Regression
    b. Rationalization   d. Sublimation

30. Critical incident stress debriefing is most helpful for which of the following?
    a. New employees after every critical patient situation
    b. Selected high-risk employees with psychological problems
    c. Mass casualty incidents involving more than 10 patients
    d. Situations in which a high degree of stress is perceived

31. When dealing with the family of a patient who is dying, you can best interact with them by doing which of the following?
    a. Reassuring them that no one you ever care for dies
    b. Changing the subject every time someone brings up death
    c. Allowing the family to remain with the patient if possible
    d. Avoiding direct communication with the immediate family

32. Which response to the death of a close family member would not be expected in a preschool child?
    a. The child acts as though nothing has happened.
    b. The child asks when the family member will come back.
    c. The child fears that other family members will also die.
    d. The child thinks that he or she was responsible for the death.

33. School-age children (7 to 12 years old) feel that death:
    a. Is temporary and reversible
    b. Happens to others, not themselves
    c. Is a punishment for their bad thoughts
    d. Is the same as severe illness

34. Which of the following is an appropriate action to take after a needle-stick injury of the finger?
    a. Complete the exposure report and turn it in at the end of your shift.
    b. Determine whether the patient is high risk to decide whether you need to report the incident.
    c. Report the exposure to your supervisor and the receiving facility immediately.
    d. Squeeze out as much blood as possible and suck on your finger.

WRAP IT UP

Today is your worst nightmare. At about 1430 you are dispatched to a government building for a report of an explosion. It's your third day of a 72-hour shift, and you were just joking about taking the world record for most hours without sleep. En route, you see a plume of thick black smoke in the direction you are headed, and dispatch updates that there have been multiple calls and it appears there is major damage. You begin to review triage principles in your head, and you notice that your mouth is dry and you can feel your own heart pounding—sensations you haven't felt since your first rides as a paramedic student. Arriving on the scene, you see a multistory commercial structure with half of the side blown off. Command directs you and your partner to begin triage. There is mass confusion; people are moving all over the place. You attempt to set up a triage area, but bystanders are everywhere, rushing out with patients. Seven long hours later, 125 patients, some critically injured, have been triaged, treated, and transported. Among the casualties were your overweight captain, who was taken to the hospital with chest pains, and an out of shape co-worker, who strained his shoulder trying to free a trapped patient.

After the incident, things just got worse. One of your best friends just seems to be falling apart; she's drinking too much and in jeopardy of losing her job because of tardiness, frequent "sick" call-ins, and poor work performance. She keeps blaming everything on others and won't admit that she has a problem. The first few days after the incident, everyone pulled together, but now the stress level at work is high. Some people just keep to themselves; others are blaming co-workers for things that go wrong; and many of your colleagues don't even want to talk about the call.

1. What caused the dry mouth and palpitations that the paramedic experienced en route to this call?
   a. Cardiac irregularity
   b. Panic attack
   c. Parasympathetic release
   d. Stress reaction
2. After the incident, which defense mechanisms were observed in the paramedic's co-workers? (Check all that apply.)

   _____ Compensation   __X__ Denial
   __X__ Isolation   __X__ Projection
   _____ Rationalization   _____ Reaction formation
   _____ Regression   _____ Repression
   _____ Substitution

3. What wellness activities may have reduced the chance of workplace illness or injury on this call?
   a. Balanced diet
   b. Cardiovascular endurance exercises
   c. Stretching and weight training
   d. All of the above
4. What stress reduction techniques might be helpful

   a. Before a call such as this:

   _____

   b. After a call such as this:

   _____

5. What strategies can paramedics use to increase their chance of sleep between calls on long shifts?

   _____

   _____

CHAPTER 2 ANSWERS

REVIEW QUESTIONS

1. h
2. e
3. i
4. b
5. d
6. g
   (Questions 1-6: Objective 8)

7. a. To reduce the risk of acquiring an infectious disease, the paramedic should obtain appropriate immunizations, maintain good personal health and hygiene, use universal precautions during patient care (in this case gloves, goggles/mask, and gown if there is a risk of splash or spray), avoid recapping needles, dispose of contaminated sharps in an appropriate container, wash hands thoroughly after completing patient care, and appropriately dispose of soiled linens, equipment, and trash.
   b. To reduce the risk of injury from moving and lifting this patient, the paramedic should maintain good physical conditioning, obtain assistance in moving the patient if the person's size is too great for the paramedic and a partner, pay attention when walking, move forward when possible, take short steps, bend at the knees and hips, lift with the legs, keep the load close to the body, keep the patient's body in line when moving, and use the appropriate device for the situation (e.g., stair chair versus long back board).
   c. To reduce the risk of injury when providing care in a hostile environment, the paramedic should coordinate activities with law enforcement, scan the area for the fastest escape route, stay alert and move the patient out of the hostile area as quickly as possible, and leave the area if the situation becomes too dangerous. The best policy is to avoid entering the scene until the police have it under control.
   d. To ensure maximum safety when leaving this scene and transporting the patient to the hospital, the paramedic should use lights and sirens as dictated by local policy, proceed carefully through intersections, and maintain due regard for the safety of others.
   (Objectives 5, 11)

8. (a.) The pituitary gland releases adrenocorticotropic hormone, stimulating the sympathetic nervous system. (b.) Adrenal glands release epinephrine and norepinephrine, which (c) cause a rise in blood pressure by increasing systemic vascular resistance; (d) slow the digestive tract; (e) dilate the bronchioles, allowing deeper breathing; (f) stimulate glucose production in the liver; (g) dilate the pupils; and (h) increase the rate and strength of the heart's contractions.
   (Objective 7)

9. Good physical conditioning permits rapid movement of the patient out of this hostile situation with reduced risk of injury to the paramedic. Good emotional health practices facilitate the use of healthy coping mechanisms in dealing with the personal stressors involved in this call.
   (Objective 2)

10. Situations that pose a threat to rescuers' lives may be perceived as stressful, depending on the situation and the individuals involved. Having a critically injured patient who is a close relative or acquaintance often creates a very stressful situation.
    (Objective 10)

11. Individual consultation may be necessary if only one person was overwhelmed by the call. If the event was perceived as very stressful by the whole group, defusing immediately after the incident, critical incident stress debriefing within 24 to 72 hours, and follow-up services after debriefing may be needed.
    (Objective 9)

12. a. Working in hazardous situations; dealing with injured or dying children; working in an uncontrolled, unpredictable environment; dealing with emotionally upset, unpredictable patients; needing to make life and death decisions quickly. b. Physical illness of oneself or a close family member; loss of a job or starting a new job; personal financial troubles; the death of a loved one; and marital troubles, among others.
(Objective 7)

13. Irritability, apathy, chronic fatigue, feelings of not being appreciated, difficulty sleeping, drinking or drug abuse, decline in social activities, appetite changes, desire to quit work, and physical complaints.
(Objective 7)

14. Early recognition of signs and symptoms of stress, awareness of personal limitations, peer counseling, group discussions, proper diet, sleep, exercise, and pursuit of positive activities outside EMS.
(Objective 8)

15. a. Bargaining: The mother is bargaining her life for her son's life. b. Denial: The wife is denying the severity of the problem. c. Anger: The brother's anger is directed at the EMS personnel.
(Objective 10).

16. You should tell the family that the patient is critically ill and that you are going to do everything possible to help him. Remain calm and try to let the family remain close if patient care is not compromised. Assign tasks to the angry brother (e.g., stay with his mother and care for her).
(Objective 10)

17. Paramedics should be encouraged to talk about particularly distressing situations with other crew members and to avail themselves of resources available through medical direction and employee assistance programs.
(Objective 8)

18. a. Yes. Use accessible sharps containers and safety lancets.
    b. Yes. Wear a mask, eye protection, and gown when there is a risk of splash or spray.
    c. No exposure involved. You should wash your arm thoroughly.
    d. Yes. Do not place objects in your mouth when biohazards are present.
    (Objective 11)

19. a. Wash the area thoroughly.
    b. Document the exposure.
    c. Immediately report to the appropriate personnel.
    d. Complete the medical follow-up.
    (Objective 12)

STUDENT SELF-ASSESSMENT

20. d. Cellular function depends on a fluid environment. Amino acids are essential for body growth and cellular life and are not produced by the body. Polyunsaturated fats can help reduce high blood cholesterol levels if included as part of a low-fat diet.
(Objective 1)

21. b. An increase in muscle mass, metabolism, and resistance to injury should be anticipated with a carefully planned fitness program. Fitness programs can be tailored to accommodate the needs of individuals with preexisting medical conditions (e.g., arthritis, heart disease) and are encouraged.
(Objective 1)

22. b. Cigarette smoking should be eliminated to reduce the risk of heart disease. The triglyceride level should not exceed 200 to 300 mg/dL, and the LDL cholesterol level should be below 160 mg/dL.
(Objective 4)

23. a. The other signs listed by the American Cancer Society are a sore throat, unusual bleeding or discharge, thickening or a lump in the breast or elsewhere, obvious change in a wart or mole, and a nagging cough or hoarseness.
(Objective 4)

24. b. Annual skin testing is an excellent measure for detecting exposure to tuberculosis so that it can be appropriately treated; however, it does not prevent infection. Needle recapping is never advised because this greatly increases the risk of injury and exposure. Body substance isolation measures should be used for all patients, not just those that might be high risk.
(Objective 5)

25. a. To minimize the risk of injury, you should also hold the load close to your body, lift with your legs (not your back), and move forward rather than backward when possible.
(Objective 5)

26. b. Lying about using a substance indicates guilt about using the substance; this is a warning sign.
(Objective 6)

27. d. Environmental stress results from factors such as siren noise and weather. Personality stress relates to the way individuals feel about themselves. Managerial stress is not a distinct entity.
(Objective 7)

28. a. *Phobias* are unrealistic fears. *Reaction formation* is a defense mechanism in which unacceptable desires are suppressed by accentuating opposite behaviors. *Stress* is a generalized response to certain situations.
(Objective 7)

29. b. *Projection* occurs when one's own undesirable feelings are attributed to someone else. *Regression* is a return to an earlier stage of emotional adjustment. *Sublimation* occurs when unacceptable urges are modified to become socially acceptable.
(Objective 7)

30. d. New paramedics may be at greater risk for high stress after a critical call; however, veterans will continue to be vulnerable to unusually stressful calls. Multiple patient situations may not always trigger stress responses in rescuers; it depends on the individual situation. A high-risk employee with psychological problems probably will require care in addition to the critical incident stress debriefing program.
(Objective 9)

31. c. If the family raises the issue of death, a realistic description of the seriousness of the patient's condition should be briefly given. Direct eye contact and touch, if appropriate, may be used to convey concern and caring.
(Objective 10)

32. a. The family should watch for behavioral changes at home and at school, as well as difficulty eating or sleeping, and should encourage the child to express his or her feelings.
(Objective 10)

33. b. School-age children have begun to understand the concept of the finality of death; however, they still feel that it happens only to others.
(Objective 10)

34. c. All needle-stick injuries should be reported immediately so that appropriate source testing and follow-up can be completed in a timely manner.
(Objective 12)

WRAP IT UP

1. d. These are normal sympathetic responses to stress.
   (Objective 7)

2. Denial, rationalization, and substitution (the paramedic who shows poor performance); isolation (co-workers who keep to themselves); and repression (responders who don't want to talk about the call).
   (Objective 7)

3. d. Diet and exercise can reduce weight and improve cardiovascular fitness. Musculoskeletal injuries can be reduced by improving strength and flexibility.
   (Objective 3)

4. a. Exercise, meditation, and positive social connections can help in the management of stress on a daily basis.
   b. Critical incident stress debriefing, one-on-one counseling, exercise, reframing, controlled breathing, progressive relaxation, guided imagery, proper diet, and sleep are all techniques that may assist in the management of stress.
   (Objective 8)

5. Take some quiet time to relax before trying to sleep (reading, meditation, exercise); avoid stimulants; eat simple carbohydrates to release serotonin; select a dark sleeping area; try to pick a "normal" nap time (often difficult at work).
   (Objective 2)

Injury Prevention

READING ASSIGNMENT
Chapter 3, pages 42-53, in *Mosby's Paramedic Textbook,* ed. 3

OBJECTIVES
Upon completion of this chapter, the paramedic student will be able to do the following:
1. Identify roles of the emergency medical services community in injury prevention.
2. Describe the epidemiology of trauma in the United States.
3. Outline the aspects of the emergency medical services system that make it a desirable resource for involvement in community health activities.
4. Describe community leadership activities that are essential to enable the active participation of emergency medical services in community wellness activities.
5. List areas with which paramedics should be familiar to participate in injury prevention.
6. Evaluate a situation to determine opportunities for injury prevention.
7. Identify resources necessary to conduct a community health assessment.
8. Relate how alterations in the epidemiological triangle can influence injury and disease patterns.
9. Differentiate among primary, secondary, and tertiary health prevention activities.
10. Describe strategies to implement a successful injury prevention program.

SUMMARY
- EMS providers are members of the community's health care system. They can be an important resource for injury prevention.
- Unintentional injuries are the fifth leading cause of death, exceeded only by heart disease, cancer, stroke, and chronic obstructive pulmonary disease.
- The United States has more than 600,000 EMS providers. This valuable human resource plays a major role in public education, a component of health promotion that seems only fitting.
- EMS workers play an active role in protecting and promoting the health of a community. The community, in turn, must protect EMS workers from injury. It also must provide them with a strong education in their field. Furthermore, the community should support and promote the collection and use of injury data. In addition, it must obtain resources for primary injury prevention activities. The community must empower EMS workers to provide primary injury prevention.
- All EMS workers must have a basic knowledge of personal injury prevention. They also should know about maladies and injuries common to various age groups, recreational activities, workplaces, and other facilities in the community.
- Paramedics must be able to identify the signs and symptoms of abuse and abusive situations. They also must be able to recognize potentially dangerous situations.
- Paramedics should identify and use outside community resources. They also should properly document primary injury data. They should be able to recognize and use the teachable moment.

- EMS providers must maximize their time and resources. Therefore they should identify targets for community health education. They can do this by performing a community health assessment.
- To identify community education goals, the paramedic must understand that illness and injury are influenced by several factors: (1) the degree of exposure to an agent; (2) the strength of the agent; (3) the susceptibility of the individual (host); and (4) the biologic, social, and physical environment.
- *Primary* injury prevention is characterized by efforts to prevent the occurrence of an injury. *Secondary* prevention and *tertiary* prevention involve efforts to help prevent the development of further problems from an event that has already occurred.
- A good injury prevention program must serve the whole target population in a community. An effective program also takes into account reading level and age. These are the marks of a successful program. The EMS provider can present community health education in diverse ways. These can include verbal, written/static material, and dynamic visual presentations.

REVIEW QUESTIONS

Questions 1 to 9 pertain to the following case study:

At 1400 the tones sound, and you are dispatched to the home of an elderly resident who has slipped and fallen. On arrival at the emergency department, the physician confirms your suspicion—the patient's hip is broken. As you ride back to the base, you remark to your partner how this is the fourth patient you've transported this month with a broken hip. These calls really bother you, because your own grandmother was institutionalized and then died of pneumonia shortly after a similar injury just 6 months ago. By the time you arrive back at your station, you have resolved to do something about the problem. You approach the chief, who listens to your idea. He tells you to return when you have some solid information about the target population, the magnitude of the problem, your goals, and the cost involved.

1. Injury accounts for about what percentage of emergency department (ED) visits in the United States?

_____

2. The initial visit to the emergency department for this type of injury has a high price. List two other "costs" associated with this type of injury.

_____

_____

3. Give at least three reasons why EMS is ideally suited to perform community prevention activities with the elderly.

   a.

   b.

   c.

4. What additional information would you need to be able to provide prevention for this type of injury in this group?

_____

5. What will you need from your boss before moving ahead with this project?

_____

6. List three community resources you may need to contact to identify the number of elderly individuals living in your district, the incidence of hip fractures, the morbidity and mortality rates associated with this injury, and costs associated with such fractures.

   a.

   b.

   c.

7. You decide that the causes of fall injury in the elderly are most likely the result of the host and environmental factors of the epidemiological triangle. List two host and two environmental factors that may contribute to falls in the elderly.

Host:

a. _____

b. _____

Environmental:

a. _____

b. _____

After careful evaluation of the problem, you decide that the best plan would be to have EMS crews visit elderly residents' homes with a checklist that would identify risk factors for falls in the home. A brief educational pamphlet with specific recommendations would then be given to the resident.

8. Is your plan an example of a primary, secondary, or tertiary intervention?

_____

9. List at least four factors you should consider in preparing the written educational materials to be distributed to the community.

_____

_____

Each of the examples in questions 10 to 18 represents a factor that could cause or increase susceptibility to illness and injury. Indicate whether the example is an *agent* factor (causative), a *host* factor (influences exposure, susceptibility, or response to agents), or an *environmental* factor (influences existence of the agent, exposure, or susceptibility).

Example	Agent, Host, or Environmental Factor
10. Fatigue	
11. Firefighter	
12. Carbon monoxide	
13. Gender	
14. Hepatitis	
15. Malnutrition	
16. Poor personal hygiene	
17. Flood	
18. Cholesterol	

19. List at least four injury prevention strategies a paramedic might use to help reduce neurological injury.

a.

b.

c.

d.

STUDENT SELF-ASSESSMENT

20. A total of 10 people in your EMS district have been killed in motor vehicle collisions thus far this year. Where do deaths from unintentional causes such as this rank in the United States?
   a. First
   b. Third
   c. Fifth
   d. Seventh

21. The number of drownings in your community rose last year. The health department asks your EMS agency to assist with an educational plan to help reduce the incidence of drowning. Why are EMS providers ideal for this type of program?
   a. They have more time than other health care providers to teach these programs.
   b. Paramedics and EMTs will be welcomed into homes and public places to present educational programs.
   c. EMS agencies have abundant financial resources to fund these programs.
   d. EMS providers are the best authorities on preventing such tragedies.

22. How can EMS safety be enhanced during emergency care and transportation?
   a. Educate the public to pull to the right when they see emergency traffic
   b. Ticket people who fail to yield to emergency traffic
   c. Establish a policy of parking upwind from all HAZMAT spills
   d. Ensure that police assume all responsibility for scene safety

23. How can EMS agencies promote the involvement of staff members in community wellness programs?
   a. Penalize those who decline to participate
   b. Ask everyone on duty to participate
   c. Offer it as an alternative to a less desirable chore
   d. Provide a salary for off-duty injury prevention work

24. You respond to a call for domestic violence. You find a woman with bruising around her face, and she and her husband are yelling at each other. She screams at you to leave her alone when you try to examine her, and he is staggering and cursing at you. What is your primary goal in this situation?
   a. To restrain the patient and ask medical direction for permission for involuntary transport
   b. To ask the police to arrest both of them so that they can be contained in a controlled space
   c. To maintain the safety of your crew and to diffuse the situation calmly without violence
   d. To forcibly remove the man from the situation so that the woman will not be afraid of treatment

25. Which of the following patient situations would likely present a teachable moment?
   a. A hysterical mother being transported with her child, who just fell down a flight of stairs
   b. An elderly patient who refuses care after falling in a dimly lit stairway and injuring her wrist
   c. A child with minor injuries who was struck by a car that crossed the median onto the sidewalk
   d. A cyclist without a helmet who fell off his bike during a race and is confused during transport

26. You believe that you are running many more calls related to heart problems in the elderly. What community resources can you use as sources of information to determine whether the makeup of your community is changing?
   a. Census data
   b. Chamber of commerce
   c. Fire service
   d. Local newspaper

27. It is a cold, wintry day, and the trees are glistening after the ice storm last night. Your crew alone has run four calls to the local sledding hill to care for patients with injuries ranging from broken extremities to lumbar fractures. Which element in the epidemiological triangle is most likely having the greatest influence on the injuries you are seeing in this situation?
   a. Physical environment
   b. Social setting
   c. Strength of the agent
   d. Susceptibility of the host

28. Which of the following is an example of a primary health prevention activity with which a paramedic may be involved?
   a. You check the blood pressure of residents diagnosed with hypertension each week.
   b. You coordinate a stop smoking program for a group of your fellow employees.
   c. You coordinate a drunk-u-drama at the high school before prom week.
   d. You arrange a support group for EMS personnel recovering from alcohol abuse.
29. You are preparing a presentation on drug use for the young people in your area. How can you make sure your audience will understand your message?
   a. You test it on a teen patient during an EMS call.
   b. You ask your crew if it appeals to them.
   c. You include slides to increase the likelihood of retention.
   d. You make sure the language and reading level suit the audience.
30. Which of the following injury prevention strategies is associated with the greatest reduction in injury and death after a vehicle crash?
   a. Automatic airbag deployment on crash impact
   b. Driver education programs for senior citizens
   c. Fines for driving without wearing seatbelts
   d. Television advertising promoting safe driving techniques

WRAP IT UP

As you arrive on the scene of a "pedestrian struck" call, you observe a child whose life has changed forever. The 8-year-old boy, who had been riding his bike without a helmet, had careened down a hill into an intersection and was struck by a small truck. The distraught driver tells you that the boy flew up and hit the windshield with his head. You note that the windshield is starred and that the front quarter panel of the truck is dented. It's immediately evident that the child is seriously injured. He has a forehead laceration and is combative. You quickly immobilize him and load him into the ambulance while maintaining the airway. En route to the local trauma center, you continue your assessments, intubate the trachea, insert an intravenous (IV) line, and notify the trauma team of your assessment and your estimated time of arrival (ETA). The boy's condition worsens as you roll him into the trauma room. Later, during the postincident review, you are told that although he survived, he will have severe cognitive impairment. He is in rehabilitation, and it is unclear whether he will ever function normally again. You are angry and frustrated. You have many long discussions about the call with your captain. After much thought, and with the captain's approval, you decide to start a helmet program in your community. You plan to hold clinics at which you will properly fit helmets for those who have one and sell helmets for $5 (your cost to buy them) to those who don't. You also plan to develop brochures and deliver presentations in the local elementary schools.

1. a. What is the goal of a program such as this?

   _____

   _____

   b. Is this goal consistent with the mission of an EMS organization? _____

   _____

   _____

2. Why would EMS providers be suitable professionals to initiate such a program?

   _____

   _____

3. Where can you find information to justify the cost of this program to your chief?

_____

_____

4. Could you tie in on-scene education to a program like this?

_____

_____

5. Place a ✔ beside the components of a community health assessment that could be helpful in your research for this program.

_____ Population demographics	_____ Morbidity statistics
_____ Mortality statistics	_____ Crime and fire information
_____ Community resource allocation	_____ Hospital data
_____ Senior citizen needs	_____ Education standards
_____ Recreational facilities	_____ Environmental conditions
_____ Other factors	

6. Would this program be a primary, secondary, or tertiary community health intervention?

_____

_____

7. Where can you seek funding to support your program?

_____

_____

8. What must you consider in developing your brochure and your presentation?

_____

_____

CHAPTER 3 ANSWERS

REVIEW QUESTIONS

1. About 42% of ED visits are related to injury.
   (Objective 2)

2. In addition to the initial ED visit, other costs related to injury include lost quality of life, loss of income, and long-term hospitalizations/care.
   (Objective 2)

3. EMS providers are ideally suited for educating elderly people in their community because they are welcomed into the home. Also, they are viewed as experts who are medically educated; they are considered to have people's best interests at heart; and they may be the first to identify situations that pose a risk.
   (Objectives 1, 3)

4. Injury prevention material specific to falls in the elderly would need to be obtained.
   (Objective 4)

5. You will need financial support, endorsement of your agency, and possibly assistance from your boss to identify other community resources.
   (Objective 4)

6. Census data should reflect the number of elderly; the area health department should have statistics on mortality and injury frequency and type; your own EMS system could provide information about the number of elderly patients transported as a result of fall-related injuries; and national agencies such as the Centers for Disease Control and Prevention (CDC) and the National Safety Council can provide cost data and are accessible either through the Internet or the library.
   (Objective 7)

7. Host: Poor eyesight, impaired balance secondary to medication use, decreased sensation. Environmental: poor lighting, loose area rugs, absence of or poorly maintained railings, icy walkways.
   (Objective 8)

8. This is a primary intervention if it involves people who have not had injuries from a fall.
   (Objective 8)

9. You will need to consider the following factors: the cost of the materials (who will pay for them); whether someone in the community already has materials you could use (e.g., hospital, health department); the reading levels of the audience; whether you need to prepare bilingual materials if you have a large group that does not read English; and the type size of the material (to accommodate clients with poor vision).
   (Objective 10)

10. Host. Fatigue may result in a shortened attention span, which may lead to an injury.
11. Environment. Firefighters are placed in hostile environments by their work, which increases their susceptibility to injury or illness.
12. Agent. Carbon monoxide is a poisonous gas that can cause illness or death.
13. Host. Certain diseases are more prevalent in one gender than the other (e.g., rheumatoid arthritis is more prevalent in women).
14. Agent. Hepatitis is a virus that causes disease.
15. Host. Malnutrition deprives the body of essential nutrients necessary to maintain health.
16. Host. Poor personal hygiene predisposes an individual to infection.
17. Environmental. Floods may cause water contamination and increase the risk of the epidemic spread of disease.
18. Agent. Excess cholesterol is associated with an increased risk of heart disease.
    (Questions 10-18: Objective 8)

19. Helmet, seatbelt, senior fall prevention, safe bicycle riding programs

20. c. Unintentional injuries are the top cause of death for persons between 1 and 38 years of age and the fifth leading cause of death overall. (Objective 2)

STUDENT SELF-ASSESSMENT

21. b. Residents of a community usually have a high level of trust in EMS providers and will let them in to speak about these issues. The amount of time paramedics have in any given EMS system depends on the call volume and other commitments, such as training or other departmental duties. EMS agencies do not always have financial resources but may have a community partner to fund the support materials for the program. EMS providers often have baseline knowledge about injury prevention but can be educated on specific injury prevention materials.
(Objective 3)

22. a. Ticketing people who fail to yield may be helpful, but it affects only those who may have caused injury to EMS providers or their patients. Education is more desirable.
(Objective 4)

23. d. Penalizing personnel or forcing them to participate in an activity may be necessary, but it does not promote maximum participation in activities. Rewards and incentives are helpful.
(Objective 4)

24. c. Situations involving domestic violence are volatile and complicated. Measures to diffuse, rather than escalate, the situation should be used unless the circumstances pose an immediate danger to your crew, your patient, or the police.
(Objective 5)

25. b. This patient is calm and cooperative, but she probably realizes that her injury could have been more serious. A few words about appropriate lighting and specific recommendations for accomplishing it would likely be taken quite seriously at that moment. For the child hit by a car, calming may be a greater priority, and there is no evidence of a need to teach him anything specific to relate to this incident. In *a* and *d,* the parent or patient is not in an appropriate mental state to be taught.
(Objective 6)

26. a. Census data, which may be obtained through the Internet or the library, provide information about population demographics, including age and income levels. The area health department can give you specific information about deaths in your community and their causes. The local paper may refer you to information sources but won't likely have specifics. Fire departments have very specific call data related to fires and whether they also provide EMS and illness or injury information. The chamber of commerce has economic data and information about industry, religious organizations, and cultural opportunities in a community.
(Objective 7)

27. a. The icy conditions undoubtedly are having the greatest influence on the situation. The ice prevented the host from controlling the speed or direction of the sled, and it caused the crash.
(Objective 8)

28. c. The drunk-u-drama will attempt to teach students how to prevent injuries from occurring. You are performing secondary interventions on the hypertensive group and the smokers; both these groups already have a condition you are attempting to control or stop. Tertiary activities, designed to rehabilitate, would include the support group activities.
(Objective 9)

29. d. Although brief opportunities for teaching occur during an EMS call, a formal educational plan wouldn't be appropriate. Your crew members may think the program is great, but the target audience may not relate to it at all. Slides are appropriate, but depending on your audience and your message, they may not be desirable or possible. For example, if your program is to be delivered to youth groups on a street corner, you would have to choose a different method.
(Objective 10)

30. a. Engineering safety controls, which do not offer the user a choice whether to use them, are more effective.

WRAP IT UP

1. a. The goal would be to reduce injury and death for those riding bicycles and other wheeled recreational toys.
   b. For most EMS agencies, this goal should be consistent with their mission, which is to reduce death and disability.
   (Objective 1)

2. EMS providers are medically educated, are high-profile role models, are welcome in schools and homes, and are considered "experts" on injury and prevention. Therefore they are ideal providers of injury prevention programs.
   (Objective 3)

3. Information on the costs of unintentional injuries can be obtained from National Safety Council statistics, some state data, trauma centers, and trauma organizations.
   (Objective 7)

4. On-scene education could be included in such a program by (1) giving helmets to children who have been in collisions while on bikes, scooters, or roller blades; (2) by offering to properly fit them for a helmet; or (3) by encouraging them to wear their helmet (or wear it properly).
   (Objective 9)

5. Population demographics, mortality statistics, morbidity statistics, hospital data, recreational facilities (e.g., a skateboard park in your district), and other factors (e.g., funding sources, a local police bicycle rodeo at which you could implement your program) could be helpful in creating your presentation.
   (Objective 7)

6. This is mainly a primary injury prevention program; it prevents the injury from happening.
   (Objective 9)

7. Funding could be sought through federal grants, local service clubs (Kiwanis, Lions, Optimists, Rotary), SafeKids coalitions, and hospitals. If you can establish the program with seed money and then sell your helmets for cost, the program may perpetuate itself, with little additional funding needed.
   (Objectives 7, 10)

8. In developing the materials for your program, you must consider (1) the money available; (2) the reading level of the target audience; (3) the likes and dislikes of the target audience; (4) the attention span of the target audience; and (5) ethnic, cultural, and religious considerations for the target audience. After the program has been put together, someone from your target audience should "preview" the material and give you their opinion.
   (Objective 10)

Medical/Legal Issues

READING ASSIGNMENT
Chapter 4, pages 54-71, in *Mosby's Paramedic Textbook,* ed. 3

OBJECTIVES
Upon completion of this chapter, the paramedic student will be able to do the following:
1. Describe the basic structure of the legal system in the United States.
2. Relate how laws affect the paramedic's practice.
3. List situations that the paramedic is legally required to report in most states.
4. Describe the four elements involved in a claim of negligence.
5. Describe measures paramedics may take to protect themselves from claims of negligence.
6. Describe the paramedic's responsibilities regarding patient confidentiality.
7. Outline the process for obtaining expressed, informed, and implied consent.
8. Describe legal complications relating to consent.
9. Describe actions to be taken in a refusal-of-care situation.
10. Describe legal considerations related to patient transportation.
11. Outline legal issues related to specific resuscitation situations.
12. List measures the paramedic should take to preserve evidence when at a crime or accident scene.
13. Detail the components of the narrative report necessary for effective legal documentation.
14. Define common medical/legal terms that apply to prehospital situations involving patient care.

SUMMARY
- The structure of the legal system in the United States is composed of five types of law: legislative law, administrative law, common law, criminal law, and civil law.
- To safeguard against litigation, the paramedic must be knowledgeable of legal issues. The paramedic also must know about the effects of these issues.
- Paramedics and health care workers may be required by law to report some cases. These include cases of abuse or neglect of children and older adults and spouse abuse. They also include cases that involve rape, sexual assault, gunshot wounds, stab wounds, animal bites, and some communicable diseases.
- Lawsuits that have to do with patient care usually result from civil claims of negligence. This refers to the failure to act as a reasonable, prudent paramedic would act in such circumstances.
- Most legal authorities stress that protection against claims of negligence has three elements. The first is training. The second is competent patient care skills. The third is full documentation of all patient care activities.
- Some state and federal regulations provide protection for the paramedic with respect to notification of infectious disease exposure, immunity statutes, and special crimes against EMS personnel.

- Confidential information is threefold. For the most part, confidential information includes any details about a patient that are related to the patient's history. Any assessment findings also are included. Any treatment given is included as well. As a rule, the release of these details requires written permission from the patient or legal guardian. (There are some exceptions.)
- A mentally competent adult has the right to refuse medical care. This is the case even if the decision could result in death or permanent disability.
- Four other legal complications related to consent are abandonment, false imprisonment, assault, and battery.
- A competent patient has certain rights. The patient has the right to decide what medical care (and transportation) to receive. This is a basic concept of law and medical practice.
- Legal responsibilities for the patient continue until patient care is transferred to another member of the health care system (or it is clear that the patient no longer requires care). Legal issues related to patient transport include level of care during transportation, use of the emergency vehicle operating privileges, choice of patient destination, and payer protocols.
- Resuscitation issues that relate directly to EMS include withholding or stopping resuscitation, advance directives, potential organ donation, and death in the field.
- Emergency medical services play two important roles when responding to crime scenes: (1) focusing on patient care and (2) preserving evidence at the scene when possible.
- In the legal field the general belief is that "if it was not written down, it was not done." Thus thoroughness and attention to detail are vital in documentation.

REVIEW QUESTIONS

Match the legal term in column II with its definition in column I. Use each answer only once.

Column I

1. ____ Forcefully restraining the arm of an alert, competent patient while an intravenous line is placed

2. ____ As a joke, advising the emergency department staff that the patient is a prostitute

3. ____ Telling a friend that you treated a nurse you both know for a drug overdose

4. ____ Restraining an alert, conscious adult with an obvious fracture and transporting him by ambulance against his will

5. ____ Documenting that the patient is homosexual and remarking, "Now let's see them get insurance"

6. ____ Leaving a patient in the emergency department to go on another call before you have an opportunity to give a report to the nurse or physician on duty

Column II

a. Abandonment
b. Assault
c. Battery
d. False imprisonment
e. Libel
f. Invasion of privacy (libel)
g. Malpractice
h. Slander

7. Violations of state motor vehicle codes by a paramedic can result only in civil lawsuits. True/False. If you answered false, explain why.

_____

_____

8. Good Samaritan legislation may protect off-duty EMS providers from litigation if no negligence or reckless disregard is involved. True/False. If you answered false, explain why.

_____

_____

9. Group insurance policies protect EMS providers from lawsuits arising from negligent acts. True/False. If you answered false, explain why.

_____

_____

10. List four situations that most states require a paramedic to report to the authorities.

   a. ChiD ABuse

   b. CRIME SCENE - gunshot , STABS

   c. RAPE

   d. ElDER ABuSE

11. List the four elements necessary to prove negligence.

   a. Duty to Act

   b. Breach of Duty

   c. DAMAgE to pAtient,

   d. Proximate cAuSe

12. A 40-year-old patient involved in a motor vehicle collision complains of mild neck pain and tingling in her fingers. She is quickly assessed and signs a refusal of care form at the urging of the paramedic crew. Later that day she loses sensation and movement in all extremities, stops breathing, and dies. Which, if any, of the four elements in question no. 11 could be used to prove negligence in this situation and why?

_____

_____

_____

13. Name three effective means by which the paramedic can avoid claims of liability when providing patient care.

   a. DelvERINg competeNt pAtient CARe

   b. Proper DocumeNtAtioN

   c.

14. You are called to treat an alert, 72-year-old patient who is experiencing chest pain. The patient exhibits classic signs and symptoms of myocardial infarction. You explain to him that he needs to go to the hospital because you feel that his symptoms could be those of a heart attack, and proper medicine could be given to help his condition. He states that he wants his wife to drive him instead of going by ambulance. You advise him that if his condition worsens in the car, his wife would be unable to help him and he might die. You again urge him to come with you. Fill in the blanks below with the type of consent that best applies to the situation.
The patient can now make a(n)

   a. _____ consent. He tells you that he has decided to go in the ambulance. This constitutes a(n)

   b. _____ consent. If he had lost consciousness before agreeing to ambulance transport, his consent is said to be a(n)

   c. _____ consent, and treatment could be rendered.

15. You respond to the scene of an automobile collision, where you find an awake, alert, 24-year-old man complaining of neck pain and tingling in his right arm. His vital signs are stable. The patient's vehicle was struck from behind and sustained considerable damage. The patient refuses transport to the hospital. What five things should be done or explained to this patient and documented on the patient care report regarding his refusal of care?

a.

b.

c.

d.

e.

Questions 16 to 21 refer to the following case study:

You are dispatched to an expensive rural home for an "accidental injury." When you arrive, you find two patients, a man and a woman. The man, who appears to be approximately 30 years old, apparently had been shot in the head at close range. He had been found pulseless and breathless by a family member, who found both patients 20 minutes before your arrival. The male patient has a large exit wound with brain matter extruding. After your initial assessment, you decide not to resuscitate him. The female patient is a woman whom you recognize as a local celebrity. She has a gunshot wound to the abdomen, is unconscious, and has no radial pulse. You note a plastic bag of white powder and a hypodermic needle next to her. A handgun is lying on the floor next to the man. The family wants you to take the woman to the closest local hospital so that they can "keep things quiet." The nearest trauma center is an equal distance away.

16. What type of consent applies in this situation?

_____

17. List four facts you must document about the male patient to ensure legal compliance.

a.

b.

c.

d.

18. Describe actions you should take to preserve evidence at this scene with regard to the following:

a. Clothing

_____

b. Weapon

_____

c. Blood on the floor

_____

d. Documentation of the scene

_____

e. Positioning of the ambulance

_____

19. Should you transport the patient to the hospital the family wants or to the trauma center? Explain your answer.

_____

_____

20. Why shouldn't you document, "Drugs found lying next to patient"?

_____

_____

21. To which of the following personnel is it appropriate to tell the facts of this case?
    a. Police officers assigned to the case   Yes/No
    b. A paramedic from another service   Yes/No
    c. The press   Yes/No
    d. Medical personnel caring for the patient   Yes/No
    e. Hospital staff in the smokers' area   Yes/No

STUDENT SELF-ASSESSMENT

22. Which branch of law is also referred to as _tort law_?
    a. Administrative law   **c.** Criminal law
    b. Civil law   **d.** Legislative law

23. In which of the following situations may abandonment be alleged when a paramedic relinquishes care to an EMT?
    a. A patient being transferred with an infusion of blood
    b. A patient going from a nursing home to a hospital for a wrist injury
    c. A hysterical, uninjured patient from a mass casualty situation
    d. A dialysis patient being transported for routine care

24. Which of the following is necessary for successful prosecution of a criminal law case?
    a. Criminal intent must be proved.
    b. Injury must be demonstrated.
    c. A patient must sue for financial gain.
    d. A statute must be violated.

25. You are called to a private residence, where you find an elderly man suffering from heat-related illness. The family evidently left this chronically confused individual at home with no air conditioning and all the windows closed. What legal issue must you remember on this call?
    a. You should not remove the patient's clothes so that you can preserve the chain of evidence.
    b. This patient can't give consent, therefore you must contact the next of kin before transport.
    c. Writing the neighbors' statements in the patient care report may constitute libel.
    d. You are required to report this situation to the appropriate legal or social agency.

26. The Ryan White Act provides protection for the paramedic with regard to which of the following?
    a. Good Samaritan acts   **c.** Infectious disease
    b. Governmental immunity   **d.** Violent acts

27. A paramedic finds an unconscious patient who has a strong odor resembling alcohol on the breath. No care is initiated, and during transport the patient aspirates. On arrival at the hospital, the patient is found to have a dangerously low blood sugar level, and a lengthy hospitalization ensues. Why could this patient claim negligence?
    a. The paramedic violated a law while providing care.
    b. The paramedic committed malfeasance while providing care.
    c. The patient suffered damage from the negligent act.
    d. Evidence existed of conflicting views of causation.

28. Patient confidentiality would be breached in most states if a paramedic discussed the patient's comments and care with which of the following?
    a. Lawyers in court
    b. Emergency department personnel
    c. Personal friends
    d. A quality assurance committee
29. When a patient agrees to treatment verbally or in writing, it is known as which of the following?
    a. Expressed consent
    b. Implied consent
    c. Informed consent
    d. Referred consent
30. You are caring for an elderly patient who experienced a syncopal episode. He now refuses care. What actions must you take to ensure legal compliance during this refusal process?
    a. Force the patient to sign the refusal form before release.
    b. Tell the patient that if he changes his mind, he can call you again for transport.
    c. Do not give the patient any additional advice or you may be liable.
    d. Transport the patient against his will because his condition involved a loss of consciousness.
31. What do EMS traffic right-of-way privileges usually include?
    a. The right to travel as fast as necessary to get to the hospital quickly
    b. The ability to proceed without slowing through intersections
    c. The right to override the directions of a traffic officer
    d. Definitions of appropriate use of lights and sirens
32. According to the American Heart Association, what criteria must be met to stop resuscitation in the prehospital setting after you have initiated advanced life support procedures?
    a. Persistent asystole or agonal rhythm is present and no reversible causes are identified.
    b. The family assures you that there is a "do not resuscitate" order, but it can't be found.
    c. Endotracheal intubation and IV access can't be established, therefore you are unable to give drugs.
    d. Trauma is a factor, and your transport time will be 20 minutes or longer.
33. You respond to a stabbing at a local bar. What actions should you take during your care of the patient to preserve evidence?
    a. Cut the clothing through the knife hole to minimize other damage
    b. Give the clothes to a bystander so that evidence will remain at the scene
    c. Move the knife, if present, so that EMS personnel will not step on it
    d. Follow the same path to and from the ambulance and patient
34. Which of the following should be included in the narrative portion of the patient care report?
    a. Care rendered
    b. History
    c. Physical findings
    d. All of the above

WRAP IT UP

Your ambulance is dispatched at 0500 to a party at a local bar. The patient is a 35-year-old woman who was involved in a fight. She has a large laceration, made by a broken bottle, that extends into her eye. You control the bleeding with 5 × 9 dressings and a Kerlix wrap. The patient is awake, alert, and oriented to person, place, and time. She refuses transport. You recognize the seriousness of her wound due to its depth and involvement with her eye, and you attempt at length to persuade her to be transported. She is rude and belligerent and persistently refuses care. You decide to take her forcibly because of the seriousness of her wound. You and your partner pick her up and carry her to the ambulance, secure her with straps and soft wrist restraints, and take her to the hospital. Patients are lined up three deep in the halls in the emergency department (ED). You wait 30 minutes to give a report to a nurse, but they are all busy. Finally, because it is a busy night and you must get back into service, you give the patient care report and your verbal report to the registration clerk, along with your phone number so that the nurse can contact you with any questions. You call an acquaintance whom you know is a co-worker of this patient, because you know that the woman will need a ride home from the hospital because of her impaired vision. After you leave the ED, the patient, whom you left restrained supine, vomits and aspirates. This results in pneumonia, which requires a 2-week hospitalization.

1. Were the actions of the paramedic within his or her scope of practice?

_____

_____

_____

2. Is the paramedic protected under the Good Samaritan rules in this case? If not, why not?

_____

_____

_____

3. Is the paramedic protected by immunity statutes in this case? If not, why not?

_____

_____

_____

4. Is this a mandatory reportable situation under most state laws?

_____

_____

_____

5. Place a ✔ beside any term that may describe a legal rule the paramedic may have violated in this situation. Explain each violation.

_____ Abandonment   _____ Negligence
_____ Assault   _____ Battery
_____ False imprisonment   _____ Libel
_____ Slander   _____ Civil rights violation

CHAPTER 4 ANSWERS

REVIEW QUESTIONS

1. c. Physical force against individuals against their will and without legal justification is battery.
2. h. Making statements about a person with malicious intent is slander.
3. f. You released information about the nurse that could cause ridicule, embarrassment, or notoriety.
4. d. Forcible restraint and confinement against one's will is false imprisonment.
5. e. Making false written statements about a person with malicious intent is libel.
6. a. Failure to appropriately turn over care of the patient to a qualified individual may be considered abandonment.

   (Questions 1-6: Objectives 7, 8, 14)

7. False. If a criminal law is violated, a paramedic could be charged under that statute as well. For example, in the past, EMS personnel have been charged with manslaughter when someone died as a result of a vehicular collision involving the ambulance.

   (Objective 2)

8. True.

   (Objective 4)

9. False. The lawsuit may be filed regardless of the presence of insurance. However, the insurance may protect the paramedic's personal assets. This is controversial; some sources advise against carrying insurance.

   (Objective 6)

10. Child abuse or neglect; elder abuse or neglect; rape; animal bites; gunshot or stab wounds.

    (Objective 3)

11. Duty to act; breach of duty; damage to the patient; and proximate cause are the four elements that must be proven to win a negligence suit.

    (Objective 5)

12. Duty to act: The unit was on duty and was called to care for this patient.

    Breach of duty: The standard of care would have indicated immobilizing and transporting this patient; the crew failed to act as the standard of care dictated.

    Damage to the patient: The patient lost movement, stopped breathing, and died after being abandoned by the paramedic crew.

    Proximate cause: The patient apparently died from spinal cord damage; the paramedic crew did not immobilize and protect the cervical spine, which might have prevented death.

    (Objective 5)

13. The paramedic may reduce the risk of liability claims by obtaining appropriate training, delivering competent patient care, and ensuring thorough documentation.

    (Objective 6)

14. a. Informed
    b. Expressed
    c. Implied

    (Question 14: Objective 8)

15. You must document the following: the patient's level of consciousness (awake and alert); that you explained to the patient the risks of refusing care, including paralysis or death; that you had the patient sign a refusal form, noting any witnesses; any follow-up instructions you gave the patient; and that you told the patient to call EMS again if his condition worsened or he changed his mind.

    (Objective 9)

16. Implied consent is assumed because the patient is unconscious.
(Objective 8)

17. The absence of a heart rate (ECG) strip in several leads; the absence of respirations, pulse, and spontaneous movement; fixed and dilated pupils; and the condition of the body (specifically the wounds) should be documented. In addition, the known time that the patient was breathless and pulseless with no care before your arrival should be documented.
(Objective 11)

18. a. You should take care not to cut the clothing through the bullet hole. If the clothes are removed, you should not shake them. If removed on the scene, the clothes should be given only to the police. If removed in the ambulance, the clothes should be placed in a paper bag and given to a police officer at the hospital, if possible. b. You should not touch the weapon unless it poses a danger to your crew. c. Try not to step in the blood on the floor, if possible. d. Carefully and objectively document your findings on the scene. Note the specific location and position of both patients and the location of the weapon. Any other unusual scene findings should also be listed. e. Your ambulance should be parked away from any obvious evidence if it does not interfere with scene safety.
(Objective 12)

19. Typically you may override a family's wishes for specific cases when state protocols indicate that patients may be taken to specialty centers such as trauma centers, which are known to improve survival for specific injuries.
(Objective 10)

20. Unless you have proof that the bag contains drugs, you should note only what you specifically observed; that is, that a bag containing a white powdery substance and a syringe with a needle were found to the right of the patient.
(Objective 13)

21. a. Yes
    b. No, not unless the paramedic has a legitimate medical or legal reason to know the information.
    c. No. Specific department regulations about information to be released to the press should be followed.
    d. Yes. Medical direction needs to know the facts of the case for quality improvement reasons.
    e. No. Only hospital staff directly involved in the patient's care should be informed of the details of the case.
    (Objective 7)

STUDENT SELF-ASSESSMENT

22. b. *Administrative law* refers to regulations that are developed by a government agency to provide details about the process of the law. *Criminal laws* are enacted by federal, state, or local government to protect society. *Legislative laws* are made by legislative branches of government and are determined by statutes and constitutions.
(Objective 1)

23. a. A patient who needs continuing advanced care should not be released by a paramedic to someone with lesser training.
(Objective 2)

24. d. Criminal law violations need not involve injury or criminal intent. The patient sues for damages in civil suits. A criminal law violation is based on proof that a statute has been violated.
(Objective 1)

25. d. If you have any suspicion of elder abuse or neglect, you are obligated to report it. You should remove clothing if necessary for care. Implied consent is indicated on this call.
(Objective 3)

26. c. The Ryan White Comprehensive AIDS Resources Emergency Act of 1990 (PL 101-381) describes reporting requirements for hospitals to EMS providers who have been exposed to certain communicable diseases and lists other organizational responsibilities for infectious disease reporting.
(Objective 4)

27. c. The patient suffered damage, as evidenced by the long hospitalization. This could result in loss of income if the person was employed. This was more likely a breach of duty or nonfeasance (failure to perform a required act or duty) rather than malfeasance (performing a wrongful or unlawful act). Although the potential exists that the paramedic's actions violated EMS law, the failure to provide standard of care is usually not legislated.
(Objective 5)

28. c. Privileged patient information should never be given to personnel with no legal right to know it.
(Objective 7)

29. a. *Implied consent* permits a paramedic to render lifesaving care if the patient is unable to agree because of a lack of mental competence. *Informed consent* means that the patient has been told the implications of the injury and illness, the treatment needed, and potential complications. There is no such thing as referred consent.
(Objective 8)

30. b. You should ask the patient to sign a refusal of care form; however, if he refuses to do so, document his refusal and witness it. Be sure to advise the patient about further care for his condition. If he is awake and alert now, he may legally refuse transport.
(Objective 9)

31. d. EMS agencies are typically permitted to travel moderately faster (often 10 mph) than regular traffic; however, excessive speed is hazardous. Crews should slow down or stop until they are certain that traffic has stopped and then proceed cautiously though intersections. Traffic officers' instructions should be followed. If a dispute occurs, supervising officers should be contacted immediately.
(Objective 10)

32. a. In most cases a written rather than verbal "do not resuscitate" order is required to stop resuscitation. If airway or IV access can't be established, resuscitation efforts should not be terminated in the field. In some cases specific time limits may be placed on the provision of resuscitation; these should be determined in cooperation with medical direction, and they usually are used only with very long transports.
(Objective 11)

33. d. Do not cut through the stab hole. Do not give clothing to bystanders other than authorized law enforcement personnel. Do not move the knife unless it is essential for crew safety.
(Objective 12)

34. d. The patient care report should be as detailed as possible to paint a picture of the clinical findings and the care given.
(Objective 13)

WRAP IT UP

1. The care of the patient's wound was within the scope of practice; however, the actions related to the patient's consent were not.
(Objective 2)

2. No. Good Samaritan protections do not typically extend to those on duty.
(Objective 5)

3. No. Immunity statutes typically apply only to government agencies and do not always protect individual employees of those agencies.
(Objective 5)

4. No. Most states would not consider this type of assault "reportable"; however, for the safety of the EMS crew, it is prudent to have law enforcement present on all scenes that involve a violent crime.
(Objective 3)

5. Abandonment: The paramedic crew left the patient in the care of a clerical employee, not a person of equal or higher license.
Negligence: The paramedics had a duty to act (monitor a restrained patient until relieved by a qualified person); they breached that duty (turned the patient over to the registration clerk); there was injury (pneumonia secondary to aspiration); and there was proximate cause (the plaintiff likely could prove that the injury was caused by the paramedics' restraint and abandonment of the patient).
Assault: The paramedics told the patient they would transport her against her will.
Battery: The paramedics forcibly restrained the patient against her will.
False imprisonment: The paramedics restrained the patient to the stretcher against her will.
Slander: The paramedic called the patient's co-worker to tell her of the situation.
(Objectives 4, 6, 14)

Ethics

READING ASSIGNMENT
Chapter 5, pages 72-79, in *Mosby's Paramedic Textbook*, ed. 3

OBJECTIVES
Upon completion of this chapter, the paramedic student will be able to do the following:
1. Define ethics and bioethics.
2. Distinguish between professional, legal, and moral accountability.
3. Outline strategies to use to resolve ethical conflicts.
4. Describe the role of ethical tests in resolving ethical dilemmas in health care.
5. Discuss specific prehospital ethical issues including allocation of resources, decisions surrounding resuscitation, confidentiality, and consent.
6. Identify ethical dilemmas that may occur related to care in futile situations, obligation to provide care, patient advocacy, and the paramedic's role as physician extender.

SUMMARY
- Ethics is the discipline relating to right and wrong, moral duty and obligation, moral principles and values, and moral character. Bioethics is the science of medical ethics. Morals refers to social standard or customs.
- Paramedics must meet a standard established by their level of training and regional practice. Paramedics must abide by the law when ethical conflicts occur.
- A paramedic must act in a way that is seen as morally acceptable.
- The rapid approach to ethical issues is a process. The process involves reviewing past experiences; deliberation (if possible); and performing the impartiality test, universalization test, and interpersonal justifiability test to reach an acceptable decision.
- Two concepts of ethical health care are to provide patient benefit and to do no harm.
- All resources must be allocated fairly. This is an accepted bioethical value.
- Advance directives, living wills, and other self-determination documents can help the paramedic to make decisions about the appropriateness of resuscitation in the prehospital setting.
- A health care professional is not allowed to reveal details supplied by the patient to others without the patient's consent. This is the principle of confidentiality.
- In some cases, patients refuse lifesaving care. These cases can produce legal and ethical conflicts.
- Other areas that are likely to raise ethical questions in the prehospital setting include providing care in futile situations, the paramedic's obligation to provide care, patient advocacy, and the paramedic's role as physician extender.

REVIEW QUESTIONS

Match the term in column II with its description in column I. Use each term only once.

	Column I		Column II
1. _B_	Working to benefit others	a.	Autonomy
2. _E_	The study of right, wrong, and morality	b.	Beneficence
3. _f_	To do no harm	c.	Bioethics
4. _A_	A person's ability to make rational decisions independently	d.	Confidentiality
5. _C_	Moral duty or obligation related to medicine	e.	Ethics
6. _D_	Maintaining the privacy of personal patient information	f.	Nonmaleficence
		g.	Rationality

Questions 7 to 9 pertain to the following case study.

> A fellow paramedic who is a close friend calls you and is very upset. Her daughter was involved in a vehicle collision. She is fine, but a person in the other car was injured and has been taken to the hospital. You transported the injured patient, and your friend wants to know the extent of injuries, what the patient said, and details related to the crash.

7. **a.** What should you tell your friend about the patient's injuries?

Nothing, this would be in conflict with Confidentiality issues

b. Is your decision ethically correct with regard to the patient and your friend?

_____

Your friend's daughter has been charged with reckless driving. You believe that the patient you transported was intoxicated; in fact, he admitted to using alcohol and cocaine before the incident. Despite his serious injuries, he was laughing and making inappropriate comments.

8. Will this affect your decision about disclosing patient information? Why or why not?

_No_

_____

9. Did you make your decision about this problem based on professional, legal, or moral accountability?

Legal obligation prevents you from doing so

_____

10. Think about how you would respond to each of the following situations and state whether *professional*, *legal*, or *moral* accountability issues would prompt your actions.

a. You are leaving the hospital after transporting a patient. You notice that your partner has picked up some towels, although you didn't use any on the patient. He says, "Oh, these are for me. I want to wash my car this afternoon."

Legal, moral, professional

_____

b. As you depart from a scene, you hear your partner make an inappropriate racial comment about the patient.

Proffessional, moral

_____

c. You notice that an on-duty co-worker has an alcoholic drink while attending your annual department awards banquet.

Legal , Proffessional , Moral

d. Your partner administers a slightly different dose of pain medicine than that ordered by medical direction because he feels that the doctor was being "too conservative."

Proffessional + Moral

e. Your teenage niece is experiencing severe vomiting in her first trimester of pregnancy. It is clear that she needs IV fluids to relieve her dehydration, but she has no insurance, and you know it will cost your brother hundreds of dollars if she is seen in the emergency department. He asks whether you can get some supplies from work and come to the house to give her the fluids.

Legal , Ethical , Moral

Question 11 pertains to the following case study:

> You and your partner are caring for a 55-year-old patient who is in respiratory arrest. You have called for assistance and are told it will be 10 minutes. After intubation, the patient is stable as long as you ventilate regularly. You are preparing for transport when suddenly your partner collapses and is pulseless.

11. a. The circumstances allow you to care for only one patient or the other. Who will you choose to resuscitate? Why?

b. How did you reach the above decision? Try using the ethical tests in the rapid approach to emergency medical problems to see whether they would assist you in this situation.

   (1) Have you experienced a similar problem in the past?

   (2) Can you buy time for deliberation or to consult with others?

   (3) Would you accept the action if you were in the patient's place?

   (4) Would you feel comfortable having the action performed in all similar circumstances?

   (5) Can you provide good reasons to justify and defend your actions to others?

12. State which of the following factors is the cause of the ethical dilemma in each of the following situations. Then give an action you could take.

Allocation of resources	Care in futile situations
Decisions regarding resuscitation	Obligation to provide care
Confidentiality	Physician extender role
Consent	

a. You request pain medicine to care for your patient's very painful single extremity injury. On-line medical direction refuses.

Cause of ethical dilemma: _____

Possible action: _____

_____

b. Your patient has a severe headache, is vomiting, and has a numb right hand. Blood pressure is 220/140 mm Hg. Despite your detailed explanations, the patient is refusing treatment or transport.

Cause of ethical dilemma: _____

Possible action: _____

_____

c. You are triaging at a mass casualty situation. You evaluate a child, the same age as yours, whose skin is warm. Bystanders say she just stopped breathing a few moments ago.

Cause of ethical dilemma: _____

Possible action: _____

_____

d. You respond to a private residence. The patient has a legally executed living will. Hysterical family members are begging you to resuscitate the patient.

Cause of ethical dilemma: _____

Possible action: _____

_____

STUDENT SELF-ASSESSMENT

13. What are the standards of honorable behavior to which paramedics are expected to conform in the EMS profession?
  a. Certifications
  b. Ethics
  c. Laws
  d. Morals

14. Which of the following determines moral accountability in the practice of EMS?
  a. Laws and regulations
  b. Personal beliefs and values
  c. Professional licensure
  d. Standards related to education and skills

15. During a call, you find yourself in a situation that involves an ethical dilemma. What strategy can you use to resolve the problem?
  a. Let the patient's family tell you what to do.
  b. Ask yourself which action you would prefer if you were in the patient's place.
  c. Abide by your partner's opinion in the situation.
  d. Rely on your policies and procedures for guidance.

16. Which of the ethical tests can help correct for your personal bias about a situation?
  a. Would you accept the action if you were in the patient's place?
  b. Would you feel comfortable having this action performed under similar circumstances?
  c. Can you justify and defend your actions to others?
  d. Have you experienced a similar problem in the past?

17. On a call, you are faced with an unusual situation that falls just on the fringe of your legal and professional boundaries. You decide to take action because you are able to provide clear reasons explaining and defending your actions to others. What type of ethical test have you used?
    a. Autonomy
    b. Impartiality
    c. Interpersonal justifiability
    d. Universalizability
18. Which of the following situations involves an ethical decision? The patient has a living will and is pulseless.
    a. The family asks you to abide by the living will.
    b. The patient is cold and has rigor mortis.
    c. A signature is in the wrong place on the living will document.
    d. The nursing home staff think that a living will exists but cannot locate it.
19. You are transporting a patient and her doctor from an outpatient surgery center to the hospital because a complication has occurred. The patient's respirations are very slow, and her chest is barely moving. You note the need to ventilate, but the physician strongly disagrees. If you elect to proceed, you are acting on which ethical principle?
    a. Allocation of resources
    b. Autonomy
    c. Care in futile situations
    d. Patient advocacy

WRAP IT UP

You are dispatched at 1500 to a home in a quiet residential neighborhood to "check the welfare with possible forcible entry." Out of town adult family members report that they have been unable to contact their father for a day and a half, and they are concerned for his health. On arrival you note that the man's car is in the garage. Two newspapers are in the driveway, and neighbors tell you that they haven't seen him in 2 days. You circle the home, knocking loudly and looking in windows. Through the kitchen window, you are able to see feet protruding from behind the counter. The captain elects to force a door to gain entry. Once in, you find a 79-year-old man who tells you he slipped and fell 2 days ago and is unable to get up. You examine him and are unable to find any injuries, although he appears somewhat dehydrated, his heart rate is elevated, and his clothing is soaked with urine. He is very thin, and when you check the refrigerator and cabinets, you find little food.

The patient is alert and oriented; however, he seems slow to respond, his speech is slightly slurred, and he has weakness on the left side. He tends to repeat information. He adamantly refuses to be transported. According to your protocol, you can't forcibly transport him based on the information you have provided. Repeated attempts to reach medical control are not successful. You decide to transport the patient anyway.

1. Why does this call present an ethical conflict?

_____

_____

2. Answer all the tests of ethical decision making to see how they would apply to this situation. Explain your answers.

    a. Impartiality test: Would you accept this action if you were in the patient's place?

_____

_____

    b. Universalizability test: Would you feel comfortable having this action performed in all relevantly similar circumstances?

_____

_____

    c. Interpersonal justifiability test: Are you able to provide good reasons to justify and defend your actions to others?

_____

_____

3. Answer the following ethical questions regarding this call.
    a. What is the patient's best interest?
    b. What are the patient's rights?
    c. Does the patient understand the issues at hand?
    d. What is the paramedic's professional, legal, and moral accountability?

    a. _____

    b. _____

    c. _____

    d. _____

4. a. Put a ✔ beside the bioethical values you would be following if you leave the patient unattended at the scene.
    b. Put an ✗ beside the bioethical values you would be following if you arrange either for someone to come and provide temporary care for the patient or for the Division of Aging to come and evaluate him within 12 hours.

_____ Autonomy		_____ Beneficence	
_____ Confidentiality		_____ Allocation of resources	
_____ Nonmaleficence		_____ Personal integrity	

REVIEW QUESTIONS

1. b
(Objective 4)

2. e
(Objective 1)

3. f
(Objective 4)

4. a
(Objective 4)

5. c
(Objective 4)

6. d
(Objective 1)

7. a. You can disclose nothing about the patient's injuries except what is permitted by departmental policy.
b. Your feelings about whether this is ethical will be personal.

8. Your legal obligation would not change regardless of your decision.

9. Your legal obligation prevents you from disclosing information. (Questions 7 to 9: Objective 2)

10. a. Legal (theft), professional, and moral conflicts may come into play here.
b. Professional and moral conflicts may be involved as you make a decision about how to respond to this situation.
c. Legal (working/driving while under the influence), professional, and moral standards are involved in the paramedic's actions and in your response to them.
d. Professional and moral issues are involved in this situation.
e. Legal (theft of equipment), professional (actions without medical direction), and moral (allocation of resources) issues are involved in this situation.
(Objective 2)

11. The answers to each of these questions are personal. Discuss your answers with a fellow student. How do your views compare?
(Objective 3)

12. a. Physician extender role. Possible actions: Clarify and repeat request for orders. Ask for a call review/critique to discuss the issue.
b. Consent. Possible actions: Have on-line medical direction speak to the patient. Talk to the family to see if they can convince the patient. If not, provide detailed follow-up instructions and try to leave the patient in the supervised care of family or friends.
c. Allocation of resources. Possible actions: Reevaluate your resources to determine whether resuscitation should proceed. Ask for a change of assignment if possible.
d. Decisions regarding resuscitation. Possible actions: Contact medical direction. Remove the family from the area and calmly explain the wishes of their loved one.
(Objectives 3-5)

STUDENT SELF-ASSESSMENT

13. b. Certification is a professional standard. Laws are legal standards. Morals are social standards.
(Objective 1)

14. b. Laws and regulations relate to legal accountability. Professional licensure and standards relate to education. Skills relate to professional accountability.
(Objective 2)

15. b. This is known as the impartiality test.
(Objective 3)

16. b. This is known as the universalizability test.
(Objective 3)

17. a. The impartiality test can correct partiality or personal bias. The universalizability test helps eliminate moral decision difficulty. The interpersonal justifiability test requires reasons for your actions and approval from others of those reasons.
(Objective 4)

18. c. If the family concurs and the living will is legal, no ethical question exists. If the patient has obvious signs of death, no ethical dilemma exists. If the living will document cannot be produced, legally it cannot be recognized.
(Objective 5)

19. d. Allocation of resources is an issue when the patient's health care needs can't be met because of inadequate resources. Autonomy is a person's ability to make decisions. Care in futile situations arises when the care you are about to give serves no purpose.
(Objective 6)

WRAP IT UP

1. An ethical conflict exists because a disparity clearly exists between what you can legally do and what you know needs to be done for this man.
(Objective 2)

2. a. Assuming the patient is lucid, he may not accept it.
b. This is a question each student should answer individually.
c. Could you justify your actions? What rationale would you use? Are other options available?
(Objective 4)

3. a. Do you have enough information to determine whether this is in the patient's best interest?
b. An alert, oriented patient has the right to refuse care. Are other social service agencies available that you could involve that might help make the determination whether the patient is presently competent to make this decision? Can local police assist you?
c. Did you explain and have the patient verbalize his understanding of the risks of leaving him alone?
d. Professionally you have a responsibility to care for patients and to ensure their safety; however, you also have a responsibility to follow protocols. Legally your state law and your local protocols may state that the patient has the right to refuse. Moral questions will be answered individually. Involve medical direction to help resolve the situation on-line.
(Objective 2)

4. a. Autonomy, possibly personal integrity
(Objective 5)
b. Beneficence, nonmaleficence
(Objective 5)

PART TWO

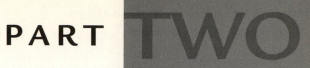

IN THIS PART

Review of Human Systems

READING ASSIGNMENT

Chapter 6, pages 80-149, in *Mosby's Paramedic Textbook,* ed. 3

OBJECTIVES

Upon completion of this chapter, the paramedic student will be able to do the following:

1. Discuss the importance of human anatomy as it relates to the paramedic profession.
2. Describe the anatomical position.
3. Properly interpret anatomical directional terms and body planes.
4. List the structures that compose the axial and appendicular regions of the body.
5. Define the divisions of the abdominal region.
6. List the three major body cavities.
7. Describe the contents of the three major body cavities.
8. Discuss the functions of the following cellular structures: the cytoplasmic membrane, the cytoplasm (and organelles), and the nucleus.
9. Describe the process by which human cells reproduce.
10. Differentiate and describe the following tissue types: epithelial tissue, connective tissue, muscle tissue, and nervous tissue.
11. For each of the 11 major organ systems in the human body, label a diagram of anatomical structures, list the functions of the major anatomical structures, and explain how the organs of the system interrelate to perform the specified functions of the system.
12. For the special senses, label a diagram of the anatomical structures of the special senses, list the functions of the anatomical structures of each sense, and explain how the structures of the senses interrelate to perform their specialized functions.

SUMMARY

- The paramedic must understand human anatomy fully. This understanding will help the paramedic to organize a patient assessment by body region. Knowledge of anatomy also will help the paramedic to communicate well with medical direction and other members of the health care team.
- The anatomical position refers to a patient standing erect with the palms facing the examiner.
- Directional terms are expressed in anatomical terminology. Examples of these are *up* or *down, front* or *back,* and *right* or *left*. These terms always refer to the patient, not the examiner. Internal body structure is classified into anatomical planes of the human body. These planes can be thought of as imaginary straight-line divisions.

- The appendicular region of the body includes the limbs, or extremities. The axial region consists of the head, neck, thorax, and abdomen.
- The abdomen usually is divided into four quadrants: upper right, lower right, upper left, and lower left.
- The three major cavities of the human body are the thoracic cavity, the abdominal cavity, and the pelvic cavity.
- The thoracic cavity contains the trachea, esophagus, thymus, heart, great vessels, lungs, and the cavities and membranes that surround them. The abdominopelvic cavity is surrounded by membranes and contains organs and blood vessels.
- The cytoplasmic membrane encloses the cytoplasm. The membrane forms the outer boundary of the cell.
- Cytoplasm lies between the cytoplasmic membrane and the nucleus. Specialized structures in the cell (organelles) are located in the cytoplasm. These organelles perform functions key to the survival of the cell. The nucleus is a large, membrane-bound organelle. It ultimately controls all other organelles in the cytoplasm.
- All human cells, with the exception of the reproductive (sex) cells, reproduce by a process known as mitosis. In this process, cells divide to multiply.
- Four main types of tissue make up the many organs of the body. These are epithelial, connective, muscle, and nervous. Epithelial tissue covers surfaces and forms structures. Connective tissue is made of cells separated from each other by intercellular material. This material is known as the extracellular matrix. Muscle tissue is contractile tissue and is responsible for movement. The nervous tissue has the ability to conduct electrical signals. These signals are known as action potentials.
- A system is a group of organs arranged to perform a more complex function than any one organ can perform alone. The eleven major organ systems in the body are the integumentary, skeletal, muscular, nervous, endocrine, circulatory, lymphatic, respiratory, digestive, urinary, and reproductive.
- The integumentary system consists of the skin and accessory structures such as hair, nails, and a variety of glands. The functions of the integumentary system include protecting the body against injury and dehydration, defense against infection, and temperature regulation.
- The skeletal system consists of bone and associated connective tissues, including cartilage, tendons, and ligaments. The skeletal system provides a rigid framework for support and protection. It also provides a system of levers on which muscles act to produce body movements.
- The three primary functions of the muscular system are movement, postural maintenance, and heat production.
- The nervous and the endocrine systems are the major regulatory and coordinating systems of the body. The nervous system rapidly sends information. It does this by means of nerve impulses conducted from one area of the body to another. The endocrine system sends information more slowly. It does this by means of chemicals secreted by ductless glands into the bloodstream.
- The heart and cardiovascular system are responsible for circulating blood throughout the body. Blood transports nutrients and oxygen to tissues. Blood carries carbon dioxide and waste products away from tissues. In addition, blood carries hormones produced in endocrine glands to their target tissues. Blood also plays a key role in temperature regulation and fluid balance. Blood also protects the body from bacteria and foreign substances.
- The lymphatic system includes lymph, lymphocytes, lymph nodes, tonsils, spleen, and thymus gland. The lymphatic system has three basic functions. The first is to help maintain fluid balance in tissues. The second is to absorb fats and other substances from the digestive tract. The third is to play a role in the immune defense system of the body.
- The organs of the respiratory system and the cardiovascular system move oxygen to cells. They move carbon dioxide from cells to where it is released into the air. The entrance to the respiratory tract begins at the nasal cavity and includes the nasopharynx, oropharynx, laryngopharynx, and larynx. Below the glottis are the structures of the lower airway and lungs. These structures include the trachea, the bronchial tree, the alveoli, and the lungs.
- The digestive system provides the body with water, electrolytes, and other nutrients used by cells. The gastrointestinal tract is an irregularly shaped tube. Associated accessory organs (mainly glands) secrete fluid into the digestive tract.
- The urinary system works with other body systems to maintain homeostasis. It does this by removing waste products from the blood. It also does this by helping to maintain a constant body fluid volume and composition. The contents of the urinary system include two kidneys, two ureters, the urinary bladder, and the urethra.
- The purpose of the male reproductive system is to make and transfer spermatozoa to the female. The purpose of the female reproductive system is to make oocytes and to receive the spermatozoa for fertilization, conception, gestation, and birth. The male reproductive system consists of the testes, epididymis, ductus deferens, urethra, seminal vesicles, prostate gland, bulbourethral glands, scrotum, and penis. The female reproductive

organs consist of the ovaries, uterine (or fallopian) tubes, uterus, vagina, external genital organs, and mammary glands.

- Senses provide the brain with information about the outside world. Four senses are recognized as special senses: smell, taste, sight, and hearing and balance.

REVIEW QUESTIONS

Match the cellular structure from column II with its definition in column I. Use each answer only once.

Column I	Column II
1. _D_ Cytoplasmic "canals" that transport proteins and other substances	a. Centrioles
	b. Cytoplasm
2. _C_ Phospholipid layer that forms the outer boundary of the cell	c. Cytoplasmic membrane
3. _f_ Organelles that contain enzymes capable of digesting proteins and lipids	d. Endoplasmic reticulum
4. _B_ Mass of a cell that lies between the cytoplasmic membrane and nucleus	e. Golgi apparatus
	f. Lysosomes
5. _e_ Sacs that package materials for secretion from the cell	g. Mitochondria
	h. Nucleus
6. _h_ Control center of the cell; contains genetic material	i. Ribosomes
7. _i_ Structures composed of ribonucleic acid and protein that manufacture enzymes	
8. _G_ Powerhouse of the cell, responsible for production of adenosine triphosphate	

9. Label Fig. 6-1 with the appropriate cellular structures listed in column II of question 8.

   a. ~~Lysosomes~~ CENTRIOLE S

   b. ~~Endoplasmic Reticulum~~ RIBOSOMAS

   c. golgiapparatus

   d. Nucleus

   e. ~~Ribosomes~~ ENDOPLASMR RETICULM

   f. Lysosome

   g. Mitochondria

10. All human cells divide by the process of mitosis throughout the life of a human organism. True/False. If this is false, explain why.

FALSE.

_____

_____

11. Describe the anatomical position.

STANDING, feet flat, Palms forward

12. Circle the appropriate directional terms in boldface in the following sentences.

   a. The wrist lies **distal**/**proximal** to the elbow.

   b. The right nipple is located **medial**/**lateral** to the sternum.

   c. The cervical spine is **superior**/**inferior** to the lumbar spine.

   d. The umbilicus is located on the **dorsal**/**ventral** surface of the body.

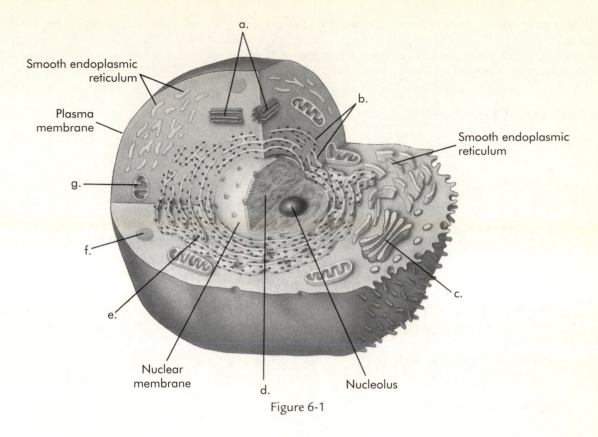

Figure 6-1

13. List the structures that make up the following regions of the body.

    a. Appendicular region:

EXTREMITIES AND THEIR GIRDLES

    b. Axial region:

HEAD, NECK thorax AND Abdomen

14. Name the anatomical landmarks that divide the abdomen into four quadrants.

Questions 15 to 19 pertain to the following case study:

You respond to a call for a burn. You determine that the scene is safe and then approach the patient. She is lying on her right side, moaning, and has burned sites over several areas. You begin your assessment and care and roll her supine. As you carefully remove her clothing, you can better observe the burns, as shown in Fig. 6-2.

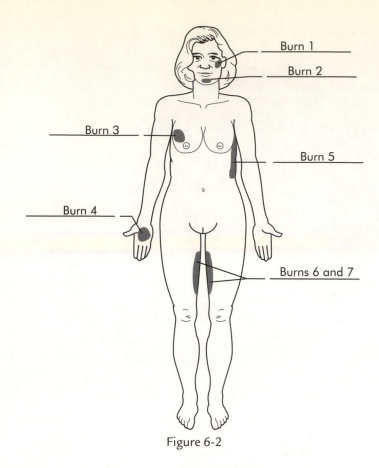

Figure 6-2

15. What directional term describes the patient's position when you arrived?

Right lateral recumbent

16. Using appropriate directional terms, describe where

a. Burn (1) is located relative to the left eye

Inferior to (L) eye

b. Burn (2) is located relative to the mouth

Inferior to mouth

c. Burn (3) is located relative to the nipple

Superior / lateral

d. Burn (4) lies relative to the right hand

Anterior palm

e. Burn (5) lies relative to the axilla

f. Burns (6 and 7) are located

Medial aspect of thigh, bilateral

17. Burn (5) encroaches on what abdominal quadrant?

_____

18. List the major body cavities under each wound.

    a. Burn (3)

Thoracic cavity _____

    b. Burn (5)

_____

19. Have these wounds affected the axial or appendicular regions of the body?

_____

20. For each of the following subgroups of tissues, list the tissue type (epithelial, connective, muscle, or nervous), one area of the body where it is found, and at least one specialized function it performs.

Subgroup	Type	Body Area	Function
Striated voluntary tissue			
Bone			
Epithelium			
Adipose tissue			
Hemopoietic tissue			
Striated involuntary tissue			
Neurons			
Cartilage			
Areolar tissue			
Nonstriated involuntary tissue			
Neuroglia			

21. List the 11 major body systems.

    a. Respiratory

    b. Circulatory

    c. Lymphatic

    d. Urinary

    e. Integumentary

    f. Skeletal

g. ENDOCRINE

h. Digestive

i. REPRODUCTIVE

j. NERVOUS

k.

22. Label the structures of the skin shown in Fig. 6-3 and list two functions of each.

	Structure	Functions
a.		
b.		
c.		

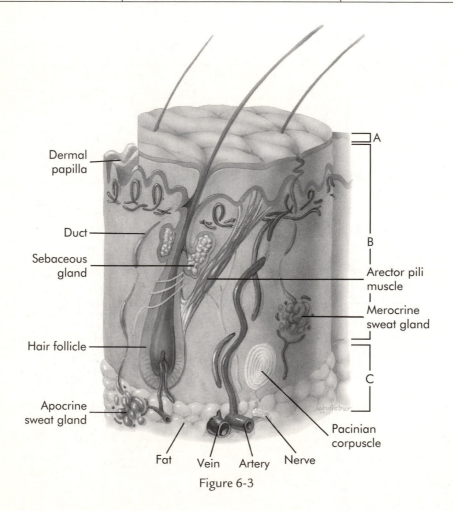

Figure 6-3

23. List three functions of the glands located in the skin.

a.

b.

c.

24. Describe the effect on the skin's function of a large, third-degree (full-thickness) burn that destroys all the layers of the dermis.

inAbility to Regulate temperature, innability to protect feen bata

25. Label the bones of the human skull shown in Fig. 6-4.

a. *Parietal*

b. *Temporal*

c. *Frontal*

d. *Occipital*

e. *Sphenoid*

f. *Ethmoid*

g. *Maxilla*

h. *Mandibe*

i. *Zygoma*

j. *Nasal*

k. *Lacrimal*

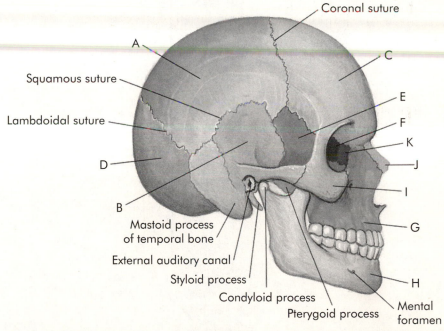

Figure 6-4

26. Label the bony regions of the vertebral column shown in Fig. 6-5 and indicate the number of vertebrae in each region.

Region   **Number of Vertebrae**

   a. CERVICAl

   b. Thoracic

   c. LumbAR

   d. SacrAl

   e. COcyXX

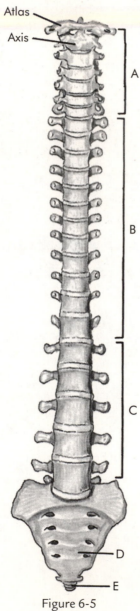

Atlas

Axis

A

B

C

D

E

Figure 6-5

27. List two functions of the thoracic cage.

   a. PROtect Ribs

   b. MAINtENANce of lung inflatior

28. Label the structures of the thoracic cage shown in Fig. 6-6.

a. MANUBRIUM

b. BODY

c. STERNUM

d. XHIPHOID PROCESS

e. JUGULAR NOTCH

f. STERNAL ANGLE

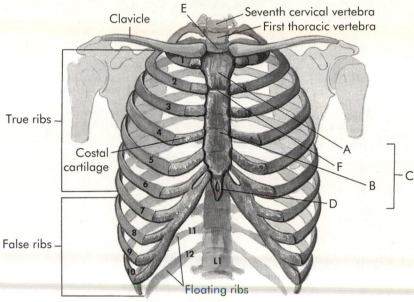

Clavicle

E

Seventh cervical vertebra

First thoracic vertebra

True ribs

Costal cartilage

A

F

B

C

D

False ribs

11

8

12

9

L1

10

Floating ribs

Figure 6-6

29. What problems can occur when a patient sustains a traumatic injury that results in a fractured sternum and multiple fractured ribs?

IMPAIRED VENTILATIONS, BLOOD LOSS, INJURY TO UNDERLYING ORGANS

30. Complete the following sentences, which relate to the skeletal system.

The pectoral girdle is composed of the **(a)** SCAPULA and **(b)** CLAVICLE. Its function

is to **(c)** ATTACH UPPER EXTREMITY TO AXIAL SKELETON.

The point of attachment of the appendicular and axial skeleton occurs at the **(d)** STERNO-CLAVICULAR

joint.

31. Label the diagram of the upper extremity shown in Fig. 6-7.

a.

b.

c.

d.

e.

f.

g.

h.

i.

j.

k.

l.

m.

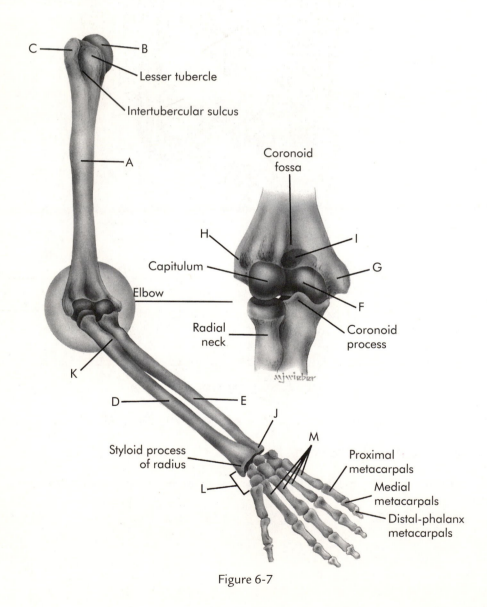

Figure 6-7

32. Label the parts of the pelvic girdle shown in Fig. 6-8.

a.

b.

c.

d.

e.

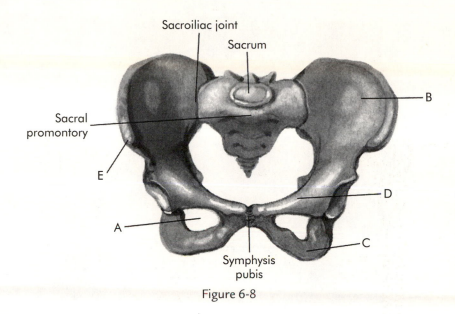

Figure 6-8

33. What are the functions of the pelvic girdle?

_____

_____

34. Label the bones of the lower extremity shown in Fig. 6-9.

a.

b.

c.

d.

e.

f.

g.

h.

i.

j.

k.

l.

m.

n.

o.

p.

q.

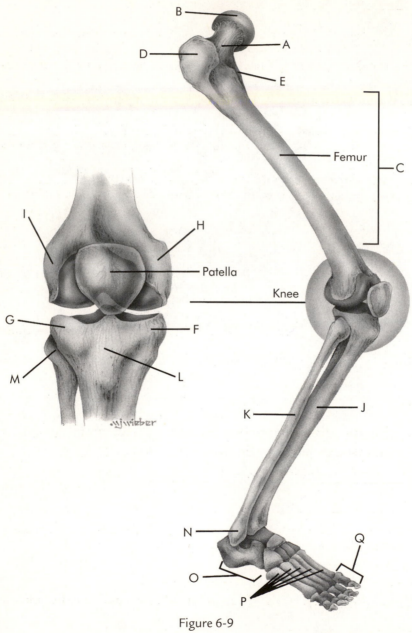

Figure 6-9

35. Complete the blanks in the following statements about joints.

The three major classifications of joints are **(a)** _____, _____, and

_____. Fibrous joints have **(b)** _____ movement. Fibrous joints can

be further divided into sutures, found in the **(c)** _____, syndesmoses found between the

(d) _____ and _____, and a gomphosis joint, which consists of a peg in

a socket, such as the joints between (e) _____ and _____. A synchondrosis is
a cartilaginous joint that allows only slight movement. One can be found in the chest between the ribs and the

(f) _____. Symphysis joints, another example of cartilaginous joints, can be found in the

chest at the (g) _____ _____, in the pelvis at the (h) _____ _____, and in the spine at the

(i) _____ _____. Synovial joints are classified into six divisions, all of which contain (j) _____

_____. Joints consisting of two opposed, flat surfaces, such as the articular processes between vertebrae,

are (k) _____ joints. Joints that consist of two saddle-shaped, articulating surfaces that allow

movement in two planes (e.g., the carpometacarpal joint in the thumb) are (l) _____ _____. Joints
that consist of a convex cylinder of bone that fits into a corresponding concavity in another bone and permit

movement in one plane, such as the elbow and knee, are known as (m) _____ joints. A cylindri-
cal bony process that rotates within a ring composed of bone and ligament, such as the head of the radius where

it articulates with the ulna, is a(n) (n) _____ joint. A wide range of motion is permitted by
shoulder and hip joints, where the head of one bone fits into the socket of an adjacent bone. These are known as

(o) _____ _____ _____ joints. The atlantooccipital joint is an example of a modified

ball and socket joint known as a(n) (p) _____ joint.

36. Replace the boldface words in the following sentences with the correct terms from the following list. Use each
term only once.

Abduction	Excursion	Opposition
Adduction	Extension	Pronation
Depression	Flexion	Rotation
Eversion	Inversion	Supination

a. The patient has sustained an injury to his elbow and is unable to **rotate his forearm so that the anterior surface is up** or **rotate his forearm so that the anterior surface is down**.

_____ or

_____

b. To determine whether the patient had intact neurological function, the paramedic had **her move her
thumb and little finger toward each other.**

_____

c. After he injured his knee, the soccer player had pain when he **bent** and **stretched out** his lower leg.

_____ and

_____

d. An older woman with a hip fracture has a leg that looks shortened and shows **external movement about its
axis.**

_____

e. A person with a shoulder separation has limited ability to **move the arm from the midline.**

_____

f. A patient with a posterior hip dislocation has the following physical findings: the leg is shortened, internally rotated, and slightly **moved toward the midline.**

_____

g. Ankle sprains are frequently produced by turning the ankle **inward** or turning it **outward.**

_____   or

_____

h. Newer splints for the foot can sometimes make casting unnecessary when the desired effect is to prevent **movement from side to side.**

_____

i. The blow to the head with a baseball bat **produced movement of the temporal bone in an inferior direction.**

_____

37. List the three primary functions of the muscular system.

a.

b.

c.

38. Complete the following sentences pertaining to the muscular system.

The specialized contractile cells of the muscles are called **(a)** _____. Each muscle fiber is filled

with thick and thin threadlike structures known as **(b)** _____. These are composed of the

proteins **(c)** _____ and _____. The contractile unit of skeletal muscle fibers

is the **(d)** _____. During muscle contraction, the two myofilaments slide toward each other and

shorten the sarcomere fueled with energy from **(e)** _____.

39. Define the following terms.

a. Isometric muscle contraction:

_____

b. Isotonic muscle contraction:

_____

c. Muscle tone:

_____

40. Describe the role the muscular system plays in maintaining body temperature.

_____

_____

41. Briefly describe the function of the nervous system.

_____

_____

42. List the primary components of the following:

   a. Central nervous system:

_____

   b. Peripheral nervous system:

_____

43. List the two subdivisions of the efferent division of the nervous system and briefly describe the function of each.

   a. _____

   b. _____

44. Label the parts of the brain shown in Fig. 6-10.

   a.

   b.

   c.

   d.

   e.

   f.

   g.

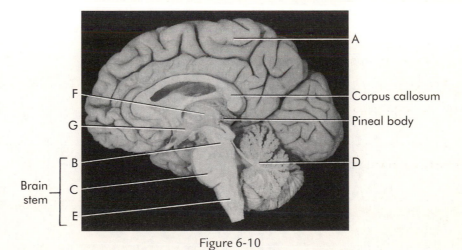

Figure 6-10

45. Briefly describe the functions of each of the following areas of the brain stem.

   a. Medulla:

_____

b. Pons:

_____

c. Midbrain:

_____

d. Reticular formation:

_____

e. Hypothalamus:

_____

f. Thalamus:

_____

46. Label the parts of the cerebrum shown in Fig. 6-11 and list one important function of each area.

Area	Function
a.	
b.	
c.	
d.	

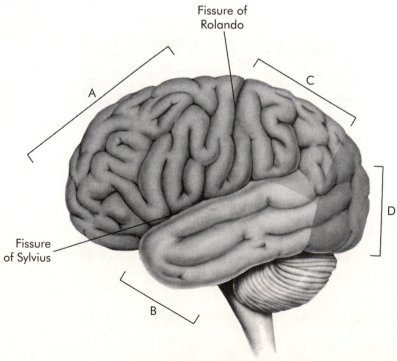

Figure 6-11

47. Briefly describe the major functions of the cerebellum.

_____

_____

48. List two functions of the spinal cord.

a.

b.

49. Complete the following sentences about the meninges.

Cerebrospinal fluid bathes and cushions the **(a)** _____ and _____ . It is

formed in a network of brain capillaries known as the **(b)** _____ .

50. List the three functional categories of the 12 cranial nerves.

a.

b.

c.

51. For each of the following organs or body systems, describe the effects of stimulation by each division of the autonomic nervous system.

Affected Organ	Sympathetic	Parasympathetic
Heart		
Lungs		
Pupils		
Intestine		
Blood vessels		

52. Describe the function of the endocrine system.

_____

_____

53. For each of the following hormones, list the primary target tissue and one action the hormone may have on that tissue.

Hormone	Target	Action
Epinephrine		
Aldosterone		
Antidiuretic hormone		
Parathyroid hormone		
Calcitonin		
Insulin		
Glucagon		
Testosterone		
Thymosin		
Oxytocin		
Thyroid hormone		

54. Describe how hormones reach their target tissues.

_____

_____

55. List five functions of the circulatory system.

a. TRANSPORTS NUTRIENTS

b. CARRIES HORMONES

c. TRANSPORTS WASTE

d. Regulates temp & fluid Balance

e. Provides Protection from Bacteria

56. Complete the following sentences regarding the components of blood.

About 95% of the formed elements in blood are red blood cells, also known as **(a)** _____.

The primary component of red blood cells is **(b)** _____. This gives blood its red color and allows it

to transport **(c)** _____ from the lungs to the tissues and to transport

(d) _____ from the tissues to the lungs. The remaining 5% of the formed elements in

blood consists of white blood cells, called **(e)** _____ and platelets, known as

(f) _____. The primary function of white blood cells is

(g) _____. Platelets help prevent blood loss by activating the formation of

(h) _____ to seal off wounds in the blood vessels. The pale yellow fluid that surrounds these

formed elements is **(i)** _____.

57. Label the structures of the heart indicated on Fig. 6-12 and draw arrows to show the path taken by the blood
from the point where it enters the heart from the body until it returns to the body from the heart.

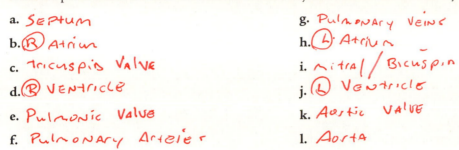

a. SEPTUM

b. Ⓡ Atrium

c. Tricuspid VALVE

d. Ⓡ VENtricle

e. Pulmonic Valve

f. Pulmonary Arteies

g. Pulmonary Veins

h. Ⓛ Atrium

i. Mitral / Bicuspid

j. Ⓛ Ventricle

k. Aortic VALVE

l. Aorta

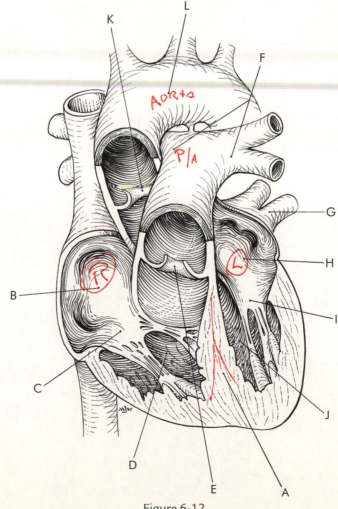

Figure 6-12

58. Name the branches of the circulatory system from the aorta to the cellular level and back to the vena cava.

_____

_____

59. Briefly describe the characteristics of blood vessels that permit vasodilation and vasoconstriction.

_____

_____

60. What structural feature of some veins inhibits the back flow of blood?

_____

61. What is the purpose of an arteriovenous anastomosis (arteriovenous shunt)?

_____

_____

62. List the three basic functions of the lymphatic system.

   a.

   b.

   c.

63. Describe the flow of lymph from its beginning in the tissues until it empties into the circulatory system.

_____

_____

_____

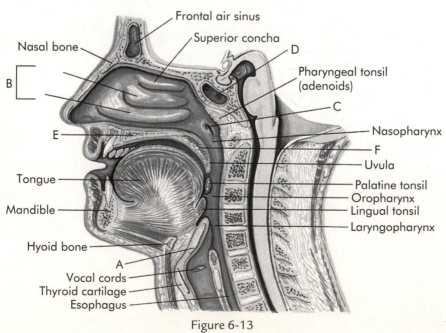

Figure 6-13

64. Label the parts of the upper airway shown in Fig. 6-13 and list one function of each structure.

Structure	Function
a. EPiGlotHis	Protection of Lower AirWAy
b. ConchAE + turbsinates	WARMinG + filtering of Are
c.	
d.	
e.	
f.	

65. Label the parts of the larynx shown in Fig. 6-14.

a. Epiglottis
b. ThyRoid cartilage
c. Cricoid Cartilage
d. hyoid Bone
e. Vocal cords folds

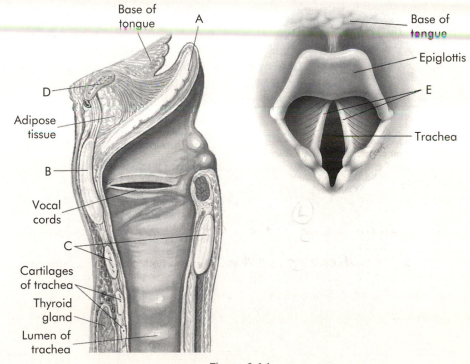

Figure 6-14

66. Label the parts of the lower airway shown in Fig. 6-15.

a. TRACHEA

b. Bronchi

c. Alveoli

d. CARINA

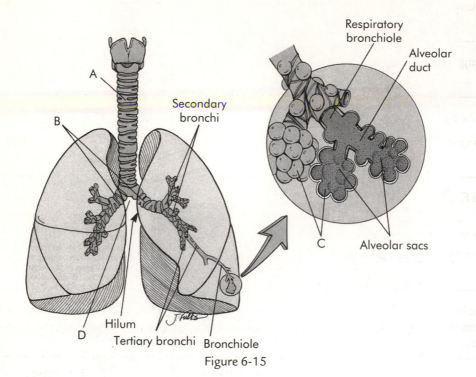

Respiratory
bronchiole

Alveolar
duct

Secondary
bronchi

A

B

C

Alveolar sacs

Hilum

D

Tertiary bronchi   Bronchiole

Figure 6-15

67. Describe how the structure of the trachea protects the airway.

_____

_____

68. Describe what happens to the bronchioles that causes wheezing during an asthma attack.

Smooth muscle surrounding the Bronchioles Become irritation constriction causes wheezing when Airw passes through tight space,

69. Describe the anatomical feature of the alveoli that performs the following functions.

a. Permits the movement of oxygen to the blood and carbon dioxide (CO_2) from the blood:

_____

b. Prevents collapse of the alveoli:

Pulmonary Surfactant

70. Describe the location of the lungs in the chest cavity.

_____

_____

71. List the divisions of the following:

    a. Right lung:

_____

    b. Left lung:

_____

72. Describe the functions of the following:

    a. Pleural space:

_____

    b. Pleural fluid:

_____

73. List the functions of the digestive system.

_____

74. As a cheeseburger passes through the digestive tract, many digestive juices act on it to convert the food into a usable form for the body. For each area of the digestive tract listed, name a digestive juice excreted and briefly describe its function.

Area	Digestive Juice	Function
Mouth		
Stomach		
Pancreas		
Liver		
Large intestine		

75. List the functions of the urinary system.

_____

_____

76. List two specific functions of the kidneys in addition to urine production.

    a.

    b.

77. The basic functional unit of the kidney is the **(a)** _____. It produces urine by a three-step

process: **(b)** _____, **(c)** _____, and **(d)** _____.

78. State whether each of the following increases or decreases urine production.

   a. Aldosterone:

   b. Atrial natriuretic factor:

   c. Large increase in blood pressure:

   d. Shock:

79. Label the parts of the male reproductive system shown in Fig. 6-16.

   a.

   b.

   c.

   d.

   e.

   f.

   g.

   h.

   i.

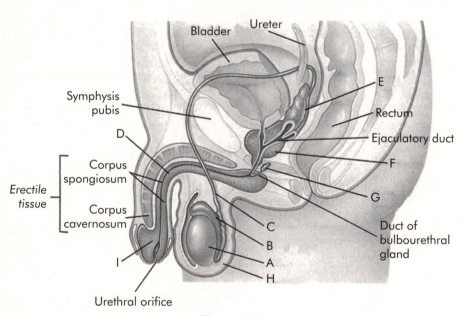

Figure 6-16

80. Label the parts of the female reproductive system shown in Fig. 6-17.

   a.

   b.

   c.

   d.

   e.

   f.

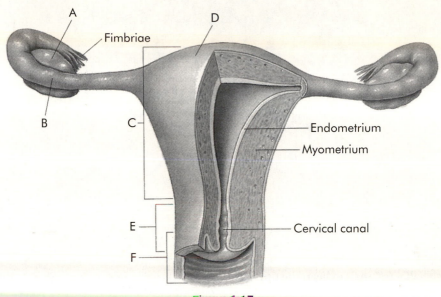

Figure 6-17

81. Label the parts of the female perineum shown in Fig. 6-18.

   a.

   b.

   c.

   d.

   e.

   f.

   g.

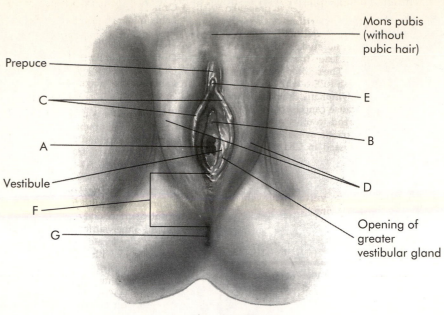

Prepuce

Mons pubis (without pubic hair)

C

E

A

B

Vestibule

D

F

Opening of greater vestibular gland

G

Figure 6-18

82. Complete the following sentences pertaining to the olfactory sense.

Receptors for the olfactory nerves lie in the upper part of the **(a)** _____ cavity. When olfactory cells

are stimulated by airborne molecules, the nerve impulses travel in the olfactory bulb and **(b)** _____.

The brain interprets the impulses as specific odors in the **(c)** _____ and **(d)** _____ centers.

83. Complete the following sentences pertaining to the sense of taste.

Sensory structures that detect taste stimuli in the mouth are **(a)** _____ _____.

Taste buds are most commonly found in the mouth on the **(b)** _____. However, they are also

found on the **(c)** _____, _____, and _____. The four basic tastes

that are detected are **(d)** _____, _____, _____, and

_____.

84. Complete the following sentences pertaining to the sense of vision.

The sensation of vision is transmitted from the eye to the brain by way of the **(a)** _____ nerve.

Impulses that travel from the brain to control the movements of the eye are relayed by the **(b)** _____

nerve. The avascular, transparent structure that bends and refracts light as it enters the eye is the **(c)** _____ .

The size of the pupil and therefore the amount of light that enters the eye through it is controlled by the

(d) _____. The inner sensory layer of the retina contains two types of photoreceptor cells. The receptors responsible for night vision are the (e) _____, and the receptors that permit daytime and color vision are the (f) _____. The eye has two compartments. The anterior chamber is filled with (g) _____ humor, and the posterior chamber contains (h) _____ humor. The humor in both chambers helps maintain (i) _____ _____.

85. List the function of each of the following accessory structures of the eye.

   a. Eyebrows:

   _____

   b. Eyelids:

   _____

   c. Lacrimal glands:

   _____

86. Complete the following sentences pertaining to the tissues associated with hearing and balance.

   The external and middle ear are involved in (a) _____, and the inner ear plays a role in

   (b) _____ and _____. The senses of hearing and balance are transmitted by the

   (c) _____ nerve. Sound is picked up by the external ear prominence, known as the

   (d) _____, and transmitted through the external auditory meatus into the (e) _____

   canal. At the end of the canal, vibration of the (f) _____ _____ is produced. These vibrations are

   picked up and transmitted to the oval window by the auditory ossicles of the middle ear. These three bones are

   the (g)_____, _____, and _____. Finally, in the inner ear inside the

   cochlea lies the hearing sense organ, called the (h)_____. The two other structures in the inner

   ear involved in balance are the (i) _____ and (j) _____ _____.

STUDENT SELF-ASSESSMENT

87. You find your patient lying face up on his back. This is which position?
   a. Anatomical
   b. Lateral recumbent
   c. Prone
   d. Supine
88. A teenage football player has collapsed after a sharp blow to the left upper quadrant of the abdomen. You suspect injury to which of the following?
   a. Appendix
   b. Gallbladder
   c. Liver
   d. Spleen

89. Which of the following structures is located in the mediastinum?
    a. Diaphragm
    b. Lungs
    c. Thyroid
    d. Trachea
90. Cardiac muscle cells are which of the following?
    a. Striated voluntary
    b. Striated involuntary
    c. Nonstriated voluntary
    d. Nonstriated involuntary
91. The actual conducting cells of the nervous system are which of the following?
    a. Dendrites
    b. Neuroglia
    c. Neurons
    d. Synapses
92. Which of the following is a function of the integumentary system?
    a. Collection of lymph
    b. Movement
    c. Production of vitamin C
    d. Temperature regulation
93. The scapula and clavicle make up which of the following?
    a. Pectoral girdle
    b. Pelvic girdle
    c. Thorax
    d. Vertebral disks
94. An indoor soccer player has sustained an injury resulting in marked swelling and pain at the inner aspect of the ankle. You would describe this to an on-line physician as pain and swelling in which area?
    a. Lateral malleolus
    b. Medial malleolus
    c. Olecranon
    d. Patella
95. Muscle fiber contractions are initiated when stimulated by which of the following?
    a. Actin and myosin
    b. Motor neurons
    c. Myofilaments
    d. Sarcomeres
96. Which of the following is the primary action of the frontal lobe of the cerebral cortex?
    a. To receive and integrate visual input
    b. To evaluate olfactory and auditory input
    c. To receive and interpret sensory information
    d. To initiate voluntary motor function
97. The spinal cord ends at which vertebra?
    a. Twelfth thoracic
    b. Second lumbar
    c. Sacral
    d. Coccygeal
98. What is the innermost meningeal layer (mater), which adheres to the brain and spinal cord?
    a. Arachnoid
    b. Choroid
    c. Dura
    d. Pia
99. Which component of the endocrine system transmits information from the gland to its target body part?
    a. Enzyme
    b. Hormone
    c. Neurotransmitter
    d. Synapse
100. Which of the following is the formed element in blood that contains hemoglobin and carries oxygen?
    a. Erythrocyte
    b. Immunoglobulin
    c. Leukocyte
    d. Platelet
101. Which blood vessel (or vessels) carry blood from the heart to the systemic circulation?
    a. Aorta
    b. Pulmonary arteries
    c. Pulmonary veins
    d. Vena cava
102. Cardiac electrical impulse conduction is normally initiated in which of the following structures?
    a. Atrioventricular node
    b. Bundle of His
    c. Purkinje fibers
    d. Sinoatrial node
103. Lymph nodes filter foreign substances and are located in all the body regions listed below except which?
    a. Axillary
    b. Cervical
    c. Inguinal
    d. Temporal
104. Which of the following is the airway division that is involved in the production of speech and that serves as a protective sphincter to prevent liquids and solids from entering the lungs?
    a. Larynx
    b. Retropharynx
    c. Pharynx
    d. Trachea

105. The functional unit of the respiratory system where gas exchange occurs between the lungs and the blood is which of the following?
   a. Alveolus
   b. Bronchus
   c. Capillary
   d. Trachea

106. The major site of nutrient absorption in the intestines is which of the following?
   a. Colon
   b. Duodenum
   c. Ileum
   d. Jejunum

107. Liver function includes all the following actions except:
   a. Bile production
   b. Drug detoxification
   c. Hormone secretion
   d. Plasma protein synthesis

108. Which of the following statements is true with regard to renal function?
   a. All fluid filtered from the glomerulus becomes urine.
   b. Healthy people produce 180 L of urine per day.
   c. Water and other nutrients are reabsorbed in the tubules.
   d. Potassium and ammonia are secreted into the blood.

109. Which of the following hormones influences urine production?
   a. Aldosterone
   b. Glucagon
   c. Oxytocin
   d. Testosterone

110. Where does sperm production occur?
   a. Epididymis
   b. Prostate
   c. Seminal vesicle
   d. Testes

111. When the nasal receptors of the olfactory neurons are stimulated, messages are sent for interpretation to the olfactory and_____centers of the brain.
   a. Frontal
   b. Medullary
   c. Pontine
   d. Thalamic

112. The hearing sense organ is which of the following?
   a. Cochlea
   b. Organ of Corti
   c. Semicircular canal
   d. Vestibule

WRAP IT UP

You are dispatched to a rural emergency department to transfer a patient to the regional trauma center. The nurse gives you the following patient report: The 27-year-old female was thrown off her all-terrain vehicle (ATV) and struck a tree. She is lying on her back in full spinal immobilization. She has a laceration on her forehead above her right eyebrow; a fracture of her right forearm; a fracture in her right upper thigh; a pelvic fracture; several rib fractures on the left anterior side of her chest; and possible internal abdominal injuries. The nurse also tells you that the patent's erythrocyte count is low; her urine output is 10 mL/hour, which is draining through the urinary catheter; she has a nasogastric tube because she vomited earlier; and she is receiving high-concentration oxygen because her oxygen saturation level dropped and she was dyspneic. The woman is conscious but slightly confused and can't feel anything below her umbilicus. She is unable to move below her waist but can bend and straighten her arms.

1. Fill in the appropriate anatomical terms to describe this patient.

   She is lying (a) _____ on the long spine board. Her laceration is (b) _____to her

   eyebrow. Her forearm fracture is (c) _____ to her elbow and could be in one of two long bones,

   the (d) _____ or _____. The fracture in her upper thigh is in the

   (e)_____, and the bones of the pelvis that could be fractured are the (f) _____,

   _____, _____, or _____.

2. What structures underlie the fractured ribs that could also be injured?

_____

3. List the abdominal organs that could be involved if the patient's injuries are in the following places.

    a. Upper right quadrant: _____

    b. Upper left quadrant:_____

    c. Lower right quadrant:_____

    d. Lower left quadrant: _____

4. What region of the brain lies under her facial injury? _____

5. a. What are erythrocytes?

_____

    b. What is the significance of a low erythrocyte count?

_____

6. The loss of sensation below her umbilicus signals likely injury to what level of the spinal cord?

_____

7. a. Is she producing too much, too little, or a normal amount of urine?

_____

    b. What could cause a change in urine output?

_____

_____

8. The urinary catheter passes through what anatomical structures?

_____

9. What medical terms could you substitute for "can bend and straighten her arms"?

_____

10. Put a ✔ beside the body systems that are affected in some way by this patient's condition (either directly or by the body's compensatory mechanisms).

    _____Integumentary system   _____Skeletal system
    _____Muscular system   _____Nervous system
    _____Endocrine system   _____Circulatory system
    _____Lymphatic system   _____Digestive system
    _____Urinary system   _____Reproductive system
    _____Respiratory system

CHAPTER 6 ANSWERS

REVIEW QUESTIONS

1. d
2. c
3. f
4. b
5. e
6. h
7. i
8. g
   (Questions 1-8: Objective 8)

9. a. centrioles; b. ribosomes; c. Golgi apparatus; d. nucleus; e. endoplasmic reticulum; f. lysosome; g. mito-chondrion
   (Objective 8)

10. False. Some cells, such as those of the nervous system, divide only until birth.
    (Objective 9)

11. The person is standing erect with palms and feet facing the examiner.
    (Objective 2)

12. a. Distal; b. lateral; c. superior; d. ventral
    (Objective 3)

13. a. Extremities and their girdles; b. head, neck, thorax, and abdomen
    (Objective 4)

14. Horizontally through the umbilicus and vertically from the xiphoid process through the symphysis pubis
    (Objective 5)

15. You initially found the patient in the right lateral recumbent position.
    (Objective 3)

16. a. Burn (1) is inferior and lateral to the left eye.
    b. Burn (2) is inferior to the mouth.
    c. Burn (3) is superior and lateral to the right nipple.
    d. Burn (4) is on the ventral aspect (or palmar surface) of the hand.
    e. Burn (5) is inferior to the axilla.
    f. Burns (6) and (7) are on the medial aspect of both thighs.

17. Burn (5) encroaches on the left upper quadrant of the abdomen.
    (Objective 5)

18. a. Burn (3) overlies the thoracic cavity.
    b. Burn (5) overlies the thoracic and abdominal cavities.

19. The wounds affect both the axial and appendicular regions of the body.
    (Objective 4)

20. Conduction of action potentials

Subgroup	Type	Body Area	Function
Striated voluntary tissue	Muscle	Skeletal muscle	Movement of bones
Bone	Connective	Bones of body	Support and protection
Epithelium	Epithelial	Skin, glands	Protection, lining of body cavities
Adipose tissue	Connective	Subcutaneous tissue	Insulation, protection, storage of energy
Hemopoietic tissue	Connective	Marrow cavities, spleen, tonsils	Formation of blood and lymph cells
Striated involuntary tissue	Muscle	Cardiac muscle	Contraction of the heart
Neurons	Nervous	Nervous system	Conduction of action potentials
Cartilage	Connective	Articulating surface	Smooth movement of bones; ear, nose
Areolar tissue	Connective	Around organs, under skin	Cushioning and affixing
Nonstriated involuntary tissue	Muscle	Smooth muscle of viscera	Vegetative muscle functions
Neuroglia	Nervous	Nervous system	Support cells, nourishment, protection, insulation

(Objective 10)

21. Integumentary, skeletal, muscular, nervous, endocrine, circulatory, lymphatic, respiratory, digestive, urinary, and reproductive
(Objective 11)

22. a. Epidermis: barrier against infection, protection, prevention of fluid loss
b. Dermis: sense organ, contains sweat glands
c. Subcutaneous layer: insulation, storage of energy, shock layer, absorption
(Objective 11)

23. Lubrication to prevent drying, excretion of water and wastes, and temperature regulation
(Objective 11)

24. Decreased ability to perceive pain, decreased ability to regulate temperature, and decreased ability to preserve body fluids
(Objective 11)

25. a. Parietal; b. temporal; c. frontal; d. occipital; e. sphenoid; f. ethmoid; g. maxilla; h. mandible; i. zygomatic; j. nasal; k. lacrimal
(Objective 11)

26. a. Cervical spine (7); b. thoracic spine (12); c. lumbar spine (5); d. sacrum (1 fused); e. coccyx (1 fused)
(Objective 11)

27. Protection for the organs of the thorax (and some abdominal organs) and maintenance of lung inflation
(Objective 11)

28. a. Manubrium; b. body; c. sternum; d. xiphoid process; e. jugular notch; f. sternal angle
(Objective 11)

29. Injury to underlying organs, impaired ventilation, and blood loss
(Objective 11)

30. a. Scapula; b. clavicle; c. attach the upper extremity to the axial skeleton; d. sternoclavicular joint
(Objective 11)

31. a. Humerus; b. head; c. greater tubercle; d. radius; e. ulna; f. trochlea; g. medial epicondyle; h. lateral epicondyle; i. olecranon; j. styloid process; k. radial tuberosity; l. carpals; m. metacarpals
(Objective 11)

32. a. Obturator foramen; b. ilium; c. ischium; d. pubis; e. anterior superior iliac spine
(Objective 11)

33. Protection of the pelvic organs and point of attachment for the lower extremity to the axial skeleton
(Objective 11)

34. a. Neck; b. head; c. shaft; d. greater trochanter; e. lesser trochanter; f. medial condyle; g. lateral condyle; h. medial epicondyle; i. lateral epicondyle; j. tibia; k. fibula; l. tibial tuberosity; m. head of fibula; n. lateral malleolus; o. tarsal bones; p. metatarsals; q. phalanges
(Objective 11)

35. a. Fibrous, cartilaginous, synovial; b. little or no; c. skull; d. radius, ulna; e. teeth, mandible (or maxilla); f. sternum; g. sternal angle; h. symphysis pubis; i. intervertebral disks; j. synovial fluid; k. plane (or gliding); l. saddle joints; m. hinge; n. pivot; o. ball and socket; p. ellipsoid
(Objective 11)

36. a. Supinate (supination) or pronate (pronation); b. opposition; c. flexion and extension; d. rotation; e. abduction; f. adduction; g. inversion or eversion; h. excursion; i. depression
(Objective 11)

37. Movement, muscle tone, and heat production
(Objective 11)

38. a. Muscle fibers; b. myofilaments; c. actin, myosin; d. sarcomere; e. adenosine triphosphate (ATP)
(Objective 11)

39. a. Isometric muscle contraction maintains constant length of the muscles in the body. b. During an isotonic contraction, the amount of muscle tension is constant, but the length of the muscle changes, causing movement of a body part. c. Muscle tone is the constant tension of muscles responsible for posture and balance.
(Objective 11)

40. Excess energy from adenosine triphosphate in a muscle contraction is released as heat. If the body temperature falls below a certain level, muscles begin shivering, which can increase heat production up to 18 times the normal resting level.
(Objective 11)

41. Regulation and coordination of the body to maintain homeostasis
(Objective 11)

42. a. Brain and spinal cord; b. nerves and ganglia
(Objective 11)

43. The somatic division transmits impulses from the central nervous system to skeletal muscle. The autonomic division transmits impulses from the central nervous system to smooth muscle, cardiac muscle, and certain glands.
(Objective 11)

44. a. Cerebral cortex; b. midbrain; c. pons; d. cerebellum; e. medulla; f. thalamus; g. hypothalamus
(Objective 11)

45. a. Serves as conduction pathway for ascending and descending nerve tracts and regulates heart rate, blood vessel diameter, breathing, swallowing, vomiting, coughing, and sneezing. b. Ascending and descending nerve tracts pass through and relay information from cerebrum to cerebellum and sleep and respiratory center. c. Involved in hearing and visual reflexes, regulates some automatic functions, such as muscle tone. d. Important for arousal and consciousness, sleep/wake cycle. e. Temperature regulation, water balance, sleep cycle control, appetite, sexual arousal. f. Relays information from sense organs to cerebral cortex, influences mood.
(Objective 11)

46. a. Frontal lobe: voluntary motor function, motivation, aggression, and mood. b. Temporal lobe: olfactory and auditory input, memory. c. Parietal lobe: reception and evaluation of sensory information (except smell, hearing, and vision). d. Occipital lobe: reception and integration of visual input.
(Objective 11)

47. Coordination, balance, and smooth, flowing movement
(Objective 11)

48. Reflex center; also transmits impulses to and from the brain and the rest of the body
(Objective 11)

49. a. Brain, spinal cord; b. choroid plexus
(Objective 11)

50. Sensory, somatomotor and proprioception, and parasympathetic
(Objective 11)

51. Affected

Affected Organ	Sympathetic	Parasympathetic
Heart	Increased rate, contractility	Decreased rate and electrical activity contractility conduction speed
Lungs	Bronchodilation	Bronchoconstriction
Pupils	Dilation	Constriction
Intestine	Decreased peristalsis	Increased peristalsis
Blood vessels	Constriction	No effect

(Objective 11)

52. Coordinates with the nervous system to regulate and control multiple body functions, including metabolic activities and body chemistry
(Objective 11)

53.

Hormone	Target Tissue	Action
Epinephrine	Heart, blood vessels, liver, lungs	Increases heart rate, contractility, blood flow to heart, and release of glucose and fatty acids into blood Bronchodilation
Aldosterone	Kidneys	Regulates water and electrolyte balance
Antidiuretic hormone	Kidneys	Stimulates water retention by kidneys
Parathyroid hormone	Bone, kidney	Increases bone breakdown, helps maintain blood calcium levels
Calcitonin	Bone	Decreases breakdown of bone; maintains blood calcium levels
Insulin	Liver	Promotes glucose entry into cells
Glucagon	Liver	Increases blood glucose by glycogenolysis
Testosterone	Most cells	Produces male sex characteristics, behavior, spermatogenesis
Thymosin	Immune tissues	Promotes development of immune system
Oxytocin	Uterus, mammary gland	Causes uterine contractions, milk expulsion from breasts
Thyroid hormone	Most cells	Increases metabolic rate

(Objective 11)

54. Hormones are secreted into blood and travel to all tissues of the body but act only on the target tissues.
(Objective 11)

55. Transports nutrients, carries hormones, transports wastes, regulates temperature and fluid balance, and provides protection from bacteria
(Objective 11)

56. a. erythrocytes; b. hemoglobin; c. oxygen; d. carbon dioxide; e. leukocytes; f. thrombocytes; g. defense; h. clots; i. plasma
(Objective 11)

57. a. septum; b. right atrium; c. tricuspid valve; d. right ventricle; e. pulmonic valve; f. pulmonary arteries; g. pulmonary veins; h. left atrium; i. mitral or bicuspid valve; j. left ventricle; k. aortic valve; l. aorta
(Objective 11)

58. Aorta, smaller arteries, arterioles, capillaries, venules, veins, venae cavae, and right atrium
(Objective 11)

59. Blood vessels have smooth muscle walls; this allows them to dilate (increasing their diameter) or constrict (decreasing their diameter). This allows blood flow to be directed away from less vital organs to the heart and brain during emergencies.
(Objective 11)

60. Many veins, especially in the lower extremities, have valves that prevent the back flow of blood in this low-pressure system.
(Objective 11)

61. The arteriovenous shunt can selectively allow blood to bypass the capillaries. This is useful to help maintain body temperature.
(Objective 11)

62. Maintains tissue fluid balance, absorbs fats and other substances from the digestive tract, and enhances the body's defense system.
(Objective 11)

63. Lymph is gathered from the tissues by lymph capillaries that have one-way valves to prevent the back flow of lymph into tissues. It flows to larger lymph capillaries that resemble veins. Then it passes through the lymph nodes (in the groin, axilla, and neck), where microorganisms and foreign substances are removed. The lymph vessels meet to enter the right or left subclavian vein, where the lymph reenters the blood.
(Objective 11)

64. a. Epiglottis: protection of lower airway; b. conchae and turbinates: warming and filtering of air; c. eustachian and auditory tube: joining of nasopharynx to ear; d. sinuses: production of sound and mucus; e. hard palate: separation of oropharynx from sinuses; f. soft palate: prevents food from entering nasal cavities.
(Objective 11)

65. a. Epiglottis; b. thyroid cartilage (or Adam's apple); c. cricoid cartilage; d. hyoid bone; e. vocal folds
(Objective 11)

66. a. Trachea; b. bronchi; c. alveoli; d. carina
(Objective 11)

67. Cartilage rings maintain patency of the airway. Goblet cells in the ciliated epithelium of the trachea sweep mucus, bacteria, and other small particles toward the larynx.
(Objective 11)

68. The small bronchioles are surrounded by smooth muscle. Irritants cause constriction of that muscle, the airway size decreases, and a wheeze is produced as air is forced through a very tight airway.
(Objective 11)

69. a. Alveoli are only one cell thick, allowing gases to diffuse easily from within them into the pulmonary capillaries. b. Pulmonary surfactant reduces surface tension in the alveoli, which inhibits collapse of the alveoli.
(Objective 11)

70. The bases of the lungs rest on the diaphragm; the apex extends to a point 2.5 cm superior to the clavicles.
(Objective 11)

71. a. Three lobes, which are further divided into 10 lobules; b. Two lobes, which are further divided into nine lobules
(Objective 11)

72. a. A potential space that forms a vacuum and causes the lung to adhere to the chest wall and remain expanded; b. a lubricant that allows the pleural membranes to slide across one another and that helps the visceral and parietal pleurae to adhere to one another.
(Objective 11)

73. Provides the body with water, nutrients, and electrolytes
(Objective 11)

74.

Area	Digestive Juice	Function
Mouth	Salivary amylase	Begins digestion of carbohydrates
Stomach	Hydrochloric acid, mucus	Produces chyme (intrinsic factor, gastrin, semisolid mixture), pepsinogen
Pancreas	Amylase, sodium bicarbonate	Neutralizes stomach acid, continues digestion
Liver	Bile	Dilutes stomach acid, emulsifies fat
Large intestine	Mucus	Aids movement of feces

(Objective 11)

75. Removes wastes from the body and helps maintain normal body fluid volume and composition
(Objective 11)

76. Control of red blood cell production and vitamin D metabolism
(Objective 11)

77. a. Nephron; b. filtration; c. reabsorption; d. secretion
(Objective 11)

78. a. Decreases; b. increases; c. increases; d. decreases
(Objective 11)

79. a. Testis; b. epididymis; c. ductus deferens and vas deferens; d. urethra; e. seminal vesicles; f. prostate gland; g. bulbourethral glands; h. scrotum; i. penis
(Objective 11)

80. a. Ovary; b. fallopian tube; c. uterine body; d. fundus; e. cervix; f. vagina
(Objective 11)

81. a. Vagina; b. urethra; c. labia minora; d. labia majora; e. clitoris; f. clinical perineum; g. anus
(Objective 11)

82. a. Nasal; b. olfactory tract; c. thalamic; d. olfactory
(Objective 12)

83. a. Taste buds; b. tongue; c. palate, lips, throat; d. sweet, sour, bitter, salt
(Objective 12)

84. a. Optic; b. oculomotor; c. cornea; d. iris; e. rods; f. cones; g. aqueous; h. vitreous; i. intraocular pressure
(Objective 12)

85. a. Shade eyes from direct sun and prevent perspiration from entering eyes; b. protect against foreign objects; c. moisten the eye, lubricate the eyelids, and wash away foreign objects
(Objective 12)

86. a. Hearing; b. hearing, balance; c. vestibulocochlear; d. pinna; e. auditory; f. tympanic membrane; g. incus, stapes, malleus; h. organ of Corti; i. vestibule; j. semicircular canals
(Objective 12)

STUDENT SELF-ASSESSMENT

87. d. The anatomical position is standing erect with palms forward. A person lying in the lateral recumbent position is reclining on the right or left side. The prone position refers to a patient who is lying on the stomach.
(Objective 2)

88. d. The liver and gallbladder are located in the right upper quadrant, and the appendix is in the right lower quadrant.
(Objective 5)

89. d. The lungs are found in the thoracic cavity, and the diaphragm separates the thoracic cavity from the abdominal cavity. The thyroid gland is found in the neck.
(Objective 7)

90. b. Striated voluntary muscle is skeletal muscle, and nonstriated involuntary muscles are found in the viscera. Nonstriated muscles are always involuntary.
(Objective 10)

91. c. A *dendrite* is a component of the neuron. *Neuroglia* are types of nerve cells that support the cells in the nervous system. *Synapses* are the gaps or spaces between nerve cells or effector tissues.
(Objective 10)

92. d. Lymph is collected by the lymphatic system and drains into the circulatory system. Movement is a function of the musculoskeletal system. Vitamin C is ingested by food sources. A form of vitamin D is produced in the skin when exposed to light.
(Objective 11)

93. a.
(Objective 4)

94. b. The lateral malleolus is on the outside of the ankle, the olecranon is at the elbow, and the patella is over the knee.
(Objective 3)

95. b. *Actin* and *myosin* are the actual myofilaments (thin, threadlike structures) that pull together to cause movement. A *sarcomere* is the contractile unit that contains actin and myosin.
(Objective 10)

96. d. The other actions described are attributed to the occipital lobe (a), temporal lobe (b), and parietal lobe (c).
(Objective 11)

97. b
(Objective 11)

98. d. The layers, from innermost to outermost, are the pia, arachnoid, and dura. The choroid plexus is where the cerebrospinal fluid is manufactured.
(Objective 11)

99. b
(Objective 11)

100. a. Immunoglobulins are antibodies, leukocytes are white blood cells, and platelets are cell fragments that aid in hemostasis.
(Objective 11)

101. a. Pulmonary arteries carry deoxygenated blood from the heart to the lungs. Pulmonary veins carry oxygenated blood from the lungs to the heart, and the vena cava carries blood from the systemic circulation to the heart.
(Objective 11)

102. d. Sinoatrial node impulses travel to the atrioventricular node, the bundle of His, and then to the Purkinje fibers.
(Objective 11)

103. d.
(Objective 11)

104. a.
(Objective 11)

105. a. The trachea and bronchus convey air to the alveoli. The capillary is not part of the respiratory system.
(Objective 11)

106. d. Absorption occurs in the other areas of the small intestine (duodenum and ileum) and to a much lesser extent in the colon; however, the primary site of absorption is the jejunum.
(Objective 11)

107. c
(Objective 11)

108. c. Roughly 180 L per day is filtered from the glomerulus; however, all but approximately 2 L of this is reabsorbed into the blood. Potassium and ammonia are secreted from the blood into the urine.
(Objective 11)

109. a. Glucagon promotes conversion of glycogen stored in the liver back to glucose. Oxytocin is a female sex hormone that stimulates uterine contractions and plays a role in lactation. Testosterone is the male sex hormone responsible for male sexual characteristics.
(Objective 11)

110. d. Final maturation (but not production) of the sperm occurs in the epididymis. The prostate and seminal vesicle produce seminal fluid.
(Objective 11)

111. d. Thalamic
(Objective 12)

112. b. The organ of Corti lies within the cochlea. The semicircular canals and vestibule are involved in balance.
(Objective 12)

WRAP IT UP

1. a. supine; b. superior; c. distal; d. radius, ulna; e. femur; f. sacrum, pubis, ilium, ischium
(Objectives 2, 3, 11)

2. aorta, lungs, heart, spleen
(Objective 7)

3. a. liver, intestines; b. spleen, stomach, liver, pancreas, intestines; c. intestines; d. intestines
(Objectives 5 through 7)

4. Frontal
(Objective 11)

5. a. red blood cells; b. A drop in the number of red blood cells reduces the blood's ability to carry oxygen to the cells. It is an indication of blood loss.
(Objective 11)

6. Injuries to the lower thoracic or upper lumbar vertebrae can cause these symptoms.
(Objective 11)

7. a. There is too little urine output. Normal urine output should be approximately 40 to 80 mL/hour (1 to 2 L/day).
b. Urine production could be reduced by increased secretion of aldosterone or antidiuretic hormone (ADH); by a drop in arterial blood pressure; or by sympathetic nervous stimulation.
(Objective 11)

8. The urinary catheter passes through the urethra and into the urinary bladder.
(Objective 11)

9. Flex and extend
(Objective 3)

10. Integumentary system (wound above her eye); skeletal system (fractures); muscular system (damage surrounding fractures); nervous system (motor/sensory deficit in lower extremities); endocrine system (hormone secretion to limit urine output); lymphatic system (if splenic injury is present); respiratory system (increased respiratory rate to compensate for decrease in red blood cells and circulatory shock); digestive system (decreased peristalsis); urinary system (decreased urinary output)
(Objective 11)

General Principles of Pathophysiology

READING ASSIGNMENT

Chapter 7, pages 150-195, in *Mosby's Paramedic Textbook,* ed. 3

OBJECTIVES

Upon completion of this chapter, the paramedic student will be able to do the following:

1. Describe the normal characteristics of the cellular environment and the key homeostatic mechanisms that strive to maintain an optimal fluid and electrolyte balance.
2. Outline pathophysiological alterations in water and electrolyte balance and list their effects on body functions.
3. Describe the treatment of patients with particular fluid or electrolyte imbalances.
4. Describe the mechanisms in the body that maintain normal acid-base balance.
5. Outline pathophysiological alterations in acid-base balance.
6. Describe the management of a patient with an acid-base imbalance.
7. Describe the changes in cells and tissues that occur with cellular adaptation, injury, neoplasia, aging, or death.
8. Outline the effects of cellular injury on local and systemic body functions.
9. Describe changes in body functions that can occur as a result of genetic and familial disease factors.
10. Outline the causes, adverse systemic effects, and compensatory mechanisms associated with hypoperfusion.
11. Describe the ways in which the inflammatory and immune mechanisms respond to cellular injury or antigenic stimulation.
12. Explain how changes in immune status and the presence of inflammation can adversely affect body functions.
13. Describe the impact of stress on the body's response to illness or injury.

SUMMARY

- Two facts illustrate the importance of body water. First, body water is the medium in which all metabolic reactions occur. Second, the precise regulation of the volume and composition of body fluids is essential to health. Water follows osmotic gradients established by changes in sodium concentrations. Thus, sodium and water balance are closely related.
- Two abnormal states of body-fluid balance can occur. If the water gained exceeds the water lost, a state of water excess, or overhydration, exists. If the water lost exceeds the water gained, a state of water deficit, or dehydration, exists.
- In addition to fluid imbalances, disturbances in the balance of electrolytes (other than sodium) may occur. These electrolytes include potassium, calcium, and magnesium. Imbalances of these electrolytes can interfere with neuromuscular function. They may even cause cardiac rhythm disturbances.

- The treatment of isotonic dehydration may include volume replacement with isotonic or occasionally hypotonic solutions. The treatment of hypotonic dehydration may involve intravenous replacement with normal saline or lactated Ringer solution. Occasionally hypertonic saline (e.g., in seizures caused by hyponatremia) is used. Interventions for overhydration depend on the cause. These interventions may include water restriction, administration of a diuretic, or, if hyponatremia is present, administration of saline.
- In-hospital treatment of hypokalemia involves intravenous or oral potassium replacement. Management of hyperkalemia may involve potassium restriction, enteral administration of a cation exchange resin, or intravenous administration of glucose and insulin, sodium bicarbonate, calcium, or nebulized albuterol.
- Treatment of hypocalcemia involves intravenous administration of calcium ions. The management of hypercalcemia may include controlling the underlying disease, hemodialysis, hydration, and, occasionally, drug therapy such as with furosemide and other calcium-lowering drugs.
- Hypomagnesemia typically is corrected by the administration of intravenous magnesium sulfate. The most effective treatment for hypermagnesemia is hemodialysis. Saline and furosemide may be administered until dialysis can be performed. Calcium salts that antagonize magnesium may also be given.
- The healthy body is sensitive to changes in the concentration of hydrogen ions (pH). It tries to maintain the pH of extracellular fluid at 7.4. This is accomplished through three interrelated compensatory mechanisms: carbonic acid–bicarbonate buffering, protein buffering, and renal buffering.
- Metabolic acidosis occurs when the amount of acid generated exceeds the body's buffering capacity. The four most common forms of metabolic acidosis encountered in the prehospital setting are lactic acidosis, diabetic ketoacidosis, acidosis resulting from renal failure, and acidosis caused by ingestion of toxins. Treatment for metabolic acidosis is aimed at correcting the underlying cause.
- Loss of hydrogen is the initial cause of metabolic alkalosis. This may be caused by vomiting (hydrochloric acid loss), gastric suction, or increased renal excretion of hydrogen ion in the urine. Treatment is directed at correcting the underlying condition. Volume depletion, if present, should be corrected with isotonic solutions.
- Respiratory acidosis is caused by the retention of carbon dioxide. This leads to an increase in the Pco_2. This condition usually is caused by an imbalance in the production of carbon dioxide and its elimination through alveolar ventilation. Treatment for respiratory acidosis involves improving ventilation quickly to eliminate carbon dioxide.
- Hyperventilation may produce respiratory alkalosis by decreasing the Pco_2. Treatment of respiratory alkalosis is directed at correcting the underlying cause of the hyperventilation. An initial approach is to place the patient on low-concentration oxygen. Another is to provide calming measures to assist the patient with slow, controlled breathing.
- An understanding of the processes of disease is crucial. This requires a knowledge of the structural and functional reactions of cells and tissues to injurious agents. Changes in cells and tissues can be caused by adaptation, injury, neoplasia, aging, or death.
- An injured cell may have an abnormal physical shape or size. Cell injury has both cellular and systemic indications.
- Certain factors cause disease. For the most part, these factors may be classified as genetic or environmental. However, a strong interaction occurs between the two.
- The term *hypoperfusion* is used to describe inadequate tissue circulation. Hypoperfusion may result from decreased cardiac output. Decreased cardiac output can lead to shock, multiple organ dysfunction syndrome, and other disease states associated with impaired cellular metabolism. Negative feedback mechanisms important in maintaining cardiac output and tissue perfusion are baroreceptor reflexes, chemoreceptor reflexes, the central nervous system ischemia response, hormonal mechanisms, reabsorption of tissue fluids, and splenic discharge of stored blood.
- The external barriers are the body's first line of defense against illness and injury. These barriers include the skin and the mucous membranes of the digestive, respiratory, and gastrointestinal tracts. When these barriers are breached, chemicals, foreign bodies, or microorganisms are allowed to penetrate cells and tissues. Then the second and third lines of defense are activated. These are the inflammatory response and the immune response. Both the external barriers and the inflammatory response respond to all organisms using the identical nonspecific mechanism. The immune response is specific to individual pathogens.
- Immune responses usually are protective. They help to protect the body from harmful microorganisms and other injurious agents. At times these responses may be inappropriate. They may even have undesirable effects. Examples of inappropriate responses include hypersensitivity and immunity or inflammation deficiencies.
- Many immune-related conditions and diseases are associated with stress. However, the exact cause of these illnesses has not yet been clearly defined. It is believed that the immune, nervous, and endocrine systems communicate through complex pathways. They may be affected by factors involved in the stress reaction.

REVIEW QUESTIONS

Match the mechanism of cellular injury in column I with the appropriate cause in column II.

Column I		Column II
1. _G_	Inadequate perfusion of oxygenated blood to an organ	**a.** Aerobic
2. _F_	Group of proteins that kill or help kill bacteria	**b.** Afterload
3. _A_	Presence of air or oxygen	**c.** Anerobic
4. _I_	Amount of blood returning to the ventricle	**d.** Anion
5. _B_	Total resistance against which blood is pumped	**e.** Antigen
6. _C_	Substance that causes an antibody to form	**f.** Complement system
7. _h_	Osmotic concentration of a solution	**g.** Ischemia
8. _D_	Ion with a negative charge	**h.** Osmolality
9. _J_	Volume of blood ejected from a ventricle with each heart beat	**i.** Preload
		j. Stroke volume

Match the mechanism of cellular injury in column I with the appropriate cause in column II.

Column I		Column II
10. _A_	Skin burns resulting from prolonged contact with gasoline	**a.** Chemical injury
11. _G_	Bruising caused by a blow from a tire iron	**b.** Genetic factors
12. _F_	Unconsciousness resulting from a drop in blood sugar	**c.** Hypoxic injury
13. _E_	Death secondary to septic shock	**d.** Immunological injury
14. _C_	Tissue death in a leg after occlusion of a blood vessel	**e.** Infectious injury
15. _D_	Severe wheezing that develops after a bee sting	**f.** Nutritional imbalances
		g. Physical agents

16. Complete the following sentences, which refer to the fluid compartments of the body.
The water found outside the cells that includes the water in plasma, bone, tendon, and fascia is the

(a) _Extracellular_ fluid. The water outside the vascular bed that lies between the tissue cells is known as
Interstitial
(b) ~~Intracellular~~ fluid. The fluid found inside the cells of the skeletal muscle, intestine, viscera, bone

marrow, glands, and red blood cells is the (c) _Intracellular_ fluid.

17. For each of the following ions, state its name, indicate whether it is a cation or an anion, and state where it is most plentiful in the body (extracellular fluid [ECF] or intracellular fluid [ICF]).

Ion	Name	Cation or Anion	ECF or ICF
PO_4^-	Phosphate	Anion	Intracellular
K^+	Potassium	Cation	Intracellular
Na^+	Sodium	Cation	Extracellular
HCO_3^-	Bicarbonate	Anion	Extracellular
Mg^{++}	Magnesium	Cation	Intracellular
Cl^-	Chloride	Anion	Extracellular

18. Briefly define the following terms:

   a. Cell membrane permeability:

_____

_____

   b. Diffusion:

_____

_____

   c. Concentration gradient:

_____

_____

   d. Osmosis:

_____

_____

   e. Active transport:

_____

_____

   f. Facilitated diffusion:

_____

_____

19. For each of the following patient situations, choose the suspected fluid or electrolyte imbalance from the list provided and describe appropriate assessments and/or interventions.

   a. You are transporting an older patient for chest pain. After an intravenous (IV) line has been inserted, 500 mL is accidentally infused rapidly. The patient becomes very short of breath, and evaluation reveals moist crackles in the lungs.

   Imbalance: Hyponatremia, hypermagnesemia, or overhydration?

   OVERHYDRATION - SALINE TKO

   Management:

   SALINE - TKO

   b. Your patient is a 65-year-old adult who complains of vomiting and diarrhea. Home medications include a diuretic. The physical examination reveals a blood pressure of 100/70 mm Hg, a weak pulse, decreased reflexes, and shallow respirations.

   Imbalance: Hyperkalemia, hypocalcemia, or hypokalemia?

_____

Management:

LACTATED RINGERS TKO - ↑flow O² ,

In hospital tx - POTASSIUM

c. You are called to the airport to evaluate an obviously malnourished child flown to the United States from India for adoption. The chaperone reports that the child has shown abnormal behavior and complains of muscle cramps, abdominal cramps, and tingling of the extremities. As you begin to assess the vital signs, the patient has a grand mal seizure.
Imbalance: Hypernatremia, hypocalcemia, or hypomagnesemia?

HYPOCALCEMIA

Management:

POSSIBLY the Calcium Chloride IV, Anticonvulsant

d. A father calls you to evaluate an infant who has been vomiting for 36 hours. The father states that the child has not had a wet diaper in 8 hours. The anterior fontanelle is depressed, and the skin and mucous membranes are dry.
Imbalance: Hypercalcemia, hypermagnesemia, or isotonic dehydration?

ISOTONIC DEHYDRATION

Management:

ASSES ABC'S , ASSES for SHOCK , Bolus of ISOTONIC Fluid

e. Your patient is a 13-year-old bulimic girl who admits to frequent use of water enemas for weight control. You were called for a chief complaint of abdominal pain; however, on arrival you find the patient diaphoretic with a rapid, thready pulse and cyanosis. There is no indication of bleeding.
Imbalance: Hyperkalemia, hyponatremic dehydration, or overhydration?

HYPONATREMIC DEHYDRATION

Management:

LR OR NS

f. The family of an older patient with chronic renal failure says that she is confused and very weak. The physical examination reveals shallow, slow respirations that become progressively worse.
Imbalance: Hypermagnesemia, hypocalcemia, or hypokalemia?

HYPERMAGNESIA ,

Management:

FUROSEMIDE.

20. Describe the mode of action of the three acid-base buffer systems in the body. Begin with the fastest mechanism and end with the slowest one.

a. _____

b. _____

c. _____

_____

_____

21. For each case presented, indicate which one of the four acid-base disturbances listed below is the cause. State at least one prehospital intervention for management of the imbalance.

Respiratory acidosis   Respiratory alkalosis
Metabolic acidosis   Metabolic alkalosis

a. A 17-year-old student complains of dizziness and tingling in the hands and around the mouth during a college entrance examination. The medical history and physical examination are unremarkable. The respiratory rate is 28 breaths/min and deep.

Imbalance: _RESPIRATORY Alkalosis_____
Intervention:

_TREAT UNDERLYING HYPERVENTILATION_____

b. A 72-year-old resident of an extended care facility has been treated with gastric suction.

Imbalance: _Metabolic Alkalosis_____
Intervention:

_I.V.   LR or NS_____

c. A 30-year-old diabetic woman has had influenza. She has taken no insulin in 2 days and appears dehydrated. Respirations are deep and rapid.

Imbalance: _____
Intervention:

_____

d. A 46-year-old patient who took an overdose of a barbiturate has shallow respirations at a rate of 8 breaths/min.

Imbalance: _RESPIRATORY ACIDOSES_____
Intervention:

_____

22. The following arterial blood gas values were obtained in a patient who had had a stroke. State whether each is normal or abnormal. Discuss any action that may be taken in the field to correct any abnormalities identified.

a. pH: 7.25   Normal/Abnormal
   Actions: _____

b. Po_2: 60 mmHg   Normal/Abnormal
   Actions: _____

c. Pco_2: 53 mmHg   Normal/Abnormal
   Actions: _____

23. For each of the following cellular adaptations, give the cause, the effect on the cell, and an example.

Adaptation	Cause	Effect on Cell	Example
Atrophy		DECREASE IN cell SIZE	Shrinkage of muscle iN CASTED limb
Dysplasia	Chronic Irritation	Abnormal changes in cell	Precancerous changes
Hyperplasia			
Hypertrophy			
Metaplasia			

24. For each of the following situations, explain why cardiac output will increase or decrease in an otherwise healthy individual.

   a. The patient has had a myocardial infarction with necrosis of 50% of the heart muscle.

_____

_____

   b. A dehydrated patient is given 500 mL of normal saline intravenously.

_____

_____

   c. The patient's normal heart rate is 80 and suddenly drops to 40.

_____

_____

   d. A paramedic student enters a testing station.

_____

_____

25. Describe the physiological effects of the baroreceptor response to compensate in each of the following situations.

   a. A 47-year-old adult has a sudden increase in blood pressure to 170/110 mm Hg.

_____

_____

   b. A 22-year-old adult is thrown from a horse and suffers a pelvic fracture. The paramedic's findings are significant internal bleeding and a sudden drop in blood pressure to 60 mm Hg systolic by palpation.

_____

_____

26. Describe the physiological effects of chemoreceptor stimulation in the following situations.

a. A 36-year-old adult has a massive hemothorax from a gunshot wound. Blood pressure is 76/60 mm Hg.

_____

_____

b. A 17-year-old patient who took a drug overdose has a shallow respiratory rate of 8 breaths/min. Arterial blood gas tests reveal a Pco_2 of 60 mm Hg

_____

_____

27. A 47-year-old man who suffered a large inferior myocardial infarction has progressively deteriorated. He is now unconscious and has a weak carotid pulse and no obtainable blood pressure. Describe the physiological effects that ensue when the central nervous system ischemia response is initiated.

_____

_____

28. A 65-year-old alcoholic man states that he had a sudden onset of vomiting. The emesis contains bright red blood, and he continues to vomit. Vital signs are: blood pressure, 94/78 mm Hg; pulse, 132 beats per minute (bpm); and respirations, 28 breaths/min. Describe the effects of the following three hormonal mechanisms, which will be activated.

a. Adrenal medullary mechanism

_____

_____

b. Renin-angiotensin-aldosterone mechanism

_____

_____

c. Vasopressin mechanism

_____

_____

29. Multiple organ dysfunction syndrome (MODS) begins with **(a)** _____ _____ damage

caused by **(b)** _____ and _____, which are released into the circulation. This causes the

vascular **(c)** _____ to become **(d)** _____, which allows fluid and cells to leak into the

(e) _____ spaces, increasing **(f)** _____ and _____. Three plasma enzyme cascades

are then activated. They are **(g)**_____, _____, and _____/_____.

Phagocytes cause further damage to the endothelium, causing uncontrolled **(h)** _____ and the

formation of microvascular **(i)** _____ and tissue ischemia. Bradykinin contributes to low

(j) _____ _____ _____. The overall effect of the three complement systems is **(k)** _____ formation, **(l)** _____, and **(m)** _____ _____. Initially the body compensates for these changes, but ultimately tissue hypoxia causes **(n)** _____ _____, _____ _____. Finally, multiple **(o)** _____ failure occurs.

30. Your partner is off sick with a diagnosis of strep throat. Describe whether the following signs and symptoms experienced during this illness are local or systemic and give at least one inflammatory mechanism that causes the sign or symptom.

Sign or Symptom	Local or Systemic Response	Cause
Edematous throat		
Purulent drainage		
Fever		
Red throat		
Difficulty swallowing		

31. For the following patient blood types, list all safe donor types.

Blood Type	Donors
a. A positive	
b. O negative	
c. AB positive	
d. B negative	

32. For each statement below, note which one of three types of altered immunological reaction has occurred: allergy, autoimmunity, or isoimmunity.

   a. Your patient is agitated and complains of severe low back pain a few moments after you begin to transfuse a unit of blood. _____

   b. You are dispatched to a private residence to care for a 46-year-old woman who began to experience dyspnea, a swollen face, and hives after taking a penicillin tablet prescribed by her dentist. _____

   c. You are transferring a patient to a dialysis center for care after his body rejected his kidney transplant. _____

   d. You notice that your eyes water and get puffy and your hands become very red and itchy when you wear Latex gloves at work. _____

e. Your patient, a 30-year-old woman, is having chest pain. The family tells you she has systemic lupus erythematosus with cardiac and pulmonary involvement. _____

Match the probable cause of immune suppression in column II with the statement in column I.

Column I	Column II
33. _B_ An elderly woman develops pneumonia several months after the death of her husband.	a. Acquired immune deficiency
34. _D_ A cancer patient becomes septic after a course of chemotherapy.	b. Deficiencies caused by stress
35. _E_ A young girl suffering from anorexia nervosa repeatedly becomes ill with viral illness.	c. Deficiencies caused by trauma
36. _A_ A patient infected with the human immunodeficiency virus (HIV) develops Kaposi sarcoma.	d. Iatrogenic deficiencies
	e. Nutritional deficiencies

37. Fill in the missing information relating to the stress response.

Hormone or Receptor	Location	Action
a.	Found in plasma	Stimulates gluconeogenesis; suppresses immune cell activity
Alpha-1 receptors	Postsynaptic located on effector organs	b. VASOCONSTRICTION
Beta-1 receptors	c. HEART	Increased pulse rate
d. BETA-2 receptors	Lungs and arteries	Bronchodilation

38. For each of the following diseases, list a factor that may contribute to its development. Identify whether the factor is environmental or genetic.

Disease	Factor	Environmental or Genetic
Stroke	HTN, ↑cholesterol, smoking	Environmental
Cervical cancer	Gonorreah	Environmental
Oral cancer	Chewing tobacco	Environmental
Melanoma (skin cancer)		
Depression		

STUDENT SELF-ASSESSMENT

39. Which mechanism of cellular transport moves substances against a concentration gradient and requires the use of energy?
    a. Active transport
    b. Diffusion
    c. Facilitated diffusion
    d. Osmosis

40. Which of the following electrolytes is found predominantly in the intracellular fluid?
    a. Bicarbonate
    c. Potassium
    b. Chloride
    d. Sodium
41. A solution that has a concentration of solute particles equal to that inside the cells is a(n) _____ solution.
    a. Atonic
    c. Hypotonic
    b. Hypertonic
    d. Isotonic
42. Which of the following causes the normal flow of fluid through the interstitial space?
    a. Capillary hydrostatic pressure filters fluid from the interstitial space through the capillary wall.
    b. Oncotic pressure exerted by blood proteins attracts fluid from the vascular space back into the interstitial space.
    c. Capillary permeability determines the ease with which fluid can pass through the capillary wall.
    d. The lymphatic channels close to prevent entry of capillary fluid pushed out by hydrostatic pressure.
43. Your patient is being transferred from a nursing home to a hospital for admission for an intestinal obstruction. His skin is dry, and his tongue has furrows. What fluid and electrolyte imbalance do you suspect?
    a. Hypernatremic dehydration
    c. Isotonic dehydration
    b. Hyponatremic dehydration
    d. Osmotic dehydration
44. You are called to transport a 56-year-old patient with a history of renal failure who missed his last dialysis session. He complains of nausea, abdominal distention, weakness, and irritability. Which of the following do you suspect?
    a. Hypercalcemia
    c. Hypernatremia
    b. Hyperkalemia
    d. Hyperuria
45. Which of the following is true regarding hypomagnesemia?
    a. It is often accompanied by hypercalcemia.
    b. It results from antacid abuse.
    c. It causes hypoactive reflexes.
    d. It causes cardiac dysrhythmias.
46. Your patient has metabolic acidosis. Which of the following compensatory mechanisms uses proteins in an attempt to rapidly restore normal acid-base balance?
    a. Carbonic acid–bicarbonate buffering
    b. Excretion of hydrogen ions to acidify the urine
    c. Exhalation of excess carbon dioxide
    d. Recovery of bicarbonate in the renal tubules
47. Which acid-base disturbance would you anticipate in a patient with severe flail chest?
    a. Metabolic acidosis
    c. Respiratory acidosis
    b. Metabolic alkalosis
    d. Respiratory alkalosis
48. Lactic acidosis is harmful to the body because it
    a. Increases the basal metabolic rate
    b. Decreases the force of cardiac contraction
    c. Increases the response to catecholamines
    d. Can cause severe hypertension
49. Increasing the rate of ventilations for a patient with metabolic acidosis and inadequate stroke volume typically causes which of the following?
    a. Decreased pH and decreased Pco_2
    b. Decreased pH and increased Pco_2
    c. Increased pH and decreased Pco_2
    d. Increased pH and increased Pco_2
50. Which cellular change, which may occur with aging, results in shrinkage of the brain and may cause a delay in the signs and symptoms associated with subdural hematoma (blood clot on the brain).
    a. Atrophy
    c. Metaplasia
    b. Dysplasia
    d. Hypertrophy
51. The process of cellular self-destruction is known as _Autolysis_
    Autolysis
    Necrosis
    MODS
    Osmosis

52. Which of the following changes would be expected early after cellular injury?
    a. Accelerated cellular reproduction
    b. Decreased intracellular hydrostatic pressure
    c. Increased intracellular oxygen accumulation
    d. Swelling of cells from increased osmosis
53. Sympathetic vasoconstriction during shock results in which of the following?
    a. Tachycardia
    b. Pupil dilation
    c. Increased container size
    d. Pale, cool skin
54. The central nervous system ischemic response is initiated when
    a. Blood pressure falls below 90 mm Hg systolic.
    b. Aortic and carotid chemoreceptors are stimulated.
    c. Bradycardia and vasodilation are present.
    d. Blood flow decreases in the vasomotor center.
55. Which of the following hormonal mechanisms increases urine production?
    a. Adrenal medullary mechanism
    b. Atrial natriuretic mechanism
    c. Renin-angiotension-aldosterone mechanism
    d. Vasopressin mechanism
56. An elderly patient calls 9-1-1 complaining of chest discomfort and difficulty breathing. Electrocardiographic changes on arrival at the hospital are consistent with acute myocardial infarction. The patient is showing signs of hypoperfusion. What type of shock does this likely represent?
    a. Anaphylactic
    b. Cardiogenic
    c. Hypovolemic
    d. Septic
57. Which of the following situations represents natural immunity in a fellow paramedic?
    a. Immunity to feline leukemia virus
    b. Immunity to measles after immunization
    c. Immunity to chicken pox after having them
    d. Immunity to hepatitis after immunoglobulin administration
58. Which of the following is true regarding hypersensitivity?
    a. It occurs only when the body encounters foreign antigens.
    b. The response always occurs immediately after exposure to the antigen.
    c. It may produce either minor or life-threatening consequences.
    d. It is a normal immune response resulting from exposure to an antigen.
59. Which hormone increases the level of blood glucose and acts as an immunosuppressant by reducing the number of selected leukocytes?
    a. Cortisol
    b. Dopamine
    c. Epinephrine
    d. Norepinephrine

WRAP IT UP

You are dispatched to an industrial accident where people reportedly are trapped. When you arrive, the incident commander tells you that a floor collapsed during erection of a high-rise building. A worker is trapped under the rubble, and the rescue squad is attempting to free him. The commander allows one person to approach the scene. You ask your partner to set up the ambulance and then meet you with a stretcher as close as he can approach the scene. You take the long spine board, immobilization supplies, an airway kit, and your primary resuscitation bag and move carefully toward the patient. He is conscious but very pale, and complains of a burning pain in his lower extremities. The extrication is dangerous; with every piece of debris removed, the entire pile becomes unstable. It is 4 hours before the patient is released. You immobilize him and quickly move him to the ambulance. His skin is pale and cool, he is breathing rapidly, and he has a puncture wound of unknown depth over his right upper abdomen. His lower extremities are gray and pale, but no crepitus or deformity is noted. His vital signs are: BP, 80/56 mm Hg; P, 136/min; R, 32/min; and an oxygen saturation (Sao_2) that won't register a reading. The monitor shows a sinus tachycardia with tall-tented T waves. You administer oxygen by nonrebreather mask at 15 L/min; initiate two large-bore IVs and infuse them at a rapid rate; and quickly begin transport to the trauma center.

1. What fluid should be started on this patient? Explain your answer.
   a. D_5W
   b. D_5NS
   c. LR
   d. NS
   Explanation:

   _____

   _____

2. a. If the electrocardiographic (ECG) change indicates excessive amounts of potassium in the blood, what additional signs or symptoms might this patient experience?

   WEAKNESS, PARALYSIS, NAUSEA, CARDIAC DISTURBANCES

   b. What could explain this patient's hyperkalemia?
      (1) Abdominal puncture releases potassium into the blood.
      (2) Crushed cells release potassium into the blood.
      (3) Lack of oxygen related to shock causes the release of potassium.
      (4) Potassium production is stimulated during hypoperfusion.

3. What acid-base imbalance will this patient most likely experience? Explain your answer.
   a. Metabolic acidosis
   b. Metabolic alkalosis
   c. Respiratory acidosis
   d. Respiratory alkalosis
   Explanation:

   _____

   _____

4. How will the body attempt to compensate for this acid-base imbalance?

   _____

   _____

5. For each of the following compensatory mechanisms used by the body during shock, put a ✔ on the line if the mechanism directly increases heart rate or contractility; put an ✕ if it acts directly on the blood vessels to cause constriction; and put a ★ if it conserves body water.
   _____ Parasympathetic stimulation   _____ Sympathetic stimulation
   _____ Adrenal medullary mechanism   _____ Renin-angiotensin-aldosterone mechanism
   _____ Vasopressin mechanism   _____ Tissue fluid reabsorption
   _____ Splenic discharge of blood

6. What stage of shock does this patient's signs and symptoms appear to indicate?
   a. Compensated
   b. Multiple organ dysfunction syndrome
   c. Terminal
   d. Uncompensated

CHAPTER 7 ANSWERS

REVIEW QUESTIONS

1. g
   (Objective 10)

2. f
   (Objective 11)

3. a
   (Objective 5)

4. i
   (Objective 10)

5. b
   (Objective 10)

6. c
   (Objective 11)

7. h
   (Objective 1)

8. d
   (Objective 5)

9. j
   (Objective 10)

10. a
11. g
12. f
13. e
14. c
15. d
   (Questions 10-15: Objective 7)

16. (a) Extracellular; (b) interstitial; (c) intracellular (Objective 1)

17. PO_4^-: phosphate, anion, intracellular; K+: potassium, cation, intracellular; Na+: sodium, cation, extracellular; HCO_3^-: bicarbonate, anion, extracellular; Mg^{++}: magnesium, cation, intracellular; Cl^-: chloride, anion, extracellular (Objective 1)

18. a. The property of a cell membrane that freely permits the passage of water but selectively allows the passage of solute particles. This permits the cell to maintain a relatively constant internal environment. b. A passive process that allows molecules or ions to move from an area of higher concentration to an area of lower concentration in an attempt to achieve a state of equilibrium. c. A situation in which the solute concentration is greater at one point than another in a solvent. Solutes diffuse from the area of higher concentration to the area of lower concentration until equilibrium is achieved. d. The diffusion of water across a selectively permeable membrane from an area of higher water concentration to an area of lower water concentration. e. A rapid, carrier-mediated process that can move a substance across a selectively permeable membrane from an area of low concentration to an area of high concentration. This process requires energy. f. A carrier-mediated process (faster than diffusion) that can move a substance from an area of higher concentration to an area of lower concentration. This process does not require energy. (Objective 1)

19. a. Overhydration; fluid restriction, normal saline given intravenously to keep the vein open.

b. Hypokalemia; lactated Ringer solution given intravenously to keep the vein open, preparation to assist ventilations, and high-flow oxygen. In-hospital treatment may include oral or IV potassium.

c. Hypocalcemia; possibly calcium ions (calcium chloride) given intravenously, airway management, seizure precautions, IV anticonvulsant therapy.

d. Isotonic dehydration; evaluation of airway, breathing, and circulation; assessment for shock, IV therapy with an isotonic solution.

e. Hyponatremic dehydration; evaluation of the effectiveness of ventilations, high-flow oxygen, IV therapy with lactated Ringer solution or normal saline, and evaluation of vital signs. Occasionally hypertonic saline may be administered.

f. Hypermagnesemia; open airway, assistance with ventilations as necessary, high-flow oxygen, evaluation of vital signs, IV line with normal saline, furosemide 1 mg/kg if dialysis is not available, and possibly IV calcium salts. The most effective treatment is hemodialysis. (Objective 2)

20. a. Buffers produce an immediate response to changes in the hydrogen ion concentration (pH). They represent the body's ability to adjust the concentration of bicarbonate and carbon dioxide in the blood to maintain a relationship of 1 mEq of carbonic acid to 20 mEq of base bicarbonate. If this relationship is maintained, the pH stays within normal limits.

b. The respiratory system can increase alveolar ventilation within minutes in response to an increase in the hydrogen ion concentration. Hydrogen ions combine with bicarbonate to form carbonic acid, which in turn breaks down into carbon dioxide and water. Therefore, by increasing the amount of carbon dioxide the body eliminates, the process can be accelerated and the hydrogen ion concentration reduced.

c. The renal system takes hours to days to act. It restores normal pH by reabsorbing or excreting bicarbonate or hydrogen ions. (Objective 4)

21. a. Respiratory alkalosis; treat cause of underlying hyperventilation.

b. Metabolic alkalosis; initiate IV administration of lactated Ringer solution or normal saline.

c. Metabolic acidosis; initiate IV administration of normal saline.

d. Respiratory acidosis; assist ventilations. (Objectives 5, 6)

22. a. Abnormal; for acidosis caused by an increase in the Pco_2, increase ventilations. b. Abnormal; increase oxygen delivery to the patient. c. Abnormal; increase rate of ventilations.
(Objective 6)

23.

Adaptation	Cause	Effect on Cell	Example
Atrophy	Diminished function, inadequate hormonal or nervous stimulation, reduced blood supply	Decrease or shrinkage in cellular size	Shrinkage of muscle size in a casted limb or from neuro-muscular disease; brain atrophy in old age
Dysplasia	Chronic irritation or inflammation	Abnormal changes in mature cells	Precancerous changes of the cervix or lungs
Hyperplasia	Response to an increase in demand	Increase in the number of cells in a tissue or organ	Cellular or endometrial hyperplasia
Hypertrophy	Increased demand for work by a cell	Increase in the size (but not number) of cells	Large muscles of a body builder or enlarged heart or kidneys
Metaplasia	Cellular adaptation to adverse conditions	Conversion or replacement of normal cells by other cells	Bronchial metaplasia secondary to cigarette smoke

(Objective 7)

24. a. Muscle is lost, therefore contractility and stroke volume decrease, lowering cardiac output.
b. The additional fluid volume improves preload, thereby increasing stroke volume and cardiac output.
c. A sudden drop in the heart rate results in a decrease in cardiac output.
d. Fear and anxiety cause a rise in heart rate and stroke volume, which in turn increases cardiac output.
(Objective 10)

25. a. The vasoconstrictor center of the medulla is inhibited, and the vagal center is excited, resulting in peripheral vasodilation and a decrease in heart rate and the strength of contraction. This results in a decrease in blood pressure.
b. Vagal stimulation is reduced, resulting in a sympathetic response that causes an increase in peripheral vasoconstriction and in the heart rate and strength of contraction. This results in an increase in blood pressure.
(Objective 10)

26. a. The low pressure results in a decrease in oxygen to the chemoreceptor cells; this in turn stimulates the vasomotor center of the medulla, resulting in peripheral vasoconstriction.
b. Chemoreceptors are also stimulated by an increase in the P_{CO_2}, which causes vasoconstriction and an increase in blood flow to the lungs, enhancing their ability to eliminate carbon dioxide. (Objective 10)

27. The central nervous system ischemic response is initiated when blood pressure drops below 50 mm Hg; it triggers intense vasoconstriction in an attempt to improve perfusion to the brain. If the ischemia lasts longer than 10 minutes, the vagal center may be activated, resulting in peripheral vasodilation and bradycardia.
(Objective 10)

28. a. Increased sympathetic stimulation causes the adrenal medulla to release epinephrine and norepinephrine, which results in an increase in heart rate, stroke volume, and vasoconstriction.
b. Low flow to the kidneys results in a release of renin, which by a series of chemical reactions causes plasma proteins to synthesize angiotensin II. Angiotensin II causes vasoconstriction and initiates the release of aldosterone. Aldosterone causes increased retention of sodium and water by the kidneys.
c. The hypothalamic neurons are stimulated by a drop in blood pressure or an increase in plasma solutes, and the secretion of antidiuretic hormone (vasopressin) is increased. This results in vasoconstriction and a decreased rate of urine production.
(Objective 10)

29. (a) vascular endothelial
(b) endotoxins, inflammatory mediators
(c) endothelium
(d) permeable
(e) interstitial
(f) hypotension, hypoperfusion
(g) complement, coagulation, kallikrein/kinin
(h) coagulation
(i) thrombus
(j) systemic vascular resistance
(k) edema
(l) cardiovascular instability
(m) clotting abnormalities
(n) cellular acidosis, impaired cellular function
(o) organ
(Objective 10)

30.

Sign or Symptom	Local or Systemic Response	Cause
Edematous throat	Local	Cellular accumulation of sodium causes edema. Also, hyperemia increases filtration pressure and capillary permeability, causing fluid to leak into interstitital spaces.
Purulent drainage	Local	Bacteria are destroyed by phagocytosis. Then macrophages clear and destroy tissues of dead cells. Destruction of leukocytes is initiated by phagocytosis. Dead tissues plus dead leukocytes plus fluid that leaks into the area form pus.
Fever	Systemic	Mast cell degranulation and an increase in the metabolic rate caused by the inflammatory process
Red throat	Local	Dilation of arterioles, venules, and capillaries in the area of cellular injury
Difficulty swallowing	Local	A consequence of the edema described above

(Objective 11)

31. a. O positive, O negative, A positive, A negative; b. O negative; c. O positive, O negative, A positive, A negative, B positive, B negative, AB positive; AB negative; d. O negative, B negative
(Objective 11)

32. a. Isoimmunity. The body is reacting to beneficial foreign cells.
b. Allergy. The body is responding to the introduction of a foreign protein (antigen) that it recognizes as harmful.
c. Isoimmunity. The body rejects helpful foreign tissue that it sees as harmful.
d. Allergy. The body may be reacting to the protein (antigen) in the Latex.
e. Autoimmunity. It is thought that systemic lupus erythematosus and other diseases such as dermatomyositis, periarteritis nodosa, scleroderma, and rheumatoid arthritis may be caused by an autoimmune response.[1]
(Objective 12)

33. b. Prolonged emotional or psychological stress can result in physical illness.
34. d. Patients undergoing chemotherapy or radiation therapy for cancer may experience significant suppression of the immune system.
35. e. Severe deficits in calorie or protein intake can seriously impair the immune system.
36. a. The human immunodeficiency virus (HIV) attacks the immune system, making the body easy prey for opportunistic infections and malignancies. (Questions 25-28: Objective 10)
37. a. Cortisol
b. Vasoconstriction
c. Heart
d. Beta-2 receptors

Anderson KN, Anderson LE, Glanze WD: *Mosby's medical nursing and allied health dictionary,* ed 6, St Louis, 2002, Mosby.

38.

Disease	Factor	Environmental or Genetic
Stroke	Hypertension, high cholesterol, smoking	Environmental
Cervical cancer	Infection with gonorrhea	Environmental
Oral cancer	Chewing smokeless tobacco	Environmental
Melanoma (skin cancer)	Excessive exposure to sun	Environmental
Depression	Familial tendency	Genetic
	Metabolic disturbance, drug reaction, nutritional disorder, situational crisis	Environmental

(Objective 9)

STUDENT SELF-ASSESSMENT

39. a. Diffusion is a passive process involving the movement of molecules from an area of high concentration to an area of lower concentration. Facilitated diffusion uses a carrier molecule to move molecules rapidly down a concentration gradient. Osmosis is a process that causes the movement of fluid from an area of low solute concentration to an area of high solute concentration.
(Objective 1)

40. c. All others are found chiefly in the extracellular fluid.
(Objective 1)

41. d. *Atonic* means without tone. A *hypertonic* solution has a greater solute concentration than that inside the cells; a *hypotonic* solution is less concentrated than that inside the cells.
(Objective 1)

42. c. Capillary hydrostatic pressure filters fluid from the blood through the capillary wall. Oncotic pressure exerted by blood plasma proteins attracts fluid from the interstitial space into the blood. The lymph channels open and collect some of the fluid forced out of the capillaries by hydrostatic pressure and return it to the circulation.
(Objective 2)

43. c. Hypernatremic dehydration is associated with an intake of sodium that exceeds sodium losses. Hyponatremic dehydration typically manifests with cramps, seizures, a rapid, thready pulse, diaphoresis, and/or cyanosis. There is no such classification as osmotic dehydration.
(Objective 3)

44. b. A patient in renal failure is frequently hypocalcemic, not hypercalcemic.
(Objective 2)

45. d
(Objective 2)

46. c. Both hydrogen and carbon dioxide bind to hemoglobin, which carries them to the lungs for exhalation. (Objective 4)

47. c. Ventilation (due to a reduced tidal volume) is frequently severely decreased in these patients. This inhibits the excretion of carbon dioxide from the lungs, causing an increase in carbonic acid and a decrease in the pH. (Objective 5)

48. b. Lactic acid reduces the peripheral response to catecholamines and can cause severe hypotension. (Objective 5)

49. c. A decreased pH and increased Pco_2 are signs of respiratory acidosis. An increased pH and decreased Pco_2 are signs of respiratory alkalosis. An increased pH and increased Pco_2 are signs of metabolic alkalosis. (Objective 6)

50. a. The decrease in cell size that occurs secondary to atrophy of brain cells causes the brain to shrink in size. *Dysplasia* is an abnormal change in a mature cell. *Metaplasia* is the substitution of one cell type for another. *Hypertrophy* is an increase in cell size that results in an increase in organ size. (Objective 7)

51. Autolysis. *MODS* is the progressive failure of two or more organ systems secondary to severe illness or injury. *Necrosis* refers to the cellular changes that occur after local cell death. *Osmosis* is the movement of water across a semipermeable membrane. (Objective 7)

52. d. Sodium rushes into the injured cells, increasing the osmotic pressure, which draws more water into the cell. (Objective 8)

53. d. Tachycardia and pupil dilation are sympathetic responses but do not occur secondary to vasoconstriction. The container size should decrease because of vasoconstriction. (Objective 10)

54. d. When blood flow to the vasomotor center of the medulla is reduced to the point of ischemia, this response initiates profound vasoconstriction. (Objective 10)

55. b. All other mechanisms decrease urinary output to conserve blood volume. (Objective 10)

56. b. If sufficient cardiac muscle is destroyed in myocardial infarction, the stroke volume and therefore cardiac output can be markedly decreased. Anaphylactic shock occurs secondary to exposure of a sensitized individual to an allergen, resulting in dyspnea, wheezing, shock, urticaria, erythema, angioedema, and other dramatic signs and symptoms. Septic shock occurs secondary to a bacterial infection that releases harmful endotoxins. (Objective 10)

57. a. Feline leukemia virus is a disease to which humans have a natural immunity. Acquired immunity occurs after immunization for measles and after having chicken pox (for most patients). Temporary acquired immunity is conferred if hepatitis B immunoglobulin is administered, but vaccination is needed to ensure acquired long-term immunity. (Objective 11)

58. c. Hypersensitivity can occur secondary to foreign antigens (allergy, isoimmune reactions) or, in the case of autoimmunity, when the body attacks its own tissues. The response may be immediate or delayed up to several days. Hypersensitivity represents an abnormal immune response. (Objective 12)

59. a. Dopamine exerts effects on the blood vessels. It causes renal and mesenteric dilation at low levels, beta effects at midrange levels, and strong alpha stimulation at high levels. Epinephrine stimulates alpha and beta cells, causing an increase in the heart rate and contractility and in bronchiolar dilation; it also increases blood glucose by glycogenolysis. It does not suppress white blood cells, as cortisol does. Norepinephrine exerts effects similar to those of epinephrine; however, its alpha effects predominate.
(Objective 13)

WRAP IT UP

1. d. Normal saline (NS) is an isotonic fluid that remains in the intravascular space, available for the heart to pump longer than either of the fluids containing dextrose (D$_5$W, D$_5$NS). Lactated Ringer solution (LR) contains potassium, which would not be indicated in this patient.
(Objective 3)

2. a. Cardiac conduction disturbances, irritability, abdominal distention, nausea, diarrhea, oliguria, weakness or paralysis.
(Objective 3)

   b. (2). Intracellular potassium levels are very high. When cells break open, such as during an extensive crush injury or electrical injury, large amounts of potassium are released into the blood.
(Objective 3)

3. a. The prolonged crush forces create an accumulation of lactic acid in the tissues that is released into the general circulation when the patient is freed. In addition, the presence of systemic hypoperfusion creates anaerobic metabolism in some tissues, resulting in the production of lactic acid.
(Objective 5)

4. The respiratory rate will increase, the kidneys will excrete hydrogen ions, and the carbonic acid–bicarbonate buffering system will try to compensate for the metabolic acidosis.
(Objective 4)

5. Parasympathetic stimulation: None
Sympathetic stimulation: Increases heart rate and contractility, constricts blood vessels
Adrenal medullary mechanism: Increases heart rate and contractility, constricts blood vessels
Renin-angiotensin-aldosterone mechanism: Constricts blood vessels, conserves body water
Vasopressin mechanism: Constricts blood vessels, conserves body water
Tissue fluid reabsorption: Moves fluid from interstitial to intravascular space (doesn't conserve it)
Splenic discharge of blood: Releases blood from spleen (doesn't conserve it) (Objective 10)

6. d. The blood pressure is low, therefore the compensatory mechanisms are no longer sufficient to resolve the patient's hypoperfusion.
(Objective 10)

Life Span Development

READING ASSIGNMENT
Chapter 8, pages 196-211, in *Mosby's Paramedic Textbook*, ed. 3

OBJECTIVES
Upon completion of this chapter, the paramedic student will be able to:
1. Describe the normal vital signs and body system characteristics of the newborn, neonate, infant, toddler, preschooler, school-aged child, adolescent, young adult, middle-aged adult, and older adult.
2. Identify the psychosocial features of the infant, toddler, preschooler, school-aged child, adolescent, young adult, middle-aged adult, and older adult.
3. Explain the effect of parenting styles, sibling rivalry, peer relationships, and other factors on a child's psychosocial development.
4. Discuss the physical and emotional challenges faced by the older adult.

SUMMARY
- The newborn is a baby in the first hours of life. A neonate is a baby younger than 28 days. An infant is a child 28 days to 1 year of age.
- The newborn normally weighs 3 to 3.5 kg (7 to 8 pounds). This weight typically triples in 9 to 12 months. The infant's head accounts for about 25% of the total body weight.
- At birth, structures unique to fetal circulation constrict and normally close within the first year of life. Fluid is expelled from the lungs during the first few breaths. Respiratory muscles and alveoli are not fully developed.
- Infants are born with protective reflexes related to breathing, eating, and stress or discomfort.
- At birth the anterior and posterior fontanelles are open. Bone growth occurs at the epiphysis of the bones.
- Some passive immunity is conferred at birth and through the mother's breast milk.
- The caregiver is the major factor in the infant's psychosocial development.
- Temperament is a person's behavioral style. It is the way the person interacts with the environment.
- Toddlers are children 1 to 3 years of age. Preschoolers are 3 to 5 years of age.
- The hemoglobin level in toddlers and preschoolers approaches that of adults. The brain in this age group is about 90% of the adult brain weight. Muscle mass and bone density increase. Walking occurs by age 2, and fine motor skills develop. Control of bowel and bladder is achieved.
- Parenting styles can be described as authoritarian, authoritative, or permissive.
- Sibling rivalry, peer relationships, divorce, and exposure to aggression and violence affect a child's development.

- School-aged children range from 6 to 12 years of age. Physical growth slows, but brain function and the ability to learn quickly develop in this age group. Many children reach puberty during this time. Self-esteem and moral development are critical at this age.
- Adolescents are 13 to 19 years of age. The growth of bone and muscle mass is nearly complete in this age group. Reproductive maturity has been reached. Adolescence often involves some emotional turmoil, and antisocial behavior may be seen.
- Early adulthood spans the period from 20 to 40 years of age. Lifelong habits and routines develop. Body systems are at their optimal performance.
- Middle adulthood extends from 41 to 60 years of age. The physiological aspects of aging become more apparent in this age group. Menopause in women occurs during this stage.
- People reach late adulthood at 61 years of age. Body system changes vary widely from person to person, but the systemic changes of aging become apparent. Some adults in this age group face financial, physical, and emotional challenges.

Match the age range in Column I with the appropriate age in Column II.

Column I		Column II
1. _C_ Infant		a. First few hours of life
2. _B_ Neonate		b. Younger than 28 days
3. _A_ Newborn		c. 28 days to 1 year
4. _e_ Preschool		d. 1 to 3 years
5. _f_ School age		e. 3 to 5 years
6. _D_ Toddler		f. 6 to 12 years

Match the reflex in Column II with the appropriate description in Column I.

Column I		Column II
7. _E_ Head turns toward facial stimulation.		a. Babinski's
8. _G_ Lips pucker when mouth contacts nipple.		b. Babkin
9. _A_ Toes spread up and out when sole stroked.		c. Moro
10. _B_ Mouth opens if palm is pressed when supine.		d. Palmar grasp
11. _C_ Infant stretches and then hugs self after loud noise.		e. Rooting
		f. Stepping
		g. Sucking

Circle toddler (1 to 3 years) or preschooler (3 to 5 years) to indicate the most common age that children achieve the following social milestones.

12. Can state name of friend   Toddler or Preschooler
13. Speech is understandable to strangers   Toddler or Preschooler
14. Follows directions   Toddler or Preschooler
15. Shows sympathy when appropriate   Toddler or Preschooler
16. Points to a named part of the body   Toddler or Preschooler

17. Fill in the blanks related to the physiological changes associated with late adulthood.

Blood pressure rises as blood vessels (a) _____, (b) _____ resistance increases, and

(c) _____ sensitivity decreases. Blood flow to organs (d) _____. Increased workload

on the heart causes (e) _____, changes in the mitral and aortic (f) _____,

and decreased (g) _____ elasticity. The number of pacemaker cells in the heart (h) _____,

resulting in (i) _____. Blood volume, red blood cells, and platelet count (j) _____.

Lung function and lung capacity (k) _____. Pain (l) _____ and reaction

(m) _____ decrease. Secretion of (n) _____ and gastric juices decreases. Intestinal

sphincters lose (o) _____. About 50% of the nephrons in the (p) _____ are lost.

18. List two causes of each of the following stressors that affect the older adult's lifestyle.
   a. Financial burdens:

_____

_____

   b. Physical and emotional challenges:

_____

_____

19. A heart rate of 140 beats per minute at rest would be considered normal for what age range?
   a. Newborn
   b. Preschool
   c. School age
   d. Toddler

20. Which of the following physiological changes occurs at birth?
   a. Ductus venosus dilates.
   b. Pulmonary vascular resistance decreases.
   c. Right ventricular pressure increases.
   d. Systemic vascular resistance decreases.

21. Which is true regarding the infant's respiratory system?
   a. Bones are the primary chest support.
   b. Body heat and fluids can be lost through respirations.
   c. The number of alveoli is close to the adult.
   d. Tracheal bifurcation occurs lower than the adult.

22. Which is a protective survival reflex in the infant?
   a. Babinski's
   b. Moro
   c. Palmar grasp
   d. Rooting

23. For which type of temperament might low intensity of reactions and a negative mood be observed?
   a. Difficult
   b. Easy
   c. Slow to warm up
   d. Temperamental

24. Which statement is true regarding the toddler?
   a. Hemoglobin approaches adult levels.
   b. Ear, nose, throat structures are similar to the adolescent.
   c. Passive immunity protects children of this age.
   d. Visual acuity averages 20/20.

25. Which parenting style tends to produce children who are responsible, assertive, and self-reliant?
   a. Authoritarian
   b. Authoritative
   c. Permissive
   d. Traditional

26. Which is true regarding the development of peer relationships in the toddler/preschool age group? They are formed with others _____.
   a. At the same age level
   b. Of same school age
   c. Who are adult caregivers
   d. Younger than they are

27. Which is true regarding the school-age child?
    a. Growth rates are faster than toddlers.
    b. Lymphatic tissue is small relative to adults.
    c. Primary tooth growth is beginning.
    d. Skull growth is 95% complete.
28. Conventional reasoning is a stage in which phase of the psychosocial development of a child?
    a. Moral
    b. Peer relationships
    c. Self-concept
    d. Self-esteem
29. What stimulates the release of hormones that initiate the physical changes of puberty in girls?
    a. Gonadotropin
    b. Follicle-stimulating hormone
    c. Luteinizing hormone
    d. Progesterone
30. Which is true regarding psychosocial issues in teenagers?
    a. Anorexia nervosa is a depressive disorder seen in this age group.
    b. Appearance is not a major concern for teens.
    c. Suicide is the leading cause of death in gay and lesbian teens.
    d. Depression rarely is seen in this age group.
31. On which developmental issue do early adults often focus?
    a. Losing weight
    b. Health concerns
    c. Retirement planning
    d. Selecting a mate
32. Which health-related concern is common in the middle-aged adult?
    a. Dementia
    b. Diverticulitis
    c. Hypercholesterolemia
    d. Stroke

WRAP IT UP

You find yourself in a difficult situation. You are the only paramedic on the rescue squad at the scene of a fire at a home day care and have been assigned to care for a group of children until the next ambulances arrive; ETA is 20 to 30 minutes. The caregiver, a 60-year-old woman, and one child sustained significant smoke inhalation and are being rushed to the hospital. You are left with four children: a 5-week-old infant, a 13-month-old boy, a 3-year-old girl, and a 5-year-old girl. The baby is sleeping quietly, and the other children are upset and crying. You manage quickly to obtain the following vital signs with the help of another firefighter:

5-week-old: BP 78/60 mm Hg, P 124/min, R 28/min, SaO_2 99%
13 month-old: BP 80/64 mm Hg, P 120/min, R 28/min, SaO_2 100%
3-year-old: BP 94/66 mm Hg, P 112/min, R 24/min, SaO_2 98%
5-year-old: BP 96/68 mm Hg, P 104/min, R 20/min, SaO_2 98%

When you examine the baby, you note that he is pink with a 1-second capillary refill and is using abdominal muscles to breath, and you can feel a soft diamond-shaped depression at the top of his skull that appears to pulsate with each heartbeat. When he awakens, he turns his face toward you and tries to suck when you stroke his cheek, but he does not cry or seem upset.

The 13-month-old wants nothing to do with you. He screams when you approach him and tries to run, but falls, striking his head on the corner of the bench on which you are seated. His abdomen is protruding, and you note that he has a wet diaper.

The 3-year-old is calmed by the time you try to examine her. She asks what happened to her caregiver, "mo-mo," and you explain that there was a fire and the smoke made her sick.

The 5-year-old girl is trying to be helpful, watching the younger children. She denies feeling sick or hurt and wants her parents to come. You explain that you will call them to come and get her as quickly as they can, but it may take a few minutes.

As you complete your exam, a bystander comes over and explains that she saw the smoke coming from the basement and ran in and got these kids from the family room upstairs where there was no smoke or fire. By then, the children's caregiver ran up the stairs from the basement with the other child and collapsed on the lawn. You continue to monitor the children until the ambulance arrives. In consultation with medical direction and the children's parents, it is decided to leave the children in the care of their parents with detailed follow-up instructions.

1. Place a check mark beside the age groups for which you were responsible on this call.
   a. _____ Newborn   d. _____ Toddler
   b. _____ Neonate   e. _____ Preschooler
   c. _____ Infant   f. _____ School age
2. Identify the abnormal findings that you encountered in each of the following children:
   a. 5-week-old

   _____

   b. 13-month-old

   _____

   c. 3-year-old

   _____

   d. 5-year-old

   _____

3. Which of the following is true regarding the 5-week-old child's behavior?
   a. He should have cried when he awoke and did not recognize you.

   _____

   b. He should be able to track your finger with his eyes.

   _____

   c. He should grasp your finger if you place it in his hand.

   _____

   d. He should be saying some single-syllable words.

   _____

   _____

CHAPTER 8 ANSWERS

REVIEW QUESTIONS
1. c
2. b
3. a
4. e
5. f
6. d
(Objective 1)

7. e
(Objective 1)

8. g
(Objective 1)

9. a
(Objective 1)

10. b
(Objective 1)

11. c
(Objective 1)

12. Preschooler
(Objective 2)

13. Preschooler
(Objective 2)

14. Toddler
(Objective 2)

15. Preschooler
(Objective 2)

16. Toddler
(Objective 2)

17. a. Thicken
(Objective 1)

b. Peripheral
(Objective 1)

c. Baroreceptor
(Objective 1)

d. Decreases
(Objective 1)

e. Cardiomyopathy
(Objective 1)

f. Valves
(Objective 1)

g. Myocardial
(Objective 1)

h. Decreases
(Objective 1)

i. Dysrhythmias
(Objective 1)

j. Decrease
(Objective 1)

k. Decreases
(Objective 1)

l. Perception
(Objective 1)

m. Time
(Objective 1)

n. Saliva
(Objective 1)

o. Tone
(Objective 1)

p. Kidney
(Objective 1)

18. a. Reduced income at retirement; increased health care costs (insurance, drugs); costs of assisted living needs
(Objective 4)

b. Decreased mobility; disease processes; cognitive loss; death of a companion (Objective 4)

19. a. The heart rate for each of the other ages can increase to 140 beats/min during serious illness or injury.
(Objective 1)

20. b. The ductus venosus constricts, right ventricular pressure decreases, and systemic vascular resistance increases at birth.
(Objective 1)

21. c. The bones are not fully formed, and so muscles provide much support to the chest. The infant has significantly fewer alveoli than the adult. The tracheal bifurcation is higher in the infant.
(Objective 1)

22. d. Rooting reflex allows the baby to move toward food.
(Objective 1)

23. c. Easy children are characterized by regularity of body functions and acceptance of new situations. Difficult children display intense reaction and withdrawal from new stimuli.
(Objective 2)

24. a. The ear, nose, and throat structures are shorter and more susceptible to infection than the adolescent's. Passive immunity wanes early in infancy. Visual acuity is typically 20/30 in this age group.
(Objective 1)

25. b. Authoritarian parenting style tends to produce children who have low motivation and self-esteem. Children reared by permissive parents may be discontented, distrustful, and self-centered.
(Objective 3)

26. a. Peer relationships are formed with children near the same age and level of maturity.
(Objective 2)

27. d. Growth rates are slower than infants and toddlers. Lymphatic tissue is larger relative to adults until about age 10. Primary teeth are lost, and replacement with permanent teeth begins.
(Objective 1)

28. a. One theory of moral development lists three stages: preconventional reasoning, conventional reasoning, and postconventional reasoning. Self-concept, self-esteem, and peer relationships are also critical in the development of children.
(Objective 2)

29. b. Gonadotropin is released from the hypothalamus and subsequently stimulates the release of luteinizing and follicle-stimulating hormones from the pituitary. These in turn stimulate the release of progesterone (breast development and menstrual cycle) and estrogen (female secondary sex characteristics).
(Objective 1)

30. c. Suicide is the third leading cause of death for teens 15 to 19, but gay and lesbian teens are 2 to 3 times more likely to attempt suicide. Anorexia nervosa is an eating disorder. Depression is common. Appearance is important to teens.
(Objective 1)

31. d. Other key issues in this age group include rearing children, managing a home, finding a social group, leisure activities, and selecting a stable occupation.
(Objective 2)

32. c. Dementia, diverticulitis, and stroke can occur in this age group but are much more common in older adults.
(Objective 2)

WRAP IT UP

1. c, d, e, f
(Objective 1)

2. No abnormal findings were identified in any of the children.
(Objectives 1 and 2)

3. c. This is known as the palmar grasp reflex.
(Objective 1)

PART THREE

IN THIS PART

Therapeutic Communications

READING ASSIGNMENT
Chapter 9, pages 214-225 in *Mosby's Paramedic Textbook*, ed. 3

OBJECTIVES
1. Define therapeutic communication.
2. List the elements of effective therapeutic communication.
3. Identify internal factors that influence effective communication.
4. Identify external factors that influence effective communication.
5. Explain the elements of an effective patient interview.
6. Summarize strategies for gathering appropriate patient information.
7. Discuss methods of assessing the individual's mental status during the patient interview.
8. Describe ways the paramedic can improve communication with a variety of patients. Such patients include (1) those who are unmotivated to talk; (2) hostile patients; (3) children; (4) older adults; (5) hearing-impaired patients; (6) blind patients; (7) patients under the influence of drugs or alcohol; (8) sexually aggressive patients; and (9) patients whose cultural traditions are different from those of the paramedic.

SUMMARY
- Therapeutic communication is a planned act. It is also a professional act. The paramedic, working with the patient, obtains information that is used to meet patient care goals.
- Communication is a dynamic process. It has six elements: the source, encoding, the message, decoding, the receiver, and feedback.
- To effectively communicate with patients, paramedics must genuinely like people. They must be able to empathize with others. They also must have the ability to listen.
- Good communication calls for a favorable physical environment. Factors such as privacy, interruption, eye contact, and personal dress are external influences. These factors can be controlled. This allows the paramedic to better communicate with the patient.
- The patient interview often decides the direction of the physical examination. Good care means that the paramedic sees each patient as an individual. It also means that the patient's needs are met in a caring, concerned, and receptive way.
- Open-ended and closed (direct) questions can be used to get information from the patient. Techniques include resistance, shifting focus, recognizing defense mechanisms, and distraction.

- The first step with any patient is to assess mental status. This can be done by observing the patient's appearance and level of consciousness. The paramedic also can look for normal or abnormal body movements. During normal conversation, the patient should be able to show clear thinking, a normal attention span, and the ability to concentrate on and understand the discussion. The patient's responses to the environment (i.e., affect) should be appropriate to the situation.
- Difficult interviews generally arise from four situations: (1) the patient's condition may affect the ability to speak; (2) the patient may fear talking because of psychological disorders, cultural differences, or age; (3) a cognitive impairment may be present; or (4) the patient may want to deceive the paramedic.

REVIEW QUESTIONS

Match the communication response in column II with the description in column I. Use each response only once.

Column I	Column II
1. _____ Making associations or implying a cause	a. Clarification
2. _____ Paraphrasing a patient's words	b. Confrontation
3. _____ Pausing for several moments	c. Empathy
4. _____ Reviewing with open-ended questions	d. Explanation
5. _____ Having the patient rephrase a word	e. Interpretation
6. _____ Providing information	f. Reflection
7. _____ Refocusing on one aspect of the interview	g. Silence
	h. Summary

8. Identify selected elements of the communication process in the following example:

You tell your patient that you plan to take his temperature. He says, "Where are you going to take it to?" You clarify that you are going to put a thermometer under his tongue to see whether he has a fever.
a. Who is the source?
b. Who did the encoding in the initial message?
c. Was the decoding effective?
d. Who was the receiver?
e. Why was feedback needed?

9. You are caring for a patient who is very emotionally upset. List six actions you can use to convey that you are actively listening to the patient.

a.

b.

c.

d.

e.

f.

10. A patient was assaulted and is found in the midst of a large crowd. How can you control external factors to enable effective communication with this patient?

_____

_____

11. Rewrite the following questions into an open-ended format:

    a. Do you feel bad?

_____

    b. Does your chest hurt here?

_____

    c. Did this problem start today?

_____

    d. Are you taking any medicine on a daily basis?

_____

12. Can you identify the problem in each of the following statements if they were made by a paramedic?

    a. I know you can't move your legs right now, but don't worry; everything will be just fine.

_____

    b. You know you won't have this trouble breathing if you quit smoking.

_____

    c. We believe your substernal chest pain may be causing an ischemic area in your myocardium that is going to result in myocardial infarction.

_____

    d. Why didn't you take your blood pressure medicine?

_____

13. You are called to a residence for a woman who fell down the stairs. You begin your assessment and patient management, and by the time you get in the back of the ambulance, you realize that her injuries are not consistent with the mechanism of injury she describes. The patient is reluctant to give you much information, and you strongly suspect domestic violence was the cause of her injuries.

    a. What reasons may this patient have for resistance regarding information?

_____

    b. What statements might you make to begin to talk about this issue?

_____

    c. If she tells you she was beaten up by her husband but doesn't want to leave him or have him arrested, how should you respond?

_____

14. You are called to a college dorm for an "overdose." As you arrive on the scene, the patient is walking toward you.

    a. What is the first step in your mental status examination of this patient?

_____

    b. As you begin your conversation with the patient, what observations will you make regarding mental status?

_____

15. For each of the following difficult situations, identify three strategies that you may use to attempt to communicate with the patient.
   a. A 72-year-old man has paralysis on the right side. He appears to be awake and alert, but he is not responding to your questions appropriately.

   _____

   b. You have been called to a jail to care for a patient who has expressed a wish to kill a number of people. He is sitting with his arms folded, and his voice is getting progressively louder.

   _____

16. Describe your approach when interviewing a 3-year-old and his father.

   _____

17. You are caring for a patient in the ambulance who makes inappropriate and sexually suggestive remarks. What should you do?

   _____

STUDENT SELF-ASSESSMENT

18. Which of the following best describes therapeutic communication?
   a. Verbal and nonverbal behavior that conveys a message
   b. Planned act to communicate and obtain information
   c. Spoken or written words to express ideas or feelings
   d. Decoding and encoding from a messenger to a receiver
19. When a message is put into an understandable format, it is considered which of the following?
   a. Decoded   c. Received
   b. Encoded   d. Sourced
20. When you try to see the situation from another person's point of view, you are demonstrating which of the following?
   a. Cultural imposition c. Ethnocentrism
   b. Empathy   d. Sympathy
21. Which of the following would convey a confident, open attitude during the patient interview in the prehospital setting?
   a. Speaking loudly and quickly
   b. Standing with your arms folded on your chest
   c. Looking into the patient's eyes as the patient speaks
   d. Not invading the patient's personal space
22. Which of the following would demonstrate an effective patient communication strategy?
   a. Beginning questions with "How"
   b. Demonstrating personal bias
   c. Interrupting to get to the point
   d. Using medical terminology
23. Which of the following is a normal finding during the mental status examination?
   a. The patient demonstrates long pauses and rapid shifts in conversation.
   b. The patient has an upright posture and is well groomed.
   c. You repeat questions several times before the patient understands you.
   d. The patient is trembling and clenching and unclenching the fists.
24. Which of the following is the most effective method for communicating with a hearing-impaired patient in the prehospital setting?
   a. Lipreading
   b. Sign language
   c. Whatever method the patient prefers
   d. Note writing

WRAP IT UP

You are working on LSV 4097 and are dispatched to a quiet residential neighborhood for an "unknown nature." The local police community officer meets you on the scene and says that he is worried about the resident. The officer has been working with the resident to improve his living conditions. A month ago, he found the 70-year-old patient living without electricity or running water. He was using the nearby creek for toileting, and he used candles to light his home. Currently the patient is living in a nearby community while trying to clean up his home. This morning a sore on his leg began to bleed, and he is unable to control the bleeding. You note a dirty, ulcerated wound that is red and swollen on the patient's lower leg. He tells you that he is diabetic and not to worry, he will take care of it. He then walks over to a dirty basin of water in the yard and begins to clean the wound with a dirty rag.

You take a short history and do a brief physical examination. You determine that the patient needs to be transported for care of his wound. His compliance with his diabetic medicines is questionable, and you are unsure how well his basic nutritional and hygiene needs are being met. The patient adamantly refuses transport; he is afraid he won't ever be able to come home. Your partner begins to argue with him, and the patient becomes progressively more angry and agitated.

1. What message were you trying to encode to the patient?

   _____

2. What information did he decode from your message?

   _____

3. What strategy do you think will be most successful for communicating with this patient?
   a. Empathy
   b. Pity
   c. Sympathy
   d. Threats

4. How can you show that you are listening effectively?
   a. Look for weak spots in his arguments that you can debate
   b. Prepare your answer while you listen so you can respond fast
   c. Try to ignore the body language, voice tone, and just listen to his words
   d. Summarize the patient's statements to clarify meaning if you are unsure

5. What are six techniques that you can use from the beginning of the patient interview to improve the chance for an effective patient encounter?
   a.
   b.
   c.
   d.
   e.
   f.

6. Which of the following statements would likely be most effective in this situation?
   a. "Living like this isn't healthy for a human being. You should find somewhere else to live. We need to take you to the hospital to get you to a cleaner place."
   b. "Why are you living in these conditions? Don't you know this isn't healthy?"
   c. "The impaired circulation secondary to your diabetes will prohibit normal mechanisms of healing, leading to possible sepsis. You need immediate medical interventions."
   d. "It looks as though you need some help to heal this wound. Let's take you to the doctor so you can get better quickly and get back to your work here at home."

7. Which of the statements in question 6 appear judgmental?

8. Which of the following would not be helpful in responding to this patient's anger?
   a. "I know you're angry because it seems as if we're telling you what to do. We would just like you to get some care for your wound so you can get home quickly."
   b. You ignore the patient's anger and continue more forcefully with your attempts to make him go to the hospital
   c. "It seems as though you're angry because you're worried you won't be able to come home if you go to the hospital. Our goal is just the opposite; we know how important your home is to you, and we want you to be healthy so you can stay here."
   d. "You seem really angry; can you tell us why? We'd like to be here to help you solve your problem."

The patient responds to your partner with a raised voice and tells him he has no business coming on his property and telling him what to do.

After you calmly sit with the patient for a few minutes and clearly explain your concerns, as well as the actions the hospital may take to get the patient home quickly, he agrees to be transported for care.

CHAPTER 9 ANSWERS

REVIEW QUESTIONS

1. e
2. f
3. g
4. h
5. a
6. d
7. b

8. a. You (the paramedic) are the source.
   b. You did the encoding.
   c. No, the patient did not interpret the message in an appropriate manner.
   d. The patient was the receiver of the first message.
   e. Feedback was needed to clarify the message.
   (Objective 2)

9. a. Face the patient when he or she speaks.
   b. Maintain eye contact.
   c. Avoid crossing your legs or arms.
   d. Avoid distracting body movements.
   e. Nod in acknowledgment at appropriate times.
   f. Lean toward the patient.
   (Objective 3)

10. Move the patient into the ambulance as quickly as possible for more privacy. Try to avoid interruptions until the interview is finished.
   (Objective 4)

11. a. "How do you feel?"
   b. "Describe (or show me) where your chest hurts."
   c. "Tell me when this problem began."
   d. "What medicines do you take on a daily basis?"
   (Objective 5)

12. a. You shouldn't offer false reassurance.
   b. Showing disapproval and offering unsolicited advice impair effective communication.
   c. Using professional jargon impairs the patient's ability to understand you.
   d. "Why" questions may be viewed as accusations.
   (Objective 5)

13. a. Her resistance may be related to personal pride, fear of loss of self-esteem, or fear of retribution.
   b. Shifting the focus temporarily to her injuries and making statements such as, "I've seen this pattern of injuries before in women who have been hurt by their husbands or boyfriends," may allow her to respond to your comments.
   c. Explain that you recognize she is in a dangerous situation and that you are worried about her. Then give her some information about social service agencies that can provide support or help if she changes her mind later. Report your observations to the hospital staff.
   (Objective 6)

14. a. Observe the patient's appearance, level of consciousness, and gait. Note how he or she is dressed and groomed. Look for any defensive or aggressive postures.

b. Talk to the patient to see if he or she is oriented to person, place, and time. Note the quality of speech and the ability to think clearly, maintain a normal attention span, and concentrate on the discussion.
(Objective 7)

15. a. Consider whether the patient's present illness or a preexisting condition may prevent him from speaking. Tell him that you are there to help. Question family members. See whether the patient can nod to answer questions if he is unable to respond verbally.

b. Make sure you are positioned close to an exit and that law enforcement officers are close by. Try to use normal interviewing techniques. Set limits. Follow protocols for restraint if the patient's behavior becomes violent.
(Objective 8)

16. Ask the father questions first. Offer a distraction to the child and gradually approach and start talking to him. Speak at eye level in a calm, quiet voice. Use short sentences with concrete explanations.
(Objective 8)

17. Inform the patient of your professional role and the inappropriate nature of the comments. Document the situation; if possible, have another caregiver ride in the patient compartment with you.
(Objective 8)

18. b. Each of the other answers describes communication. Therapeutic communication is a planned, deliberate act that uses specific techniques to build a positive relationship and share information to achieve goals for the patient.
(Objective 1)

19. b. Decoding involves interpretation of a message.
(Objective 2)

20. b. *Cultural imposition* means to impose your beliefs or values on people from other cultures. *Ethnocentrism* is viewing your own life as the most acceptable, the best, or superior to others. *Sympathy* is the expression of your feelings about another person's predicament.
(Objective 3)

21. c. Folding your arms may indicate a closed, defensive feeling. Although you need to be aware of a patient's personal space, in the prehospital setting you need to make close contact on most calls to perform an effective examination.
(Objective 5)

22. a. Demonstrating personal bias that leads the patient in an unwanted direction can hamper communications. Interruptions occasionally may be necessary if a life-threatening condition exists, but a more appropriate action is to allow the patient to proceed uninterrupted. Excessive use of medical terminology with patients may impair their ability to understand you.
(Objective 5)

23. b. This observation is just one clue in the examination. All other choices reflect possible abnormal mental status exams.
(Objective 7)

24. c. The paramedic's abilities (regarding sign language) and the circumstances of the call determine which method can be used. Whenever possible, the method that the patient chooses should be used.
(Objective 8)

WRAP IT UP

1. You are trying to encode a message that the patient has a specific medical problem that needs to be cared for in the hospital.
   (Objective 2)

2. The message he has decoded tells him that your efforts to get him to go to the hospital will mean that he may never come home again.
   (Objective 2)

3. a. Telling the patient that you understand his fear and then clarifying the issues may be effective.
   (Objective 2)

4. d. You want him to know that you are listening carefully. You also want to make sure that you understand the meaning of his words.
   (Objective 6)

5. Six strategies you can use include the following: face the patient; maintain eye contact; look attentive (don't cross your arms and legs); avoid distracting movements; nod to acknowledge important points; lean toward the speaker.

6. d. You want to use nonthreatening language and acknowledge the patient's chief concern about getting home.
   (Objective 6)

7. Responses (a) and (b) sound very judgmental and may make the patient even more angry.
   (Objective 6)

8. b. The other answers acknowledge the patient's emotions.
   (Objective 6)

History Taking

READING ASSIGNMENT
Chapter 10, pages 226-233, in *Mosby's Paramedic Textbook,* ed. 3.

OBJECTIVES
Upon completion of this chapter, the paramedic student will be able to:
1. Describe the purpose of effective history taking in prehospital patient care.
2. List components of the patient history as defined by the Department of Transportation.
3. Outline effective patient interviewing techniques to facilitate history taking.
4. Identify strategies to manage special challenges in obtaining a patient history.

SUMMARY
- Obtaining a patient history offers structure to the patient assessment. The history often sets priorities in patient care as well.
- Content of the patient history includes date and time, identifying data, source of referral, history, reliability, chief complaint, present illness, past medical history, and review of body systems.
- The paramedic should ensure patient comfort. Several methods are available to accomplish this. The paramedic should avoid entering the patient's personal space. Sensitivity to the patient's feelings and watching for signs of uneasiness also are important. The paramedic should use appropriate language and ask open-ended and direct questions. The paramedic should use therapeutic communications techniques as well.
- Many challenges can affect history taking. One of these challenges is silent or talkative patients. Another is patients with multiple symptoms. Then there are anxious, angry, or hostile patients. The paramedic also may see intoxication, crying, depression, and sexually attractive or seductive patients. False reassurance is a major issue to consider. Patient may present confusing behaviors and histories. Two other issues are developmental disabilities and communication barriers. With these last two, the issue of talking with family and friends can be complex as well.

REVIEW QUESTIONS

Questions 1 and 2 pertain to the following case study:

> You are dispatched to a home to care for a 75-year-old woman who is having chest pain.

1. What additional questions will you need to ask related to her history?

   a. Present illness:

b. Significant medical history:

_____

c. Personal habits and environmental conditions:

_____

d. Family history:

_____

2. What is her chief complaint?

3. Your elderly patient fell and has a painful wrist. Discuss any finding in each of the following elements of the SAMPLE history that may explain a reason for her fall.

S—

A—

M—

P—

L—

E—

4. For each of the following patient complaints, list any personal habits and environmental conditions that are important to know during the patient history:

a. A 4-year-old child awakens suddenly with a sore throat, fever, muffled voice, dysphagia, and pain on swallowing:

_____

b. A 25-year-old soldier complains of fever, night sweats, weight loss, and hemoptysis:

_____

c. A 40-year-old is injured in a motor vehicle collision:

_____

d. An 18-year-old woman is complaining of abdominal pain:

_____

e. A 72-year-old has slurred speech:

_____

f. A 45-year-old is complaining of depression:

_____

g. A 27-year-old has a heart rate of 50 beats/min:

_____

h. A 77-year-old is dirty and has bruises in various stages of healing on the back and arms:

_____

    i. A 16-year-old is extremely thin and frail looking:

_____

5. Describe one technique to use when dealing with each of the following situations during the patient interview:

    a. Your elderly patient clearly is distraught and has a lengthy pause in his conversation as he relates a painful story to you:

_____

    b. The patient begins a long and complex history in much more detail than necessary:

_____

    c. Within the first 60 seconds of your interview, your patient has related at least five different problems of varying severity:

_____

    d. The patient is trembling and tearful despite a relatively minor injury:

_____

    e. The patient asks you to tell her everything will be all right, when you know her condition is critical, and perhaps even lethal:

_____

    f. A patient is verbally venting his anger and frustration about his illness:

_____

    g. The patient strokes your leg in a sexually suggestive manner:

_____

    h. The patient does not speak or understand your language:

_____

STUDENT SELF-ASSESSMENT

6. What is the purpose of obtaining a patient history?
    a. To obtain billing information
    b. To detect signs of injury
    c. To establish priorities of patient care
    d. To make the patient comfortable

7. Which of the following is a routine component of the patient history?
    a. Age   **c.** Religion
    b. Insurance information   **d.** Vital signs

8. Which of the following is true regarding the chief complaint in the patient history?
    a. It is always stated by the patient.
    b. It is usually the reason that emergency medical services was called.
    c. It includes significant medical history.
    d. It will remain the same throughout the call.

9. What might be a good question to ask while taking the history of present illness for a patient who is experiencing difficulty breathing?
   a. Did it start today?
   b. Is your difficulty breathing pretty bad?
   c. Where is your difficulty breathing?
   d. What makes your breathing better or worse?

10. Your patient is complaining of headache and chest tightness after an exposure to an unknown gas at work. What personal habits should you ask about for this patient?
    a. Exercise
    b. Immunizations
    c. Sleep patterns
    d. Smoking history

11. You plan to administer ketorolac tromethamine (Toradol) to a patient. You will not give it if your patient reports anaphylactic reaction to which drug?
    a. Acetaminophen (Tylenol)
    b. Aspirin
    c. Meperidine (Demerol)
    d. Penicillin

12. In which of the following situations is determination of last oral intake important?
    a. An adult with a corneal abrasion
    b. An adult with a small laceration on the forearm
    c. An adult with dizziness
    d. An adult with shoulder pain

13. Which of the following illnesses is not hereditary?
    a. Diabetes
    b. Kidney disease
    c. Sickle cell anemia
    d. Tuberculosis

14. You are called to care for a patient who is very depressed. Which statement may be most helpful?
    a. "Don't worry, we'll take good care of you."
    b. "Everything will be okay when we get you to the hospital."
    c. "My friend was depressed, and he's just fine now."
    d. "It seems as though you are really sad. I'm here to listen."

15. What is a good approach when you are managing the angry or intoxicated patient who does not pose an immediate danger to self or the emergency medical services crew?
    a. Physical restraint
    b. Set limits
    c. Threaten
    d. Yell

16. When interviewing the patient who has developmental delays, you should do which of the following?
    a. Clarify answers.
    b. Not ask the patient.
    c. Omit most questions.
    d. Speak loudly.

WRAP IT UP

At 0900 on a warm spring morning, you are dispatched to a call for "chest pain." On arrival you find a 45-year-old black woman who is complaining of diffuse chest and abdominal pain. She is pale, cool, and diaphoretic. Her husband called you because he was concerned when she said she was too ill to go to work at her law firm, which she had never done before. She is conscious, alert, and oriented and tells you that this began about an hour ago. She is unable specifically to describe the pain but says it is a gnawing sensation sometimes in her chest and left shoulder, and other times in the left lower quadrant of her abdomen. She is nauseated as well. Nothing seems to make the pain change in severity (rated as a 5 to 7), character, or location. She says she is normally healthy, takes Humulin 70/30 insulin for her diabetes, which she was diagnosed with at the age of 6 years. She indicates that she has taken her insulin, has eaten her regular breakfast, and had a normal dinner last evening. Just before your arrival, she says her blood sugar was 80 mg/dL, a normal value for her at this time of day. Her allergies include aspirin and shellfish. She reports no trauma, major surgeries, or hospitalizations since her initial diagnosis of diabetes. She has not traveled recently nor had any occupational exposures to anything unusual. She has two teenage children and is premenopausal with irregular periods (last period 5 weeks ago) and uses rhythm method for birth control. A normal bowel movement was reported this morning. Her parents are both deceased: her father died of an abdominal aneurysm at 48 and her mother of a heart attack at 45 years of age. Vital signs are BP 98/58, P 110, and R 24/min; oxygen saturation is 93%; blood glucose 82 mg/dL; and her electrocardiogram shows a sinus tachycardia. Her physical exam reveals some mild tenderness in the abdomen not specifically localized. Peripheral pulses are weak in all extremities. You apply oxygen at 4 L/min by nasal cannula, initiate an IV of normal saline TKO, and begin transport to the hospital while continuing to monitor the patient's vital signs and level of pain.

1. Which of the following illnesses is a possibility based on the history that she has given to you? List the reasons for your response.

Illness	Yes	No	Reasons (Family History, Signs and Symptoms, Medications)
a. Myocardial infarction			
b. Stroke			
c. Appendicitis			
d. Ectopic pregnancy			
e. Abdominal aortic aneurysm			
f. Urinary tract infection			
g. Gastroenteritis			
h. Hypoglycemia			

2. What could be the significance of neglecting to ask about the following?
   a. Allergies
   b. Menstrual history
   c. Family history

3. Why might the patient be reluctant to call 911 with her history and symptoms?

4. What can you say to the patient if she wants to know what is wrong with her?

CHAPTER 10 ANSWERS

HISTORY TAKING

1. a. Does anything make the pain better or worse? What does the pain feel like? Show me where the pain is. Does it go anywhere else? On a scale of 1 to 10, with 1 being the least and 10 being the worst, where do you rate your pain? When did you first notice your pain?

   b. How is your health in general? Have you been hospitalized for any major illness or injury? Are you having any other signs or symptoms today (difficulty breathing, nausea, vomiting, dizziness, or palpitations)? Do you have any allergies? What medicines do you take? Have you taken anything today? What significant medical history do you have (heart disease, lung disease, high blood pressure, diabetes)? When did you last eat? Was it anything unusual? What were you doing when you first noticed this pain?

   c. Do you smoke? Do you use alcohol or any other drugs?

   d. Are your parents living? Do (Did) they have any heart disease or other major medical problems?
   (Objective 3)

2. Chest pain
   (Objective 2)

3. S—Does the patient have any associated signs or symptoms that may suggest a cardiac or other medical reason for the fall?

   A—Allergies or allergic reactions are unlikely to explain a fall unless the patient becomes hypotensive because of anaphylaxis, loses consciousness, and then falls.

   M—Some daily medicines can cause hypotension (especially orthostatic hypotension) that could lead to a fall. Other sedative, hypnotic, and psychotropic drugs may impair judgment or level of consciousness and predispose a person to a fall. Medications also can suggest preexisting medical conditions such as diabetes, heart disease, or neurological illness that may cause a fall.

   P—Pertinent past medical history may include factors such as heart disease (dysrhythmias), neurological disease (stroke with neurological deficit), diabetes (hypoglycemia), recent surgery, and other conditions that could alter balance, judgment, or consciousness and cause a fall.

   L—If the last meal was not timed correctly and the patient is diabetic or hypoglycemic, a fall could result.

   E—Did the patient have chest pain, visual disturbances, dizziness, palpitations, or any medical reason that could have caused the fall?
   (Objective 3)

4. You should ask about the following:

   a. Immunizations

   b. Tobacco use, alcohol use, screening tests (for tuberculosis), immunizations, home situation, exposure to contagious diseases, travel to other countries

   c. Alcohol or other drugs, use of safety measures (restraint devices)

   d. Diet, exercise, sexual history (possibly physical abuse)

   e. Alcohol and other drugs

   f. Alcohol and other drug use, sleep patterns, home situation, significant other (abuse or violence), sexual history, daily life, patient outlook, and economic condition

   g. Alcohol, drugs, and related substances, exercise and leisure activities

   h. Tobacco use, alcohol, other drugs and related substances, diet, home situation and significant other, physical abuse or violence, daily life, housing, and economic condition

   i. Tobacco use, alcohol, other drugs and related substances, sleep patterns, diet and exercise, and leisure activities
   (Objective 3)

5. a. Remain attentive and listen. Reflect on some of the emotions you sense the patient may be experiencing.

   b. Let the patient talk for a few minutes. Summarize his comments.

   c. Summarize the comments, and ask the patient to select the most pressing ones on which to focus in your examination.

d. Remain calm and caring, and reassure the patient.

e. Reassure the patient that you are listening to her fears, that you are there to care for her, and that you understand her condition.

f. Remain calm and set limits about ways he can express his feelings in an appropriate manner. Be alert for signs of escalation so you can maintain the safety of the patient, yourself, and your crew.

g. Be clear that you are in a caring role and you feel the behavior is unacceptable. If it persists, consider trading roles with your partner if appropriate.

h. Determine whether a family member can translate, or use a translating resource if available.

(Objective 4)

6. c. The history can provide structure and guidance during the physical examination, where you hope to find signs of the illness or injury.
(Objective 1)

7. a. Vital signs are part of the physical assessment.
(Objective 2)

8. b. The patient often states the chief complaint but may not be able to do so if he or she is unconscious. Obtain the medical history after the chief complaint. It may change during the call if the patient's condition changes.
(Objective 3)

9. d. "Did the difficulty start today?" is not an open-ended question. A better way to ask about time of onset is, "Tell me when you noticed that you were having trouble breathing." Answer b. also is not an open-ended question. Asking about location is inappropriate with this chief complaint.
(Objective 3)

10. d. Lung function and laboratory values can be affected by smoking and are important information for this patient.
(Objective 3)

11. b. Allergy to other nonsteroidal antiinflammatory drugs also is a contraindication.
(Objective 3)

12. c. Lack of food intake could lead to hypoglycemia and dizziness.
(Objective 3)

13. d. Tuberculosis may be found in family members because of transmission by close contact.
(Objective 3)

14. d. Offering false reassurances does not benefit the patient.
(Objective 3)

15. b. Establish limits for acceptable behavior.
(Objective 4)

16. a. Use phrases and words that can be understood easily.
(Objective 4)

WRAP IT UP

1. a. Signs and symptoms of present illness, family history of myocardial infarction at early age, diabetes

b. Signs and symptoms do not suggest stroke; however, diabetic and family history are strong for vascular disease.

c. Signs and symptoms vaguely suggest an abdominal condition that may require emergency surgery but may be masked by patient's diabetic history.

d. Ectopic pregnancy is a possible: irregular periods, high-risk birth control method, abdominal pain with radiation to shoulder.

e. Abdominal aneurysm is a possibility based on family history, race (but male sex would be higher risk), weak pulses, diabetes.

f. Urinary tract infection is a high risk in diabetic patients, but you have no report of urinary frequency. Dysuria could be masked by diabetes.

g. Gastroenteritis: mild abdominal symptoms, nausea but no vomiting, no diarrhea reported
(Objective 1)

h. Hypoglycemia: the patient's blood glucose is within the normal range. She does not appear to have other signs or symptoms of hypoglycemia (except tachycardia)

2. a. If myocardial infarction was suspected and aspirin was given without knowledge of the patient's allergy to it, a severe allergic reaction could occur.

b. If a menstrual history was not obtained, the possibility of pregnancy and ectopic pregnancy might not be considered. Patient could have received radiographs and medications harmful to early fetal development, or the possibility of life-threatening ectopic pregnancy might not be considered.

c. The family history is strongly suggestive of two lethal vascular diseases: myocardial infarction and aortic aneurysm. Without the knowledge of this, certain diagnostic tests could be overlooked and the diagnosis missed.
(Objective 1)

3. The patient may be reluctant to call because of fear or denial of illness.
(Objective 4)

4. Tell her your concerns based on her symptoms, history, and physical findings, and explain that further diagnostic tests only available at the hospital will be needed to pinpoint the specific nature of her problem.
(Objective 3)

CHAPTER 1

Techniques of Physical Examination

READING ASSIGNMENT
Chapter 11, pages 234-279, in *Mosby's Paramedic Textbook,* ed. 3

OBJECTIVES
Upon completion of this chapter, the paramedic student will be able to:
1. Describe physical examination techniques commonly used in the prehospital setting.
2. Describe the examination equipment commonly used in the prehospital setting.
3. Describe the general approach to physical examination.
4. Outline the steps of a comprehensive physical examination.
5. Detail the components of the mental status examination.
6. Distinguish between normal and abnormal findings in the mental status examination.
7. Outline the steps in the general patient survey.
8. Distinguish between normal and abnormal findings in the general patient survey.
9. Describe physical examination techniques used for assessment of specific body regions.
10. Distinguish between normal and abnormal findings when assessing specific body regions.
11. State modifications to the physical examination that are necessary when assessing children.
12. State modifications to the physical examination that are necessary when assessing the older adult.

SUMMARY
- The examination techniques commonly used in the physical examination are inspection, palpation, percussion, and auscultation.
- Equipment used during the comprehensive physical examination includes the stethoscope, ophthalmoscope, otoscope, and blood pressure cuff.
- The physical examination is performed in a systematic manner. The exam is a step-by-step process. Emphasis is placed on the patient's present illness and chief complaint.
- The physical examination is a systematic assessment of the body that includes mental status, general survey, vital signs, skin, head, eyes, ears, nose, throat, chest, abdomen, posterior body, extremities, and neurological examination.
- The first step in any patient care encounter is to note the patient's appearance and behavior. This includes assessing for level of consciousness. This may include assessment of posture, gait, and motor activity; dress, grooming, hygiene, and breath or body odors; facial expression; mood, affect, and relation to person and things; speech and language; thought and perceptions; and memory and attention.

- During the general survey, the paramedic should evaluate the patient for signs of distress, apparent state of health, skin color and obvious lesions, height and build, sexual development, and weight. The paramedic also should assess vital signs.
- The comprehensive physical examination should include an evaluation of the texture and turgor of the skin, hair, and fingernails and toenails.
- Examination of the structures of the head and neck involves inspection, palpation, and auscultation.
- A full knowledge of the structure of the thoracic cage is needed. This knowledge aids in performing a good respiratory and cardiac assessment. Air movement creates turbulence as it passes through the respiratory tree. Aire movement produces breath sounds during inhalation and exhalation. In the prehospital setting the paramedic must examine the heart indirectly. However, the paramedic can obtain details about the size and effectiveness of pumping action through a skilled assessment that includes palpation and auscultation.
- The four quadrants of the abdomen and their contents provide the basis for inspection, auscultation, percussion, and palpation of this body region.
- An examination of the genitalia of either sex can be awkward for the patient and the paramedic. The paramedic should inspect the genitalia for bleeding and signs of trauma (if indicated).
- Examination of the anus is indicated in the presence of rectal bleeding or trauma to the area.
- When examining the upper and lower extremities, the paramedic should direct his or her attention to function. The paramedic also should pay attention to structure.
- Assessment of the spine begins with a visual assessment of the cervical, thoracic, and lumbar curves. The assessment continues with a region-by-region examination for pain, swelling, and range of motion.
- A neurological examination may be organized into five categories: mental status and speech, cranial nerves, motor system, sensory system, and reflexes.
- When approaching the pediatric patient, the paramedic should remain calm and confident. The paramedic should observe the child before beginning the physical examination. The paramedic also should make sure to avoid separation of the child and parent. Moreover, the paramedic must establish a rapport with parents and child and must be honest. One caregiver should be assigned to the child.
- The paramedic should not assume that all older adults are victims of disorders related to aging. Individual differences in knowledge, mental reasoning, experience, and personality influence how these patients respond to examination.

REVIEW QUESTIONS

Match the sign in column II with its definition in column I. Use each answer only once.

Column I

1. _____ Persistent respiratory rate less than 12 breaths/min

2. _____ Normal breath sounds heard over most lung fields

3. _____ Low-pitched, rumbling expiratory sounds
4. _____ Crowing sound associated with upper airway narrowing
5. _____ Crescendo-decrescendo sequence of respirations followed by apnea
6. _____ Irregular respirations interrupted by apneic periods
7. _____ End-inspiratory sounds associated with fluid in the small airways
8. _____ High-pitched airway noise resulting from lower airway narrowing

Column II

a. Biot
b. Bradypnea
c. Cheyne-Stokes
d. Crackles
e. Rhonchi
f. Stridor
g. Vesicular
h. Wheezes

Match the term in column II with the appropriate statement in column I. Use each answer only once.

Column I

9. _____ The child with Down syndrome had a slanted opening between the upper and lower eyelids.
10. _____ The patient said the aliens were controlling him.
11. _____ Third-degree burns affect the skin's resiliency.
12. _____ Malnutrition had caused the man to be very thin.
13. _____ The older patient staggered when he tried to walk.
14. _____ The paralyzed patient had a persistent erection.
15. _____ A semicircle of blood is seen over the iris.
16. _____ The patient's cirrhosis made him look pregnant.
17. _____ After her stroke the woman had trouble making the muscles of her mouth form words.
18. _____ The alcoholic's wife told you that the history he gave you was untrue.

Column II

a. Affect
b. Ascites
c. Ataxia
d. Confabulation
e. Delusions
f. Dysarthria
g. Emaciated
h. Hyphema
i. Hypopyon
j. Macula
k. Palpebral fissures
l. Priapism
m. Turgor

19. Describe the correct method of performing each of the following patient assessment techniques:

   a. Inspection:

   _____

   b. Palpation:

   _____

   c. Auscultation:

   _____

20. For each of the following deviations from normal pupil response, list a cause:

   Abnormality   **Cause**
   a. Dilated/unresponsive
   b. Constricted/unresponsive
   c. Unequal/one dilated and unresponsive
   d. Dull/lackluster

21. Your patient is a teenage assault victim who was struck repeatedly on the head with a baseball bat.

   a. List the 10 steps in the comprehensive physical examination.
      (1)
      (2)
      (3)
      (4)
      (5)
      (6)
      (7)
      (8)
      (9)
      (10)

b. List the components of the mental status examination for this patient.

_____

_____

_____

c. Describe your physical examination of this patient's head and neck, detailing specific examination techniques and the types of normal or abnormal findings you would look for (include ophthalmoscopic and otoscopic examination techniques).

_____

_____

_____

22. You are called to evaluate a patient whose chief complaint is difficulty breathing. Explain your assessment of the thorax.

_____

_____

23. Your 56-year-old patient has a history of right upper quadrant abdominal pain, malaise, nausea, and vomiting. He is jaundiced and complains of itching. Past history reveals heavy alcohol use. You suspect hepatitis. Describe your physical examination of this patient's abdomen.

_____

_____

24. You are examining a patient involved in a motor vehicle collision whose automobile was struck on the side. The patient complains of considerable pain in the pelvic area. The primary survey has been completed. The patient's pulse is elevated, but blood pressure is within normal limits. Describe your examination of this patient's pelvic area.

_____

_____

25. Your crew arrives at the home of an older patient whose family states that she complained of weakness on one side, stumbled, and fell down five steps. No life-threatening conditions are found in the primary survey, and vital sign assessment reveals a moderately elevated blood pressure and pulse. The patient is slightly confused but cooperative. You suspect a stroke. Describe your assessment of this patient's extremities.

_____

_____

26. A painter has fallen approximately 20 feet, striking a scaffold rail with his lower back. Primary survey and vital signs are normal. Outline your physical examination of this patient's back.

_____

_____

27. Provide the information that is missing in the following table, which outlines examination techniques for cranial nerves.

Cranial Nerve Number	Cranial Nerve Name	Assessment Technique
I		Test smell with ammonia inhalants
II		
	Optic	
III	Oculomotor	Test extraocular movements (EOMs) by asking the patient to look up and to the left and right, and diagonally up and down to down, the left and right
IV VI	Trochlear	
V		
	Facial	Note facial symmetry, tics, or abnormal movement; have patient raise eyebrows, frown, show upper and lower teeth, smile, and puff out cheeks; have patient close eyes tightly and resist while you try to open lids
VIII		
IX X		
	Spinal accessory	
XII		

28. List four general guidelines that are helpful when approaching a pediatric patient.

   a.

   b.

   c.

   d.

29. Describe two specific developmental differences that influence patient assessment for the children in each of the following age groups:

   a. Birth to 6 months:

_____

   b. 7 months to 3 years:

_____

   c. 4 to 10 years:

_____

d. Adolescence:

---

30. Describe two special considerations and techniques that may be useful when caring for an older patient.

STUDENT SELF-ASSESSMENT

31. Auscultation is the examination technique that involves which of the following?
    a. Listening with a stethoscope
    b. Feeling for masses and assessing for crepitus
    c. Looking for signs of illness
    d. Tapping the body with your finger

32. Which instrument is used to evaluate the retina, macula, and optic nerve disc?
    a. Ophthalmoscope   **c.** Penlight
    b. Otoscope   **d.** Sphygmomanometer

33. Using an adult blood pressure cuff to evaluate a child's blood pressure can result in which of the following?
    a. False low reading   **c.** Normal reading
    b. False high reading   **d.** Inability to inflate cuff

34. What is the most important information to guide your physical examination of the patient?
    a. Medications and specific doses
    b. Past medical history
    c. Present illness and chief complaint
    d. Vital signs, including blood pressure

35. Which of the following is a component of the comprehensive physical examination?
    a. Chief complaint   **c.** Vascular access
    b. History of present illness **d.** Vital signs

36. Which of the following is a component of the mental status examination?
    a. Distal pulses   **c.** Speech and language
    b. Pupil reaction   **d.** Visual acuity

37. Which of the following is the clearest way to report an altered level of consciousness?
    a. The patient is obtunded.
    b. The patient is semiconscious.
    c. The patient is stuporous.
    d. The patient is unresponsive to pain.

38. Patient memory and attention can be assessed with which of the following?
    a. AVPU method   **c.** General survey
    b. Digit span   **d.** Glasgow coma scale

39. Your patient walks with a limp. What is this known as?
    a. An abnormal gait   **c.** Bizarre posture
    b. Ataxia   **d.** Cranial nerve palsy

40. An odor of acetone on the breath is associated with which condition?
    a. Alcohol use   **c.** Diabetic conditions
    b. Bowel obstruction **d.** Poor dental hygiene

41. A patient who tells you that he is very depressed and suicidal but has an expressionless face may be said to have which condition?
    a. Altered affect   **c.** Altered attention
    b. Altered appearance **d.** Altered emotion

42. Which sign of distress may be found in a patient who has cardiorespiratory insufficiency, pain, or anxiety?
   a. Bradycardia
   b. Cough
   c. Sweating
   d. Wincing

43. Skin color is best assessed by observing the skin on what part of the body?
   a. Arms
   b. Face
   c. Legs
   d. Nail beds

44. When you are taking an axillary temperature using a standard mercury thermometer, what is the minimum time the thermometer should be in place to obtain an accurate temperature?
   a. 4 minutes
   b. 5 minutes
   c. 8 minutes
   d. 10 minutes

45. What is the proper sequence for examination of the abdomen?
   a. Auscultation, inspection, palpation
   b. Inspection, palpation, auscultation
   c. Inspection, auscultation, palpation
   d. Auscultation, palpation, inspection

46. Which of the following findings during examination of the nails is consistent with chronic respiratory or cardiac disease?
   a. Beau lines
   b. Clubbing
   c. Paronychia
   d. Terry nails

47. What should you do to verify that vision is present?
   a. Assess bilateral pupil response to light.
   b. Ask the patient to count fingers at a distance.
   c. Lightly touch the cornea with a cotton swab.
   d. Palpate the globe for firmness.

48. To perform an effective otoscopic examination of the ear, you should pull the ear in what direction?
   a. Down and back in adults
   b. Down and forward in adults
   c. Down and back in infants
   d. Down and forward in infants

49. What physical finding may be encountered in patients who are pregnant, have leukemia, or are taking phenytoin?
   a. Enlarged gums
   b. Nasal bleeding
   c. Swollen eyelids
   d. Tonsillar exudate

50. Chest wall diameter may be increased in patients with what condition?
   a. Heart disease
   b. Implanted cardiac pacemaker
   c. Obstructive pulmonary disease
   d. Rib fractures

51. Which sound may be heard during percussion if hyperinflation due to pulmonary disease, pneumothorax, or asthma is present?
   a. Dullness
   b. Flatness
   c. Resonance
   d. Hyperresonance

52. Which of the following is true regarding assessment of breath sounds?
   a. Normal breath sounds are louder on exhalation.
   b. The stethoscope bell is used to auscultate the lungs.
   c. The patient's mouth should be open.
   d. The patient should be in the supine position.

53. For maximal effectiveness, where should heart sounds be auscultated?
   a. Over the left anterior axillary line
   b. Over the left fifth intercostal space
   c. Over the sternal angle
   d. Over the xiphoid process

54. Simultaneous palpation of the apical and carotid pulses in which each apical beat is not transmitted is known as which of the following?
   a. Mean arterial pressure
   b. Pulse deficit
   c. Pulsus paradoxus
   d. Pulse pressure

55. All of the following may cause muffled heart sounds except which one?
   a. Cardiac tamponade
   b. Obesity
   c. Obstructive lung disease
   d. Myocardial infarction

56. What is a palpable tremor over a blood vessel called?
   a. Bruit
   b. Murmur
   c. Thrill
   d. Vibration

57. During the vascular examination, the anterior surface of the foot should be palpated to detect which pulse?
   a. Brachial pulse
   b. Dorsalis pedis pulse
   c. Popliteal pulse
   d. Posterior tibial pulse

58. If a deformity and point tenderness are noted on examination of the pelvis, what condition should you consider?
   a. Appendicitis
   b. Internal hemorrhage
   c. Ruptured ectopic pregnancy
   d. Spinal cord injury

59. To evaluate motor function in the lower extremities, you should instruct the patient to do what?
   a. Flex and extend the feet and lower and upper legs
   b. Lift and hold both legs in the air while lying supine
   c. Move the legs laterally as far as possible bilaterally
   d. Push the soles of the feet against the paramedic's palms

60. Which of the following is an example of a test to evaluate gait?
   a. Have the patient hop in place.
   b. Have the patient do the Romberg test.
   c. Have the patient touch each heel to the opposite shin.
   d. Have the patient touch the finger to the nose, alternating hands.

61. Your patient is a 2-year-old in respiratory distress. Level of consciousness, spontaneous movement, respiratory effort, and skin color can be most effectively evaluated when the child is in which position?
   a. Held by the paramedic
   b. Held by the parent
   c. On the stretcher
   d. Sitting in a chair

62. A young child has an obviously fractured lower leg. Which of the following statements is *false* regarding the care of this patient?
   a. Remain calm and confident.
   b. Separate the parents from the child.
   c. Establish rapport with the parents.
   d. Be honest with the child and parents.

63. Which of the following statements is *true* regarding the physical examination of a 2-year-old child?
   a. Abdominal breathing is normal in this age group.
   b. Patient modesty should be a primary concern.
   c. Explanations should be given for each activity.
   d. Separation anxiety will not be a problem.

64. When examining an older patient, what should you do?
   a. Always speak loudly, because most of these patients are deaf.
   b. Assume that memory impairment is present.
   c. Anticipate numerous health problems and medications.
   d. Not expect any variation in the examination.

WRAP IT UP

You are called to a small home for a "person fallen." You arrive on the scene and find an elderly man who has fallen and is lying naked, trapped between the toilet and the bathtub. He is awake but confused. He has cool skin and some injuries to his head and shoulders from trying to wriggle out of his confined space. His family tells you they couldn't get him on the phone for 24 hours so they came by this morning to see what was wrong. You find that he is wedged tightly and you are unable to free him, and a rescue unit is dispatched. They bring hand tools and carefully remove the commode without breaking it to avoid making sharp shards of porcelain that may injure your patient. You extricate him onto the back board after applying a cervical collar and move him to the ambulance. During the rescue your partner checks around the house, looking for medications, signs of drug or alcohol use, or anything unusual, but finds nothing.

The patient's vital signs are: BP 100/60, P 112 irregular, R 20. Oxygen saturation is not detected because of the coolness of the man's extremities, so you administer oxygen by nonrebreather mask at 12 L/min. Your thermometer reads a temp of 97.6° F (36.4° C). The patient's pupils are 4 mm, equal, round, and react to light. Inspection of his head reveals abraded areas where you suspect he was moving his head to free himself. You palpate no deformities or crepitus of the head or face. He follows commands and can move his eyes in the cardinal fields of gaze. There is no tenderness, swelling, or deformity around the nose or frontal or maxillary sinuses. His lips are pale and cracked, as is his tongue. The trachea is midline, neck veins are flat, and the patient denies pain to the posterior aspect of his neck. However, you do not ask him to move it because of your concern about spinal trauma. Inspection of the chest reveals some redness to the left posterior and lateral aspect in a linear fashion. There is considerable tenderness when those areas are palpated. Respiration excursion seems slightly shallow; breath sounds are clear but diminished in all fields. Heart sounds are auscultated with the patient supine, and a normal S1 and S2 are audible. Percussion of the abdomen reveals tympany and dullness in the appropriate locations. The patient winces when his abdomen is palpated but does not seem to be able to localize the pain. His liver and spleen are not palpable. His penis is flaccid, and there is no blood at the urinary meatus. His left shoulder has an abraded area that is tender, but no deformity or crepitus is noted. His hands, wrists, and arms appear to have normal range of motion, but the joints seem somewhat enlarged. Examination of the lower extremities is normal. Palpation of the spine is negative. The patient remains confused and unable to tell you what happened but is cooperative. You ask him to smile, and it exaggerates the facial droop that you noticed earlier in your exam. You also detect some slurring of his speech. Evaluation of muscle strength demonstrates some weakness in his right arm and leg. You initiate an IV TKO, determine that his blood glucose is 110 mg/dL, and monitor his vital signs en route to the hospital. He is later diagnosed with a stroke; however because of his fall and the unknown time of onset, he is not a candidate for fibrinolytic therapy. At the time of follow-up, he is in rehabilitation.

1. Why was it difficult to focus your physical exam on any one area on this patient?

_____

2. Why was a temperature assessment indicated in this patient, even though he was found in the house?

_____

3. How can you tell whether this patient's confusion is new or normal for him?

_____

4. Put a ✔ by each area of the cranial nerve examination where an abnormality was detected and fill in the name of the nerve(s) listed.

Cranial Nerve Number	Cranial Nerve Name(s)
_____Cranial nerve I	
_____Cranial nerve II	
_____Cranial nerves II and III	
_____Cranial nerves III, IV, and VI	
_____Cranial nerve V	
_____Cranial nerve VII	
_____Cranial nerve VIII	
_____Cranial nerves IX and X	
_____Cranial nerve XI	
_____Cranial nerve XII	

5. Why were the liver and spleen not palpable?

_____

CHAPTER 11 ANSWERS

REVIEW QUESTIONS

1. b
2. g
3. e
4. f
5. c
6. a
7. d
8. h
9. k
10. e
11. m
12. g
13. c
14. l
15. h
16. b
17. f
18. d
(Questions 1-18: Objective 10)

19. a. Observe the environment (scene), general patient appearance, and specific body regions to gather data. b. Use the palmar surface of the hands and fingers to feel for texture, mass, fluid, temperature, and crepitus in various body regions. c. Use a stethoscope or the unaided ear to assess sounds generated by the movement of air or gases within the body.
(Objective 1)

20.

Abnormality	Cause
a. Dilated/unresponsive	Cardiac arrest, hypoxia, drug use or misuse
b. Constricted/ unresponsive	Injury or disease of the central nervous system, narcotic drug use, use of eye medications
c. Unequal/one dilated	Cerebrovascular accident, direct trauma to the eye, use of eye medications, use of an ocular prosthesis
d. Dull/lackluster	Shock or comatose states

(Objective 6)

21. a. (1) Mental status; (2) general survey; (3) vital signs; (4) skin; (5) head, eyes, ears, nose, and throat (HEENT); (6) chest; (7) abdomen; (8) posterior body; (9) extremities; (10) neurological examination.
(Objective 7)

b. Assess whether the patient is alert and responsive to touch and verbal and painful stimuli. Assess the patient's general appearance and behavior. Note verbal and motor responses. If the patient is ambulatory when you arrive, note posture, gait, and motor activity. Observe dress and hygiene and note any body odors, such as alcohol. Note facial expression and determine whether it is appropriate for the situation. Is the patient's affect appropriate for the situation? Is the speech understandable and moderately paced? Assess the quality, rate, loudness, and fluency of the patient's speech. Determine whether the patient has organized thoughts. Determine whether the patient is oriented to person, place, and time. Assess remote and recent memory.
(Objective 5)

c. Inspect for shape and symmetry of the skull and facial bones. Note bleeding, trauma, deformity, or drainage around the face or from the ears or nose. Inspect the mouth for bleeding and loose or missing teeth. Observe for pupil response to light and assess to see whether the patient's vision is intact. Examine the conjunctiva and sclera by asking the patient to look up while both lower lids are depressed with the thumbs. Palpate the lower orbital rims to determine structural integrity. Use the ophthalmoscope to check the cornea for lacerations, abrasions, or foreign bodies; to check for hyphema in the anterior chamber; to assess the fundus; to see retinal vessels, the optic nerve, and retina; and to assess the vitreous. Palpate the scalp and face for deformities, swelling, indentations, or bleeding, noting pain or tenderness. Inspect the external ear for signs of bruising, deformity, or discoloration. Look for bleeding in the ear canal. Palpate the bones around the ear to see whether the patient feels discomfort. Look for discoloration on the mastoid process. Assess gross auditory acuity by covering one ear at a time and asking the patient to repeat short test words spoken in soft and loud tones. Pull the auricle up and back to perform the otoscopic examination and look at the eardrum. Before applying the cervical collar but while still maintaining cervical immobilization, inspect to ensure that the trachea is midline and note tracheal tugging or obvious symptoms of trauma. Palpate the anterior and posterior neck, noting pain, deformity, malalignment, or subcutaneous emphysema.
(Objective 9)

22. Inspect for chest shape, symmetry, expansion, and the use of accessory muscles. Note the rate, depth, and pattern of respirations. Palpate for tenderness, bulges, depressions, unusual movement, crepitus, and chest expansion. Place both thumbs on the xiphoid process with palms lying flat on the chest wall and palpate for symmetry. Assess the posterior chest wall by placing the thumbs along the spinous processes at the level of the tenth rib. Percuss the chest to detect resonance (normal), hyperresonance (hyperinflation), or dullness or flatness (fluid or pulmonary congestion). Auscultate bilaterally (anterior and posterior) with the patient upright if possible and ask the patient to breathe in and out slowly through the open mouth, noting diminished or adventitious sounds. Palpate the apical impulse. Auscultate the heart at the fifth intercostal space to note frequency, intensity, duration, and timing as well as abnormal sounds such as murmurs.
(Objective 9)

23. Inspect for symmetry, jaundice, or distention and look for surgical scars. Look for smooth movement of the abdomen during respiration. Auscultate all four quadrants for rumblings. Palpate for tenderness, masses, skin temperature, and rigidity and observe for guarding. Percuss all four quadrants of the abdomen to assess for tympany (normal over stomach and intestines) and dullness (over organs and solid masses). Percuss the liver by beginning just above the umbilicus in the right midclavicular line in an area of tympany. Continue in an upward direction until the change from tympany to dullness occurs (usually slightly below the costal margin, which indicates the upper border of the liver). During palpation of the liver the patient should be supine and relaxed. Stand on the patient's right side and place the left hand under the patient in the area of the eleventh and twelfth ribs. Place your right hand on the abdomen, with the fingers pointing toward the patient's head, resting just below the edge of the costal margin. As the patient exhales, press the hand under the patient upward while pushing your right hand gently in and up. If you can feel the liver, it should be firm and nontender. (A healthy adult liver usually cannot be palpated.)
(Objective 9)

24. Inspect for obvious trauma, deformity, symmetry, or bleeding, especially from the urethra. Place the hands on each anterior iliac crest and press down and out, noting movement or crepitus. Place the heel of the hand on the symphysis pubis and press down to determine stability. Palpate the femoral pulses.
(Objective 9)

25. For each extremity, inspect for position, deformity, and obvious signs of trauma, and compare the right extremity with the left. Palpate for structural integrity. Assess grips; have the patient push and pull the paramedic's hands against force, and have the patient push the feet against the opposing force of the paramedic's hands bilaterally to note muscle strength and tone. Assess distal pulse and sensation in all extremities.
(Objective 9)

26. Log roll patient with cervical immobilization. Inspect the neck for midline position. Inspect the back for signs of injury, swelling, discoloration, and open wounds. Palpate the spine, beginning at the neck and proceeding to the sacrum, noting point tenderness or deformity. Place the palm of your hand over the costovertebral angle and strike the hand with your fist, noting any painful reaction.
(Objective 9)

27.

Cranial Nerve Number(s)	Cranial Nerve Name(s)	Assessment Technique
I	Olfactory	Test smell with ammonia inhalants
II	Optic	Test for visual acuity
II	Optic	Inspect the size and shape of the pupils; assess the pupil's response to light
III	Oculomotor	Test EOMs by asking patient to look up and down, to the left and right, and diagonally up and down to the left and right
IV	Trochlear	
VI	Abducens	
V	Trigeminal	Ask patient to clench the teeth while you palpate the temporal and masseter muscles; touch the forehead, cheeks, and jaw to determine sensation
VII	Facial	Note facial symmetry, tics, or abnormal movement; have patient raise eyebrows, frown, show upper and lower teeth, smile, and puff out cheeks; have patient close eyes tightly and resist while you try to open lids
VIII	Acoustic	Assess hearing acuity
IX	Glossopharyngeal	See whether patient can swallow easily and produce saliva and normal voice sounds; ask patient to hold breath and then assess for slowing of the heart rate; test for gag reflex
X	Vagus	
XI	Spinal accessory	Ask patient to raise and lower shoulders and turn the head
XII	Hypoglossal	Ask patient to stick out the tongue and move it in several directions

28. Remain calm and confident; do not separate the parents and child unless absolutely necessary; establish rapport with the parents and child; be honest with the child and parents; if possible, assign one caregiver to stay with the child; observe the patient before the physical examination.
(Objective 11)

29. a. The child is not frightened, the child needs care to maintain body temperature, the child is in constant motion, the child is an abdominal breather, and the paramedic can use the fontanelles to assess overhydration and underhydration. b. Separation anxiety occurs, the child has a fear of strangers, and the paramedic should explain procedures in short sentences. c. The child has a capacity for rational thought, the child can provide a limited history, the paramedic should allow participation in care, the child has a limited understanding of the body, the child fears intrusion into private areas, and the paramedic must explain everything completely. d. The

teenager is concerned about body image and privacy is a major concern, the paramedic should treat the teenager like an adult, and the paramedic must consider sexually transmitted diseases, pregnancy, and drug and alcohol use.
(Objective 11)

30. The patient may have sensory loss that impairs communication, may experience memory loss and confusion, often has numerous health problems that require him or her to take a number of home medications, may have decreased sensory function that can conceal symptoms, and may have fears regarding hospitalization.
(Objective 12)

STUDENT SELF-ASSESSMENT

31. a. Inspection involves looking, palpating involves feeling the body, and selected body areas are tapped during percussion.
(Objective 1)

32. a. The otoscope is used for examining the ears, the penlight can be used to evaluate pupil response, and the sphygmomanometer is used to measure blood pressure.
(Objective 2)

33. a. Blood pressure cuffs that are too wide give a false low reading, and those that are too narrow give a false high reading.
(Objective 2)

34. c. Although all the other information is important, the chief complaint and history of the present illness guide the physical examination and allow the paramedic to focus on key areas.
(Objective 3)

35. d. Chief complaint and history of present illness are historical findings. Vascular access is an intervention.
(Objective 4)

36. c
(Objective 5)

37. d. The other terms are vague and may be interpreted in a variety of ways.
(Objective 3)

38. b. Ask the patient to count from 1 to 10 using only odd numbers. Asking the patient to count by serial sevens or spell a word backward also can be used.
(Objective 5)

39. a. *Ataxia* is a staggering gait, and postural imbalance is associated with central nervous system lesions. Cranial nerve palsy does not cause a limp.
(Objective 6)

40. c. Diabetic ketoacidosis is associated with an odor of acetone on the breath.
(Objective 6)

41. a
(Objective 6)

42. c. Tachycardia, not bradycardia, is a common trait for all three. Cough is not present with pain or anxiety. Wincing is not associated with cardiorespiratory insufficiency.
(Objective 8)

43. d. This area has less pigmentation, and pallor or cyanosis is easier to see.
(Objective 7)

44. b. Oral thermometers should be left in place for 5 to 7 minutes and rectal thermometers for 5 minutes.
(Objective 7)

45. c. Palpation of the abdomen may create sounds that falsely indicate normal bowel function when none exists.
(Objective 10)

46. b. *Beau lines* are transverse depressions in the nail that inhibit growth and are associated with systemic illness, severe infection, and nail injury. *Paronychia* is an inflammation of the skin at the base of the nail that may result from local infection or trauma. *Terry nails* are transverse white bands that cover the nail except for a narrow zone at the distal tip and are associated with cirrhosis.
(Objective 10)

47. b. Pupil response and corneal touch test the cranial nerves. Palpation of the globe is used to assess for dehydration.
(Objective 9)

48. c. For the adult examination, the auricle should be pulled gently up and back.
(Objective 9)

49. a. This also may be noted if the patient is going through puberty.
(Objective 9)

50. c. This barrel-shaped appearance develops because of air trapping.
(Objective 10)

51. d. Dullness or flatness is heard when fluid is present or pulmonary congestion has occurred. Resonance is usually heard over normal lungs.
(Objective 10)

52. c. Normal breath sounds are louder on inspiration. The diaphragm is used to auscultate the lungs. Ideally, the patient should be sitting if the condition permits.
(Objective 9)

53. b. Ideally, the patient should be sitting up and leaning slightly forward or should be in the left lateral recumbent position.
(Objective 9)

54. b. *Mean arterial pressure* is the diastolic pressure plus one third of the pulse pressure. *Pulsus paradoxus* is a fluctuation in the systolic blood pressure with respiration. *Pulse pressure* is the systolic blood pressure minus the diastolic blood pressure.
(Objective 10)

55. d
(Objective 10)

56. c. *Murmurs* are prolonged extra sounds auscultated with a stethoscope. A *bruit* is an abnormal sound audible over the carotid artery or an organ or gland. A thrill may feel like a tremor or vibration.
(Objective 9)

57. b. The brachial pulse is on the arm, the popliteal pulse is behind the knee, and the posterior tibial pulse is on the medial aspect of the ankle, behind the tibia.
(Objective 9)

58. b. Pelvic fractures are often accompanied by substantial hemorrhage.
(Objective 10)

59. d
(Objective 9)

60. a. Point-to-point movements are evaluated using the heel to shin and finger to nose tests. Stance and balance are tested with the Romberg test.
(Objective 9)

61. b. Anxiety is usually minimized while the child is in the parent's arms. This can minimize respiratory effort and distress and allow for a more effective assessment.
(Objective 11)

62. b. Anxiety can usually be decreased and cooperation increased if the parent and child remain together.
(Objective 11)

63. c
(Objective 11)

64. c. These numerous illnesses can confuse the clinical picture and complicate the paramedic's examination of the patient.
(Objective 12)

WRAP IT UP

1. No history was available, therefore it was unclear whether this was a medical, trauma, or combination call and where the exam should be focused.
(Objective 3)

2. Patients can become hypothermic or hyperthermic in their residence, especially with injury or severe illness.
(Objective 3)

3. Ask relatives and neighbors or call the office of the man's physician if you can find a name on a prescription bottle.
(Objective 3)

4. CN I—not tested—olfactory
CN II, III—normal—optic and oculomotor
CN III, IV, VI—normal—oculomotor, trochlear, abducens
CN V—not tested—trigeminal
CN VII—abnormal (facial droop)—facial
CN VIII—not tested—acoustic
CN IX, X—not tested—glossopharyngeal and vagus
CN XI—not tested—spinal accessory
CN XII—not tested—hypoglossal
(Objective 10)

5. The liver and spleen should not be palpable in a normal adult.
(Objective 10)

Patient Assessment

READING ASSIGNMENT
Chapter 12, pages 280-289, in *Mosby's Paramedic Textbook,* ed. 3

OBJECTIVES
Upon completion of this chapter, the paramedic student will be able to:
1. Identify the components of the scene size-up.
2. Identify the priorities in each component of patient assessment.
3. Outline the critical steps in initial patient assessment.
4. Describe findings in the initial assessment that may indicate a life-threatening condition.
5. Discuss interventions for life-threatening conditions that are identified in the initial assessment.
6. Identify the components of the focused history and physical examination for medical patients.
7. Identify the components of the focused history and physical examination for trauma patients.
8. List the components of the detailed physical examination.
9. Describe the ongoing assessment.
10. Distinguish priorities in the care of the medical versus trauma patient.

SUMMARY
- Sizing up the scene consists of the initial steps performed on every emergency medical services response. These steps help to ensure scene safety. They also provide valuable information to the paramedic.
- Patient assessment comprises five priorities: initial assessment, resuscitation, focused history and physical examination, detailed physical examination, and ongoing assessment.
- The initial assessment includes the paramedic's general impression of the patient, the assessment for life-threatening conditions, and the identification of priority patients requiring immediate care and transport.
- Assessment of life-threatening conditions entails a systematic evaluation of the patient's level of consciousness, airway, breathing, and circulation.
- The paramedic begins resuscitative measures such as airway maintenance, ventilatory assistance, and cardiopulmonary resuscitation immediately after recognizing the life-threatening condition that necessitates each respective maneuver.
- The focused history and physical examination for medical patients are dictated by the patient's overall condition and level of consciousness.
- The paramedic performs a focused history for a trauma patient to reconstruct the mechanism of injury. The paramedic should perform a rapid trauma examination on all patients with a significant mechanism of injury to identify life-threatening conditions.
- The detailed physical examination should be specific to the patient. The exam also should be specific to the injury. The exam should include an assessment of mental status, a general survey, a head-to-toe examination, and baseline vital signs.
- The ongoing assessment is a repeat of the initial assessment.

REVIEW QUESTIONS

Questions 1 to 15 pertain to the following case study:

> You are dispatched from your base on a cold, snowy winter night to a motor vehicle crash with injuries on the highway.

1. After ensuring safety, list five priorities during your scene size-up/assessment on this call.

    a.

    b.

    c.

    d.

    e.

> You find one patient, the driver of a car involved in a single-car collision. He was not restrained and has been ejected about 15 feet from the car. You find him lying motionless in a safe location.

2. What are three goals of your initial assessment of this patient?

    a.

    b.

    c.

3. What information have you already gathered to form your general impression of this patient?

_____

4. What mnemonic can you use to quickly assess his level of consciousness?

_____

> As you approach the patient, you see some slight movement and note a gurgling sound in his mouth. He responds to pain only.

5. What could be causing gurgling in his airway?

_____

_____

6. What personal protective equipment should you be wearing?

_____

_____

7. What measures will you use to secure this patient's airway?

_____

_____

8. How should you evaluate his breathing?

_____

_____

The patient has a dusky color and slow, agonal respirations.

9. What care should you initiate based on this finding?

_____

_____

_____

10. What assessment techniques will you use in the initial assessment to evaluate circulatory status?

_____

_____

You palpate a rapid carotid pulse but *cannot* detect a radial pulse. His skin is pale and cool, and capillary refill is slow.

11. What criteria for priority patients does this patient meet?

_____

_____

12. List the components of the focused history and physical examination that you will perform on this patient.

_____

_____

You note numerous facial lacerations and crepitus of the facial bones. He has an abrasion on the lateral chest and abdominal area. His left lower arm is deformed, and his left ankle is swollen.

13. What care should you provide before transport for this patient?

_____

14. What should be your goal for scene time on this type of call?

_____

15. Outline the components of the reassessment and the time interval at which they should be performed.

_____

Questions 16 to 20 pertain to the following case study:

You are dispatched to a home for a call of a patient with "difficulty breathing." Your initial scene assessment reveals no hazards, and you enter the patient's bedroom to begin your assessment and care.

16. What information will you gather as you enter the room that will help form your general impression of the patient?

_____

_____

The patient, an elderly black woman, is awake and appears to be in respiratory distress.

17. How will you further assess the following to determine her condition?

a. Airway

_____

b. Breathing

_____

c. Circulation

_____

You note that the patient is speaking in broken sentences because she must stop often to catch her breath. She has wheezes throughout her lungs and intercostal muscle retractions, and her mucous membranes and nail beds are blue. Her pulse is 124 (regular and strong in the radial artery), and her skin is damp.

18. List two criteria that she meets indicating that she is a priority patient who needs stabilization and rapid transport.

a.

b.

19. List four types of information you should gather in the focused history portion of this patient's examination.

a.

b.

c.

d.

20. How might the care of this patient differ from that given to a critically ill trauma patient?

_____

STUDENT SELF-ASSESSMENT

21. You arrive on the scene of a rollover motor vehicle crash involving a small sports car. Which of the following is a component in scene size-up/assessment on this call?
  a. Begin definitive patient care activities.
  b. Contact medical direction with an initial report.
  c. Initiate a mass casualty plan if indicated.
  d. Notify dispatch to send more resources if needed.

22. During which phase of the patient assessment will the first vital signs be assessed?
  a. Detailed physical examination
  b. Focused physical examination
  c. Initial assessment
  d. Ongoing assessment

23. During the initial assessment of a trauma patient, what is the most appropriate method to assess the neurological status?
  a. AVPU
  b. Determination of extraocular muscle function (EOM)
  c. Pupil assessment
  d. Reflex examination

24. Which of the following patient situations represents a life threat identified in the initial assessment of an adult?
  a. Blood pressure in the right arm is much greater than in the left arm.
  b. Heart rate increases by 30 beats/min when the patient stands up.
  c. Stridor is audible.
  d. Temperature is 105.8° F (41° C).

25. You detect that the patient has agonal respirations and a radial pulse during your initial assessment. How should your care and assessment proceed?
   a. Auscultate the chest to determine the proper intervention.
   b. Continue assessment and then manage respiratory failure.
   c. Initiate airway management and ventilation and then proceed.
   d. Treat the respiratory difficulty, and transport with no further examination.

26. What should be the primary determinant of the extent of the focused history and physical examination of the patient?
   a. Patient's overall condition and level of consciousness
   b. Age and preexisting illness
   c. Response time to the closest appropriate hospital
   d. Results of the initial vital sign assessment

27. You respond to a call to aid a person who has fallen 25 feet and is complaining of severe pain in the finger. Which of the following is a component of the focused history and physical examination for this patient?
   a. Continued spinal immobilization
   b. Detailed examination of the finger
   c. Initiation of intravenous fluid therapy
   d. Otoscopic examination of the eyes

28. In which of the following cases is the paramedic most likely to perform a detailed physical examination?
   a. A 2-year-old is acutely dyspneic and cyanotic.
   b. A pale 40-year-old was shot in the chest.
   c. A 59-year-old is weak and diaphoretic.
   d. A 67-year-old patient is in cardiac arrest.

29. What should be included in the ongoing assessment of a patient?
   a. Detailed physical examination
   b. Head-to-toe examination
   c. Repetition of the initial assessment
   d. Vital sign assessment only

30. _____ should *not* be included in the scene management of the critical trauma patient.
   a. Airway control   c. Major fracture stabilization
   b. Intravenous fluid therapy   d. Spinal immobilization

WRAP IT UP

You are dispatched to respond to a snowmobile collision. On arrival you find a 17-year-old boy who struck a boating dock submerged under the powdery snow while traveling at a high rate of speed. You don the appropriate protective gear and cautiously evaluate the ice conditions and then with great difficulty approach the patient through the waist deep snow. He was not wearing a helmet, and you recognize immediately that he has significant head and facial injuries. His eyes are closed, he is not arousable to voice, and his arms and legs extend when you apply painful stimulus. You radio dispatch and request a rescue unit to assist in extricating him across the snowy lake, and for a helicopter because it is clear that he will need transport to the regional trauma center, located 70 miles away. As you await the rescue, you apply a cervical collar and secure the patient to the long spine board. The patient has a gag reflex and adequate respirations, so you begin high-concentration oxygen administration. You can feel a slow, strong radial pulse, and his pupils are 4 mm, are equal, and react to light. You are unable to remove any of his clothing to perform further assessments because of the frigid conditions. You radio the rescue unit on the truck frequency and instruct them to prepare their stokes unit with sled skids and ask them to set up a landing zone on the road for the incoming helicopter. Dispatch updates you that the air unit has a 7-minute ETA, and you ask them to relay your patient's condition, which you continually reevaluate, to the flight crew. The patient is packaged onto the sled and pulled using a rope and winch to the shore where the flight crew is waiting. You give them a report and help them move the patient into their aircraft. They immediately perform rapid sequence intubation, and noting that one of his pupils is now dilated and nonreactive, begin to hyperventilate the patient. Eight minutes after you give them a report, they are in flight to the trauma center. Later you are told that the patient survived for 2 days in the ICU, was declared brain dead, and donated eyes, bone, skin, liver, heart, and lungs for transplantation.

1. What type of protective gear would be indicated for this situation?

_____

2. Why was it necessary to pause and check ice conditions before proceeding to the patient?

_____

3. What is your highest priority in the scene size-up and assessment?
   a. Forming a general impression
   b. Evaluating resources
   c. Initial patient assessment
   d. Scene safety determination

4. Why were resources called for before patient interventions began?

_____

5. What do you know about the patient's blood pressure?

_____

6. Why was an IV not established or rapid sequence intubation attempted before the patient was moved?

_____

7. Why was a detailed physical examination not performed initially on this patient?

_____

CHAPTER 12 ANSWERS

REVIEW QUESTIONS

1. a. Determine the mechanism of injury.
    b. Find out the number of persons injured.
    c. Determine the need for rescue or hazardous materials resources and request these from dispatch if needed.
    d. Determine the best access for responders you request.
    e. Secure the area, clearing unnecessary persons from the scene.
    (Objective 1)

2. a. Form a general impression of the patient.
    b. Assess for life-threatening conditions.
    c. Identify him as a patient who needs immediate care and transport.
    (Objective 2)

3. The patient is male; has been ejected from a vehicle (a mechanism that is associated with severe injuries); and is not moving, which may indicate severe injury with altered mental status (or death).
    (Objective 3)

4. AVPU (alert, responds to verbal, responds to pain, or unresponsive)
    (Objective 3)

5. Facial or oral bleeding, vomiting, partial obstruction with the tongue and mucus, facial fractures, soft tissue trauma to the face
    (Objective 4)

6. Goggles, mask, gloves, and possibly a gown
    (Objective 1)

7. Open the airway with a modified jaw thrust, suction the secretions, and insert an oral airway if the patient has no gag reflex.
    (Objective 5)

8. Assess the rate, depth, and symmetry of chest movement. Expose the chest wall, inspect for accessory muscle use, and palpate for structural integrity, tenderness, and crepitus. Auscultate for bilateral breath sounds.
    (Objective 4)

9. Begin to assist ventilation with bag-valve device and supplemental oxygen. Hyperventilate and intubate while maintaining in-line cervical immobilization.
    (Objective 5)

10. Assess radial and carotid pulse. Determine skin color, temperature, moisture, and capillary refill (although this determination is not likely to be reliable because of cold environmental conditions).
    (Objective 3)

11. He has a poor general impression and decreased level of consciousness, is unresponsive, has difficulty breathing, and is in shock (likely because of numerous injuries and mechanism of injury [ejection]).
    (Objectives 4 and 7)

12. Continue spinal immobilization and perform a mental status assessment. Inspect and palpate for injuries or signs of injuries of the head, neck, chest, abdomen, pelvis, and extremities. Logroll the patient, and inspect and palpate the posterior surfaces of the body. Obtain baseline vital signs. Determine a brief patient history if anyone is on the scene to provide it.
    (Objective 7)

13. Airway control, ventilation, and spinal immobilization (for spine and fracture immobilization) are first; intravenous therapy can be initiated during transport.
(Objective 10)

14. 10 minutes
(Objective 10)

15. Because the patient is unstable (a priority patient), mental status, airway, breathing, and circulation should be reevaluated at least every 5 minutes during care and transport of this patient.
(Objective 9)

16. You will assess the patient's approximate age, sex, and race; look for obvious injury or indications of medical conditions; note the patient's general level of distress; and ask for the chief complaint.
(Objectives 2 and 3)

17. a. Ask the patient to speak and listen for stridor or gurgling.
b. Evaluate the rate, depth, and symmetry of chest movement. Expose the chest and palpate, observing for respiratory use of the accessory muscles of the neck, chest, and abdomen. Auscultate for breath sounds. Observe for cyanosis, respiratory distress, and distended neck veins. Determine the need to assist ventilations.
c. Assess the patient's skin color, moisture, and temperature, and evaluate the pulse for quality, rate, and regularity.
(Objective 3)

18. a. Poor general impression
b. Difficulty breathing
(Objective 4)

19. a. Chief complaint
b. History of present illness
c. Medical history
d. Current health status
(Objective 6)

20. The priority with the trauma patient is to secure the airway while maintaining spinal immobilization, ventilate with high-flow oxygen, and initiate rapid transport for definitive care. This patient has a patent airway but needs oxygenation and possibly assisted ventilation if the condition deteriorates. Emergency vascular access and drug administration may improve her condition rapidly and may be initiated before transport.
(Objective 10)

21. d. Patient care activities typically begin after the initial scene size-up. Medical direction should be contacted later. A mass casualty incident is unlikely in this setting.
(Objective 1)

22. c. The vital signs should be reassessed during the ongoing assessment.
(Objective 2)

23. a. The other components of the neurological examination are performed later in the assessment.
(Objective 3)

24. c. All other findings are identified later in the examination.
(Objective 4)

25. c. The life threat must be addressed before the examination can proceed.
(Objective 4)

26. a. The speed and focus of the examination are determined rapidly by the condition of the patient as noted in the initial assessment.
(Objective 6)

27. a. Detailed examination can be performed later if no life threats are identified. Otoscopic examination of the eyes is not indicated in this phase of the examination.
(Objective 6)

28. c. In each of the other patients, care in the prehospital setting generally is directed to correction of the life threats.
(Objective 8)

29. c. This should be done every 15 minutes for stable (nonpriority) patients and at least every 5 minutes for unstable (priority) patients.
(Objective 9)

30. b. Intravenous fluid therapy should be initiated only on the scene if it will not delay transport. More often intravenous therapy can be started during transport.
(Objective 10)

WRAP IT UP

1. If this lake were considered a busy traffic way, a helmet and safety goggles would be indicated. A warm turnout coat with reflective strips, slip-resistant waterproof gloves, and boots with steel insoles and steel toe protection should be worn.
(Objective 2)

2. If the ice were unsafe in any part of the scene, it would be critical to know to prevent injury or death to the rescuers and patient.
(Objective 2)

3. d. Evaluation of scene safety throughout all calls is critical.
(Objective 2)

4. Additional resources often take significant time to deploy. Activating them as early as possible is critical to expedite care and rescue.
(Objective 2)

5. A strong radial pulse is palpable, so you can surmise that his systolic blood pressure is close to 80 mm Hg.
(Objective 4)

6. In unsafe situations and in cases of environmental extremes, it is often safer for the crew and the patient to initiate most care in the ambulance. That way proper assessments, visualization, and access can be obtained safely.
(Objective 5)

7. Patient clothing would prevent a detailed physical examination. Priorities were packaging and rescue of the patient; management of the airway, breathing, and circulation; and preventing hypothermia.
(Objective 8)

Clinical Decision Making

READING ASSIGNMENT

Chapter 13, pages 290-297, in *Mosby's Paramedic Textbook,* ed. 3

OBJECTIVES

Upon completion of this chapter, the paramedic student will be able to:
1. List the key elements of paramedic practice.
2. Discuss the limitations of protocols, standing orders, and patient care algorithms.
3. Outline the key components of the critical thinking process for paramedics.
4. Identify elements necessary for an effective critical thinking process.
5. Describe situations that may necessitate the use of the critical thinking process while delivering prehospital patient care.
6. Describe the six elements required for effective clinical decision making in the prehospital setting.

SUMMARY

- The paramedic must be able to do several things at the same time. The paramedic must be able to gather, evaluate, and synthesize information. The paramedic also must be able to develop and implement appropriate patient management plans. The paramedic must apply judgment and exercise independent decision making as well. Lastly, the paramedic must be able to think and work effectively under pressure.
- Protocols, standing orders, and patient care algorithms have several limitations. They may not apply to nonspecific patient complaints that do not fit the model. They also do not address multiple disease etiologies or multiple treatment plans. Moreover, they may promote linear thinking.
- The critical thinking process includes concept formation, data interpretation, application of principle, evaluation, and reflection on action.
- For effective critical thinking, a paramedic must have a solid knowledge base. The paramedic must be able to deal with a large amount of data all at once as well. The paramedic must be able to organize those data, deal with ambiguity, and relate the situation to similar past experience. The paramedic also must be able to reason and construct arguments to support or discount the decision.
- When using assessment-based patient management, the paramedic must analyze a patient's problems, determine how to solve them, carry out a plan of action, and evaluate its effectiveness.
- Effective clinical decision making requires the paramedic to read the patient and the scene. The paramedic also must be able to react, reevaluate, and revise the management plan. Then the paramedic must be able to review performance at a run critique.

REVIEW QUESTIONS

1. List the four key elements of paramedic practice described in this chapter.

    a.

    b.

    c.

    d.

2. Why is it difficult to follow standard protocols, standing orders, and patient care algorithms in the following situations?

    a. A patient does not speak your language. He appears very ill, is pale and diaphoretic, and has a very slow, irregular heartbeat. He gets very anxious and pulls away when you attempt to establish an intravenous line to give medications.

    _____

    b. A patient with chronic obstructive pulmonary disease has signs and symptoms of heart failure and is wheezing.

    _____

    c. An elderly patient with severe kyphosis (hunchback posture) has fallen off a ladder but screams in pain when you attempt to immobilize him on the spine board.

    _____

    d. A child choked on a toy and is stridorous. Each time you approach to assess her, she begins to cry and has increased distress.

    _____

Question 3 pertains to the following case study:

> An elderly patient is complaining of chest pain that began 30 minutes ago. She tells you that it began suddenly when she was reading the paper. It is crushing and substernal, rating an "8" on a 1 to 10 scale. It does not radiate, but she feels nauseated and is diaphoretic. Your assessment reveals normal vital signs, clear breath sounds, and no other obvious clinical findings. A 12-lead ECG demonstrates ST segment elevation in leads V_1 and V_2. You and your partner recognize that her presentation is consistent with septal myocardial infarction. You immediately begin oxygen, initiate an intravenous line, and administer nitroglycerin and aspirin. You notify medical direction and transmit the ECG, anticipating the need for cardiac catheterization. You reevaluate her vital signs, breath sounds, and level of pain every 5 minutes during the 15-minute transport to the hospital. During the following shift, your supervisor gives you feedback on the patient's outcome. During the run critique, everyone agrees that the care was good but the scene time was somewhat long. During the ensuing discussion, you identify ways to reduce scene times on future calls.

3. Identify which parts of this scenario demonstrate each of the following phases of the critical thinking process:

    a. Concept formation:

    _____

    b. Data interpretation:

    _____

c. Application of principle:

_____

d. Evaluation:

_____

e. Reflection on action:

_____

4. List five steps that can help paramedics to think clearly in highly stressful situations.

   a.

   b.

   c.

   d.

   e.

5. List the six "Rs" of effective clinical decision making.

   a.

   b.

   c.

   d.

   e.

   f.

STUDENT SELF-ASSESSMENT

6. To practice effectively as a paramedic, you should be able to do which of the following?
   a. Gather, evaluate, and synthesize information
   b. Know all current medical techniques
   c. Make diagnoses and provide definitive care
   d. Teach your personal values to patients
7. Which of the following is an advantage of protocols, standing orders, and patient care protocols?
   a. They don't work well when numerous disease etiologies coexist.
   b. They may not apply to nonspecific patient complaints that do not fit the model.
   c. They promote a standardized approach to patient care for classic presentations.
   d. They promote linear thinking and cookbook medicine in all situations.
8. You recognize that a patient is hypoglycemic based on the history, physical examination, and blood analysis. What phase of the critical thinking process have you entered when you initiate an intravenous line and administer glucose?
   a. Application of principle   **c.** Data interpretation
   b. Concept formation   **d.** Reflection on action
9. In which of the following situations is a paramedic most likely to use critical thinking skills?
   a. The monitor shows ventricular fibrillation.
   b. The blood glucose strip reads 40 mg/dL.
   c. The patient stops breathing and becomes cyanotic.
   d. The trauma patient has severe neck pain but is dyspneic when supine.

10. Which of the following is *not* one of the six elements described in the text as being needed for effective clinical decision making?
  a. React
  b. Read the scene
  c. Request consultation with medical direction
  d. Review performance at a run critique

WRAP IT UP

You are dispatched to a residence for a seizure at 2300. When you arrive, you find a 2-year-old child who is drowsy but easily arousable. Her mother says she found her shaking in bed. She has a "cold" that began today but is otherwise quite healthy. The child is becoming progressively more awake, as you assess her vital signs: P 128; R 28; Sao_2 98%. You are questioning the mother when, moments later, the child seizes again. You move her to the ambulance, and you become concerned when her level of consciousness remains significantly depressed 5 minutes after the seizure, with snoring respirations noted. You insert a nasal airway and administer oxygen as your partner initiates an IV into her left antecubital fossa. You place her on an ECG monitor so that you can continuously monitor her heart rate. Her BP is 60/40 mm Hg; you know that's too low for her. Something seems out of place here. After a fluid bolus, her pressure comes up, but she is still very drowsy. You call your report while en route to the pediatric emergency department.

1. What additional measures might you have used to help with your concept formation?

2. Why would it be difficult to follow a standard protocol or algorithm for this child?

3. After interpreting the data you currently have, what are the chief life threats that concern you?

4. How did you react to the data found on this call?

CHAPTER 13 ANSWERS

REVIEW QUESTIONS

1. a. Gather, evaluate, and synthesize information. b. Develop and implement appropriate patient management plans. c. Apply judgment and exercise independent decision making. d. Think and work effectively under pressure.
(Objective 1)

2. a. The language barrier makes it impossible to explain properly to the patient what needs to be done, yet you cannot forcibly treat the patient. b. Wheezing caused by chronic obstructive pulmonary disease is treated with a beta agonist such as albuterol; however, treatment for congestive heart failure involves furosemide, nitroglycerin, and morphine. Critical thinking is required to identify subtle findings and point you to the correct treatment path for this patient. c. The correct treatment for this patient is to place him on a spine board (because of the mechanism of injury and age); however, this increases his pain and perhaps his injury because of his altered anatomy, therefore critical thinking is required to determine an acceptable compromise to meet this patient's needs. d. Standard of care requires you to perform a patient assessment on this child; however, when you attempt to do this, her condition worsens. You must determine a compromise that will not harm her.
(Objectives 2, 5)

3. a. Concept formation occurred when the patient assessment was done; b. data interpretation included interpretation of the vital signs, physical findings, history, and ECG to determine the likelihood of myocardial infarction; c. application of principle involved making the interpretation (MI), selecting the appropriate course of care (O_2, intravenous therapy, nitroglycerin, aspirin), and then delivering that care; d. reassessment of pain, vital signs, and breath sounds constitutes the evaluation phase of the process; e. the run critique provided the opportunity for reflection on action.
(Objective 3)

4. a. Stop and think; b. scan the situation; c. decide and act; d. maintain clear and concise control; e. regularly and clearly reevaluate the patient.
(Objective 4)

5. a. Read the patient; b. read the scene; c. react; d. reevaluate; e. revise patient management plan; f. review performance at run critique.
(Objective 6)

STUDENT SELF-ASSESSMENT

6. a. Paramedics must know techniques appropriate within their scope of practice that have been approved by medical direction. Paramedics are not expected to make diagnoses. Although in some cases (such as hypoglycemia) paramedics provide definitive care, in most cases definitive care is delivered at the hospital. Paramedics must recognize that their personal values may be different from those of the patient.
(Objective 1)

7. c. Each of the other choices represents a possible disadvantage of protocols, standing orders, and patient care protocols.
(Objective 2)

8. a. Concept formation involves the process of gathering elements to determine the "what" of the patient story. Data interpretation occurs when data are gathered and interpreted to form a field impression.
(Objective 3)

9. d. The patient has two concurrent serious problems, and the treatments of these conditions conflict. The paramedic must use critical thinking to resolve the problem.
(Objective 5)

10. c. In some situations medical direction is unavailable or is not available in a timely manner to provide assistance in situations that require rapid clinical decision making.
(Objective 6)

WRAP IT UP

1. Check the environment for any medicines; check her blood glucose level; check her skin temperature; complete her exam (e.g., pupils, rashes, and so on).
(Objective 3)

2. With no history of this, it is unclear what is causing the seizures. In this case general measures to ensure airway, breathing, and blood pressure and to manage recurring seizures would be followed.
(Objective 2)

3. Altered level of consciousness; partial airway obstruction; seizures; low blood pressure
(Objective 4)

4. Airway was managed (nasal airway); IV initiated; fluid bolus given; patient monitored; medical direction consulted.
(Objective 6)

Assessment-Based Management

READING ASSIGNMENT

Chapter 14, pages 298-305, in *Mosby's Paramedic Textbook,* ed. 3

OBJECTIVES

Upon completion of this chapter, the paramedic student will be able to:

1. Discuss how assessment-based management contributes to effective patient and scene assessment.
2. Describe factors that affect assessment and decision making in the prehospital setting.
3. Outline effective techniques for scene and patient assessment and choreography.
4. Identify essential take-in equipment for general and selected patient situations.
5. Outline strategies for patient approach that promote an effective patient encounter.
6. Describe techniques to permit efficient and accurate presentation of the patient.

SUMMARY

- Assessment-based management "puts it all together." This means that the paramedic gathers, evaluates, and synthesizes information. The paramedic makes proper decisions based on the information. Then the paramedic takes the appropriate actions required for the patient's care.
- Factors that can affect the quality of assessment and decision making include the paramedic's attitude, the patient's willingness to cooperate, distracting injuries, labeling and tunnel vision, the environment, patient compliance, and considerations of personnel availability.
- Promoting a coherent assessment is the goal. Thus members of the response team should have a preplan for determining roles and responsibilities.
- The paramedic crew should always be prepared for the worst event. They should carry essential equipment to manage every aspect of patient care.
- A calm and orderly manner is essential for the paramedic. This is especially the case when approaching a patient. During the initial assessment the paramedic must look actively for problems that pose a threat to life.
- Presenting the patient in the course of prehospital and hospital care is twofold. Presentation refers to the skills of effective communication. Presentation also refers to the effective transfer of patient information.

REVIEW QUESTIONS

For questions 1 to 5, what is your field impression based on the patterns described in each of the following scenarios (knowing that further assessment is necessary to confirm each)? Describe the key differences in each pair that distinguish the patterns.

1. a. A 24-year-old patient with a history of diabetes is found confused and diaphoretic with weakness on the right side.

_____

b. An 80-year-old patient with a history of hypertension is found confused and diaphoretic with weakness on the right side.

_____

c. Key differences in patterns:

_____

2. a. A 20-year-old woman whose last menstrual period was 8 weeks ago has severe right lower quadrant abdominal pain and signs of shock.

_____

b. A 12-year-old boy has severe right lower quadrant abdominal pain, fever, and vomiting.

_____

c. Key differences in patterns:

_____

3. a. A 38-year-old man has severe left lower back pain that radiates down into his testicle, and he has hematuria.

_____

b. A 70-year-old man had a sudden onset of lower back pain described as "ripping." He is pale, wants to have a bowel movement, and has a cool left foot.

_____

c. Key differences in patterns:

_____

4. a. A healthy 4-month-old infant is found pulseless, with rigor mortis, and in bed with no obvious signs of trauma.

_____

b. A healthy 16-year-old patient is found pulseless, with rigor mortis, and in bed with no obvious signs of trauma.

_____

c. Key differences in patterns:

_____

5. a. A 70-year-old man complains of crushing substernal chest pain. He is diaphoretic and having multifocal premature ventricular contractions. His history includes hypertension, smoking, and diabetes.

_____

b. A 25-year-old woman complains of crushing substernal chest pain. She is diaphoretic and having multifocal premature ventricular contractions. Her chest struck the steering wheel in a motor vehicle crash 10 minutes ago.

_____

c. Key differences in patterns:

_____

Questions 6 and 7 refer to the following case study:

You are dispatched to an address where the resident is an alcoholic who calls often for minor problems. She curses at you for taking so long to respond, and then says she fell out of bed yesterday, hit her head, and now has a headache. You note a large bruise on the temporal area of her head but no other injuries. Her speech is slurred, and she has a staggering gait. Her vital signs are BP 160/100 mm Hg, P, 64/min, and R 16/min. You advise her that she will be okay, and she declines transport. The next day she is found unconscious and is diagnosed with a large subdural hematoma that resulted in her death.

6. List factors that may have contributed to your decision in this case.

_____

_____

7. Why is this patient at increased risk for intracerebral bleeding?

_____

Questions 8 to 12 refer to the following case study:

You are dispatched to a call for a stabbing. Your patient is a 17-year-old boy who was stabbed at a street party. It is dark, and the police are trying to control a large, loud, belligerent crowd that has gathered at the scene. Your patient says he cannot breathe, and when you pull his shirt off, you note a stab wound above the right nipple. Breath sounds are equal. You apply an occlusive dressing, and you elect to move the patient to the ambulance for further assessment and care.

8. During the initial contact with this patient, what are the responsibilities for each of the following team members?

a. Team leader

_____

b. Patient care person (as described in this textbook)

_____

_____

9. Should you carry your drug box with you on a call like this? Why?

_____

10. Explain why the contemplative or the resuscitative approach would be appropriate for this call.

_____

_____

When you get in the ambulance, you talk to the patient, assess his airway and breathing, and apply oxygen. Your partner begins transport. As you begin to initiate an IV, you note blood dripping off the side of the ambulance cot. You cut the patient's clothing off and find a wound in the groin spurting blood.

11. List two factors that you think delayed detection of the patient's bleeding.

a.

b.

12. What pertinent positives should be included in your patient care report?

STUDENT SELF-ASSESSMENT

13. Which of the following terms describes the process of gathering, evaluating, and synthesizing information; making appropriate decisions based on available information; and taking the appropriate actions required for patient care?
  a. Assessment-based management
  b. Initial assessment
  c. Ongoing assessment
  d. Patient-focused care

14. Field impression of any given situation is based on which of the following factors?
  a. Information gathered before any physical examination
  b. Advice of medical direction and perception of the call
  c. The paramedic's "gut instinct" and pattern recognition
  d. The patient's chief complaint and assessment of the problem

15. What should you rule out if you encounter an uncooperative patient?
  a. Chest pain or dyspnea
  b. Hypoxia or hypoglycemia
  c. Neuromuscular disorder
  d. Personality disorder

16. Why is it important to predesignate roles for emergency medical services calls?
  a. To identify who is at fault if a problem occurs on a call
  b. To allow all paramedics to perform the skills at which they excel
  c. To ensure appropriate skills acquisition
  d. To promote coherent, efficient patient care delivery

17. What is the advantage of taking notes while obtaining the patient history?
  a. To obtain adequate billing information
  b. To provide evidence that may be used in court
  c. To prevent the need for repetitive questioning of the patient
  d. To reassure the patient that you are listening

18. In which of the following patient situations would the contemplative approach to patient care be appropriate?
  a. A large bleeding laceration
  b. Cramping abdominal pain
  c. Decreased level of consciousness
  d. Dyspnea and diaphoresis

19. You respond to a call in which you find a 24-year-old woman who is hyperventilating. What is the *last* condition for which you should assess while performing your history and physical exam?
  a. Anxiety attack
  b. Asthma
  c. Diabetic ketoacidosis
  d. Pulmonary embolus

20. You are caring for a patient who is seriously injured after a fall. What is a serious consequence of inadequately presenting your patient during your report to the hospital?
  a. Appropriate resources may not be ready.
  b. The nursing staff will be angry with you.
  c. The patient may misunderstand you.
  d. You may have an increased time out of service.

21. Which of the following is a characteristic of an effective patient presentation?
- **a.** Every assessment finding is described.
- **b.** It should last no longer than 5 minutes.
- **c.** It should include the name of the patient and the doctor.
- **d.** It should follow a standard format and be concise.

WRAP IT UP

Your partner groans as you pull up to the three-story apartment building where you are responding for a "person passed out." You know the address, you know the patient, and you know that this is probably no emergency, because you have been here many times for minor complaints of headache, constipation, and blood pressure checks. "What should we bring?" he asks wearily. "Let's bring it all," you say, grabbing the monitor, airway bag, and jump kit, even though you realize it is probably just an exercise in weight lifting. You enter the apartment, and your patient, a 70-year-old man, is semireclined on the sofa. When you ask what is going on, he tells you he must have pulled something in his back, it has been bothering him all day, and then he "fell out" and when he woke up, he called 911. "Tell me about your pain," you inquire, as vital signs are taken and his medicines (labetolol, hydrochlorothiazide (HydroDIURIL), potassium, aspirin) are recorded. "Well, it's in my back, and it's real bad, kind of like I tore something in there, and it goes down in my leg," he says, grimacing suddenly as he relates his story. You notice his skin is cool, his lips and nails are pale, and when you grab his wrist, his heart rate, while not rapid, is weak. His vital signs are BP 104/64 mm Hg, P 68/min, R 20/min, and SaO_2 93%. "That pressure's a bit low for you," your partner tells the patient as he opens a nasal cannula and places it on his face. On the physical exam, you note a tender pulsatile mass above his umbilicus to the right of the midline. Femoral pulses are weak, and you cannot feel any pulses in his cool, pale feet. You establish a line and send your partner and the police officer to retrieve the stretcher from the ambulance. Your patient is monitored, packaged, and transported to the hospital after you call report. Based on your notification, the ED resuscitation room is setup, and the patient is quickly diagnosed with abdominal aortic aneurysm. He is in surgery by the time you complete your report and is hospitalized for several weeks because of renal complications.

1. What findings fit the "pattern" of abdominal aortic aneurysm in this case study?

_____

2. How would your impression of the situation have changed if the following were true:
- **a.** The patient were 17 years old, had no medical history (no daily medications), and was unknown to the paramedics.
- **b.** The patient did not have a pulsating mass.
- **c.** You found a heart rhythm disturbance before you palpated his abdomen.
3. **a.** Which vital sign assessment did not fit the "pattern."
   b. What could explain this altered vital sign?
4. Which factor had the potential to have a negative impact on your assessment of this patient?
- **a.** Distracting environment
- **b.** Labeling and tunnel vision
- **c.** Personnel considerations
- **d.** Uncooperative patient
5. Place a check mark beside the team leader responsibilities that you observed on this call.
- **a.** _____ Accompanies patient to hospital
- **b.** _____ Establishes dialogue with patient
- **c.** _____ Obtains history
- **d.** _____ Performs physical exam
- **e.** _____ Presents the patient
- **f.** _____ Completes documentation
- **g.** _____ Team leadership

CHAPTER 14 ANSWERS

REVIEW QUESTIONS

1. a. Hypoglycemia (further assessment to rule out stroke would also be needed.)
   b. Stroke
   c. Age (Stroke is more common in the elderly.), history (Patient in *a*. had a history of diabetes); (patient in *b*. had a history of hypertension.)
   (Objective 1)

2. a. Ectopic pregnancy
   b. Appendicitis
   c. Sex (Boy in *b*. would not have gynecological complaints.), age (Appendicitis is common in this age group.), clinical signs (shock in ectopic pregnancy versus fever in appendicitis)
   (Objective 1)

3. a. Nephrolithiasis (kidney stone)
   b. Abdominal aortic aneurysm
   c. Age (Aneurysm is more common in men 60 to 70 years of age.), clinical signs/symptoms (Hematuria is common in kidney stones; urge to defecate, cool extremity, and signs of shock are consistent with aneurysm.)
   (Objective 1)

4. a. Sudden infant death syndrome or child abuse
   b. Drug or alcohol toxicity or suicide
   c. Age (Sudden infant death syndrome and abuse are more common in infants; suicide and drug abuse or overdose are more common in teens).
   (Objective 1)

5. a. Myocardial infarction
   b. Myocardial contusion
   c. Age (Myocardial infarction is more common in older patients; history of *a*. is consistent with risk factors of myocardial infarction; mechanism of injury in *b*. is consistent with myocardial injury.)
   (Objective 1)

6. Your attitude, the patient's willingness to cooperate, and labeling or tunnel vision (the expectation that her signs and symptoms were related to alcohol intoxication) may have contributed to your decision.
   (Objective 2)

7. Chronic alcoholism can impair the clotting mechanisms, putting the patient at risk for bleeding. Poor coordination caused by intoxication increases the risk of injury (falls) in alcoholic patients.
   (Objective 2)

8. a. The team leader establishes contact and begins dialogue with the patient, obtains the history, and performs the physical examination.
   b. The patient care person provides scene cover (watches the crowd), gathers scene information (size/type of weapon), obtains vital signs, and performs skills.
   (Objective 3)

9. When moving into a volatile situation such as this one, you should take the minimum amount of equipment; the drug box would not be indicated based on the dispatch information. (This may vary by agency based on size and contents of drug box.)
   (Objective 4)

10. The resuscitative approach is necessary because a life threat exists.
    (Objective 5)

11. a. The presence of distracting injuries (the chest wound)
    b. The environment (dangerous and dark)
    (Objective 2)

12. The patient is conscious, and breath sounds are present and equal bilaterally.
    (Objective 6)

13. a. Initial assessment and ongoing assessment are components of assessment-based management.
    (Objective 1)

14. c. The field impression is based on a careful history, physical examination, and then analysis and evaluation based on the paramedic's knowledge and past experiences.
    (Objective 2)

15. b. Alcohol or drug intoxication, hypovolemia, and head injury or concussion are other physiological problems that may cause a patient to be uncooperative.
    (Objective 3)

16. d. This becomes especially important when multiple units respond to a scene.
    (Objective 4)

17. c. Taking notes keeps you from forgetting critical information that will be necessary when you complete your patient care report later.
    (Objective 5)

18. b. The contemplative approach is appropriate only when immediate intervention to manage a life threat is not needed.
    (Objective 5)

19. a. All the other conditions represent life-threatening problems associated with hyperventilation; your examination therefore should be tailored to rule out those problems first.
    (Objective 5)

20. a. An inadequate or inaccurate report can result in delayed patient care related to room or resource (medical staff, equipment) unavailability.
    (Objective 6)

21. d. Ideally, the report should be concise, follow a standard format, and include pertinent positives and negatives. The patient's name should not be included if radio communication is used.
    (Objective 6)

WRAP IT UP

1. Patient age, history of hypertension (from medications), description and location of pain, pulsatile mass, location of mass, diminished pulses in extremities, hypotension, syncopal episode
   (Objective 1)

2. a. Aneurysm would be unlikely (but not impossible) in someone that age and with no previous history. The patient would still need similar interventions and urgent transport due to the physical findings (cool skin, weak pulse, low SaO_2 for age).
   b. The treatment and impression should not change. A pulsatile mass is not always palpable.
   c. The history and description of the pain should still lead you to suspect aneurysm.

3. a. Tachycardia would have been expected.
b. Patient was taking a beta-blocker, which will not permit the heart to speed up effectively to compensate for shock.
(Objective 2)

4. b. Having been to many "false alarms," it would be possible to discount the patient's complaints and, if a comprehensive exam was not done, to miss this critical condition.
(Objective 2)

5. a, b, c, d, e, f, g
(Objective 3)

Communications

READING ASSIGNMENT
Chapter 15, pages 298-317, in *Mosby's Paramedic Textbook,* ed. 3

OBJECTIVES
Upon completion of this chapter, the paramedic student will be able to:
1. Outline the phases of communications that occur during a typical emergency medical services (EMS) event.
2. Describe the role of communications in EMS.
3. Define common EMS communications terms.
4. Describe the primary modes of EMS communications.
5. Describe how EMS communications are regulated.
6. Describe the role of dispatching as it applies to prehospital emergency medical care.
7. Outline techniques for relaying EMS communications clearly and effectively.

SUMMARY
- Communications regarding EMS refers to the delivery of information. The patient and scene information is delivered to other key members of the emergency response team.
- Verbal, written, and electronic communications allow the delivery of information between the party requesting help and the dispatcher; between the dispatcher and paramedic; and between the paramedic, hospital, and direct/online medical direction.
- Emergency communications technology has industry-specific terminology.
- The primary modes of EMS communications include simplex mode, duplex mode, multiplex mode, trunking system, digital, and computer.
- In the United States, the FCC regulates communications over the radio. The paramedic must be familiar with the regulatory agencies. The paramedic must follow their guidelines as well.
- The functions of an effective dispatch communications system include receiving and processing calls for EMS assistance, dispatching and coordinating EMS resources, relaying medical information, and coordinating with public safety agencies.
- A standard format of transmission of patient information is a wise idea. The standard allows for the best use of communications systems. The standard also allows physicians to receive details quickly about the patient. In addition, the standard decreases the chance of omitting any critical details.

REVIEW QUESTIONS

Match the communication term in Column II with the appropriate definition in Column I. Use each answer only once.

Column I

1. _____ A unit of frequency equal to one cycle per second
2. _____ The ability to transmit or receive in one direction at a time
3. _____ A grouping of radio equipment that includes a transmitter and receiver
4. _____ Radio frequencies between 300 and 3000 MHz
5. _____ The ability to transmit and receive simultaneously through two different frequencies
6. _____ A unit of frequency equal to 1 million cycles per second
7. _____ Radio frequencies between 30 and 300 MHz
8. _____ A unit that receives transmissions from a mobile radio and retransmits them at higher power on another frequency

Column II

a. Base station
b. Duplex
c. Hertz
d. Kilohertz
e. Megahertz
f. Mobile station
g. Remote console
h. Repeater
i. Simplex
j. UHF
k. VHF

9. A person is stabbed with a knife. List the five phases of communications that occur on most emergency medical services calls such as this.

a.

b.

c.

d.

e.

10. A man is injured seriously at a rural site. Describe the communication process from the time of his injury until the EMS crew returns to service.

_____

_____

_____

_____

_____

11. List three common causes of interference with radio transmissions.

a.

b.

c.

12. Briefly describe four responsibilities of an EMS dispatcher.

a.

b.

c.

d.

13. List three essential pieces of information that the dispatcher must obtain from a bystander who calls in to report a motor vehicle crash.

   a.

   b.

   c.

14. Identify three ways in which the Federal Communications Commission directly influences EMS.

   a.

   b.

   c.

15. Describe six actions the paramedic may take to ensure clear and understandable radio transmissions.

   a.

   b.

   c.

   d.

   e.

   f.

Johnny Smith, a paramedic who works on City Unit 7, is called to an industrial site. He finds a 30-year-old patient lying on his back on the grass, where he landed after falling 20 feet from a painting platform. On the paramedic's arrival at 1 PM, the patient's vital signs are as follows: blood pressure, 120/80 mm Hg; pulse, 116 per minute; and respirations, 20 per minute. He states he became dizzy and fell. When Smith palpates, the patient complains of pain in the lumbar region of the back and on both heels, which are swollen. Distal pulses, sensation, and movement are present in all extremities. Lung sounds are clear and equal bilaterally. The patient gives Smith his name and knows the date and time and where he is. His skin is warm and dry. The patient weighs about 100 kg and takes ibuprofen prescribed by Dr. Jones for back pain. Smith places him on 100% oxygen via non-rebreather mask, positions him on a backboard with cervical collar, and notifies Dr. Kane, the online medical physician, of the patient's condition and the 15-minute estimated arrival time to City Hospital. Vital signs at 1:25 PM are unchanged. The patient's condition remains the same en route.

16. Write a concise, complete radio report to communicate the appropriate information regarding this patient to the base hospital.

_____

_____

_____

_____

_____

_____

_____

_____

_____

_____

_____

_____

_____

_____

STUDENT SELF-ASSESSMENT

17. What is manipulation of the intended idea for communication known as?
    a. Decoding
    c. Feedback
    b. Encoding
    d. Receiving

18. After being called to an airplane crash with two seriously injured patients, the first arriving EMS crew tells online medical direction, "There are people (meaning bystanders) everywhere." The physician interprets this to indicate a mass casualty situation and activates the mass casualty incident plan. What type of communication error occurred here?
    a. Attributes of the receiver
    c. Semantic problems
    b. Selective perception
    d. Time pressures

19. Which of the following is a component of a simple communication system?
    a. Remote console
    c. Mobile unit
    b. Microwave links
    d. Satellite receivers

20. What is a radio receiver circuit used for suppressing the audio portion of unwanted radio noises or signals called?
    a. Decibel
    c. Squelch
    b. Frequency modulation
    d. Tone

21. What is the term for the number of repetitive cycles per second completed by a radio wave?
    a. Amplitude modulation
    c. Range
    b. Frequency
    d. Wattage

22. What is transmission and reception of electrocardiograms over the radio or telephone called?
    a. Coverage
    c. Patch
    b. Hotline
    d. Telemetry

23. What are the HEAR and EACOM radios used to tie hospitals together and receive and transmit tone pulses known as?
    a. Cellular telephones
    c. Microwave transmitters
    b. Decoders and encoders
    d. Satellite dishes

24. Which component of a communication system receives transmissions from a low-power portable radio on one frequency and simultaneously retransmits it at a higher power on another frequency?
    a. Mobile transceivers
    c. Remote console
    b. Portable radios
    d. Repeaters

25. How is the strongest signal selected when numerous satellite receivers are used?
    a. Base stations
    c. Decoders
    b. Cellular lines
    d. Voting systems

26. What are dispatch services located away from base stations that facilitate communications with field personnel known as?
    a. Complex systems
    c. Portable transceivers
    b. Mobile transceivers
    d. Remote consoles

27. What is an advantage of communication with cellular telephones?
    a. They allow unlimited channel access.
    b. They permit uninterrupted communication.
    c. They provide a secure link between EMS and the hospital.
    d. They transmit simultaneous calls in disaster situations.
28. Which of the following is not a responsibility of the dispatcher?
    a. Dispatching EMS resources
    b. Coordinating with public safety services
    c. Receiving calls for assistance
    d. Providing off-line medical control
29. What is a function of prearrival instructions?
    a. To allow EMS personnel to be disregarded
    b. To determine whether the call is unfounded
    c. To provide life-saving instructions
    d. To allow the EMS crew more time to respond
30. What is the role of the Federal Communications Commission?
    a. To consult with EMS agencies regarding radio equipment
    b. To develop new radio technologies
    c. To monitor frequencies for appropriate usage
    d. To train dispatchers in prearrival instructions
31. Which of the following is a technique for effective radio communication?
    a. Speak at a range of 6 to 8 inches from the microphone.
    b. Speak slowly and clearly and enunciate words distinctly.
    c. Show emotion to demonstrate the urgency of critical situations.
    d. Take your time and include all patient information available.
32. Which is *not* a component of the SOAP format for patient reports?
    a. Assessment data   c. Patient information
    b. Objective data   d. Subjective information

WRAP IT UP

At 0130 the prealert tone sounds in your engine-house, and the lights go on as you hear the dispatcher say, "4017 respond to number 12 Avid Court, chest pain." As you roll out of your bunk, the call is repeated, and then you hear the dispatcher recite the call numbers. Your partner pulls the run direction card as a backup because the computer was down earlier. You are attending this call, so you read the directions and tap the responding key of your on-board computer screen as you pull out of the engine room. The instructions on the screen note the patient's previous heart history. You pull up the global positioning system map to ensure you are proceeding in the correct direction. The dispatcher sends you a note indicating that there is a large dog that the caller has been instructed to secure in a bedroom. You tap the arrival button on your computer screen and proceed in to care for the patient. Based on your patient assessment, you suspect the patient is having an acute myocardial infarction and perform a 12-lead ECG. Your partner connects your monitor to the telephone line, and you transmit a copy of the ECG to medical direction. Then, when you contact medical direction using the cellular telephone for orders, they agree with your interpretation of inferior myocardial infarction. You notify dispatch that you are departing the scene to transport to Central Medical Center. They notify you that the local hospital diversion program indicates that they are on diversion and cannot accept the patient, so you elect to go the other direction to a medical center an equal distance and contact them on your VHF radio with a patient report. You indicate your arrival at the hospital on your dispatch screen. After giving a verbal report to the receiving RN, you proceed to the EMS report room where the fax from dispatch with your call times is waiting. Your partner has brought in your computer, and so you complete your report following the prompts on the screen and then type in the narrative. The patient is now in the cardiac catheterization lab and unable to sign the consent and notice of receipt of the HIPAA forms, so you document that and give the privacy notice to the family member. You obtain the nurse's signature, print your report, and then touch your computer screen to notify dispatch that you are returning in service. As you pull into you station, you pop out the wireless antenna in your laptop computer, and then, when a good signal is detected, press upload, and the report now is securely in the department mainframe and accessible to only the privacy officer and a few designated officers.

1. List all the persons and/or agencies with which the EMS crew communicated on this call.

_____

_____

2. What key information did the dispatcher provide on this call?

_____

_____

3. What modes of communication were used on this EMS call?

_____

_____

4. Identify problems that could have been encountered on this call if any of the following communication errors had occurred.

Communication Error	**Potential Problems**

   a. Dispatcher fails to identify or transmit correct address.

_____

_____

   b. Dispatcher fails to give instructions regarding dog.

_____

_____

   c. Computer fails and no backup system is available.

_____

_____

   d. Incorrect or incomplete information is reported to medical direction.

_____

_____

   e. Fail to report all medications given to receiving RN.

_____

_____

   f. Forget to notify dispatch when returning in service.

_____

_____

CHAPTER 15 ANSWERS

REVIEW QUESTIONS

1. c
(Objective 3)

2. i
(Objective 3)

3. a
(Objective 3)

4. j
(Objective 3)

5. b
(Objective 3)

6. e
(Objective 3)

7. k
(Objective 3)

8. h
(Objective 3)

9. a. Occurrence of the event
   b. Detection of the need for emergency services
   c. Notification and emergency response
   d. EMS arrival, treatment (including consultation with medical direction), and preparation for transport
   e. Preparation of EMS for the next emergency response
(Objective 1)

10. Emergency medical services response is initiated by bystanders by telephone to a communications center or public safety answering point. The communications specialist obtains the necessary information (often accompanied by digital information) about the origin of the call. The call taker then passes the information by digital technology (if available) to the telecommunicator, who dispatches appropriate emergency personnel and equipment. The EMS crew notifies the communications center while en route and obtains additional information. The EMS crew notifies the communications center on arrival to scene. The EMS crew contacts medical direction for orders and reports. Care is rendered, and the patient is prepared for transport; the EMS crew notifies the communication center when they depart from the scene and arrive at the receiving facility. The ambulance is made ready for the next emergency call and communications is notified when it is available for another call.
(Objective 2)

11. Mountains, dense foliage, and tall buildings
(Objective 4)

12. a. To receive calls for EMS assistance
   b. Dispatch and coordinate EMS resources
   c. Relay medical information
   d. Coordinate with public safety agencies
(Objective 5)

13. a. Name and callback number of individual who placed the call
   b. Address of emergency and directions including specific landmarks because of the possible rural location
   c. The nature of the emergency (Is the victim trapped, how seriously is he or she injured, and is he or she accessible to the EMS crew?)
   (Objective 5)

14. Licensing and frequency allocation, establishing technical standards for radio equipment, and establishing and enforcing rules and regulations
   (Objective 6)

15. Speak 2 to 3 inches away from and across the microphone, speak slowly and clearly, speak without emotion, be brief, avoid codes (unless approved by system), and advise the receiving party when the transmission has been completed.
   (Objective 7)

16. City Unit 7, paramedic Smith calling City Hospital. We are on the scene at an industrial site with a patient who fell approximately 20 feet onto a grassy area. The patient is a 30-year-old male weighing approximately 100 kg. Patient's chief complaint is back pain. Also complaining of bilateral heel pain. Patient states he became dizzy and fell. Medical history of back pain for which he takes ibuprofen. Patient is awake, alert, and oriented times 3. Lungs are clear bilaterally; skin is warm and dry. Tenderness to palpation in lumbar region of back and bilaterally on heels. Soft tissue swelling present bilaterally at calcaneus. Distal pulse, sensation, and movement present in all extremities. V/S are BP 120/80, P 116, R 20. Patient placed on 100% oxygen by complete non-rebreather mask and immobilized on a backboard with cervical collar. Private physician is Dr. Jones. ETA will be 15 minutes. Standing by for any additional orders, over.
   (Objective 7)

17. b. Decoding is interpretation of a message. Feedback is the response to the initial idea. Receiving indicates the receiver got the message.
   (Objective 2)

18. c. The word *people* was mistakenly interpreted as *patients*.
   (Objective 2)

19. c. All other equipment listed is part of a complex system.
   (Objective 4)

20. c. A decibel is a unit of measurement for signal power levels. Frequency modulation is a deviation in carrier frequency resulting in less noise. A tone is a unique carrier wave used to signal a receiver selectively.
   (Objective 3)

21. b. Amplitude modulation is a radio frequency that fluctuates according to the applied audio. Range refers to the general perimeter of signal coverage. A watt measures power output.
   (Objective 3)

22. d. Coverage refers to the area where radio communication exists. A hotline is a dedicated line activated by merely lifting the receiver. Patching permits communication between different communication modes.
   (Objective 3)

23. b. These tones can be set to all-call for efficient disaster communication. Cellular telephones are used for ambulance-to-hospital contact in some areas. Satellite dishes and microwave transmitters extend transmission distance.
   (Objective 4)

24. d. Mobile transceivers usually are mounted on the vehicle and operate at lower outputs than base stations. Portable radios are handheld devices used when working away from the emergency vehicle. Remote center consoles are located away from base stations and are connected by dedicated telephone line, microwave, or other radio means.
(Objective 4)

25. d. Voting systems automatically select the strongest or best audio signal among numerous satellite receivers.
(Objective 4)

26. d. Remote consoles control all base station functions and are connected by dedicated telephone lines.
(Objective 4)

27. c. No dedicated cell channels exist for EMS, so lines may be busy when an emergency call is being made. In some areas the cell coverage is not good and communication may be terminated abruptly. This does not allow simultaneous communication.
(Objective 4).

28. d. This is the physician medical director's job.
(Objective 5)

29. c. Prearrival instructions complement EMS care but do not include call screening.
(Objective 5)

30. c. They also are responsible for licensure and allocation of frequencies. They establish technical standards for radio equipment and establish and enforce rules and regulations for equipment operation.
(Objective 6)

31. b. You should speak 2 to 3 inches from the microphone, converse without emotion, and be brief.
(Objective 7)

32. c. Plan of patient management is the fourth component.
(Objective 7)

WRAP IT UP

1. Partner, dispatch, patient and their family, medical direction, receiving facility, receiving RN.
(Objective 1)

2. Location of call, nature of call, previous information known about patient, presence of dog, diversion status of hospital, times
(Objective 6)

3. Radio voice, tones, light, computer (dispatch of call); fax (ECG); cellular telephone (medical direction); radio (dispatch, receiving facility); face-to-face (patient, partner, family, receiving RN)
(Objective 7)

4. a. Determining the correct location of a call is a critical element in your response time. Failure to do so could delay your response significantly.
   b. Scene safety could have been compromised.
   c. Response delays if no backup directions are available.
   d. Inappropriate and even dangerous orders may be given if the report to medical direction is not accurate.
   e. Duplicate administration of medications is possible if an incomplete report is given. This could cause serious side effects.
   f. A call might be given to a more distant unit, delaying response time and leaving their zone without coverage.
   (Objective 7)

Documentation

READING ASSIGNMENT

Chapter 16, pages 318-330, in *Mosby's Paramedic Textbook,* ed. 3

OBJECTIVES

Upon completion of this chapter, the paramedic student will be able to:
1. Identify the purpose of the patient care report (PCR).
2. Describe the uses of the patient care report.
3. Outline the components of an accurate, thorough patient care report.
4. Describe the elements of a properly written emergency medical services document.
5. Describe an effective system for documentation of prehospital patient care.
6. Identify differences necessary when documenting special situations.
7. Describe the appropriate method to make revisions or corrections to the patient care report.
8. Recognize consequences that may result from inappropriate documentation.

SUMMARY

*   The patient care report is used to document the key elements of patient assessment, care, and transport.
*   The three primary reasons for written documentation are that the medical community involved in the patient's care uses it, it is a legal record, and it is essential to data collection.
*   The PCR should include dates and response times, difficulties encountered, observations at the scene, previous medical care provided, a chronological description of the call, and significant times.
*   A properly written EMS document is accurate, legible, timely, unaltered, and free of nonprofessional or extraneous information.
*   Many approaches for writing the narrative can be used. The paramedic should adopt only one approach. The paramedic should use this approach consistently to avoid omissions in report writing.
*   Special documentation is necessary when a patient refuses care or transport. Such documentation also is needed in those cases when care or transportation is not needed. Special documentation also is needed for mass casualty incidents.
*   Most EMS agencies have separate forms for revisions or corrections to the patient care report.
*   Documentation that is inappropriate may have medical and legal implications.

REVIEW QUESTIONS

Questions 1 and 2 pertain to the following case study:

> You are a paramedic working on Unit 4017 and are dispatched to a private residence on a call for a "person down."
> On arrival at the scene at 1400, you find a 20-year-old woman lying on the lawn in front of the house. She is awake

but is saying inappropriate words. The patient's husband tells you that his wife is diabetic and takes insulin, but she missed lunch. He says he found her confused in the yard. Her skin is pale, cool, and diaphoretic; respiratory rate is 20 breaths per minute and unlabored with clear breath sounds in all fields; radial pulse is 120 per minute; and her blood pressure is 110/70 mm Hg. While your partner initates an IV in the right antecubital space at 1406, you measure the patient's blood glucose level, which is 50 mg/dL. Following your standing orders, you begin an IV of normal saline and then at 1408 administer 25 g (50 mL) of D50W through the IV. Within 2 minutes the patient looks at you and asks, "Why are you here?" She is now alert and answering appropriately, and by the time her husband reminds her what has happened, she is oriented completely to person, place, and time. She agrees to be transported to General Hospital, and the ambulance departs the scene at 1413. While en route, you call a report to Dr. Smith, and at 1416 another set of vital signs reveals the following: BP 118/74, P 96/min, R 20/min with warm, dry, pink skin. She denies allergies to medicine and states she took 10 units of regular and 20 units of Lente insulin at 0700. On arrival to the hospital at 1420, there is no change in the patient's condition, and you note that 100 mL of the IV fluid has been infused. Your partner restocks your bag with the supplies used, which include a 250-mL bag of normal saline, macrodrip IV tubing, an 18G IV catheter, and D50W.

1. Write a narrative documenting your findings on this patient as you would on your state patient care report (assuming there is no check-box format on your report).

_____

_____

_____

_____

_____

_____

_____

_____

_____

_____

_____

2. List at least four activities for which your patient care report from this call may be used.

_____

_____

_____

_____

3. Describe the appropriate method to complete documentation for each of the following situations:
   a. Your patient lacerated his hand. The wound is deep and gaping, and he cannot move two of his fingers. He is refusing care and says he will go to his doctor tomorrow.

   _____

   _____

   _____

   b. You are responding to a call for a "full arrest." Before you arrive on scene, the dispatcher notifies you to disregard the call. You go back in service and return to your station.

   _____

   _____

   _____

   c. More than 100 patients are complaining of burning eyes and throats and difficulty breathing after an industrial gas release. You are providing care in the treatment sector.

   _____

   _____

   _____

   d. You have just returned to your engine house from the hospital when you realize that you did not document some essential information about the patient's history on the patient care report.

   _____

   _____

   _____

4. What is a possible consequence of failure to document the following information in a patient care report?
   a. The trauma patient reports an allergy to tetanus vaccine. He is unconscious when you arrive in the emergency department.

   _____

   _____

   _____

   b. You administered the maximum dosage of lidocaine to a patient who was in ventricular tachycardia but neglected to document it on your patient care report.

   _____

   _____

   _____

c. The patient fell earlier in the day and is unconscious on arrival to the emergency department. You do not document that the patient takes warfarin (Coumadin) daily.

_____

_____

_____

d. You fail to note that a patient had numbness in his arm before spinal immobilization.

_____

_____

_____

STUDENT SELF-ASSESSMENT

5. What is the purpose of the patient care report?
   a. To document patient assessment
   b. To document patient care
   c. To document patient transport
   d. To document all of the above

6. Which of the following is not an appropriate use of the patient care report?
   a. Administrative and billing information
   b. Legal record of sequence of care provided
   c. Research document for the local press
   d. Supply inventory tracking

7. Which of the following should *not* be documented on the patient care report?
   a. Chronological description of events that occurred during the call
   b. Circumstances documenting that the paramedic fell during care of this patient
   c. Difficulties encountered during patient care, treatment, and transport
   d. Time of call, dispatch, arrival at scene, arrival at hospital, and back in service

8. If the respiratory rate section is not completed on the ambulance reporting form, what should the physician assume about patient respirations?
   a. They were not an important vital sign assessment.
   b. They were not pertinent in this patient section.
   c. They were not assessed specifically by the paramedic.
   d. They were within normal limits for the patient age group.

9. When a patient refuses care, what must the paramedic document?
   a. Advice given to the patient regarding the condition
   b. Nothing is needed as long as the patient was alert and oriented.
   c. The detailed physical examination
   d. The patient's insurance information

10. What should you document when your response is canceled en route to the scene?
   a. Canceling authority and time of cancellation
   b. No documentation is needed in this situation.
   c. Scene size-up information
   d. You must still respond and obtain a refusal.

11. You are leaving work and suddenly realize you forgot to document a crucial piece of information about patient care on a patient record. What should you do?
   a. Ask your supervisor to fill in the essential information.
   b. Note the date and time the correction was made on the appropriate form.
   c. Wait until you return to work after your 4-day break to finish it.
   d. You may not add anything after the report is complete.

WRAP IT UP

It seems odd that you would be nervous today. Normally, you are the one who is calm, cool, and collected even on the most serious trauma calls. As you sit waiting to testify at the deposition, you go over the details of the call in your mind. At the time you thought you'd never forget them, but after 5 years the details tend to fade. Thankfully, your attorney says that you will have the benefit of your patient care report to refer to during your testimony. The plaintiff who was thrown off of a motorcycle while apparently intoxicated is alleging that your care led to the long-term disability he is experiencing from nerve damage to his badly fractured leg. You sit around the table with your attorney, the prosecuting attorney, and a court reporter who swears you in. The attorney begins by asking you why your response to the scene of the collision was so slow based on the location from which you responded. You explain, as you documented, that traffic was diverted that evening because of highway construction, resulting in an unavoidable delay in response. He queries you about your statements that the patient was "drunk." You respond that you did not document that the patient was drunk. Rather, you noted that there was a strong odor resembling alcohol on the patient's breath, that he had slurred speech, that he repeatedly was moving his clearly fractured extremity, despite repeated requests for him to hold still so that he would not injure it further until appropriate immobilization could be completed. The attorney asks if that behavior was consistent with a head injury also, and you state that yes it would be; however, as you detailed in your report, the mechanism of injury was not consistent with head injury as evidenced by bystander reports that his leg had been pinned between the bike and a car, and his head never struck the ground. You also note that his helmet was undamaged. The attorney then makes the allegation that you did not follow proper care to his client's injured leg and wonders why you scratched out the word "traction" before splint. You state that, as you noted in your report, there was gross deformity to his lower leg and ankle; however, before, during, and after splinting, there was a good dorsalis pedis and posterior tibial pulse with the last check you noted after you moved the patient to the cot in the resuscitation room at the trauma center. Further, you review with him the policy of your department when an error is made on the report as was done here. Evidently, the word *traction* was written mistakenly, so you crossed through it with a single line and placed your initials beside the strikeout. You also had documented the numbness that the patient reported in his toes and his ability to move them during those pulse checks. In response to his questions regarding your apparently long scene time, you point to your note regarding the patient's repeated attempts to get off the cot and run away. With each series of questions, you were able to answer accurately and thoroughly based on your documentation. After the deposition, your attorney notifies you that, while his client's suit is still proceeding against the hospital, the prosecuting attorney will be dropping your name and your service from the client's claims.

1. List five uses of this patient care report aside from the one already mentioned.

_____

_____

_____

_____

_____

2. Place a check mark beside the components of an accurate, complete patient care report that were mentioned in this case.
   a. _____ Dates
   b. _____ Response times
   c. _____ Difficulties en route
   d. _____ Communication difficulties
   e. _____ Scene observations
   f. _____ Reasons for extended on scene time
   g. _____ Previous care provided
   h. _____ Time of extrication
   i. _____ Time of patient transport
   j. _____ Reason for hospital selection
3. Which is true regarding the correction of a patient care report that was done in this case?
   a. It would have been better to black out the error completely.
   b. It should have been explained thoroughly in the narrative.
   c. It was completed properly.
   d. Individual strikeouts should not be done, the entire sentence should be rewritten.

CHAPTER 16 ANSWERS

REVIEW QUESTIONS

1. At 1400, 4017 arrived to the scene of a residence. Found a 20-year-old woman supine on the lawn, saying inappropriate words. Her husband states she is a diabetic. He found her in the yard confused. Patient's skin is pale, cool, and diaphoretic. Vital signs are BP 110/70, P 120/min, R 20/min with clear breath sounds. Blood glucose determined to be 50 mg/dL. 1406 IV 250 mL NS initiated in the right antecubital space by paramedic Ward. 1408 25 g (50 mL) D50W given IVP by paramedic McKenna. 1410 Patient states, "Why are you here?" 1412 Patient is alert and oriented to person, place, and time. Patient states she took 10 units of regular and 20 units of Lente insulin at 0700 today. 1413 Ambulance en route to General Hospital. Report called to Dr. Smith. No further orders requested. 1416 BP 118/74, P 96/min, R 20/min. Skin is pink, warm, and dry. 1420 Arrival to General Hospital. 100 mL NS infused.
   On some patient report forms, check boxes or tables will permit documentation of many of the items included in this narrative report. In that instance, it is often unnecessary to repeat the information on the narrative.
   (Objectives 3, 4, 5)

2. Medical continuity of care, quality improvement, legal record, supply tracking, performance evaluation, state reporting, education, and skill tracking
   (Objective 2)

3. a. Document the patient's level of consciousness, your advice to the patient (including possible consequences of refusal) medical direction advice to the patient, signatures of the patient and/or witnesses as required in your system, a narrative description of your exam that you told patient to call 9-1-1 again if he changes his mind, and the events that occurred.
   b. Note the name of the person/agency that canceled your response, and the time the response was terminated. Ensure that this falls within the scope of your departmental policies.
   c. Document care on the appropriate mass casualty incident (MCI) forms (often on triage tags). Record patient condition and disposition on appropriate tracking form (may be done by sector leader).
   d. Note the purpose of the revision or correction and why the information did not appear on the original document as soon as possible using the appropriate departmental form. Ensure the correction is made by the original author. Send a copy of the revision to the appropriate parties.
   (Objective 6)

4. a. If tetanus vaccine is administered to the patient in the hospital, he will likely have an allergic reaction and be harmed. You could face legal repercussions.
   b. If additional lidocaine is administered at the hospital, the patient may have a toxic reaction. When the chart is audited for quality purposes, it will appear that you did not perform a procedure that was indicated. If drug inventory is tracked from the patient report, it will not be replaced, and you may run short. If the patient's bill is itemized, he or she will not be charged for this intervention, and your department may lose revenue needed for operations.
   c. The patient's condition could deteriorate quickly, and the medical staff would not recognize the increased risk of bleeding. You could face legal repercussions.
   d. If the patient alleges that the numbness developed as a result of your care, you would have no documentation to substantiate your claim that the patient was symptomatic before your care; you could be successfully sued.
   (Objective 8)

5. d. All these elements should be recorded in an accurate, legible, understandable manner.
   (Objective 1)

6. c. The records should be maintained confidentially and only released to parties other than the hospital after patient consent is given.
   (Objective 2)

7. b. This is documented on the appropriate department incident report.
   (Objective 3)

8. c. In a court of law the assumption is that if it is not documented, it was not done.
   (Objective 4)

9. a. Advice to the patient, including risks of refusal and benefits of treatment, should be noted. Additionally, you should document that the patient was instructed to call back if the condition worsened or if he or she reconsidered. A detailed examination generally is not performed on a patient who refuses (document it if it is done).
   (Objective 6)

10. a. A special form may be required to document these situations. You should always keep a record in case subsequent liability results.
   (Objective 6)

11. b. Some agencies and states require separate reports. Patient care information should be completed only by the paramedic on the call. Corrections and revisions should be made as soon as possible.
   (Objective 7)

WRAP IT UP

1. Medical audit, quality improvement, billing and administration, data collection, written record for other health care professionals to reference
   (Objective 2)

2. Dates, response times, difficulties en route, scene observations, reasons for extended on scene time, time of patient transport
   (Objective 3)

3. c. Local and state policy for report correction should be followed.
   (Objective 7)

IN THIS PART

Pharmacology

READING ASSIGNMENT
Chapter 17, pages 332-387 , in *Mosby's Paramedic Textbook,* ed. 3

OBJECTIVES
Upon completion of this chapter, the paramedic student will be able to:
1. Explain what a drug is.
2. Identify the four types of drug names.
3. Outline drug standards and legislation and the enforcement agencies pertinent to the paramedic profession.
4. Describe the paramedic's responsibilities in drug administration.
5. Distinguish among drug forms.
6. Outline autonomic nervous system functions that may be changed with drug therapy.
7. Discuss factors that influence drug absorption, distribution, and elimination.
8. Describe how drugs react with receptors to produce their desired effects.
9. List variables that can influence drug interactions.
10. Identify special considerations for administering pharmacological agents to pregnant patients, pediatric patients, and older patients.
11. Outline drug actions and care considerations for a patient who is given drugs that affect the nervous, cardiovascular, respiratory, endocrine, and gastrointestinal systems.
12. Explain the meaning of drug terms that are necessary to interpret information in drug references safely.

SUMMARY
- A drug may be defined as any substance taken by mouth; injected into a muscle, blood vessel, or cavity of the body; or applied topically to treat or prevent a disease or condition.
- Drugs can be identified by four types of names. These include the chemical name; generic or nonproprietary name; trade, brand, or proprietary name; and official name.
- The Drug Enforcement Agency is the sole legal drug enforcement body in the United States. Other regulatory bodies or services include the FDA; the Public Health Service; the Federal Trade Commission; in Canada, the Health Protection Branch of the Department of National Health and Welfare; and for international drug control, the International Narcotics Control Board.
- Paramedics are held responsible for the safe and effective administration of drugs. In fact, they are responsible for each drug they provide to a patient. They are legally, morally, and ethically responsible.
- Drug allergies can be divided into four classifications based on the mechanism of the immune reaction. They are type I (anaphylactic), type II (cytotoxic), type III (serum sickness), and type IV (contact dermatitis) reactions.
- The parasympathetic and sympathetic nervous systems function continuously. They innervate many of the same organs at the same time. The opposing actions of the two systems balance each other. In general, the sympathetic

system dominates during stressful events. The parasympathetic system is most active during times of emotional and physical calm.

- The degree to which drugs attain pharmacological activity depends partly on the rate and extent to which they are absorbed. Absorption in turn depends on the ability of the drug to cross the cell membrane. The rate and extent of absorption depend on the nature of the cell membrane the drug must cross, blood flow to the site of administration, solubility of the drug, pH of the drug environment, drug concentration, and drug dosage form.
- The route of drug administration influences drug absorption. These routes can be classified as enteral, parenteral, pulmonary, and topical.
- Distribution is the transport of a drug through the bloodstream to various tissues of the body and ultimately to its site of action. After absorption and distribution, the body eliminates most drugs. The body first biotransforms the drug and then excretes the drug. The kidney is the primary organ for excretion; however, the intestine, lungs, and mammary, sweat, and salivary glands also may be involved.
- Many factors can alter the response to drug therapy, including age, body mass, gender, pathological state, genetic factors, and psychological factors.
- Most drug actions are thought to result from a chemical interaction. This interaction is between the drug and various receptors throughout the body. The most common form of drug action is the drug-receptor interaction.
- Many variables can influence drug interactions, including intestinal absorption, competition for plasma-protein binding, biotransformation, action at the receptor site, renal excretion, and alteration of electrolyte balance.
- Narcotic analgesics relieve pain. Narcotic antagonists reverse the narcotic effects of some analgesics. Nonnarcotic analgesics interfere with local mediators released when tissue is damaged in the periphery of the body. These mediators stimulate nerve endings and cause pain.
- Anesthetic drugs are CNS depressants that have a reversible effect on nervous tissue. Antianxiety agents are used to reduce feelings of apprehension, nervousness, worry, or fearfulness. Sedatives and hypnotics are drugs that depress the CNS. They produce a calming effect. They also help induce sleep. Alcohol is a general CNS depressant that can produce sedation, sleep, and anesthesia.
- Anticonvulsant drugs are used to treat seizure disorders. Most notably they treat epilepsy.
- All CNS stimulants work to increase excitability. They do this by blocking activity of inhibitory neurons or their respective neurotransmitters or by enhancing the production of the excitatory neurotransmitters.
- Psychotherapeutic drugs include antipsychotic agents, antidepressants, and lithium. These drugs are used to treat psychoses and affective disorders, especially schizophrenia, depression, and mania.
- Several movement disorders can result from an imbalance of dopamine and acetylcholine. Drugs that inhibit or block acetylcholine are referred to as anticholinergic. Three classes of drugs affect brain dopamine: those that release dopamine, those that increase brain levels of dopamine, and dopaminergic agonists.
- The autonomic drugs mimic or block the effects of the sympathetic and parasympathetic divisions of the autonomic nervous system. These drugs are classified into four groups: cholinergic (parasympathomimetic) drugs, cholinergic blocking (parasympatholytic) drugs, adrenergic (sympathomimetic) drugs, and adrenergic blocking (sympatholytic) drugs.
- Skeletal muscle relaxants can be classified as central acting, direct acting, and neuromuscular blockers.
- Cardiac drugs are classified by their effects on specialized cardiac tissues. Cardiac glycosides are used to treat congestive heart failure and certain tachycardias. Antidysrhythmic drugs are used to treat and prevent disorders of cardiac rhythm. The pharmacological agents that suppress dysrhythmias may do so by direct action on the cardiac cell membrane (lidocaine), by indirect action that affects the cell (propranolol), or both.
- Antihypertensive drugs used to reduce blood pressure are classified into four major categories: diuretics, sympathetic blocking agents (sympatholytic drugs), vasodilators, and ACE inhibitors. Calcium channel blockers also are used to treat persons with hypertension who do not respond to other drug therapies.
- Antihemorrheologic agents are used to treat peripheral vascular disorders. These disorders are caused by pathological or physiological obstruction (e.g., arteriosclerosis). These agents improve blood flow to ischemic tissues.
- Drugs that affect blood coagulation may be classified as antiplatelet, anticoagulant, or fibrinolytic agents. Drugs that interfere with platelet aggregation are known as antiplatelet or antithrombic drugs. Anticoagulant drug therapy is designed to prevent intravascular thrombosis. The therapy decreases blood coagulability. Fibrinolytic drugs dissolve clots after their formation. These drugs work by promoting the digestion of fibrin.
- Hemophilia is a group of hereditary bleeding disorders. These disorders involve a deficiency of one of the factors needed for the coagulation of blood. Replacing the missing clotting factor can help manage hemophilia.

- Hemostatic agents speed up clot formation, thus reducing bleeding. Systemic hemostatic agents are used to control blood loss after surgery. They work by inhibiting the breakdown of fibrin. Topical hemostatic agents are used to control capillary bleeding. They are used during surgical and dental procedures.
- The treatment of choice in managing a loss of blood or blood components is to replace the sole blood component that is deficient. Replacement therapy may include transfusing whole blood (rare), packed red blood cells, fresh-frozen plasma, plasma expanders, platelets, coagulation factors, fibrinogen, albumin, or gamma globulins.
- Hyperlipidemia refers to an excess of lipids in the plasma. Antihyperlipidemic drugs sometimes are used along with diet and exercise to control serum lipid levels.
- Bronchodilator drugs are the primary form of treatment for obstructive pulmonary disease such as asthma, chronic bronchitis, and emphysema. These drugs may be classified as sympathomimetic drugs and xanthine derivatives.
- Mucokinetic drugs are used to move respiratory secretions, excessive mucus, and sputum along the tracheo-bronchial tree.
- Oxygen is used chiefly to treat hypoxia and hypoxemia.
- Direct respiratory stimulant drugs act directly on the medullary center of the brain. These drugs are analeptics. They increase the rate and depth of respiration.
- Spirits of ammonia is a reflex respiratory stimulant. The drug is administered by inhalation.
- A cough may be prolonged or may result from an underlying disorder. In such a case, treatment with antitussive drugs may be indicated.
- The main clinical use of antihistamines is for allergic reactions. They also are used to control motion sickness or as a sedative or antiemetic.
- Drug therapy for the gastrointestinal system can be divided into drugs that affect the stomach and drugs that affect the lower gastrointestinal tract. Antacids buffer or neutralize hydrochloric acid in the stomach. Antiflatulents prevent the formation of gas in the gastrointestinal tract. Digestant drugs promote digestion in the gastrointestinal tract. They do this by releasing small amounts of hydrochloric acid in the stomach. Drugs used to induce vomiting may be administered as part of the treatment of certain drug overdoses and poisonings. Drugs used to treat nausea and vomiting include antagonists of histamine, acetylcholine, and dopamine and other drugs the actions of which are not understood clearly.
- Cytoprotective agents and other drugs are used to treat peptic ulcer disease by protecting the gastric mucosa. H_2 receptor antagonists block the H_2 receptors. They also reduce the volume of gastric acid secretion and its acid content.
- Two common conditions of the lower gastrointestinal tract may require drug therapy: constipation and diarrhea. Drugs used to manage these conditions include laxatives and antidiarrheals.
- Drugs used to treat eye disorders include antiglaucoma agents, mydriatics, cycloplegics, antiinfective/antiinflammatory agents, and topical anesthetics.
- Drugs used to treat disorders of the ear include antibiotics, steroid/antibiotic combinations, and miscellaneous preparations.
- The endocrine system works to control and integrate body functions. A number of drugs are used to treat disorders of the anterior and posterior pituitary, the thyroid and parathyroid glands, and the adrenal cortex.
- The pancreatic hormones play a key role in regulating the amount of certain nutrients in the circulatory system. The two main hormones secreted by the pancreas are insulin and glucagon. Imbalances in either of these may call for drug therapy. This therapy is meant to correct metabolic derangements.
- Drugs that affect the female reproductive system include synthetic and natural substances such as hormones, oral contraceptives, ovulation stimulants, and drugs used to treat infertility.
- The male sex hormone is testosterone. Adequate amounts of this hormone are needed for normal development. Adequate amounts also are needed for the maintenance of male sex characteristics.
- Antineoplastic agents are used in cancer chemotherapy to prevent the increase of malignant cells.
- Antibiotics are used to treat local or systemic infection. This group includes penicillin, cephalosporins, and related products; macrolide antibiotics; tetracyclines; and miscellaneous antibiotic agents.
- Persons can be infected by bacterial organisms, fungi, and viruses. Examples of antifungal drugs include tolnaftate (Tinactin), fluconazole (Diflucan), and nystatin (Mycostatin).
- Few drugs exist for use in any viral infections. One antiviral drug is acyclovir (Zovirax). This drug is effective against herpes infection. Another one is zidovudine (Retrovir, AZT), which currently is used to treat human immunodeficiency virus infection.

- Drugs used to treat inflammation or its symptoms may be classified as analgesic-antipyretic drugs and non-steroidal antiinflammatory drugs. A number of medications have both properties.
- Immunosuppressant drugs reduce the activity of the immune system. They do this by suppressing the production and activity of lymphocytes. These drugs are prescribed after transplant surgery. They can help to prevent the rejection of foreign tissues. They also are sometimes given to halt the progress of autoimmune disorders.
- Immunomodulating agents are drugs that help the immune system to be more efficient. They do this by activating the immune defenses and by modifying a biological response to an unwanted stimulus.
- Serum contains agents of immunity. These are antibodies. The antibodies can protect against an organism if the serum is injected into someone else. This forms the basis for passive immunization. Vaccines are composed of killed or altered microorganisms. These are administered to a person to produce specific immunity to a disease-causing bacterial toxin, virus, or bacterium (active immunization).

REVIEW QUESTIONS

Match the appropriate drug form in Column II with its description in Column I. Use each drug form only once.

Column I		Column II
1. _H_	Semisolid medicine in a greasy base externally applied to the skin	a. Capsule
2. _B_	A sweetened alcohol and water solution	b. Elixir
3. _J_	Drug ground into loose granules	c. Emulsion
4. _i_	Drug compressed into small disks	d. Extract
5. _k_	Drug dissolved in sugar and water suspension (magma)	e. Liniment
6. _l_	Flat or round medicine held in mouth until dissolved	f. Lotion
7. _A_	Gelatin-covered, dry drug preparation	g. Aqueous
8. _c_	Suspension of fat or oil in water with an agent that decreases surface tension	h. Ointment
9. _G_	Suspension of insoluble particles in water	i. Tablets
		j. Powder
		k. Aqueous solution
		l. Troche

10. Complete the following sentences by listing the appropriate drug name:
The precise composition and molecular structure of a drug are described in its (a) _chemical NA_ name. The name that is not protected by law and denotes pharmacologically similar drugs is known as the

(b) _GENERIC_ name. The trademarked name of the drug designated by the company

that manufactures it is the (c) _TRADE_ name. The initials *USP* or *NF* follow the

(d) _Official_ name.

11. In one sentence, describe how the following drug standards or legislation influence medication administration and distribution in the United States:
   a. Pure Food and Drug Act (1906):

   _____

   b. Federal Drug and Cosmetic Act (1938):

   _____

   c. Harrison Narcotic Act (1914):

   _____

12. List the agency responsible for each of the following aspects of drug control:
   a. It has the power to suppress false or misleading advertising regarding drugs to the general public.

   _____

   b. It is responsible for enforcing the federal Food, Drug, and Cosmetic Act.

   _____

   c. It monitors the distribution of controlled substances.

   _____

   d. It regulates biological products like antitoxins.

   _____

13. Refer to the *Physician's Desk Reference* (PDR) or *Mosby's DRUGConsult,* common drug reference sources, to find the answers to the following questions.
   a. What is the indication for the drug beclomethasone?

   _____

   b. List the contraindications and side effects of this drug.

   _____

Questions 14 to 17 pertain to the following case study:

   Dispatch alerts you to respond to a call for an "accidental injury." When you arrive on the scene, you find a 35-year-old man who stumbled and fell, injuring his wrist. There is deformity, swelling, crepitus, and tenderness proximal to his right hand. After application of the appropriate splint and ice, you decide that medication for pain is indicated.

14. What eight points are critical to ensure that you meet your legal, moral, and ethical obligations for safe, effective medication administration to this patient?

   a. Expiration Date

   b. Allergies

   c. Righ meDS

   d. Right Dose

   e.

   f.

   g.

   h.

   After eliciting a careful history and consultation with medical direction, you initiate an intravenous line in the uninjured extremity and administer ketorolac tromethamine (Toradol) intravenous push. Several moments after administration, the patient becomes anxious and states that he feels like "his throat is going to close in." His skin appears flushed, and a large, flat, raised rash is erupting. The patient states he has never taken this drug before.

15. What type of reaction is this patient having?

   _____

16. List two emergency drugs that may be used to treat this patient's signs and symptoms.

   _____

After you arrive at the emergency department, the patient admits to the physician that he has had a reaction to aspirin in the past (although during your history, he denied allergic reaction). The physician tells you that there is a reported cross-reactivity between aspirin and ketorolac tromethamine.

17. How would you have known that this type of reaction was possible?

_____

18. Select the appropriate drug term from the following list to complete the sentences:

Antagonism	Potentiation
Contraindications	Side effect
Cumulative action	Stimulant
Depressant	Summation
Drug allergy	Synergism
Drug dependence	Therapeutic action
Drug interaction	Tolerance
Idiosyncrasy	Untoward effect

a. An abnormal or peculiar response to a drug that possibly is caused by a genetic deficiency is

IDIOSYNCRASY.

b. Caffeine and methylphenidate (Ritalin) are examples of drugs that exhibit a(n)

Stimulant effect.

c. A drug action caused by an immunological response to a previous exposure is a(n)

Drug Allergy reaction.

d. The desired effect of naloxone on narcotics is attributed to _Antagonism_.

e. The enhancement of the effects of one drug caused by the concurrent administration of a second drug is

Potentiation.

f. An undesirable effect of a drug that is harmful to the patient is a(n) _Side effect_.

g. The combined action of two drugs that is greater than the sum of each individual agent acting

independently is _Synergism_.

h. The intense physical or emotional disturbance possibly resulting when a narcotic is withheld from a person

who frequently uses it is a result of _Drug Dependence_.

i. A drug that diminishes a person's central nervous system function is a _Depressant_.

j. The ability of atropine to increase the heart rate is known as the desired effect, or _Therapeutic Action_

k. The list of factors used to describe situations when medication administration would be harmful is the

Contra indications.

l. Concurrent administration of drugs such that one agent modifies the actions of the other is

Drug interaction.

m. A decreased response to a drug after repetitive doses, which necessitates higher doses to achieve the desired

effect, is _Tolerance_.

n. When repeat administration of drugs results in absorption that exceeds metabolism and excretion, the increased effect that results is known as _____.

19. List six factors that influence the rate and extent to which a drug is absorbed in the body.

a.

b.

c.

d.

e.

f.

20. List four groups of drugs that are associated with a high incidence of drug-drug interactions.

a. Blood thinners tricyclic

b. Tricyclic Antidepressants

c. Amphetamines

d. Digitalis

21. You need to administer acetaminophen to a child who has been vomiting repeatedly. What enteral route will you choose?

Rectal

22. When giving epinephrine to an asthmatic patient, a slow and sustained effect is desirable to minimize side effects and prolong the effects of the drug. You will administer the drug by the Subcutaneous route.

23. Your 76-year-old patient has a heart rate of 34 and a blood pressure of 70 mm Hg by palpation. You wish to give atropine to increase the heart rate. What route will you choose? I.V.

24. A 3-month-old infant is in hemorrhagic shock after sustaining a gunshot wound to the abdomen. After intravenous attempts are unsuccessful, what route will you consider for fluid volume resuscitation?

I.O.

25. Is the rate of drug absorption by the pulmonary route faster or slower than the subcutaneous route?

faster

26. List the two physiological barriers to drug distribution within the body.

a. Placental Barrier

b. Blood-Brain Barrier

27. Circle the appropriate response regarding drug effects in children.
   a. The blood-brain barrier in infants is less/more effective than in adults; therefore the central nervous system effects of drugs will be less/more.

   b. The newborn has a(n) decreased/increased ability to metabolize drugs; therefore drug toxicity is less/more likely to occur.

28. List three physiological factors that may result in altered drug absorption, distribution, biotransformation, or elimination in the older adult.

   a.

   b.

   c.

29. You are called to a sparsely furnished, one-room apartment to care for a 79-year-old woman complaining of difficulty breathing. She states that she has a history of heart disease and "swelling," and she hands you a sack of empty medication bottles that contained furosemide, digoxin, and potassium. She thinks she last took them 5 or 6 days ago. Discuss three possible reasons for the patient's medication noncompliance.

   a.

   b.

   c.

DRUG CLASSIFICATIONS

30. When given the following description and drug name, identify the drug group to which it belongs and give one additional example of another drug from the same group.
   a. Your patient says he takes lorazepam (Ativan) to help him relax.

   Drug group: _____ Example: _____

   b. You arrive in the emergency department with a 65-year-old woman experiencing an acute myocardial infarction. Immediately, the emergency department staff administers tissue plasminogen activator in an attempt to dissolve the clot.

   Drug group: _____ Example: _____

   c. Before your Mediterranean cruise, you take dimenhydrinate (Dramamine) to prevent seasickness.

   Drug group: _____ Example: _____

   d. During a cardiopulmonary arrest or in selected cases of shock, drugs such as epinephrine (Adrenalin) may be used to stimulate the heart.

   Drug group: _____ Example: _____

   e. Your 45-year-old patient is complaining of chest pain. His only home medication is hydrochlorothiazide (HCTZ) for hypertension.

   Drug group: _____ Example: _____

   f. An older patient is taking captopril (Capoten) for her congestive heart failure.

   Drug group: _____ Example: _____

g. A 30-year-old patient with a seizure disorder is taking phenobarbital (Luminal).

Drug group: _____ Example: _____

h. A 52-year-old hospice patient is taking hydromorphone (Dilaudid) to control his pain.

Drug group: _____ Example: _____

i. Diltiazem (Cardizem) is used by a patient who states that she takes it to control a fast heart rhythm.

Drug group: _____ Example: _____

j. A person at risk for developing clots that may cause heart attack or stroke may be prescribed dipyridamole (Persantine).

Drug group: _____ Example: _____

k. Asthmatics may have a large number of home medicines that may include isoetharine hydrochloride (Bronkosol).

Drug group: _____ Example: _____

l. You observe a patient in the emergency department who is drowsy and having difficulty speaking moments after she has been given etomidate (Amidate).

Drug group: _____ Example: _____

m. You will have increased vigilance for evidence of bleeding if a patient tells you he is taking warfarin sodium (Coumadin).

Drug group: _____ Example: _____

n. A 35-year-old patient is experiencing complications following an outpatient surgical procedure. Her only home medication is pentazocine (Talwin).

Drug group: _____ Example: _____

o. Asthmatic patients may be taking a variety of drugs besides bronchodilators in an attempt to control their disease. Examples of these include cromolyn sodium (Intal), beclomethasone dipropionate (Vanceril Inhaler), and ipratropium (Atrovent).

Drug group: _____ Example: _____

p. You are dispatched to a call for an unconscious person. The patient is awake but confused and combative when you arrive and has a medication list that includes ethosuximide (Zarontin).

Drug group: _____ Example: _____

q. You are treating a young woman with a history of depression. She has taken all 20 of her fluoxetine (Prozac) in a suicide attempt.

Drug group: _____ Example: _____

r. When you arrive at the emergency department with a combative, psychotic patient in restraints, the nurse gives the patient an intramuscular injection of haloperidol (Haldol).

Drug group: _____ Example: _____

s. A patient with a chronic pain disorder is taking amitriptyline (Elavil).

Drug group: _____ Example: _____

t. Medications for management of gastroesophageal reflux disease may include esomeprazole (Nexium).

Drug group: _____ Example: _____

u. During your annual physical, a blood test reveals that you have high cholesterol. The doctor prescribes atorvastatin (Lipitor).

Drug group: _____ Example: _____

v. A patient with Parkinson's disease is taking levodopa (Larodopa).

Drug group: _____ Example: _____

w. Your patient is vomiting blood. His home medicines include ranitidine (Zantac).

Drug group: _____ Example: _____

31. List the generic name of one drug and its general mechanism of actions for each of the following groups of antidysrhythmic drugs.

Group	Generic Name	Actions
IA		
IB		
IC		
II		
III		
IV		

32. Fill in the missing information about hypertensive medications in the following table:

Classification	Generic Name	Actions
	Furosemide, hydrochlorothiazide, spironolactone with hydrochlorothiazide (Aldactazide)	
Beta-blocking agents		
		Block sympathetic stimulation, have multiple sites of action
	Diazoxide, hydralazine, minoxidil (arteriolar dilator), sodium nitroprusside, amyl nitrite, isosorbide dinitrate, nitroglycerin (arteriolar and venous dilator drugs)	
Angiotensin II receptor antagonists	Irbesartan (Avapro), losartan (Cozaar, Hyzaar), valsartan (Diovan)	
Calcium channel blockers		Decrease peripheral resistance by inhibiting blockers, decreasing the contractility of vascular smooth muscle

33. Match the drug listed in Column II with the endocrine gland that it affects in Column I. Use each drug only once.

Column I
_____ Adrenal cortex
_____ Ovary
_____ Pancreas
_____ Parathyroid
_____ Pituitary
_____ Testes
_____ Thyroid

Column II
a. Clomiphene citrate (Clomid)
b. Dexamethasone (Decadron)
c. Iodine products
d. Methyltestosterone (Metandren)
e. Glimepiride (Amaryl)
f. Vasopressin
g. Vitamin D

STUDENT SELF-ASSESSMENT

34. Any substance taken by mouth; injected into a muscle, blood vessel, or cavity of the body; or applied topically to treat or prevent a disease or condition is a(n)
    a. Antidote
    b. Drug
    c. Parenteral
    d. Vaccine

35. Morphine is regulated under the Controlled Substance Act of 1970 and is a Schedule _____ drug.
    a. I
    b. II
    c. III
    d. IV

36. The blood-brain barrier and placental barrier will allow passage of only
    a. Antibiotics
    b. Lipid-soluble drugs
    c. Undissociated drugs
    d. Water-soluble drugs

37. Agonists are drugs that do which of the following?
    a. Bind to a receptor and cause a specific response.
    b. Bind to a receptor and cause no response.
    c. Cause duplication of specific receptors.
    d. Prevent chemicals from reaching the receptor sites.

38. The measurement of the relative safety of a drug is which of the following?
    a. Biological half-life
    b. Median effective dose
    c. Median lethal dose
    d. Therapeutic index

39. Which of the following drugs is recommended for administration by endotracheal tube?
    a. Bretylium
    b. Hydroxyzine
    c. Diazepam
    d. Naloxone

40. Which of the following drug administration routes will deliver the most rapid effects?
    a. Oral
    b. Intramuscular
    c. Subcutaneous
    d. Transtracheal

41. Your patient is in profound shock following myocardial infarction. The route of choice for drug administration will be which of the following?
    a. Intramuscular
    b. Intravenous
    c. By mouth
    d. Subcutaneous

42. Which of the following is an opioid antagonist?
    a. Butorphanol tartrate
    b. Naloxone hydrochloride
    c. Oxycodone hydrochloride
    d. Pentazocine hydrochloride

43. All of the following drugs have anticonvulsant properties except which one?
    a. Diazepam
    b. Magnesium sulfate
    c. Nalbuphine
    d. Phenytoin

44. You are transporting a patient with a history of narcolepsy. What drugs might you find that he is taking to reduce his symptoms of this disorder?
    a. Methamphetamine (Desoxyn)
    b. Methylphenidate (Ritalin)
    c. Pemoline (Cylert)
    d. Phenmetrazine (Preludin)

45. Drugs such as levodopa (Larodopa) and carbidopa-levodopa (Sinemet) enhance brain dopamine levels and are used to treat which of the following?
   a. Depression
   b. Hypotension
   c. Myasthenia gravis
   d. Parkinson's disease

46. You are experiencing severe muscle spasms after injuring your back at work. Which of the following is an anti-spasmodic medication that may be prescribed for you?
   a. Carbamazepine (Tegretol)
   b. Chlordiazepoxide (Librium)
   c. Chlorpromazine (Thorazine)
   d. Cyclobenzaprine (Flexeril)

47. The drugs vecuronium (Norcuron) and succinylcholine (Anectine) may be used for rapid sequence induction of intubation in a person who has sustained severe head trauma. The primary action of these drugs in this situation is which of the following?
   a. To decrease intracranial pressure
   b. To dry oral secretions
   c. To paralyze the muscles
   d. To provide pain relief

48. An indirect-acting cholinergic drug that may be used in the management of poisoning from atropine is which of the following?
   a. Glucagon
   b. Lorazepam
   c. Physostigmine
   d. Verapamil

49. What is the chief neurotransmitter for the parasympathetic nervous system?
   a. Acetylcholine
   b. Epinephrine (Adrenalin)
   c. Metaraminol (Aramine)
   d. Norepinephrine

50. Stimulation of the beta$_2$-adrenergic receptors will cause which of the following?
   a. Negative inotropic effect on the heart
   b. Positive inotropic effect on the heart
   c. Bronchiolar dilation
   d. Peripheral vasoconstriction

51. Epinephrine has which of the following?
   a. Alpha effects only
   b. Beta effects only
   c. Alpha and beta effects
   d. Neither alpha nor beta effects

52. Drugs that increase the contractility of the heart have a positive _____ effect.
   a. Chronotropic
   b. Cholinergic
   c. Dromotropic
   d. Inotropic

53. You are called to the home of an older man who is complaining of dizziness, nausea, vomiting, weakness, and yellow vision. When questioned about his home medications, he states that he takes a small tablet to help his "weak heart." His pulse is 45 per minute. You suspect he is suffering from which of the following?
   a. Digoxin overdose
   b. Isoproterenol overdose
   c. Tricyclic antidepressant overdose
   d. Verapamil overdose

54. Which of the following is a group IV antidysrhythmic drug?
   a. Bretylium tosylate
   b. Lidocaine
   c. Procainamide
   d. Verapamil

55. The primary mechanism by which antihypertensives reduce blood pressure is by decreasing which of the following?
   a. Cardiac output
   b. Intravascular blood volume
   c. Myocardial contractility
   d. Peripheral vascular resistance

56. Which of the following drugs acts by dissolving a clot that has formed already?
   a. Aspirin
   b. Coumadin
   c. Heparin
   d. Streptokinase

57. Which of the following is a beta$_2$-specific bronchodilator?
   a. Albuterol
   b. Aminophylline
   c. Ephedrine
   d. Isoproterenol

58. All of the following are indications for antihistamines except which one?
   a. Allergic reactions
   b. Asthma
   c. Motion sickness
   d. Nausea and vomiting

59. An elderly patient has a disorder necessitating the use of pilocarpine drops. What is he suffering from?
    a. Conjunctivitis
    b. Glaucoma
    c. Keratitis
    d. Pain

60. Which of the following is true about insulin?
    a. It is secreted by the adrenal glands.
    b. It is secreted only during stress.
    c. It will increase the use of fat for fuel.
    d. It will move glucose into the cells.

61. Your patient states that she is allergic to penicillin. Which of the following drugs can she take safely?
    a. Amoxicillin (Amoxil)
    b. Cefazolin (Ancef)
    c. Dicloxacillin (Dynapen)
    d. Tetracycline (Achromycin)

62. Which of the following is an antiviral drug used in treatment of patients infected with human immunodeficiency virus?
    a. Acyclovir (Zovirax)
    b. Pyrimethamine (Daraprim)
    c. Quinine (Quinamm)
    d. Zidovudine (Retrovir)

63. Isoniazid (INH) and rifampin (Rifadin) are drugs used to treat which of the following?
    a. HIV infection
    b. Leprosy
    c. Malaria
    d. Tuberculosis

WRAP IT UP

You are dispatched to the home of an elderly male who has been "passing out." When you arrive, you find him to be conscious but confused and unable to give you any history. He is pale and sweaty, has vomited, and has the following vital signs: BP 90/54 mm Hg, P 56/min, and R 16/min. When you listen to his lungs, you hear crackles in the bases on both sides. You find a medication list that indicates he is allergic to penicillin and the following list of current medicines: digoxin (Lanoxin), atenolol, amiodarone, Humulin insulin 70/30, propoxyphene, lorazepam, sertraline, cyclobenzaprine, diltiazem, aspirin, furosemide, K-Dur (potassium), ipratropium, albuterol, ranitidine, and azithromycin.

  1. What type of medication allergy reaction is penicillin most likely to cause?
    a. Type I, anaphylactic
    b. Type II, cytotoxic
    c. Type III, serum sickness
    d. Type IV, contact dermatitis

_____

  2. Which of his home medications have an effect on the autonomic nervous system?

Atenolol

  3. Which of his home medications are given by the parenteral route?

Humulin - Insulin is Subcutaneous

  4. One of his medications, Lanoxin, has a very low therapeutic index. Why is that important for you to know?

_____

  5. What factors may contribute to medication noncompliance in an older adult?

_____

  6. Which of his home medications could be contributing to his confusion?

_____

7. Which of his medications is a(n)

   a. Antihypertensive

   b. Antidysrhythmic (list specific class)

   c. Antiplatelet

   d. Muscle relaxant

   e. Controlled substancei

   f. Bronchodilator

   g. Analgesic

   h. H_2 receptor antagonist

   i. Antibiotic

8. Because the patient is unable to give you information about his medical history, you must try to determine what medical conditions he could have based on his medication list. What conditions do you suspect he suffers from?

9. Based on this knowledge and your physical exam of the patient, what are some possible causes for his signs and symptoms today?

CHAPTER 17 ANSWERS

REVIEW QUESTIONS

1. h	**6.** l
2. b	**7.** a
3. j	**8.** c
4. i	**9.** g
5. k	

(Questions 1 to 9, Objective 5)

10. a. Chemical
b. Generic or nonproprietary
c. Trade or proprietary
d. Official
(Objective 2)

11. a. Protected the public from mislabeled drugs, prohibited the use of false and misleading claims for medications, and restricted sales of drugs with abuse potential
b. Prevented marketing of drugs until they were tested and required names of all ingredients and directions on labels
c. Controlled the sale of narcotics and established *narcotic* as a legal term
(Objective 3)

12. a. Federal Trade Commission
b. Food and Drug Administration
c. Drug Enforcement Administration
d. Public Health Service
(Objective 3)

13. a. For chronic control of bronchial asthma
b. Contraindicated in the treatment of acute episodes of asthma or status asthmaticus or if a known hypersensitivity exists (PDR)
(Objective 12)

14. A paramedic's responsibilities relative to drug administration include the following: using correct techniques; observing and documenting effects of drugs; maintaining current knowledge regarding pharmacology; maintaining professional relationships; understanding pharmacology; evaluating drug indications and contraindications; using drug reference materials; taking a patient history; and consulting with medical direction.
(Objective 4)

15. The patient is demonstrating signs and symptoms of a type I hypersensitivity allergic reaction.
(Objective 4)

16. The chemicals histamine and slow-reacting substance of anaphylaxis are released during an anaphylactic reaction. Diphenhydramine and/or epinephrine are used to treat this.
(Objective 4)

17. Sometimes patients may have an allergic reaction to a drug they have never taken that is chemically similar to another drug to which they are allergic. This information can be found in the drug profile.
(Objective 4)

18. a. Idiosyncrasy   i. Depressant
    b. Stimulant   j. Therapeutic action
    c. Drug allergy   k. Contraindications
    d. Antagonism   l. Drug interaction
    e. Potentiation   m. Tolerance
    f. Side effect   n. Cumulative action.
    g. Synergism
    h. Drug dependence
    (Objective 12)

19. The nature of the absorbing surface through which the drug must travel, the blood flow to the site of adminis-tration, the solubility of the drug, the pH of the drug environment, the drug concentration, and the drug dosage form
(Objective 7)

20. Drug-drug interactions commonly are associated with blood thinners, tricyclic antidepressants, ampheta-mines, digitalis glycosides, diuretics, alcohol, antihypertensives, and cigarette smoking.
(Objective 9)

21. Rectal
(Objective 10)

22. Subcutaneous
(Objective 11)

23. Intravenous
(Objective 11)

24. Intraosseous
(Objective 11)

25. Faster
(Objective 7)

26. Placenta and blood-brain barrier
(Objective 7)

27. a. Less, more
    b. Decreased, more
    (Objective 10)

28. Decreased renal function, altered nutrition habits, greater consumption of nonprescription drugs, reduced gas-tric acid, slowed gastric motility, decreased serum albumin, congestive heart failure, and decreased blood flow to the liver
(Objective 10)

29. Inability to pay for new drugs, forgetfulness or confusion, lack of symptoms (causing patient to become non-compliant), and other physical disabilities not mentioned
(Objective 10)

30. a. Benzodiazepines: alprazolam (Xanax), chlordiazepoxide (Librium), clorazepate (Tranxene), diazepam (Valium), flurazepam (Dalmane), lorazepam (Ativan), midazolam (Versed), temazepam (Restoril), clon-azepam (Klonopin).
    b. Fibrinolytic agents: anisoylated plasminogen streptokinase activator (Eminase), streptokinase (Streptase), reteplase (Retavase), tenecteplase (TNKase)

c. Antiemetics/antihistamines: diphenhydramine hydrochloride (Benadryl), hydroxyzine pamoate (Vistaril), meclizine hydrochloride (Antivert), promethazine hydrochloride (Phenergan)

d. Adrenergics: dobutamine (Dobutrex), dopamine (Intropin), isoproterenol (Isuprel), norepinephrine (Levophed)

e. Diuretics: furosemide (Lasix), spironolactone (Aldactone).

f. Angiotensin-converting enzyme (ACE) inhibitor: enalapril (Vasotec), benazepril (Lotensin), fosinopril (Monopril), lisinopril (Prinivil, Zestril), quinapril (Accupril)

g. Anticonvulsants, barbiturate: mephobarbital (Gemonil)

h. Narcotic analgesics: codeine, methylmorphine, meperidine (Demerol), methadone (Dolophine, Methadose), morphine sulfate (Astramorph and others), oxycodone (Percodan, Tylox, Percocet), propoxyphene (Darvon, Dolene), hydrocodone (Lortab).

i. Class IV antidysrhythmics: verapamil (Isoptin), amlodipine (Norvasc), felodipine (Plendil)

j. Antiplatelet agents: aspirin, sulfinpyrazone (Anturane), clopidogrel (Plavix), ticlopidine (Ticlid), abciximab (ReoPro)

k. Beta$_2$-selective bronchodilators: albuterol (Proventil, Ventolin), bitolterol (Tornalate), terbutaline sulfate (Brethine, Bricanyl), salmeterol (Serevent), levalbuterol (Xopenex)

l. Nonbarbiturate anesthetic agents: fentanyl (Sublimaze), sufentanil (Sufenta), alfentanil (Alfenta)

m. Anticoagulants: heparin sodium (Liquaemin)

n. Opioid agonist-antagonist agents: nalbuphine hydrochloride (Nubain)

o. Muscarinic antagonists used to treat respiratory emergencies: glycopyrrolate (Robinul)

p. Anticonvulsants (succinimides): methsuximide (Celontin), phensuximide (Milontin)

q. Selective serotonin reuptake inhibitors: sertraline (Zoloft), paroxetine (Paxil), fluvoxamine (Luvox), and citalopram (Celexa)

r. Antipsychotic agents: chlorpromazine (Thorazine), thioridazine (Mellaril), fluphenazine (Prolixin), molindone (Lidone), loxapine (Loxitane), olanzapine, resperidol

s. Tricyclic antidepressants: mirtazapine (Remeron), nortriptyline (Pamelor)

t. Proton pump inhibitors: lansoprazole (Prevacid), omeprazole (Prilosec), pantoprazole (Protonix), rabeprazole (AcipHex)

u. Antihyperlipidemic drugs: fenofibrate (Tricor), fluvastatin (Lescol), gemfibrozil (Lopid), pravastatin (Pravachol), simvastatin (Zocor)

v. Drugs that affect brain dopamine (used in treatment of Parkinson's disease): cabidopa-levodopa (Sinemet), amantadine (Symmetrel), bromocriptine (Parlodel), pergolide (Permax)

w. H$_2$-receptor antagonists: cimetidine (Tagamet), famotidine (Pepcid)

(Objective 12)

31.

Group	Drug Name	Actions
IA	Quinidine, procainamide	Decrease conduction velocity; prolong electrical potential of cardiac tissue
IB	Lidocaine, phenytoin	Increase or have no effect on conduction velocity
IC	Flecainide, encainide	Profoundly slow conduction
II	Propranolol	Beta-blockers
III	Bretylium, amiodarone	Antiadrenergic agents; positive inotropic action; terminate reentry dysrhythmias
IV	Verapamil, diltiazem	Block flow of calcium into cardiac and smooth muscle cells; decrease automaticity

(Objective 11)

32.

Classification	Generic Name	Actions
Diuretics	Furosemide, hydrochlorothiazide, spironolactone with hydrochlorothiazide (Aldactazide)	Increase renal excretion of salt and water; decrease blood volume direct effect on arterioles

Beta-blocking agents	Propranolol, acebutolol, atenolol, metoprolol, labetalol, nadolol	Decrease cardiac output; inhibit renin secretion from kidneys; beta-blockers compete with epinephrine for beta receptor sites and inhibit tissue/organ response to beta stimulation
Adrenergic inhibiting agents	Clonidine (central acting), guanethidine, reserpine (peripheral inhibitors) prazosin hydrochloride, phentolamine, phenoxy benzamine (alpha$_1$- and alpha$_2$-blocking agents, nonselective)	Block sympathetic stimulation; have multiple sites of action
Vasodilator drugs	Diazoxide, hydralazine, minoxidil (arteriolar dilator), sodium nitroprusside, amyl nitrite, isosorbide dinitrate, nitroglycerin (arteriolar and venous dilator drugs)	Act directly on smooth muscle walls of arterioles, veins, or both; lower peripheral resistance and blood pressure
Angiotensin-converting enzyme inhibitors, angiotensin II receptor antagonists	Captopril, enalapril, lisinopril, irbesartan (Avapro), losartan (Cozaar, Hyzaar), valsartan (Diovan)	Inhibit the conversion of angiotensin I to angiotensin II. Angiotensin II is a powerful vasoconstrictor that suppresses renin-angiotensin aldosterone system. Selectively inhibit angiotensin receptors that include vasoconsriction, renal tubular sodium reabsorption, aldosterone release, and stimulation of arterial and peripheral sympathetic activity.
Calcium channel blockers	Verapamil, nifedipine, diltiazem	Decrease peripheral resistance by inhibiting blockers and the contractility of vascular smooth muscle

(Objective 11)

33. b, a, e, g, f, d, c
(Objective 11)

34. b. An *antidote* is a specific drug taken to minimize the adverse effects of an ingested drug or poison. *Parenteral* refers to a drug route. A *vaccine* is an injection of drug given to prevent disease.
(Objective 1)

35. b
(Objective 3)

36. b. Only selected antibiotics pass through these barriers.
(Objective 7)

37. a. Antagonists block receptor sites and inhibit action.
(Objective 8)

38. d. Median lethal dose is the lethal dose for 50% of animals that took the drug. Median effective dose is the effective dose for 50% of animals that took the drug. Biological half-life is the time required to excrete half of the total amount of drug introduced into the body.
(Objective 7)

39. d. Atropine, lidocaine, and epinephrine also may be given by this route.
(Objective 7)

40. d. Then intramuscular, subcutaneous, and oral
(Objective 7)

41. b. All of the other routes listed give unpredictable, slow absorption because of poor perfusion in shock.
(Objective 7)

42. b. Butorphanol tartrate and pentazocine are opioid agonist-antagonists, and oxycodone hydrochloride is an opioid analgesic-agonist.
(Objective 11)

43. c. Nalbuphine is an opioid agonist-antagonist.
(Objective 11)

44. a. Methylphenidate (Ritalin) and pemoline (Cylert) are used to manage patients with attention deficit disorder and hyperactivity. Phenmetrazine is an anorexiant.
(Objective 11)

45. d. Depression usually is treated with a tricyclic antidepressant. Hypotension is treated based on the cause. Occasionally, intravenously administered dopamine will be used, but it acts in a different manner than the drugs that affect brain dopamine levels. Drugs used to treat myasthenia gravis elevate acetylcholine at the myoneural junctions.
(Objective 11)

46. d. Carbamazepine (Tegretol) is used to treat seizure disorders. Chlordiazepoxide (Librium) and chlorpromazine (Thorazine) are antipsychotic drugs. Baclofen (Lioresal) and diazepam (Valium) are also antispasmodics that may be used to manage muscle spasms.
(Objective 11)

47. c. These drugs paralyze muscles and usually are given concurrently with other drugs that decrease the intracranial pressure during intubation (lidocaine) and sedatives and/or pain relievers.
(Objective 11)

48. c. Physostigmine is used to manage poisonings. Glucagon is a pancreatic hormone that increases blood glucose, lorazepam is a minor tranquilizer, and verapamil is an antidysrhythmic drug.
(Objective 11)

49. a. Norepinephrine is the primary neurotransmitter for the sympathetic nervous system. *Adrenalin* is a trade name for epinephrine, and *Aramine* is the trade name for metaraminol.
(Objective 6)

50. c
(Objective 11)

51. c
(Objective 6)

52. d. Chronotropes increase heart rate; dromotropes increase conduction velocity. Cholinergic drugs increase parasympathetic effects.
(Objective 6)

53. a. Influenza-like symptoms and a variety of dysrhythmias are associated with digoxin toxicity. Tricyclic antidepressant or isoproterenol overdose likely would produce tachyarrhythmias. Verapamil overdose may cause bradycardias and severe hypotension.
(Objective 11)

54. d. Bretylium tosylate is a group III, lidocaine is a group IB, and procainamide is a group IA antidysrhythmic agent.
(Objective 11)

55. d. Some also decrease heart rate and contractility; however, the majority achieve their effects by decreasing vascular resistance.
(Objective 11)

56. d. All of the others prevent clot formation.
(Objective 11)

57. a. Ephedrine and isoproterenol are nonspecific beta-agonists, and aminophylline is a xanthine derivative.
(Objective 11)

58. b. Antihistamines may worsen an acute asthma attack by thickening bronchial secretions.
(Objective 11)

59. b. Antiinfective and antiinflammatory agents are used to treat conjunctivitis or keratitis. Topical anesthetic agents are used to treat pain.
(Objective 11)

60. d. Insulin is secreted continually in amounts determined by the needs of the body.
(Objective 11)

61. d. Amoxicillin and dicloxacillin are penicillin drugs. A percentage of persons who are allergic to penicillin have cross-reactivity to cephalosporins such as cefazolin.
(Objective 11)

62. d. Acyclovir (Zovirax) typically is prescribed for herpes infection (some patients infected with human immunodeficiency virus also may take this to treat opportunistic herpes infections). Pyrimethamine (Daraprim) and quinine (Qui-namm) are antimalarial drugs.
(Objective 11)

63. d
(Objective 11)

WRAP IT UP

1. a. The reaction may vary from hives to life-threatening airway compromise. Cytotoxic reactions usually involve hemolysis and result from administration of procainamide or hydralazine. Serum sickness can be caused by penicillins, iodides, sulfonamides, phenytoin, and some antitoxins and can cause a severe inflammatory reaction. Contact dermatitis results from exposure to poison ivy, sunscreens, and other topical ointments.
(Objective 6)

2. Atenolol is a beta-blocker and albuterol is a beta$_2$-selective stimulant.
(Objective 7)

3. His Humulin insulin is given by subcutaneous injection.
(Objective 7)

4. The margin between the therapeutic dose of digoxin (Lanoxin) and its lethal dose is small. Often patients experience signs and symptoms of digoxin overdose.
(Objective 8)

5. Drug cost may be too much for the older adult; confusion may cause overdosing or underdosing; visual or physical impairment can cause drug errors; or the patient may choose not to follow the prescribed medication plan. (Objective 11)

6. Propoxyphene, lorazepam, sertraline, or cyclobenzaprine could cause some confusion. If his blood sugar is low because of his Humulin insulin administration, that also could cause confusion. (Objective 12)

7. a. Atenolol, diltiazem, furosemide
   b. Digoxin (Lanoxin; cardiac glycoside), atenolol (Class II—beta-blockers); diltiazem (Class IV—calcium channel blockers); amiodarone (Class III—potassium channel blockers)
   c. Aspirin
   d. Lorazepam, cyclobenzaprine
   e. Propoxyphene, lorazepam
   f. Albuterol, ipratropium (indirectly)
   g. Propoxyphene, aspirin
   h. Ranitidine
   i. Azithromycin
   (Objective 12)

8. Based on the medication list that you have found, you can suspect that his medical history may include diabetes (Humulin), hypertension (atenolol, diltiazem, furosemide), cardiac rhythm disturbance (digoxin [Lanoxin], atenolol, amiodarone, diltiazem), risk factors for or history of myocardial infarction/stroke (aspirin); musculoskeletal pain or arthritis (propoxyphene, lorazepam, cyclobenzaprine); chronic obstructive pulmonary disease (ipratropium, albuterol); gastritis or ulcers (ranitidine); recent infection (azithromycin). (Objective 12)

9. Clues to the cause of his present illness may be found in the physical examination. He could be confused because of his drugs, sepsis, a stroke, chronic dementia, electrolyte imbalance (low sodium or potassium), hypotension and subsequent decrease in cerebral perfusion; or he could be having a stroke; he could have taken too much of his medications; or he may be hypoxic. (Objective 12)

Venous Access and Medication Administration

READING ASSIGNMENT

Chapter 18, pages 388-428, in *Mosby's Paramedic Textbook,* ed. 3

OBJECTIVES

Upon completion of this chapter, the paramedic student will be able to:

1. Convert selected units of measurement into the household, apothecary, and metric systems.
2. Identify the steps in the calculation of drug dosages.
3. Calculate the correct volume of drug to be administered in a given situation.
4. Compute the correct rate for an infusion of drugs or intravenous fluids.
5. List measures for ensuring the safe administration of medications.
6. Describe actions paramedics should take if a medication error occurs.
7. List measures for preserving asepsis during parenteral administration of a drug.
8. Explain drug administration techniques for the enteral and parenteral routes.
9. Describe the steps for safely initiating an intravenous infusion.
10. Identify complications and adverse effects associated with intravenous access.
11. Describe the steps for safely initiating an intraosseous infusion.
12. Explain drug administration techniques for percutaneous routes.
13. Identify special considerations in the administration of pharmacological agents to pediatric patients.
14. Explain the technique for obtaining a venous blood sample.
15. Describe the safe disposal of contaminated items and sharps.

SUMMARY

- Three systems for measuring drug dosage are in common use today. These are the metric system, the apothecary system, and the common household system. Each system deals with units of mass and volume. Any of these three systems may be used by a physician when ordering drugs.
- Paramedics should choose a drug calculation method that is precise. It also should be reliable. Paramedics should
- (1) Convert all units of measure to the same size and system.
- (2) Assess the computed dosage to determine whether it is reasonable.
- (3) Use one method of dose calculation consistently.

- Many drug calculations can be performed almost intuitively. Nevertheless, paramedics should never rely on intuitive calculations. Methods of calculation include the basic formula (desire over have), ratios and proportions, and dimensional analysis.
- Intravenous flow rates can be calculated using the following formula:

- Drops/min = $\dfrac{\text{Volume to be infused} \times \text{Drops/mL of infusion set}}{\text{Total time of infusion (min)}}$

- Safety procedures should be a high priority during the administration of any medication. The paramedic must make sure the *right* patient receives the *right* dose of the *right* drug via the *right* route at the *right* time.
- An incident involving a medication error may occur. In such a case, paramedics should take responsibility for their actions. They should quickly advise medical direction. They also should assess and monitor the patient for effects of the drug. They must document the error as required by local, state, and medical direction policies. In addition, they must change their personal practice to prevent a similar error in the future.
- Medical asepsis is accomplished by using clean technique, which involves hygienic measures, cleaning agents, antiseptics, disinfectants, and barrier fields.
- Enteral drugs are administered and absorbed through the gastrointestinal tract. They are given by the oral, gastric, and rectal routes. Parenteral drugs are administered outside the intestine. They are usually injected. Parenteral drugs are given by the intradermal, subcutaneous, intramuscular, intravenous, and intraosseous routes.
- In the prehospital setting, the route of choice for fluid replacement is through a peripheral vein in an extremity. The over-the-needle catheter generally is preferred in this setting.
- Several possible complications are associated with all intravenous techniques. These include local complications, systemic complications, infiltration, and air embolism.
- Cannulation of the central veins presents specific dangers. These are in addition to the complications common to all intravenous methods.
- Fluids and drugs that are infused by the intraosseous route pass from the marrow cavities into the sinusoids. Next, they pass into large venous channels and emissary veins. Then they pass into the systemic circulation. The site of choice for IO infusions in children is the tibia, one to two fingerbreadths below the tubercle on the anteromedial surface.
- Percutaneous drugs are absorbed through the mucous membranes or skin. These include topical drugs, sublingual drugs, buccal drugs, inhaled drugs, endotracheal drugs, and drugs for the eye, nose, and ear.
- Administering drugs to infants and children can be quite difficult. This often is especially true in emergency situations. Paramedics frequently calculate pediatric drug doses by using memory aids. Some of these aids include charts, tapes, and dosage books. Doses also are calculated with the advice of medical direction.
- If possible, venous blood samples should be obtained when intravenous access is established. They also should be obtained before any fluids are infused. If no IV line is to be used and a blood sample is still needed, it must be obtained with a needle and syringe (or a special vacuum needle and sleeve).
- The CDC recommends that needles not be capped, bent, or broken before disposal. Rather, they should be left on the syringe and discarded in an appropriate, clearly marked container that is puncture proof and leak proof.

MATH SKILLS

The following questions are a brief review of basic math skills necessary for drug dose calculation. The review is intended as a refresher. If the student does not understand these concepts, the student should consult references or seek tutoring before proceeding to the next section.

Fractions

A fraction is part of a whole number or one number divided by another number. A fraction consists of two parts, the numerator and the denominator:

$$\dfrac{a}{b} \quad \begin{array}{l} \text{a is the numerator} \\ \text{b is the denominator} \end{array}$$

The denominator indicates the number of equal parts into which the whole is separated. The numerator tells how many parts are being considered (Fig. 18-1).

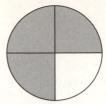

Figure 18-1

Example: $\dfrac{3}{4}$ $\dfrac{\text{Numerator is 3, so three parts are being used}}{\text{Denominator is 4 for there are four equal parts}}$

A fraction that has the same numerator and denominator equals the whole number 1 (Fig. 18-2).

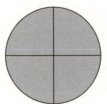

Figure 18-2

Example: $\dfrac{4}{4} = 1$

1. Identify the numerator and denominator of the following fractions.

   a. $\dfrac{7}{8}$ = ——   **b.** $\dfrac{6}{13}$ = ——

When the numerator and denominator of the fraction are multiplied by the same number, the value of the fraction remains unchanged.

Example: $\dfrac{1 \times 2}{2 \times 2} = \dfrac{2}{4} = \dfrac{1}{2}$

A fraction may be reduced to lower terms by dividing the numerator and denominator by the largest whole number that will go evenly into both of them.

Example: $\dfrac{100}{1000} \times \dfrac{100 \div 100}{1000 \div 100} = \dfrac{1}{10}$

2. Reduce the following fractions to lowest terms.
   a. $\frac{7}{28}$ **d.** $\frac{6}{36}$ **g.** $\frac{24}{120}$ **j.** $\frac{10}{25}$
   b. $\frac{3}{12}$ **e.** $\frac{25}{125}$ **h.** $\frac{5}{25}$ **k.** $\frac{17}{23}$
   c. $\frac{4}{8}$ **f.** $\frac{18}{72}$ **i.** $\frac{1000}{10,000}$ **l.** $\frac{16}{24}$

An improper fraction has a larger numerator than denominator.

Example: $\dfrac{8}{4}$

223

To change an improper fraction to a whole number, divide the numerator by the denominator:

Example: $\frac{8}{4} = 8 \div 4 = 2$ (Whole number)

           $\frac{7}{4} = 7 \div 4 = 1\frac{3}{4}$ (This is a mixed number because it has a whole number plus a fraction.)

3. Convert the following to whole numbers or mixed fractions.
    a. $\frac{7}{5}$ **b.** $\frac{24}{12}$ **c.** $\frac{12}{4}$ **d.** $\frac{15}{6}$

To change a mixed number into an improper fraction, multiply the whole number by the denominator of the fraction and add the numerator of the fraction to the result.

Example: $4\frac{1}{2} = \frac{(4 \times 2) + 1}{2} = \frac{9}{2}$

4. Change each of the following mixed numbers to improper fractions:
    a. $5\frac{3}{8}$ **b.** $1\frac{3}{4}$ **c.** $3\frac{1}{12}$ **d.** $15\frac{2}{3}$

To change a fraction to equivalent fractions in which both terms are larger, multiply the numerator and denominator by the same number.

Example: Enlarge $\frac{2}{5}$ to the equivalent fraction in tenths.

$$\frac{2}{5} \times \frac{2}{2} = \frac{4}{10}$$

5. Change the following fractions to the equivalent fraction indicated.

    a. $\frac{6}{8} = \frac{x}{24}$ **b.** $\frac{12}{15} = \frac{x}{60}$ **c.** $\frac{79}{100} = \frac{x}{100,000}$

To compare fractions with different denominators, find the lowest common denominator. The lowest common denominator is the smallest number that is divisible by the denominators.

Example 1: What is the lowest common denominator of $\frac{1}{2}$, $\frac{3}{5}$, and $\frac{7}{10}$?

The denominators are 2, 5, and 10. Because 10 is divisible by 2 and 5, it is the lowest common denominator.

Example 2: What is the lowest common denominator of $\frac{1}{3}$ and $\frac{2}{5}$? Because 5 is not divisible by 3, multiply the larger denominator by 2, 3, 4, and so on. Each time, determine whether the product is divisible by 3:

$5 \times 2 = 10$ 10 is not divisible by 3.
$5 \times 3 = 15$ 15 is divisible by 3, so 15 is the lowest common denominator.

6. Find the lowest common denominator.
    a. $\frac{1}{6}$ and $\frac{1}{8}$ **b.** $\frac{2}{3}$ and $\frac{1}{12}$ **c.** $\frac{1}{3}$, $\frac{2}{6}$ and $\frac{3}{8}$

7. Circle the correct response:
    a. $\frac{3}{8}$ is greater than, less than, or equal to $\frac{9}{24}$.
    b. $\frac{9}{8}$ is greater than, less than, or equal to $\frac{5}{6}$.
    c. $\frac{3}{5}$ is greater than, less than, or equal to $\frac{7}{10}$.

    To add or subtract fractions, do the following:
    1. Convert all fractions to equivalent fractions using the lowest common denominator.
    2. Add or subtract the numerator and place over the common denominator.
    3. Simplify to the lowest terms.

Example: $\frac{5}{9} + \frac{2}{6} = \frac{5(2)}{9(2)} + \frac{2(3)}{6(3)} = \frac{10}{18} + \frac{6}{18} \div \frac{2}{2} = \frac{8}{9}$

8. Add the following fractions and mixed numbers:
   a. ⅞ + ⅖ + ¹⁄₁₀
   b. 1¼ + 2⅔

9. Subtract the following fractions and mixed numbers:
   a. 1⅗ − ⁹⁄₁₀
   b. 2¾ − ⅚

   To multiply fractions, do the following:
   1. Change mixed numbers to improper fractions.
   2. Multiply numerators.
   3. Multiply denominators.
   4. Simplify to the lowest terms.

   Example: $\dfrac{3}{4} \times \dfrac{4}{5} = \dfrac{12}{20} \div \dfrac{4}{4} = \dfrac{3}{5}$

10. Multiply the following fractions and mixed numbers:
    a. ⁵⁄₁₆ × ¹¹⁄₁₃
    b. 8½ × 3
    c. 6⅞ × 2
    d. ⅓ × ⅞

    To divide fractions, do the following:
    1. Change mixed numbers to improper fractions.
    2. Turn the number after the division sign (÷) upside down.
    3. Follow the steps for multiplication of fractions.
    4. Simplify to the lowest terms.

    Example: $\dfrac{4}{5} \div \dfrac{2}{3} = \dfrac{4}{5} \times \dfrac{3}{2} = \dfrac{12}{10} \div \dfrac{2}{2} = \dfrac{6}{5} = 1\tfrac{1}{5}$

11. Divide the following fractions:
    a. ⅜ ÷ ³⁄₁₀
    b. 2½ ÷ ⁷⁄₁₁

Decimals

All whole numbers are to the left of the decimal; all decimal fractions are to the right of the decimal (Fig. 18-3).

12. Write the decimal notation for the following examples:
    a. 3 and 4 tenths
    b. 5 and 35 hundredths
    c. 62 thousandths

    To convert a fraction into a decimal, do the following:
    1. Divide the numerator by the denominator.
    2. Place the decimal point in the proper position.

    Example: $\dfrac{3}{5} = 3 \div 5 = 5\overline{)3.0}^{\,0.6}$

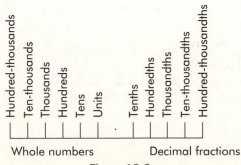

Figure 18-3

225

13. Change the following fractions to decimals:

    a. ¼   **b.** ⁷⁄₂₅   **c.** ³⁄₁₅₀

To convert a decimal to a fraction, do the following:

1. Write the numerator of the fraction as the numbers expressed in the decimal.
2. Write the denominator of the fraction as the number 1 followed by the number of zeros as there are places to the right of the decimal point.
3. Simplify the fraction to the lowest terms.

    Example: $0.234 = x$
    Numerator = 234
    Denominator = 1 + three zeros = 1000

    Simplify: $\dfrac{234}{1000} = \dfrac{234}{1000} \div \dfrac{2}{2} = \dfrac{117}{500}$

14. Change the following decimals to fractions.

    a. 0.5   **b.** 3.24   **c.** 6.007

To add or subtract decimals, do the following:

1. Line up the decimal points.
2. Add zeros to make all decimal numbers equal length.
3. Add or subtract as with whole numbers.
4. Place the decimal point in the sum.

    Example: $0.6 + 4.23 + 1.123 = x$

Line up the decimal points:	0.6
	4.23
	1.123
Add zeros:	0.600
	4.230
	1.123
Add as whole numbers:	5.953

Place the decimal point in the sum.

15. Add the following decimals.

    a. $0.03 + 0.12 + 0.32$ **b.** $0.26 + 0.01 + 0.75$

16. Subtract the following decimals.

    a. $91.5 - 62.5$ **b.** $17 - 3.42$

To multiply decimals, do the following:

1. Multiply as with whole numbers.
2. Count the total number of decimal places in the decimals multiplied.
3. Place the decimal point in the answer to the left of the total decimal places calculated in step 2.
4. When multiplying a decimal by a power of 10, move the decimal point the same number of places to the right as there are zeros in the multiplier.

    Example: $1.25 \times 3.3 = x$

    1.25   (two decimal places)
    × 3.3   (one decimal place)
    4.125   (The decimal point is placed to the left of three decimal places.)

    Example: $3.46 \times 10 = 3.4.6 = 34.6$

17. Multiply the following decimals.

    a. 3.62×0.02 **c.** 7.25×0.03 **e.** 2.9×10
    b. 27×0.04 **d.** 4.256×100 **f.** 7.052×1000

To divide decimals, do the following:
1. If the divisor (number you are dividing by) is a whole number, divide as you would with whole numbers. Place the decimal place in the answer in the same place it was in the number to be divided.
2. If the divisor (number you are dividing by) is a decimal, make it a whole number by moving the decimal place to the end of the divisor. Move the decimal in the number being divided by the same number of places.
3. If the divisor is a power of 10, move the decimal point to the left as many places as there are zeros in the divisor.

Example: $25.5 \div 5 =$ $5\overline{)25.5} = 5.1$

Example: $25.5 \div 0.5 =$ $0.5\overline{)25.5} =$ $5\overline{)255} = 51$

Example: $25.5 \div 10 = 2.55$ (2.5.5)

18. Divide the following.
   a. $0.25 \div 5$ **d.** $0.16 \div 0.04$
   b. $5.16 \div 2$ **e.** $14.237 \div 100$
   c. $4 \div 0.5$ **f.** $0.17 \div 10$

Rounding decimal fractions: Most drug calculations require rounding to the hundredth or greater. This depends on the individual example. To round off, consider the number in the next position to the right. If the number is greater than or equal to 5, increase the number being considered by 1. If it is less than 5, do not increase the number being considered.

Example: Round off 0.74 to the nearest tenths. Because the number in the hundredths column is less than 5, the answer will be 0.7.

Example: Round off 0.24555 to the nearest hundredths. Because the number in the thousandths column is 5, the answer will be 0.25.

19. Round off the following examples to the nearest tenth:
   a. 7.6245   **b.** 0.081   **c.** 0.851

20. Round off the following examples to the nearest hundredth:
   a. 0.10423   **b.** 5.6258   **c.** 892.02975

Ratios

Ratios indicate the relationship of one quantity to another. They indicate division and may be expressed as the following:

$\frac{a}{b}$, a to b, or a:b

Example: Five gallons of gas for $6 means the ratio of gas to dollars is as follows:

$\frac{5}{6}$, 5 to 6, or 5:6

21. Write the ratio for the following examples.
   a. The heart ejects approximately 5000 mL of blood every 60 seconds.
   b. Approximately 6000 mL of air is moved in and out of the lungs every 60 seconds.
   c. The intravenous line delivers 100 mL every 30 minutes.
   d. There are 100 mg of the drug in 10 mL of solution.

To simplify a ratio that compares two measures, divide the denominator into the numerator to calculate the unit rate.

Example: On a routine transfer, we traveled 120 miles in 2 hours.

$$\text{The unit rate} = \frac{120 \text{ miles}}{2 \text{ hours}} = 60 \text{ miles per hour}$$

The unit rate is 60 miles per hour.

22. Calculate the unit rate for each of the following (based on the examples in Question 21).
  a. How many milliliters of blood are ejected from the heart each second?
  b. How much air is moved in and out of the lungs each second?
  c. How much fluid is being delivered each minute?
  d. How many milligrams are in each milliliter?

A proportion shows the relationship between two different ratios. To determine whether a proportion is true (equivalent), do the following:
1. If the proportion is expressed as a fraction, ($\frac{1}{2} = \frac{2}{4}$), multiply the cross products and then determine whether the proportion is equivalent.

Example: $\dfrac{1}{2} = \dfrac{2}{4} = \dfrac{1}{2} \cdot \dfrac{2}{4} = 1 \times 4 = 4$ and $2 \times 2 = 4$;

4 = 4; therefore the proportion is true.

2. If the proportion is expressed as a ratio (2:5::4:10), multiply the two inside numbers ($5 \times 4 = 20$) and the two outside numbers ($2 \times 10 = 20$); 20 = 20; therefore the proportion is equivalent.

23. Determine whether each of the following proportions is true:
  a. $\dfrac{5}{10} = \dfrac{1}{2}$ **b.** $\dfrac{4}{6} = \dfrac{8}{10}$ **c.** $\dfrac{25}{75} = \dfrac{1}{3}$

To solve a proportion problem when one of the numbers is unknown *(x)*, do the following:
1. Use either proportion method demonstrated previously.
2. Make *x* stand alone by dividing both sides of the equation by the number on the side of *x*.
3. Solve for *x*.

Example: $\dfrac{17}{20} = \dfrac{x}{100}$ $20x = 17 \times 100 = \dfrac{20x}{20} = \dfrac{17 \times 100}{20}$

$$x = \dfrac{17 \times 100}{20}$$

$$x = 85$$

Example: 17:20::x:100 $20x = 17 \times 100$

$$\dfrac{20x}{20} = \dfrac{17 \times 100}{20}$$

24. Solve for *x* in the following problems:
  a. $\frac{2}{4} = \frac{x}{6}$ **c.** $\frac{2}{3} = \frac{7}{x}$ **e.** 3:5::x:45   **g.** x:35::80:100
  b. $\frac{1}{4} = \frac{x}{16}$ **d.** $\frac{5}{4} = \frac{x}{12}$ **f.** 4:9::16:x   **h.** 1.5:3::x:18

Simplifying a problem by cancelling common elements will make problem solving easier.

Example: $x = \dfrac{12 \times 10}{20} = 6$ Zeros cancel. Then 2 divides into 12 six times.

Example: $x = \dfrac{1 \text{ mg} \times 1 \text{ mL}}{1 \text{ mg}} = 1 \text{ mL}$ *mg* cancels *mg*. 1 mL is left.

25. Simplify the following problems as much as possible and then solve.

a. $x = \dfrac{10 \times 150}{50}$

b. $x = \dfrac{25 \times 2}{50}$

c. $x = \dfrac{2500 \times 500}{20,000}$

d. $x = \dfrac{1\,g \times 1\,L}{1\,g}$

e. $x = \dfrac{2\,mg \times 1\,mL}{10\,mg}$

f. $x = \dfrac{10\,mg \times 10\,mL}{100\,mg}$

Percentages

Percent (%) is a portion of a whole divided by 100.

1. To change a percent to a decimal, drop the percent sign and move the decimal two places to the left.
   Example: 15.0% = 0.15
2. To change a decimal to a percent, move the decimal two places to the right and add the percent sign.
   Example: 0.76 = 76%
3. To change a fraction to a percent, convert it to a decimal and follow rule 2.
   Example: ⅖ = 0.2 0.2 = 20%

26. Change the following percentages to decimals.
   a. 25%   **b.** 110%   **c.** 0.5%

27. Convert the following decimals to percentages.
   a. 0.34   **b.** 2.29   **c.** 0.07

28. Express the following as percentages:
   a. ³⁴⁄₅₀   **b.** ¹⁰⁰⁄₅₀₀   **c.** ¾

29. Rewrite the following fractions as ratios, decimals, and percentages:

Fraction	Ratio	Decimal	Percentage
a. ⅚			
b. ½₀			
c. ⁷⁄₃₃			

30. Solve the following:
   a. 15% of 75   **b.** 0.5% of 250
   This concludes the refresher.

MATHEMATICAL EQUIVALENTS AND DRUG DOSE CALCULATIONS

31. In the metric system the primary unit of volume is the (a) _____liter_____, the primary unit of mass (weight) is

the (b) _____gram_____, and the primary unit of length is the (c) _____meter_____.

32. List the four metric mass units commonly used in the prehospital environment, beginning with the largest and ending with the smallest.

a. Kg

b. g

c. mg

d. mcg

33. Each of the units listed in question 32 differs in value from the next unit by ___1000___.

34. To convert from one unit to the next smallest unit in question 32, you must move the decimal point three places to the right or left? ___R___

35. To convert from one unit to the previous unit (example unit 32d to unit 32c), you must move the decimal point three places to the right or left? ___L___

36. Convert the following units of mass to the units indicated.

a. 2 kg = __2000__ g

b. 4 mg = __4000__ mcg

c. 2 g = __2000__ mg

d. 600 mg = __.006__ kg

e. 400 mcg = __0.4__ mg

f. 350 mg = __.350__ g

g. 0.25 mg = __200.__ mcg

h. 12.5 g = __12500.0__ mg

37. Convert the following units of volume to the units indicated.

a. 1 cc = __1__ mL

b. 10 mL = __10__ cc

c. 250 mL = __.25__ L

d. 0.33 L = __330__ mL

38. The primary unit of mass in the apothecary system is the ___GAIN___.

39. The primary unit of volume in the apothecary system is the ___Minim___.

40. If the physician orders acetaminophen gr *X*, how many milligrams will you give? ___600 mg___

41. Your patient has chest pain, and medical direction orders nitroglycerin gr $\frac{1}{150}$. How many milligrams will you administer?

(a) _____

When it is time for a second nitroglycerin, the patient's blood pressure is slightly low, so this time the physician orders nitroglycerin gr $\frac{1}{200}$. How many milligrams will you give?

(b) _____

42. Convert the following measures in the household system to the units indicated:

a. 1 T = _____ tsp

b. 1 lb = _____ oz

c. 1 pt = _____ oz

d. 1 gal = _____ qt

e. 1 fl oz = _____ T

f. 1 c = _____ fl oz

43. Convert the following measures in the household system to the appropriate metric units.

a. 1 tsp = _____ mL

b. 1 T = _____ mL

c. 1 fl oz = _____ mL

d. 1 qt = _____ mL

e. 22 lb = _____ kg

f. 110 lb = _____ kg

44. Convert the following measures to the appropriate units indicated.

a. A patient's family tells you that he lost about a cup of blood from a head wound. You will relay to medical

direction that the estimated blood loss is approximately _____ mL.

b. A patient vomits about a quart of coffee-grounds emesis. This is equal to _____ mL.

c. The patient took 1 oz or _____ mL of antacid. Then she drank 16 oz of milk. This is equal to _____ mL of milk.

d. A parent reads a drug label and, instead of administering 2 mL of a drug, accidentally gives 2 oz of a drug.

How many milliliters in excess of the prescribed dose did the parent give? _____ mL

e. The human body normally contains about 5 L of blood, or _____ qt.

f. A pregnant woman states that her membranes have ruptured and about a pint of amniotic fluid leaked out.

This is equal to _____ mL.

g. A premature newborn you have just delivered weighs 2 lb, or _____ kg (_____ g).

45. Identify the following information from the drug label or package in Fig. 18-4.
   a. Drug name: **d.** Total drug:
   b. Expiration date: **e.** Concentration of drug:
   c. Total volume:

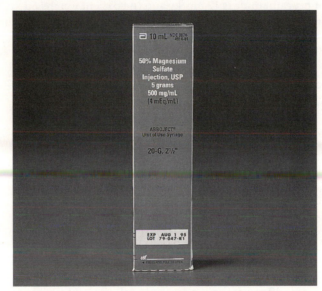

Figure 18-4

46. Convert the following drug concentrations into the total number of grams.

a. Calcium chloride 10% solution = ___10___ g in 100 mL.

b. Epinephrine 1:1000 solution = ___1___ g in 1000 mL.

c. Magnesium sulfate 10% solution = ___10___ g in 100 mL.

d. Epinephrine 1:10,000 solution = ___1___ g in 10,000 mL.

e. Lidocaine 0.4% solution = ___0.4___ g in 100 mL.

f. Mannitol 25% solution = ___25___ g in 100 mL.

g. Dextrose 50% solution = ___50___ g in 100 mL.

47. Calculate the concentration per milliliter of the following drugs using the following formula: Concentration = Total dose of drug (mg) ÷ Total volume (mL). For example, a 10-mL vial of lidocaine contains 100 mg of the drug. Concentration = 100 mg ÷ 10 mL = 10 mg/ml.
   a. A 40-mg vial of furosemide is in a 4-mL vial. Concentration = ___10mg/ml___

   b. A 10-mL vial of epinephrine contains 1 mg of the drug. Concentration = ___0.10 mg/ml___

   c. You have 25 g of D50W in 50 mL. Concentration = ___25,000mg/~~tab~~___ 500mg/mL

   d. A 2-mL vial of diphenhydramine contains 50 mg of the drug. Concentration = ___25mg./mL___

   e. A 250-mL bag contains 1 g of lidocaine. Concentration = ___4mg/ml___

48. Calculate the total dose of a drug to be administered.
   a. Lidocaine 1 mg/kg is ordered for a 100-kg patient who is having many premature ventricular contractions

      each minute. Dose = ___100___ mg.

   b. The maximum dose of procainamide is 17 mg/kg and the patient weighs 60 kg. Total dose = ___1020___ mg.
   c. Push sodium bicarbonate 1 mEq/kg during a lengthy cardiac arrest. The patient weighs 80 kg. Dose =

      ___80___ mEq.

   d. Hang a dopamine drip at 5 mcg/kg/min on a hypotensive patient who weighs 50 kg. Dose = ___250___ mcg/min.

   e. Give epinephrine 0.01 mg/kg to an 11-lb child who is in cardiopulmonary arrest. Dose = ___0.11___ mg.

   f. Administer mannitol 1 g/kg to a 176-lb patient with rising intracranial pressure. Dose = _____ g.

49. Solve the following problems using the following formula:

$$\text{Volume (x)} = \frac{\text{Desired dose (D)} \times \text{Volume on hand (Q)}}{\text{Dose on hand (H)}}$$

   a. You wish to give furosemide 20 mg. It is supplied in a 4-mL vial containing 40 mg of the drug.

      Volume = ___2___ mL.
   b. You wish to administer morphine 3 mg. You have a 1-mL Tubex containing 10 mg of the drug.

      Volume = ___.3___ mL.

   c. You wish to give amiodarone 300 mg. You have a 3-mL vial containing 150 mg of the drug. Volume = ___6___ mL.

   d. You must give 2.5 mg of diazepam. It is supplied in a 2-mL vial containing 10 mg. Volume = ___0.5___ mL.

   e. You have 50 mg of meperidine in a 1-mL Tubex. You need to give 12.5 mg of the drug.

      Volume = ___.25___ mL.
   f. Your patient needs 0.3 mg of epinephrine (1:1000). You have a 1-mL vial containing 1 mg.

      Volume = ___.05___ mL.
   g. Your patient needs 0.5 mg of dopamine. You have a 500-mL bag containing 400 mg of the drug.

      Volume = ___.625___ mL.

50. Solve the following drug dose problems using the following equation:
Desired dose:Desired volume::Dosage on hand:Volume on hand.

Example: Give 50 mg of procainamide. It is supplied in a 10-mL vial containing 1000 mg.

$$50 \text{ mg:}x = 1000 \text{ mg:}10 \text{ mL} \quad \text{Set up the ratio.}$$

$$\frac{1000 \text{ mg} \times x}{1000 \text{ mg}} = \frac{50 \text{ mg} \times 10 \text{ mL}}{1000 \text{ mg}} \quad \text{Multiply inside (means) and then outside (extremes) numbers.}$$

$$x = \frac{50 \text{ mg} \times 10 \text{ mL}}{1000 \text{ mg}} \quad \text{Solve for } x.$$

$$x = 0.5 \text{ mL}$$

a. Administer adenosine 6 mg. It is supplied in a 2-mL vial containing 6 mg of the drug. Desired volume =

___2___ mL.

b. Administer diphenhydramine 25 mg. You have a 2-mL vial containing 50 mg of the drug. Desired volume =

___1___ mL.

c. Give 2.5 mg of verapamil. It is supplied in a 2-mL vial containing 5 mg of the drug. Desired volume =

___1___ mL.

d. Give 1000 mg of mannitol. You have a 20% solution. Desired volume = __200__ mL.

51. Calculate the drops per minute needed to deliver the following volumes of fluid over the required time.
a. The physician orders an intravenous fluid to run at 30 mL/hr (drop factor, 60 drops/mL). Drops/min =

__30__.

b. You want to give a fluid challenge of 200 mL over 20 minutes (drop factor, 10 drops/mL). Drops/min =

__100__.

c. You need to infuse a drug mixed in 50 mL of fluid over 15 minutes (drop factor, 15 drops/mL). Drops/min =

__50__.

d. Online medical direction orders 150 mL of lactated Ringer's solution to infuse in 2 hours (drop factor, 15

drops/mL). Drops/min = _____.

e. You are told to give 275 mL over 2 hours (drop factor, 10 drops/mL). Drops/min = _____.

f. The intravenous drug must run in at 0.5 mL/min (drop factor, 60 drops/mL). Drops/min = _____.
g. You have delivered a baby, and medical direction advises you to add 10 units (1 mL) of oxytocin to 1000 mL

of normal saline and infuse it at 200 mL/hr (drop factor, 10 drops/mL). Drops/min = _____.
h. You have added magnesium sulfate to D$_5$W for a total volume of 100 mL. You must infuse it over 2 minutes

to treat your patient's ventricular arrhythmia (drop factor, 10 drops/mL). Drops/min = _____.
i. A severely acidotic patient needs bicarbonate. You have added 50 mEq of sodium bicarbonate (50 mL) to

1000 mL of normal saline and are to infuse it over 2 hours (drop factor, 15 drops/mL). Drops/min = _____.
j. You have added 2 mg (2 mL) of epinephrine to a 250-mL bag of normal saline and wish to infuse it at 1

mL/min to your severely bradycardic patient (drop factor, 60 drops/mL). Drops/min = _____.
k. Your patient has just converted from ventricular fibrillation. You are hanging a lidocaine drip at 3 mg/min.
You have mixed 1 g of lidocaine in 250 mL normal saline. How many drops per minute will you set your IV to

deliver the 0.75 mL/min necessary for this dose of drug (drop factor, 60 drops/mL)? Drops/min = _____.

52. Calculate the following problems using any of the methods demonstrated. Ensure that all units are compatible. If the dosage is given in milligrams per kilogram, make the appropriate calculation.

a. You wish to give lidocaine 1 mg/kg to a 75-kg man. The lidocaine is supplied in a 10-mL syringe containing 100 mg of the drug. How many milliliters will you administer?

b. You must give amiodarone 300 mg to a 60-kg woman. You have a 2-mL vial containing 150 mg of the drug. How many mL will you give?

c. You must give 0.5 mg of glucagon to a 90-kg patient. When you mix it up, you have 1 mg in 1 mL of solution. How much will you give?

d. You have diluted your phenobarbital so that you have 130 mg in 10 mL. You need to give 100 mg. The patient weighs 100 kg. How much will you give?

e. You must give 1 g/kg of mannitol. The patient weighs 70 kg. You have a 20% solution. How many milliliters will you give?

f. You need to administer 150 mg of aminophylline. You have 500 mg in a 20-mL ampule. How many milliliters will you give?

g. Your patient needs a dopamine drip at 5 mcg/kg/min. He weighs 100 kg. You have 400 mg of dopamine in 500 mL of D_5W. How many milliliters per minute will you administer and at how many drops per minute will you set the microdrip intravenous line?

h. You wish to administer a lidocaine drip at 2 mg/min. You have an intravenous bag containing a 0.4% solution of lidocaine. How many milliliters will you give each minute, and how fast will you set your microdrip tubing to deliver this rate?

53. For each of the following situations, calculate the correct volume of solution to be administered using the drug package information illustrated.

a. Give 0.5 mg of atropine (Fig. 18-5). Desired volume = _____ mL.

b. Give 0.3 mg of epinephrine (Fig. 18-6). Desired volume = _____ mL.

c. Give lidocaine 0.5 mg/kg to an 80-kg patient (Fig. 18-7). Desired volume = _____ mL.

54. After determining the correct volume of drug to be administered in the following examples, shade the corresponding syringe in Fig. 18-8 to illustrate the proper amount to be given.

a. Adenosine 6 mg must be given to a patient with paroxysmal supraventricular tachycardia. You have a 2-mL vial containing 3 mg/mL of the drug. How many milliliters will you give?

b. Your patient has had a seizure and needs phenytoin 200 mg. You have a 5-mL vial containing 250 mg of the drug. How much will you give?

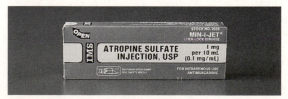

Figure 18-5

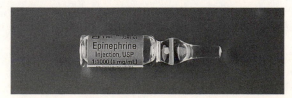

Figure 18-6

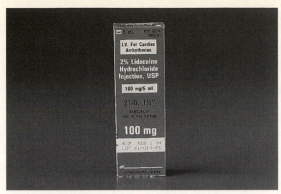

Figure 18-7

   c. You have a 10-mL vial of furosemide containing 10 mg/mL of the drug. A total of 70 mg is indicated for your patient, who is in congestive heart failure. What volume will you administer?
   d. You wish to administer epinephrine 0.3 mg to a patient experiencing an allergic reaction. The epinephrine is supplied in a 1-mL ampule containing 1 mg of a 1:1000 solution of the drug. How much will you give?

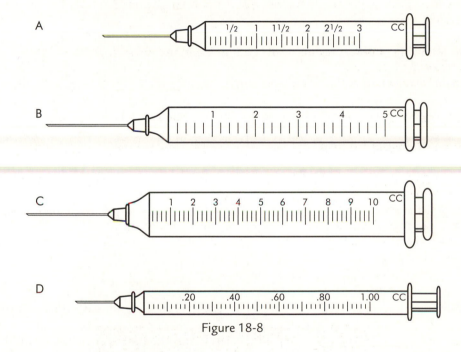

Figure 18-8

DRUG ADMINISTRATION

55. List at least 10 general steps to be taken when administering any drug to avoid errors.

   a.

   b.

   c.

   d.

   e.

   f.

   g.

h.

i.

j.

56. You intended to deliver the lidocaine drip at 1 mL/min during your 15-minute transport, but when you look at the 250-mL bag, the roller clamp has been opened, and almost 150 mL has been infused. List five actions that you should take after this error.

a.

b.

c.

d.

e.

57. List two methods to ensure medical asepsis when you administer an intramuscular injection.

a.

b.

58. Complete the following sentences regarding drug administration routes:

Oral medications should be given with the patient in the (a) _____ position. The drug should be swallowed with (b) _____ oz of fluid to ensure that it reaches the (c) _____. Sublingual medications should be placed under the (d) _____ and allowed to (e) _____. They should not be (f) _____ because this will delay action of the drug. Parenteral drug administration may cause (g) _____, (h) _____, or (i) _____. The correct needle length and size are important. For subcutaneous injections a (j) _____-inch, (k) _____-gauge needle should be used. When administering an intramuscular shot, you should select a (l) _____-inch, (m) _____-gauge needle. To minimize the risk of needle stick injury, you should understand that the use of two-handed needle recapping is (n) _____. Also, all sharp items, including needles, should be placed in (o) _____. When withdrawing medication from a multidose vial, you should cleanse the stopper with alcohol and then inject the same amount of (p) _____ as drug to be withdrawn before aspirating the appropriate amount of medicine into the syringe. To minimize the risk of glass particles entering the injection when aspirating from a glass ampule, use a (q) _____ needle. Subcutaneous injections should be administered at a (r) _____-degree angle. Sites of administration for this route include (s) _____, _____, and _____. Intramuscular injections should be administered at a (t) _____-degree angle. Administration sites for this route include the (u) _____ and

_____. To prevent drug effects on the rescuer, you should always wear (v) _____ when administering transdermal medicines. Dilution with at least (w) _____ mL of fluid is recommended to ensure maximum absorption of drugs administered by the endotracheal route. Two advantages of drugs administered by inhalation are (x) _____ and fewer _____.

59. List three complications of intravenous line placement for each of the following approaches:
   a. Peripheral site:

_____

   b. Internal jugular and subclavian sites:

_____

   c. Femoral site:

_____

60. You respond to care for a 3-year-old child who is in cardiac arrest. Attempts to intubate and secure intravenous access are unsuccessful, so you elect to attempt intraosseous infusion. After applying gloves and preparing your equipment, you select the preferred site, located (a) _____ _____. You then insert the needle using a (b) _____ motion and advance it until (c) _____. The next step involves aspirating marrow into a syringe. Then you use a syringe filled with (d) _____ to ensure that free flow occurs without resistance. If you detect correct placement, you connect the (e) _____ and infuse the drug at the appropriate rate. To prevent the needle from being dislodged, you should (f) _____ the needle.

STUDENT SELF-ASSESSMENT

61. Your patient's mother states that her child's temperature is 38.5° C. What is her temperature in degrees Fahrenheit?
   a. 69.9   **c.** 101.3
   b. 99.6   **d.** 103.6

62. You must administer a drug that is calculated based on milligrams per kilogram. The patient tells you that he weighs 144 lb. How many kilograms does that convert to (rounded to the nearest kilogram)?
   a. 65   **c.** 80
   b. 72   **d.** 86

63. You wish to administer mannitol 500 mg/kg to a 100-kg woman. You have a 10% solution of the drug. How many milliliters will you give?
   a. 2   **c.** 20
   b. 5   **d.** 500

64. You are going to give epinephrine 0.01 mg/kg to a 6-kg child. The epinephrine is supplied as 1 mg in a 10-mL syringe. How many milliliters will you administer?
   a. 0.006   **c.** 0.6
   b. 0.06   **d.** 6.0

65. Which syringe will you use to withdraw the drug volume that you calculated in question 64?
   a. 1 mL   **c.** 5 mL
   b. 3 mL   **d.** 10 mL

66. Which measure should be taken to ensure safe administration of drugs?
    a. Learn a rapid dose calculation method that you can always perform in your head.
    b. Set unlabeled syringes in a consistent place so that you will know what is in them.
    c. Verify the label of the drug selected once before administration.
    d. Monitor the patient closely for drug effects for the first 5 minutes after you give them.
67. Your patient suddenly vomits and has chest pain after you administer epinephrine intravenously instead of subcutaneously as ordered for his anaphylaxis. How should this be recorded in the patient care report?
    a. Document the correct route only.
    b. Document the route ordered and the incorrect route.
    c. Document the incorrect route only.
    d. Omit the route in the report.
68. What parenteral route would you use to test for allergies?
    a. Intradermal   c. Intravenous
    b. Intramuscular   d. Subcutaneous
69. Which muscle is appropriate for an intramuscular injection in a 2-year-old child?
    a. Deltoid   c. Ventrogluteal site
    b. Dorsogluteal site   d. Vastus lateralis
70. You suspect that your patient has a ruptured ectopic pregnancy. She is in profound shock. Which intravenous catheter will you select?
    a. 14 gauge, 1½ inch   c. 18 gauge, 1½ inch
    b. 14 gauge, 3 inch   d. 18 gauge, 3 inch
71. You are transferring a patient with a jugular central line. Suddenly, the patient becomes unconscious, cyanotic, and tachycardic. You note that the intravenous tubing has been disconnected from the central line catheter. The patient should be positioned immediately on his
    a. Left side with his head down   c. Right side with his head down
    b. Left side with his head up   d. Right side with his head up
72. You wish to administer normal saline intravenously at 30 mL/hr. The infusion set delivers 60 drops/mL. How fast will you run it?
    a. 1 drop/min   c. 100 drops/min
    b. 30 drops/min   d. 400 drops/min
73. A 200-mL fluid challenge is to be infused over 15 minutes. The drop factor is 10 drops/mL. How fast will you run it?
    a. 35 drops/min   c. 133 drops/min
    b. 75 drops/min   d. 150 drops/min
74. Which of the following statements is true regarding intraosseous infusion?
    a. It generally is recommended for children between 1 and 3 years of age.
    b. It is associated with a risk of air embolism if the tubing is disconnected.
    c. Absorption of drugs is irregular and slow through this route.
    d. The procedure should be considered only in critically ill patients.
75. Which of the following is true regarding sublingual drug administration?
    a. The patient may have a sip of water after administration.
    b. This route should not be used if the patient is nauseated.
    c. The drug should be permitted to dissolve under the tongue.
    d. Swallowing the drug will increase its effects.
76. When administering medication into a 2-year old child's ear, you should pull the ear
    a. Down and back   c. Up and back
    b. Down and forward   d. Up and forward
77. Which is true regarding administration of medication to young children?
    a. Tell the child to cry and make noise.
    b. Avoid any physical restraint.
    c. Give injections slowly and firmly.
    d. Be honest about painful techniques.

78. Which of the following describes an appropriate procedure for obtaining a blood sample for glucose on an adult patient?

   a. Disconnect the intravenous infusion, insert the vacutainer into the hub of the intravenous catheter, and withdraw.
   b. Insert the intraosseous needle, flush with normal saline, attach a syringe, and pull back.
   c. Enter the vein with a 24-gauge needle attached to a syringe and withdraw.
   d. Push blood collection tubes into the barrel of the vacutainer and allow to fill.

WRAP IT UP

Case Study: Venous Access and Medication Administration

You are dispatched to a school for an allergic reaction. On arrival you find a 66-lb 7-year-old who was stung by a bee and is having an anaphylactic reaction. She has hives, her eyes are swollen, and she is wheezing. You and your partner apply oxygen, and you draw up and administer epinephrine 0.5 mg subcutaneously; give diphenhydramine (1.25 mg/kg) intramuscularly (you carry 50 mg/mL vials); and albuterol by nebulizer treatment. You initiate an IV and reevaluate her vital signs. Her wheezing has cleared almost completely, and the hives are beginning to dissipate, but she is anxious and tachycardic. Your partner asks how much epinephrine you gave, and you realize that you administered a dose in excess of the 0.01 mL/kg (1:1000) maximum 0.3 mL indicated in your protocol.

1. Convert this child's weight to the metric system. _____

2. a. Compute the correct dose of epinephrine that should have been given. _____

   b. How much did you overdose or underdose this patient? _____

3. a. Compute the correct dose of diphenhydramine. _____

   b. How many milliliters should be administered? _____

   c. In what location should the intramuscular injection of diphenhydramine be given? _____

4. What steps should have been taken before giving the drugs to ensure safe administration? (Five rights of drug administration)

_____

5. Now that you recognize an error has been made, what should you do?

_____

6. Fill in the information missing in the table:

Injection Site	Angle of Administration	Volume to Be Given
Intradermal		
Subcutaneous		
Intramuscular		

7. Which of the following is true regarding vascular access on this child?
   a. Aseptic technique should be followed.
   b. External jugular would be the initial site of choice.
   c. Intraosseous infusion should be used.
   d. Vascular access is not needed in this situation.
8. Describe the procedure for administration of nebulized albuterol by aerosol mask.

_____

CHAPTER 18 ANSWERS

VENOUS ACCESS AND MEDICATION ADMINISTRATION

1. a. 7 is the numerator, 8 is the denominator.
   b. 6 is the numerator, 13 is the denominator.

2. a. 1/4; b. 3/4; c. 1/2; d. 1/6; e. 1/5; f. 1/4; g. 1/5; h. 9/25; i. 1/10; j. 2/5; k. 17/23; l. 2/3

3. a. 15; b. 2; c. 3; d. 2 1/2

4. a. 43/8; b. 7/4; c. 37/12; d. 47/3

5. a. 18/24; b. 48/60; c. 79,000/100,000

6. a. 45; b. 12; c. 24

7. a. Equal to; b. Greater than; c. Less than

8. a. 1 3/8; b. 3 11/12

9. a. 1; b. 1 11/12

10. a. 55/208; b. 25 1/2; c. 13 3/4; d. 7/24

11. a. 1 1/4; b. 3 13/14

12. a. 3.4; b. 5.35; c. 0.062

13. a. 0.25; b. 0.28; c. 0.02

14. a. 1/2; b. 3 6/25; c. 6 7/1000

15. a. 0.47; b. 1.02

16. a. 29; b. 13.58

17. a. 0.0724; b. 1.08; c. 0.2175; d. 425.6; e. 29; f. 7052

18. a. 0.05; b. 2.58; c. 8; d. 4.0; e. 0.14237; f. 0.017

19. a. 7.6; b. 0.1; c. 0.9

20. a. 0.10; b. 5.63; c. 892.03

21. a. 5000:60 (5000 mL:60 seconds); b. 6000:60 (6000 mL:60 seconds); c. 100:30 (100 mL:30 minutes); d. 100:10 (100 mg:10 mL)

22. a. 83 mL/sec; b. 100 mL/sec; c. 3 mL/min; d. 10 mg/mL

23. a. True; b. Not true; c. True

24. a. x = 3; b. x = 4; c. x = 10.5; d. x = 15; e. x = 27; f. x = 36; g. x = 28; h. x = 9

25. a. $x = \dfrac{10 \times 150}{50} = \dfrac{\cancel{10} \times \cancel{150}^{30}}{50} = 30$

b. $x = \dfrac{25 \times 2}{50} = \dfrac{^1\cancel{25} \times \cancel{2}^1}{50^1} = 1$

c. $x = \dfrac{2500 \times 500}{20{,}000} = \dfrac{\cancel{2500} \times \cancel{500}}{\cancel{20{,}000}} = \dfrac{125}{2} = 62.5$

d. $x = \dfrac{1\,g \times 1\,L}{1\,g} = \dfrac{\cancel{1\,g} \times 1\,L}{\cancel{1\,g}} = 1\,L$

e. $x = \dfrac{2\,mg \times 1\,mL}{10\,mg} = \dfrac{\cancel{2\,mg} \times 1\,mL}{^5\cancel{10}\,mg} = \dfrac{1\,mL}{5} = 0.2\,mL$

f. $x = \dfrac{10\,mg \times 10\,mL}{100\,mg} = \dfrac{\cancel{10\,mg} \times \cancel{10\,mL}}{\cancel{100\,mg}} = 1\,mL$

26. a. 0.25; b. 1.1; c. 0.005

27. a. 34%; b. 229%; c. 7%

28. a. 68%; b. 20%; c. 43%

29.

Fraction	Ratio	Decimal	Percentage
a. ⅚	5:6 or 5 to 6	0.83	83%
b. ¹⁄₂₀	1:20 or 1 to 20	0.05	5%
c. ⁷⁄₃₃	7:33 or 7 to 33	0.21	21%

30. a. 11.25; b. 1.25

31. a. Liter; b. Gram; c. Meter
(Objective 1)

32. Kilogram (kg), gram (g), milligram (mg), and microgram (mcg)
(Objective 1)

33. 1000
(Objective 1)

34. Right
(Objective 1)

35. Left
(Objective 1)

36. a. 2000 g; b. 4000 mcg; c. 2000 mg; d. 0.0006 kg; e. 0.4 mg; f. 0.35 g; g. 250 mcg; h. 12,500 mg
(Objective 1)

37. a. 1; b. 10; c. 0.25; d. 330
(Objective 1)

38. Grain (gr)
(Objective 1)

39. Minim
(Objective 1)

40. 600 mg
(Objective 1)

41. a. 0.4 mg; b. 0.3 mg
(Objective 1)

42. a. 3; b. 16; c. 16; d. 4; e. 2; f. 8
(Objective 1)

43. a. 5; b. 15: c. 30; d. 960; e. 10; f. 50
(Objective 1)

44. a. 240; b. 960; c. 30; 480; d. 58; e. 5.2; f. 480; g. 0.9 and 900
(Objective 1)

45. a. Magnesium sulfate; b. Aug. 1, 1995; c. 10 mL; d. 5g; e. 500 mg/mL (4 mEq/mL)
(Objective 2)

46. a. 10; b. 1; c. 10; d. 1; e. 0.4; f. 25; g. 50
(Objective 2)

47. a. 40 mg/4 mL = 10 mg/mL; b. 1 mg/10 mL = 0.1 mg/mL; c. 25 g/50 mL = 25,000 mg/50 mL = 500 mg/mL; d. 50 mg/2 mL = 25 mg/mL; e. 1 g/250 mL = 1000 mg/250 mL = 4 mg/mL
(Objective 2)

48. a. 100; b. 1020; c. 80; d. 250; e. 0.05 (Do not forget to convert to kilograms.); f. 80
(Objective 2)

49. a. $x = \dfrac{20\,mg \times 4\,mL}{40\,mg} = 2\,mL$

b. $x = \dfrac{3\,mg \times 1\,mL}{10\,mg} = 0.3\,mL$

c. $x = \dfrac{300\,mg \times 3\,mL}{150\,mg} = 6\,mL$

d. $x = \dfrac{2.5\,mg \times 2\,mL}{10\,mg} = 0.5\,mL$

e. $x = \dfrac{12.5\,mg \times 1\,mL}{50\,mg} = 0.25\,mL$

f. $x = \dfrac{0.3\,mg \times 1\,mL}{1\,mg} = 0.3\,mL$

g. $x = \dfrac{0.5\,mg \times 500\,mL}{400\,mg} = 0.625\,mL$
(Objective 3)

50. a. 6 mg:x::6 mg:2 mL

$$x \times 6\,mg = 6\,mg \times 2\,mL$$

$$\frac{x \times 6\,mg}{6\,mg} = \frac{6\,mg \times 2\,mL}{6\,mg}$$

$$x = 2\,mL$$

b. 1 mL

c. 1 mL
d. 1 g:x::20 g:100 mL, x = 5 mL
(Objective 3)

51. a. 30; b. 100; c. 50; d. 19; e. 23; f. 30 g. 33; h. 500; i. 130; j. 60; k. 45
(Objective 4)

52. a. 7.5 mL; b. 4.0 mL; c. 0.5 mL; d. 7.7 mL; e. 350 mL; f. 0.5 mL; g. 0.625 mL and 38 gtt/min; h. 0.5 mL and 30 gtt/min
(Objectives 3, 4)

53. a. 5; b. 0.3; c. 2.0
(Objective 3)

54.

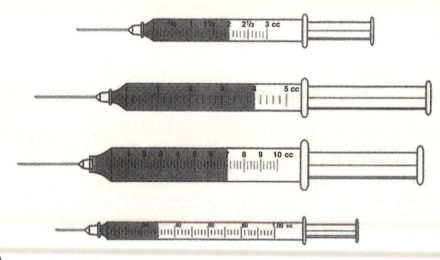

(Objective 3)

55. Avoid distractions; repeat orders to medical direction; verify that you are giving the right patient the right dose of the right drug at the right time by the right route; verify the correct drug on the label at least 3 times; verify the route of administration; ensure that the labeling information is correct for the drug you want to give; never give drugs from an unlabeled container; verify difficult calculations on paper, with a co-worker, or both; label the syringe immediately after withdrawing a drug that will not be completely administered immediately; do not give unlabeled drugs prepared by another person; do not give medications that are outdated or appear discolored, cloudy, or unusual; if the patient or a co-worker questions the drug or dose, double-check it; monitor the patient for adverse effects after administration; and document carefully.
(Objective 5)

56. a. Stop the infusion.
b. Evaluate the patient's response to the drug. Perform an assessment that includes level of consciousness, vital signs, and electrocardiogram rhythm.
c. Advise medical direction and the receiving physician of the amount of drug infused and ask for their treatment advice if you have not yet arrived at the receiving facility.
d. Document the amount of drug administered on the patient care report objectively. Document all facts surrounding the error on the appropriate confidential departmental quality improvement (incident) form.
e. Critique the situation with your crew (if appropriate), and identify measures that can be taken to prevent a similar error in the future.
(Objective 6)

57. a. Wash hands before initiating the procedure.
b. Cleanse the area with an antiseptic solution before puncturing the skin.
(Objective 7)

58. a. Upright (sitting)
  b. 4 to 8 oz
  c. Stomach
  d. Tongue
  e. Dissolve
  f. Swallowed
  g., h., and i. Infection, lipodystrophy, abscesses, necrosis, skin slough, nerve injuries, prolonged pain, and periostitis
  j. ½ or ⅝
  k. 23 or 25
  l. 1½ to 2
  m. 19 or 21
  n. Prohibited
  o. An appropriate sharps container
  p. Air
  q. Filter
  r. 45
  s. Upper arm, abdomen, thigh, and back
  t. 90
  u. Deltoid muscle, dorsogluteal site, vastus lateralis muscle, rectus femoris muscle, and ventrogluteal muscle
  v. Gloves
  w. 10
  x. Rapid onset and side effects
  (Objectives 8, 12, and 15)

59. a. Hematoma, cellulitis, thrombosis, phlebitis, sepsis, pulmonary thromboembolism, catheter embolism, fiber embolism, infiltration
  b. All complications in (a), plus air embolism, hematoma, damage to arteries or nerves, pneumothorax, hemothorax, and infiltration of fluid into the pleural space or mediastinum
  c. All complications in (a), plus hematoma, thrombosis extending to deep veins, and an inability to use the saphenous vein
  (Objective 10)

60. a. One to two fingerbreadths below the tubercle on the anteromedial surface of the tibia
  b. Boring or screwing
  c. Decreased resistance is felt (trapdoor effect)
  d. Saline
  e. Intravenous fluid infusion
  f. Secure
  (Objective 11)

61. c. To convert degrees Celsius to degrees Fahrenheit: $\dfrac{38.5 \times 9}{5} + 32 = 101.3°\,F.$

  (Objective 1)

62. a. Multiply pounds by 0.45 to convert to kilograms. $144 \times 0.45 = 64.8$. Round to 65 kg.
  (Objective 1)

63. d. $\dfrac{50\,g \times 100\,mL}{10\,g} = 500\,mL$
  (Objective 3)

64. c. $\dfrac{0.06 \times 10}{1} = 0.6$
  (Objective 3)

65. a. The 1-mL syringe will permit the most accurate measurements.
(Objective 8)

66. d. Many dose calculations can be done in your head; however, you should always write down any calculation that is difficult or that you question. Do not set down an unlabeled syringe with drug in it. Label the syringe or tape the medicine vial to it. The drug label should be verified at least 3 times before administration.
(Objective 5)

67. c. On the patient care report, only the actual action taken (the incorrect route) should be documented. The circumstances surrounding the error, including the actual correct route ordered, should be recorded in the appropriate confidential incident (quality improvement) reports.
(Objective 6)

68. a. Slower absorption and fewer systemic effects are achieved in this manner.
(Objective 8)

69. d. The other muscles are not developed adequately in the young child.
(Objective 13)

70. a. The 14-gauge, 1½-inch needle has the widest diameter and is the shortest. Both of these properties will allow rapid fluid administration.
(Objective 9)

71. a. The goal is to cause the air to stay in the right side of the heart and away from the cardiac valves.
(Objective 10)

72. b.
(Objective 4)

73. c.
(Objective 4)

74. d. Intraosseous infusion generally is recommended for children who are 6 years of age or younger. Complications include infiltration of fluid, fat embolism, osteomyelitis, periostitis at the site, infection, or fracture. Absorption of drugs and fluids from a properly placed intraosseous needle is rapid.
(Objective 11)

75. c. Swallowing a sublingual medicine will decrease its effectiveness; therefore water should not be given.
(Objective 8)

76. a. The angle of the ear canal will promote faster absorption if this technique is used.
(Objectives 12 and 13)

77. d. Recognize the child's fear and allow them to express it in appropriate ways such as crying or yelling. Use mild restraint if necessary and firmly stabilize injection sites. Give injections quickly.
(Objective 13)

78. d. Blood should not be drawn from an intravenous catheter if fluids already have been infusing (except under special circumstances and with the authorization of medical direction). Typically, a large 19- or 21-gauge needle should be used; however, in neonates a smaller needle should be used.
(Objective 14)

WRAP IT UP

1. $66 \div 2.2 = 30$ kg
   (Objective 1)

2. a. 0.01 mL/kg $\times$ 30 kg = 0.3 mL
   b. 0.5 mL given − 0.3 mL indicated = 0.2 mL overdose
   (Objective 3)

3. a. 1.25 mg/kg $\times$ 30 kg = 37.5 mg total dose
   b. 37.5 mg $\div$ 50 mg $\times$ 1 mL = 0.75 mL
   c. Diphenhydramine should be given by deep intramuscular injection into the dorsogluteal or vastus lateralis injection sites.
   (Objectives 3 and 8)

4. Ensure that the right patient gets the right dose of the right drug at the right time by the right route.
   (Objective 5)

5. After a medication error, advise medical direction and the person receiving the patient; monitor the patient; document the error according to state and local policy; determine how to prevent errors in the future.
   (Objective 6)

6. Intradermal: 15 degrees; less than 0.5 mL
   Subcutaneous: 45 degrees; less than 0.5 mL
   Intramuscular: 90 degrees; up to 5 mL (less in small children)
   (Objective 12)

7. a. Intraosseous infusion could be performed on a child in critical condition if no venous access site was readily available. A peripheral intravenous site on the arm would be preferred because of its easier access, ability to secure, and complication potential. An intravenous line is indicated to permit drug administration should the child's condition worsen.
   (Objective 9)

8. Add prescribed drug to nebulizer; attached to oxygen and mask; adjust flow meter to 6 to 10 L/min; place mask on patient; instruct patient to inhale slowly and deeply and hold breath 3 to 5 seconds before exhaling.
   (Objective 8)

PART FIVE

IN THIS PART

Airway Management and Ventilation

READING ASSIGNMENT
Chapter 19, pages 430-498, in *Mosby's Paramedic Textbook*, ed. 3

OBJECTIVES
Upon completion of this chapter, the paramedic student will be able to:
1. Distinguish between respiration, pulmonary ventilation, and external and internal respiration.
2. Explain the mechanics of respiration.
3. Explain the relationship of the partial pressures of gases in the blood and lungs to atmospheric gas pressures.
4. Describe pulmonary circulation.
5. Explain the process of exchange and transport of gases in the body.
6. Describe voluntary, chemical, and nervous regulation of respiration.
7. Discuss the assessment and management of medical or traumatic obstruction of the airway.
8. Outline the causes and effects of and preventive measures for pulmonary aspiration.
9. Outline the essential parameters for evaluating the effectiveness of the airway and breathing.
10. Describe the indications, contraindications, and techniques for delivery of supplemental oxygen.
11. Discuss methods of patient ventilation based on the indications, contraindications, potential complications, and use of each method.
12. Describe the use of manual airway maneuvers and mechanical airway adjuncts based on the indications, contraindications, potential complications, and techniques for each.
13. Describe assessment techniques and devices used to ensure adequate oxygenation, correct placement of the endotracheal tube, and elimination of carbon dioxide.
14. Explain variations in assessment and management of airway and ventilation problems in pediatric patients.
15. Given a patient scenario, identify possible alterations in oxygenation and ventilation based on a knowledge of gas exchange and the mechanics of breathing.

SUMMARY
- A key aspect of emergency care is a full understanding of the respiratory system. Another is mastery of airway management and ventilation techniques.
- The two phases of respiration are external respiration and internal respiration. External respiration is the transfer of oxygen and carbon dioxide between the inspired air and pulmonary capillaries. Internal respiration is the transfer of oxygen and carbon dioxide between the peripheral blood capillaries and the tissue cells.

- The mixture of gases that compose the atmosphere exerts a combined partial pressure of 100%, or 760 mm Hg at sea level. The composition of atmospheric gas is 21% oxygen, 0.03% carbon dioxide, and 78% nitrogen.
- The respiratory system delivers oxygen from inspired air to the blood and removes carbon dioxide.
- The 200 mL of oxygen that crosses the alveoli each minute is added to the oxygen already in the pulmonary capillaries. It is then transported to the body tissues by the circulatory system. After the body cells use the oxygen, the oxygen remaining in the blood returns to the heart and lungs. This exchange of oxygen and carbon dioxide is carried out by the passive process of diffusion.
- Respiration is controlled at any instant by a number of factors. Breathing is mainly an involuntary process. Within limits, however, the pattern of respiration can be consciously changed. The inspiratory muscles are made up of skeletal muscle. They cannot contract unless they are stimulated by nerve impulses. The activities of the respiratory centers are determined by changes in oxygen and carbon dioxide concentrations. They are also determined by the pH of the body fluids.
- The elderly cannot effectively make up for changes in airway and ventilation. Pulmonary changes that occur as a result of aging reduce vital capacity and increase physiological dead space. Po_2 also tends to decline gradually as a person ages.
- Causes of inadequate ventilation include upper airway obstruction and aspiration by inhalation. The most crucial lifesaving action for any patient who has respiratory problems from any cause is establishing and maintaining an open airway. This should always be the first priority of patient care.
- Essential parameters of airway evaluation include rate, regularity, effort, and recognition of airway problems that might indicate respiratory distress.
- The most common form of oxygen used in the prehospital setting is pure oxygen gas. This is delivered in liters per minute (LPM). Therapy regulators are used to deliver a safe pressure of oxygen to patients. Flowmeters control the amount of oxygen delivered to the patient. Several oxygen delivery devices provide supplemental oxygen to patients who have spontaneous respirations. They are the nasal cannula, simple face mask, partial rebreather mask, nonrebreather mask, and Venturi mask.
- In the prehospital setting, ventilation can be provided in several ways. These methods include rescue breathing (mouth-to-mouth, mouth-to-nose, mouth-to-stoma), mouth-to-mask breathing, use of bag-valve devices, and automatic transport ventilators.
- Emergency airway management should progress rapidly from the least to the most invasive techniques. Manual techniques for airway management include the head-tilt chin-lift method, the jaw-thrust, and the jaw-thrust without head-tilt.
- Suction catheters are used to clear the air passages of secretions and debris.
- Relief of gastric distention and/or emesis control can be accomplished through nasogastric or orogastric decompression.
- Mechanical devices for airway management include the nasal airway, oral airway, endotracheal intubation, digital intubation, nasotracheal intubation, laryngeal mask airway, multilumen airways, translaryngeal cannula ventilation, and cricothyrotomy.
- Rapid sequence intubation (RSI) involves administration of a potent sedative and a neuromuscular blocking drug at the same time. These are administered for the purpose of ET intubation.
- In the management of a child's airway, the differences in the pediatric airway must be considered. Compared to the adult airway, the child's upper airway structures have very different proportions. Their orientation to each other also differs. Smaller bag-valve devices are needed for infants and children. These reduce the chance of overinflation and barotrauma.
- End-tidal carbon dioxide detectors, pulse oximeters, and esophageal detectors can help the paramedic determine whether an ET tube has been placed correctly.

REVIEW QUESTIONS

Match the lung volume in Column II with its description in Column I. Use each answer only once.

Column I

1. __E__ The air inhaled and exhaled during a
   normal respiratory cycle (500 to 600 mL)
2. __f__ Quantity of air moved on deepest
   inspiration and expiration
3. __C__ Tidal volume multiplied by
   respiratory rate
4. __D__ Air remaining in respiratory passages
   after a forceful exhalation
5. __A__ Amount of air that can be exhaled
   forcefully after a normal breath is exhaled

Column II

a. Expiratory reserve volume
b. Inspiratory reserve volume
c. Minute volume
d. Residual volume
e. Tidal volume
f. Vital capacity

6. Pulmonary ventilation is the movement of oxygen and carbon dioxide into and out of the lungs. True/false. If this is false, why is it false?

   TRUE

7. pH is a measurement that reflects hydrogen ion concentration. True/false. If this is false, why is it false?

   TRUE

8. The pressure regulator attached to an oxygen cylinder permits administration of a specific amount of oxygen. True/false. If this is false, why is it false?

   FALSE, flow meter regulates lpm

9. Describe the *mechanical* process by which air is moved into and out of the lungs.

   _____

   _____

   _____

10. Complete the sentences in the following paragraph: At sea level, atmospheric pressure is (a) _____.

    The pressure in the alveoli is known as the (b) _____ pressure. Changes in this pressure are caused by

    changes in the (c) _____ size. During inspiration the pressure in the alveoli will (d) _____

    approximately 1 mm Hg relative to atmospheric pressure, whereas during exhalation the pressure will

    (e) _____ by 1 mm Hg. The ability of the lungs to expand during changes in pressure is known as

    (f) _____. This ability can be impaired by diseases such as (g)_____, _____,

    and _____.

11. The major blood vessels that carry deoxygenated blood to the lungs are the (a) _pulmonary arteries_. Oxygenated

    blood is carried away from the lungs by the (b) _pulmonary veins_

12. Your patient is a 70-year-old man with chronic bronchitis and emphysema who experienced an acute onset of
    shortness of breath while at the grocery store. Describe your ongoing assessment of this patient's head, neck,

chest, and abdomen. Be specific when describing the muscle groups that you will inspect to help determine his degree of distress.

_____

_____

13. The partial pressure of nitrogen = (a) _____% × atmospheric pressure (b) _____ mm Hg =

(c) _____ mm Hg. The partial pressure of oxygen (P_{O_2}) = (d) _____% × atmospheric pres-

sure (e) _____ mm Hg = (f) _____mm Hg.

14. List three physiological factors that can increase the work of breathing.

a. _____

b. _____

c. _____

15. Describe the *structural* aspects of the lung that explain the following:

a. Normal lung expansion:

_____

b. Alveolar collapse that occurs because of decreased surfactant in a premature infant:

_____

c. Poor ventilation during an asthma attack:

_____

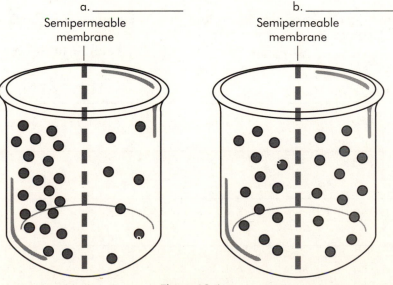

a. _____
Semipermeable
membrane

b. _____
Semipermeable
membrane

Figure 19-1

16. Each of the diagrams in Fig. 19-1 represents solutions separated by a semipermeable membrane. In each illustration, indicate whether the process of diffusion will cause a net movement of solute particles to the *left*, *right*, or *not at all*.

17. Complete the missing values for Pco_2 and Po_2 in the following. Then draw an arrow indicating the direction of movement of each of the gases across the respiratory membrane.

Alveolar Gas	Direction of Movement of Gas	Venous Blood (Pulmonary Capillaries)
Pco_2 _____ torr	Pco_2 _____ torr	
Po_2 _____ torr	Po_2 _____ torr	

18. Complete the following sentences.

    a. The primary way that oxygen is transported in the blood is by a chemical bond to __Hemoglobin__.

    b. Po_2 describes the oxygen level dissolved in blood __Plasma__.

    c. The amount of carbon dioxide present in the venous blood is influenced by the rate and type of __Metabolism__

    d. Carbon dioxide is transported in the blood in three forms: _____, _____ _____, and _____.

19. In one sentence describe the physiological basis for poor blood oxygenation in the following patients:

    a. A 23-year-old woman who is paralyzed completely from Guillain-Barré syndrome:

    _____

    b. A 52-year-old patient with pneumonia:

    _____

    c. An 8-year-old who is having an acute asthma attack:

    _____

    d. A 42-year-old with massive head trauma caused by a motor vehicle crash:

    _____

20. Briefly explain the origin or site of stimulation, location of effect, and action of each of the following mechanisms that control respiration:

Mechanism	Origin or Stimulus	Location of Effect	Action
Inspiratory centers			
Expiratory centers			
Hering-Breuer reflex			
Pneumotaxic center			
Apneustic center			

21. For each of the following scenarios, briefly explain why the patient's respirations will increase or decrease or be unchanged.

a. A 3-year-old who loses consciousness from breath-holding following a temper tantrum:

_____

b. A 34-year-old with a morphine overdose:

_____

c. A 17-year-old football player with a dislocated shoulder:

_____

d. A hostage with no apparent injuries who has just been freed:

_____

e. A student who is sleeping in class:

_____

f. An individual who suffers from chronic obstructive pulmonary disease who has fallen and for whom an oxygen level of 10 L/min is being administered by nonrebreather mask:

_____

g. A lost snow skier who has a core temperature of 84° F (28.9° C):

_____

22. Briefly describe the benefit of the following modified forms of respiration:

a. Cough:

_____

b. Sneeze:

_____

c. Hiccup:

_____

d. Sigh:

_____

23. For each of the following scenarios, identify the pathological condition or injury you would suspect, and list the signs and symptoms the patient may develop.

a. A 50-year-old man unable to speak after choking on a piece of steak:

_____

b. A nursing home patient with shortness of breath after "inhaling" some food:

_____

c. A 17-year-old hockey player who has difficulty speaking after being struck across the neck by a stick:

_____

d. A 2-year-old with croup:

_____

e. A 23-year-old who reportedly overdosed, is unconscious, and has vomitus draining from the side of her mouth.

_____

24. You are transporting a patient with severe asthma to a medical center 40 minutes away. What are the advantages of using a pulse oximeter in this scenario?

_____

25. For each of the following scenarios, circle the best oxygen-delivery device and explain why you made that selection.

a. A 76-year-old patient with chronic obstructive pulmonary disease complains of chest pain on the right side and a nosebleed after a fall. Vital signs are normal. Nasal cannula at 2 L/min oxygen or Venturi mask at 24% oxygen?

_____

b. A 25-year-old patient involved in a motor vehicle crash has ineffective respirations, cyanosis, and signs of a flail chest segment. Simple face mask at 8 L/min oxygen or bag-valve-mask with reservoir device at 15 L/min oxygen?

_____

c. A 45-year-old patient with slight chest pain (SaO_2 on room air is 98%). Simple face mask at 4 L/min oxygen or nasal cannula at 4 L/min oxygen?

_____

d. A 17-year-old patient who sustained a crush injury to the abdomen in a farming accident is pale, with cyanosis around the lips and decreased blood pressure. Simple mask at 6 L/min oxygen or complete non-rebreather mask at 10 L/min oxygen?

_____

26. For each of the following scenarios, choose the airway adjunct from the list that is most appropriate after initial manual airway maneuvers have been used. Explain why you selected your answer.

Oral airway   Nasal airway
Oral endotracheal intubation   Nasal endotracheal intubation
Percutaneous tracheal ventilation   Esophageal-tracheal combitube

a. Your patient is a 17-year-old victim of a snowmobiling accident who struck a concealed barbed wire fence, injuring his neck. The airway is not patent. All attempts to secure the airway, including oral and nasal intubation, are unsuccessful.

_____

b. You are called to evaluate a 34-year-old patient who is postictal after a single grand mal seizure. He has snoring respirations and no gag reflex.

_____

c. Your patient was pulled from a swimming pool after an unsuccessful dive into the shallow end. He has ineffective shallow respirations and flaccid paralysis of all limbs.

_____

d. A 32-year-old woman with a history of diabetes has taken her insulin but has not eaten. She has snoring respirations and can be aroused with painful stimulus.

_____

e. A 19-year-old ejected from his all-terrain vehicle has an obviously severe head injury and shallow agonal respirations.

_____

f. A 79-year-old is in cardiac arrest of medical origin.

_____

27. Describe your actions if you discover the following physical findings after endotracheal intubation of a patient:

   a. The carbon dioxide detector fades from purple to yellow as the patient exhales.

   _____

   b. Breath sounds are present bilaterally.

   _____

   c. Gurgling is auscultated over the epigastric region during ventilation.

   _____

   d. Breath sounds are diminished significantly over the left lung.

   _____

   e. The patient's color deteriorates, and the abdomen becomes distended.

   _____

   f. The bulb of the esophageal detector device fills in 8 seconds after placement on the end of the endotracheal tube.

   _____

28. Fill in the blanks with the appropriate airway adjunct(s) from the following list:

   Esophageal-tracheal Combitube (ETC)   Oral Endotracheal tube (ETT)

   Laryngeal mask airway (LMA)

   a. _____ Is available in sizes for children and adults.

   b. _____ May be used if placed in trachea or esophagus

   c. _____ Must visualize the vocal cords to insert

   d. _____ Provides best protection against aspiration

   e. _____ Requires inflation of two balloons

   f. _____ Does not enter the trachea.

29. Briefly describe each step of the orotracheal intubation procedure illustrated in Fig. 19-2.

   a.

   b.

   c.

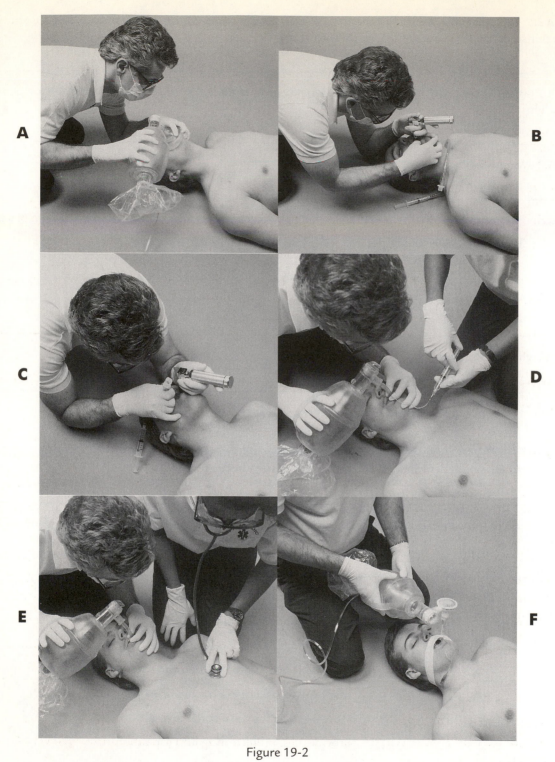

Figure 19-2

d.

e.

f.

30. List one advantage and one disadvantage for each of the following ventilation adjuncts:

Adjunct	Advantage	Disadvantage
a. Mouth to mouth		
b. Mouth to mask		
c. Bag-valve-mask		

31. List three patient situations in which use of tonsil-tip suction is indicated:

a.

b.

c.

32. What precautions should be taken to prevent complications when using a whistle-tip suction device for tracheal suctioning?

_____

33. Explain the anatomical basis for the following variations in pediatric airway management:

a. The oral airway should be inserted only with direct visualization with a tongue blade, never upside down and then rotated:

_____

b. Uncuffed endotracheal tubes should usually be used for children under 8 years of age:

_____

c. The endotracheal tube may "hang up" in the newborn, necessitating use of the Sellick maneuver to attain successful placement:

_____

34. You are called to the home of an 86-year-old patient who fell down 12 steps. Her chief complaint is rib pain and shortness of breath. On physical examination, you note crepitus and bruising on the lower rib cage. Why is it important to provide rapid, aggressive intervention for this older patient?

_____

_____

STUDENT SELF-ASSESSMENT

35. What is the term for the transfer of oxygen and carbon dioxide between the peripheral blood capillaries and tissue cells?
   a. External respiration   **c.** Pulmonary ventilation
   b. Internal respiration   **d.** Respiration

36. In what structure must continuous negative pressure be maintained to maintain lung expansion?
   a. Alveoli   **c.** Pleural space
   b. Mediastinum   **d.** Thoracic cage

37. When you arrive at the hospital, blood gasses on your 18-year-old patient indicate that the P_{O_2} is 70 mm Hg. What does this mean?
    a. Seventy percent of the hemoglobin is filled with oxygen.
    b. The patient is oxygenated adequately.
    c. Less than 3 mL of oxygen is dissolved in 1 L of blood.
    d. The blood sample must have been venous.
38. Which of the following factors will result in an *increased* energy requirement for breathing?
    a. Loss of pulmonary surfactant   c. An increase in lung compliance
    b. A decrease in airway resistance   d. Bronchodilation
39. Which of the following patients is most likely to have a decreased minute volume?
    a. A 17-year-old with deep respirations and signs of hyperventilation
    b. A 20-year-old patient with a head injury with shallow, slow respirations
    c. An alert 45-year-old with a possible myocardial infarction
    d. A 30-year-old in early shock with an increased respiratory rate
40. Your patient is on a pulse oximeter, and the reading is 100% saturation. What does this mean?
    a. The patient is on 100% oxygen by mask.
    b. The partial pressure of oxygen is 100.
    c. All hemoglobin has converted to oxyhemoglobin.
    d. The blood will not carry any more oxygen.
41. Which of the following conditions causes decreased oxygenation because of increased resistance in the airways?
    a. Asbestosis   c. Poliomyelitis
    b. Asthma   d. Tuberculosis
42. Why might the tissues of a patient with anemia not be well oxygenated?
    a. The blood does not reach all tissue to off-load oxygen.
    b. The respiratory drive in the brain is depressed.
    c. The number of red blood cells is insufficient to carry oxygen.
    d. The pulmonary vessels are not well perfused with blood.
43. Respiratory chemoreceptors in the medulla, aortic bodies, and carotid bodies are stimulated by changes in all of the following except which one?
    a. Blood pressure   c. Oxygen
    b. Carbon dioxide   d. pH
44. If a person appears to be choking but still can speak and cough, what should the rescuer do?
    a. Deliver five back blows.
    b. Perform the Heimlich maneuver.
    c. Administer five chest thrusts.
    d. Not intervene but just observe.
45. What is the most frequent cause of airway obstruction in the unconscious adult?
    a. Hot dogs   c. Tongue
    b. Steak   d. Vomitus
46. You arrive at a private residence, where you find an unconscious 52-year-old man. You open his airway and determine that he is not breathing. You attempt to ventilate his lungs, but the airflow is blocked. What is your next step?
    a. Assess the pulse.
    b. Reposition the head.
    c. Administer five abdominal thrusts.
    d. Perform a cricothyrotomy.
47. Which of the following represents the *most* effective measure to prevent aspiration of stomach contents?
    a. Applying cricoid pressure during bag-valve-mask ventilation
    b. Frequent suctioning of the mouth using a tonsil-tip suction
    c. Inserting an oropharyngeal airway and nasogastric tube
    d. Positioning the patient in the modified Trendelenberg's position
48. Your patient attempted suicide by hanging. She is hoarse and has hemoptysis and stridor. What do you suspect?
    a. Laryngeal fracture   c. Foreign body obstruction
    b. Laryngeal spasm   d. Tracheal injury

49. All of the following are potential complications of nasopharyngeal airway insertion except which one?
    a. It is poorly tolerated by sedated patients with gag reflexes.
    b. It may enter the esophagus if it is of excessive length.
    c. It may cause injury and bleeding to the nasal mucosa.
    d. It may become obstructed with blood or mucus.

50. To ensure adequate ventilation when combitube airway is used, you must be certain that
    a. The tube passes into the trachea.
    b. The mask seal is tight.
    c. The patient is less than 5 feet tall.
    d. Breath sounds are audible over the gastric area.

51. The pharyngeal tracheal lumen airway may be used successfully if the tube is placed in which structure?
    a. The esophagus
    b. The trachea
    c. The right main stem bronchus
    d. The esophagus or trachea

52. If 30 seconds have elapsed from the last ventilation and tracheal intubation has not been accomplished, what should you do?
    a. Remove the tube, hyperventilate, and try again.
    b. Continue if intubation can be done in a few more seconds.
    c. Insert an esophageal obturator airway.
    d. Have another paramedic attempt the skill.

53. Which of the following statements is true regarding percutaneous transtracheal ventilation?
    a. Demand valves may be used to provide adequate ventilations.
    b. It is a good long-term airway management device.
    c. It minimizes the risk of aspiration.
    d. The high pressures generated may cause pneumothorax.

54. Which of the following is *not* an advantage of the bag-valve-mask device?
    a. It allows delivery of high oxygen concentrations.
    b. It can give the rescuer a sense of the patient's lung compliance.
    c. It is used easily by one rescuer to deliver ventilations.
    d. It can provide a wide range of inspiratory pressures.

55. Which of the following indicates a properly placed endotracheal tube?
    a. End tidal CO_2 shows purple during ventilation.
    b. Gurgling is heard during auscultation over the stomach.
    c. Esophageal detection bulb refills in 10 seconds.
    d. Oxygen saturation changes from 79% to 94%.

56. Which of the following statements is true regarding suctioning of fluids from a patient?
    a. Preoxygenation for 2 minutes should precede suctioning.
    b. Suction should be applied for a maximum of 30 seconds.
    c. Coughing may cause decreased intracranial pressure.
    d. Suction should be set between 200 and 300 mm Hg.

57. The patient who is on a nasal cannula at 5 L/min is receiving approximately how much oxygen?
    a. 36%
    b. 40%
    c. 44%
    d. 50%

58. Your patient has been removed from a smoky building and is confused and tachycardic. What is the appropriate oxygen delivery device for this person?
    a. Nasal cannula
    b. Nonrebreather mask
    c. Simple face mask
    d. Venturi mask

59. Why might lidocaine be administered during rapid sequence induction for intubation?
    a. To minimize the potential for ventricular dysrhythmias
    b. To reduce the incidence of vomiting during the procedure
    c. To minimize the increase in intracranial pressure and prevent laryngospasm
    d. To anesthetize the airway structures and minimize the cough reflex

60. Which of the following complications related to cricothyrotomy will result in the absence of breath sounds when ventilation begins?
    a. Aspiration
    b. False passage
    c. Injury to the vocal cords
    d. Perforation of a great vessel

259

WRAP IT UP

You are dispatched to a school playground for an unconscious person. You arrive simultaneously with an ALS pumper crew and find a drowsy male who appears to be in his early 20s, lying across a playground bench. He is arousable to voice, but very drowsy and snores when not stimulated. You open his airway using the head-tilt–chin-lift method, and as you insert a nasal airway, you note some vomitus has dried partially around his mouth. Oxygen saturation readings on room air are 93%, and his lung sounds reveal sonorous wheezes (rhonchi) throughout. His pupils are midpoint and 3 mm and sluggishly react to light. Vital signs are BP 94/58 mm Hg, P 148, R 28 and shallow. Oxygen by nonrebreather mask is applied, and the patient quickly is packaged onto the stretcher and placed in the ambulance. Your partner shows you some empty pill bottles nearby, and you recognize that he likely has taken some sedatives and antipsychotic drugs. In the ambulance the patient is attached quickly to the ECG monitor, a nasogastric tube is inserted, automatic BP monitoring is set up, an IV is established, and blood glucose is checked. As you prepare to depart the scene, the patient's respirations become irregular and slow with apneic pauses. When you attempt to stimulate him, there is no response, and a glance at the monitor reveals a rapidly slowing heart rate and oxygen saturation level. You instruct your partner to set up the intubation equipment as you insert an oral airway and begin to hyperventilate with a bag-mask device. When ready, you orally intubate the patient and then verify the correct placement of the tube, secure it, and begin to ventilate using an automatic transport ventilator. His heart rate increases, oxygen saturation levels rise, and his condition remains unchanged for the 10-minute transport to the medical center.

1. Would pulmonary aspiration interfere with internal or external respiration?
2. What was the likely explanation for this patient's slow irregular respirations?
   a. Anatomical dead space increase
   b. Central nervous system depression
   c. Decreased intrapulmonary pressure
   d. Increased atmospheric pressure
3. What actions were taken to reduce the risk of further aspiration?

_____

4. Which of the following irregular patterns of breathing was this patient displaying?
   a. Air trapping
   b. Bradypnea
   c. Cheyne-Stokes
   d. Kussmaul's
5. Why was the nonrebreather mask chosen as the first oxygen delivery device?

_____

6. When the patient's respirations became irregular and slow, what acid-base disturbance most likely was occurring?
   a. Metabolic acidosis
   b. Metabolic alkalosis
   c. Respiratory acidosis
   d. Respiratory alkalosis
7. What measure was taken to correct the acid-base disturbance?

_____

8. How should the correct size of oral airway have been selected?

_____

9. a. Why was suctioning indicated before intubation?
   b. Should suctioning be performed after intubation? Yes/No. If you answered yes, describe why it would be indicated.

10. For this patient's situation, describe the finding that suggests tracheal intubation.

Method   **Finding**

   a. Auscultation over the epigastrium

_____

_____

   b. Bilateral auscultation of the lungs

_____

_____

   c. Esophageal detector device—syringe

_____

_____

   d. Esophageal detector device—bulb

_____

_____

   e. Colorimetric end-tidal CO_2 detector

_____

_____

   f. Digital end-tidal CO_2 detector

_____

_____

   g. Oxygen saturation

_____

_____

   h. Direct laryngoscopic visualization

_____

_____

11. What settings should be selected on the automatic transport ventilator?

Rate: _____/min Volume: _____mL

CHAPTER 19 ANSWERS

REVIEW QUESTIONS

1. e
   (Objective 5)

2. f
   (Objective 5)

3. c
   (Objective 5)

4. d
   (Objective 5)

5. a
   (Objective 5)

6. True
   (Objective 1)

7. True
   (Objective 3)

8. False. The pressure regulator reduces the pressure in the oxygen cylinder to 30 to 70 psi to permit safe administration. The flow meter regulates the amount of oxygen delivered.
   (Objective 10)

9. During inspiration, the dome of the diaphragm is flattened when it contracts. This causes an increase in the superior-inferior distance of the chest cavity. The intercostal muscles contract, resulting in an increase in the anteroposterior and lateral diameter of the chest cavity. This increase in the size of the chest cavity results in a pressure drop in the chest approximately 1 mm Hg below atmospheric pressure. This negative pressure causes gas to move into the lungs. During expiration the relaxation of the diaphragm and other breathing muscles results in a decrease in the size of the chest wall and an increase in pressure in the chest approximately 1mm Hg above atmospheric pressure. This positive pressure in the chest forces the gas out of the lungs.
   (Objective 2)

10. a. 760 mm Hg; b. intrapulmonic; c. thoracic; d. decrease; e. increase; f. compliance; g. asthma, emphysema, bronchitis, pulmonary edema, and lung cancer.
    (Objectives 2 and 3)

11. a. Pulmonary arteries; b. pulmonary veins
    (Objective 4)

12. Head: Inspect for cyanosis around lips and "puffing" of the cheeks; neck: inspect for the use of accessory muscles or tracheal tugging; chest: inspect for intercostal muscle use and an increased anteroposterior diameter of the chest, auscultate lung sounds; abdomen: inspect for the use of abdominal muscles when breathing.
    (Objective 9)

13. a. 79; b. 760; c. 600.2; d. 21; e. 760; f. 160
    (Objective 3)

14. Loss of pulmonary surfactant, increase in airway resistance, and decrease in pulmonary compliance
    (Objective 2)

15. a. The lungs are coated with visceral pleura that adhere to the parietal pleura that line the chest wall. In the potential space between these two membranes, negative pressure "holds" the lungs to the chest wall. Disruption of this potential space causes collapse of the lung.

b. Surfactant reduces the surface tension in the alveoli. In other words, surfactant reduces the tendency of the alveolar walls to "stick" together. In the newborn with insufficient surfactant production, extremely high airway pressures must be used to maintain inflation of the alveoli so that effective ventilation can occur.

c. The bronchioles are surrounded by smooth muscle. During an asthma attack, the smooth muscle contracts forcefully and decreases the diameter of the bronchioles, which impairs the exchange of gases.
(Objectives 2 and 15)

16. a. Right; b. not at all
(Objective 5)

17.

Alveolar Gas	Direction Movement of Gas	Venous Blood (Pulmonary Capillaries)
P_{CO_2} *0* torr	$\leftarrow$	P_{CO_2} *46* torr
P_{O_2} *100* torr	$\rightarrow$	P_{O_2} *40* torr

(Objectives 3 and 5)

18. a. Hemoglobin; b. plasma; c. metabolism; d. plasma, blood proteins, and bicarbonate ions.
(Objective 5)

19. a. Loss of function of respiratory muscles prevents ventilation from occurring without mechanical assistance.

b. Compliance of the lungs and surface area for gas exchange will decrease.

c. Resistance in the airways will increase, which will decrease the flow of gases to and from the lungs.

d. The respiratory centers may be damaged, resulting in abnormal or absent breathing. The airway may not be patent.
(Objective 15)

20.

Mechanism	Origin or Stimulus	Location of Effect	Action
Inspiratory centers	Medulla to spinal cord to phrenic and intercostal nerves	Send impulses of respiration	Stimulates muscles
Expiratory centers	Medulla	Send impulses to spinal cord to phrenic and intercostal nerves	Stimulates muscles of respiration to increase force of exhalation
Hering-Breuer reflex	Vagus nerve	Medulla discharges inhibitory impulses	Causes inspiration to cease so lungs do not overinflate
Pneumotaxic center	Pons	Inspiratory center	Inhibits inspiratory center during labored breathing
Apneustic center	Lower pons	Inspiratory center	Baseline stimulation of inspiratory neurons

(Objective 6)

21. a. The respirations increase or resume because of the increased P_{CO_2}, which stimulates the respiratory centers.

b. The respiratory rate decreases as the respiratory centers of the brain are depressed by the morphine.

c. Pain causes an increased respiratory rate.

d. The fear involved in such a situation causes an increased respiratory rate.

e. The respiratory rate slows because of the decreased metabolic rate during sleep.

f. The history of chronic lung disease may mean that the patient is operating on a hypoxic drive. If this is the case, the chemoreceptors will sense an increase in the P_{O_2} and respond by decreasing the respiratory rate.

g. During hypothermia the metabolic rate decreases, as does the respiratory rate.
(Objective 15)

22. a. The cough reflex is designed to expel foreign matter from the respiratory passages.

b. Sneezing is caused by nasal irritation and also rids the respiratory tract of unwanted irritants.

c. Hiccups serve no known useful purpose but may signal pathological conditions.

d. Sighing provides intermittent hyperinflation of the lungs to help maintain expansion of the alveoli.
(Objective 2)

23. a. Obstructed airway: The patient initially will be apneic, will lose consciousness, and finally will suffer cardiac arrest if untreated.

b. Aspiration of food and possibly gastric juices: Initially the patient may experience a cough, mucus production, decreased breath sounds, or wheezes.

c. Fractured larynx: The patient may experience localized pain, edema, or hemoptysis. Dysphagia and subcutaneous emphysema may be present if airway obstruction is imminent.

d. Croup with potential for laryngeal spasm: The patient may be anxious and have crowing respirations (stridor) because of airway tissue swelling.

e. Decreased level of consciousness may result in partial airway obstruction and aspiration of vomit.
(Objective 7)

24. The pulse oximeter permits monitoring of the effectiveness of interventions by observing the oxygen saturation and pulse rate. If the oxygen saturation does not improve, additional interventions may be needed.
(Objective 13)

25. a. Venturi mask at 24% oxygen: A nasal cannula would be ineffective because the patient has a nosebleed.

b. Bag-valve-mask with reservoir device at 15 L/min oxygen: The patient clearly is not ventilating properly and needs ventilatory assistance in addition to the highest flow of oxygen possible.

c. Nasal cannula at 4 L/min oxygen: The simple face mask should never be used with an oxygen flow set at less than 6 L/min.

d. Complete nonrebreather mask at 10 L/min oxygen: The patient is demonstrating signs of shock and decreased oxygenation, so the highest amount of oxygen possible should be administered.
(Objective 10)

26. a. Percutaneous tracheal ventilation: All other less invasive airway maneuvers have been unsuccessful, possibly because of a laryngeal injury. The patient's airway is not patent, so needle access should be attempted.

b. Oral airway: If this is an isolated seizure, the patient's level of consciousness should be improving gradually, and a more invasive airway maneuver probably can be avoided.

c. Nasal intubation: Because of the patient's spontaneous respirations, this would be selected over oral intubation because of the high probability of cervical spine injury.

d. Nasal airway: This should secure the airway quickly while glucose is administered, which should arouse the patient.

e. Oral endotracheal intubation (using manual in-line stabilization of the cervical spine): This would be chosen because of the possibility of cervical spine injury. Nasal intubation would not be an option until basilar skull fracture could be ruled out.

f. Oral intubation: This is the airway of choice in the unconscious apneic patient with no potential for cervical spine injury.
(Objective 12)

27. a. This indicates that the tube is in the correct position. The tube should be secured.
b. The endotracheal tube is in the correct position, so the tube may be secured.
c. If breath sounds are absent, the cuff should be deflated and the tube quickly removed. After hyperventilation of the patient's lungs with a bag-valve-mask and 100% oxygen, another attempt at intubation may be made.
d. The cuff should be deflated and the tube withdrawn 1 to 2 cm. The cuff should be reinflated and correct placement verified by auscultation of breath sounds bilaterally.
e. The tube is probably in the esophagus. Auscultate for breath sounds, and if they are absent or diminished, deflate the cuff and remove the tube immediately. Hyperventilate the patient's lungs with a bag-valve-mask with a reservoir at 100% oxygen.
f. The tube is probably not in the trachea. Placement should be confirmed by auscultation of lung and epigastric sounds and by direct visualization of the vocal cords and use of an end-tidal CO_2 detector.
(Objective 13)

28. a. LMA and ETC b. ETC c. ETT d. ETT e. ETC f. LMA
(Objective 12)

29. a. Hyperventilate the patient's lungs with 100% oxygen for at least 2 minutes.
b. With the laryngoscope in the left hand, insert the blade in the right corner of the mouth, displacing the tongue to the left.
c. Advance the endotracheal tube through the right corner of the mouth and, under direct vision, through the vocal cords.
d. Inflate the cuff with 5 to 8 mL of air, and ventilate the patient's lungs with a mechanical airway device.
e. Confirm endotracheal tube placement by auscultation of the abdomen and chest during ventilation.
f. Secure the endotracheal tube to the patient's head and face, and provide ventilatory support with supplemental oxygen. Continue to monitor correct placement of endotracheal tube using end-tidal CO_2 detection and other methods.
(Objective 12)

30.

Adjunct	Advantage	Disadvantage
a. Mouth to mouth	Easy to perform	Risk of infectious disease
	No equipment necessary	No supplemental oxygen
b. Mouth to mask	Easy to apply	Not possible to deliver 100% oxygen
	Can give supplemental oxygen	
c. Bag-valve-mask	Can give 100% oxygen	Mask seal difficult to maintain
	Can vary volume	Frequently requires two persons

(Objective 11)

31. Vomiting with inadequate ability to expel emesis, facial trauma with bleeding in mouth, and epistaxis (nosebleed) where blood is accumulating in the oral cavity.
(Objectives 8 and 12)

32. Place the patient on a cardiac monitor, hyperoxygenate the lungs with 100% oxygen for 5 minutes before the procedure, and apply suction for no longer than 10 seconds.
(Objective 12)

33. a. The tongue is disproportionately large in a child, and the oral airway easily can occlude the airway if it is inserted by rotation.
b. A child younger than 8 years has a circular narrowing at the level of the cricoid cartilage that serves as a functional cuff.
c. The vocal cords slope from front to back, necessitating rotation of the tube or performance of the Sellick maneuver to facilitate intubation.
(Objective 14)

34. In many older patients there is increased thoracic rigidity, decreased elastic recoil of the lungs, and diminished P_{O_2}. In addition, the chemoreceptors do not function as well, which results in a decreased ventilatory response because of compromise of the respiratory system. Therefore the patient who experiences a significant chest injury may lack the physiological capability to compensate for the injury and will need aggressive intervention by the paramedic.
(Objective 15)

35. b. External respiration is the transfer of O_2 and CO_2 between the inspired air and pulmonary capillaries. Pulmonary ventilation refers to the movement of air into and out of the lungs. Respiration is the exchange of O_2 and CO_2 between an organism and the environment.
(Objective 1)

36. c. Pressure within the lungs (including the alveolar sacs) drops approximately 1 mm Hg during inspiration to permit the entry of air but is equal to atmospheric pressure at the end of quiet exhalation. The mediastinum does not maintain inflation of the lungs. Integrity of the thoracic cage is necessary to maintain negative pressure within the pleural space.
(Objective 2)

37. c. Only 3 mL of oxgyen can be dissolved in 1 L of blood at the normal arterial P_{O_2} of 100 mm Hg. Oxygen saturation measures the amount of hemoglobin that is saturated with oxygen. Normal oxygenation for a healthy 18-year-old is indicated by a P_{O_2} of 80 to 100 or greater. Venous P_{O_2} is typically about 40 mm Hg.
(Objective 3)

38. a. Without pulmonary surfactant, alveoli tend to collapse, making the work of breathing more difficult. All other factors listed decrease the work of breathing.
(Objective 15)

39. b. Minute volume = tidal volume × respiratory rate. Anything that decreases one of these variables without a reciprocal increase in the other decreases the minute volume.
(Objective 15)

40. c. It means that all hemoglobin is saturated with oxygen. When oxygen saturation is 100%, the oxygen is typically between 80% and 100% but may vary under certain pathological conditions.
(Objective 13)

41. b. Oxygenation is impaired in all these examples by different mechanisms.
(Objective 15)

42. c.
(Objectives 5 and 15)

43. a. Only if the changes in respiratory rate alter the oxygen or carbon dioxide level or the pH will chemical receptors be triggered.
(Objective 6)

44. d. If the patient's physiological signs deteriorate, the rescuer should intervene.
(Objective 7)

45. c.
(Objective 7)

46. b. Because the tongue is the most frequent cause of airway obstruction, repositioning the airway may be the only maneuver necessary to permit air exchange.
(Objective 7)

47. a. Cricoid pressure (Sellick maneuver), if done properly, can greatly minimize the risk of aspiration during artificial ventilation until the airway is secured with an endotracheal tube. Suctioning will reduce but not eliminate the risk of aspiration. A nasogastric tube will decrease the risk of aspiration by minimizing the gastric content, but an oropharyngeal airway may stimulate the gag reflex and cause aspiration. The most appropriate position to minimize the risk of aspiration is the left lateral recumbent position.
(Objective 8)

48. a. The mechanism of injury and signs are consistent with this life-threatening emergency, which necessitates aggressive airway management.
(Objective 7)

49. a. It is a frequently underused adjunct usually well tolerated by a semiconscious patient with a gag reflex.
(Objective 12)

50. b. The tube should be in the esophagus of a patient more than 5 feet tall, and no sounds should be audible over the gastric area when the patient's lungs are ventilated.
(Objective 12)

51. d. The tube is designed to function correctly in the trachea or esophagus.
(Objective 12)

52. a. Repeat attempts should be performed after hyperventilation.
(Objective 12)

53. d. Percutaneous transtracheal ventilation is a short-term (less than 45 minutes) airway device used when other measures to secure the airway are unsuccessful. The demand valve does not provide sufficient pressure to ventilate by this method. It offers no protection from aspiration. (Objective 11)

54. c.
(Objective 11)

55. d.
(Objective 11)

56. a. Suction should be applied for no longer than 10 seconds. A cough is stimulated frequently and may increase intracranial pressure. Suction should be set between 80 and 120 mm Hg.
(Objective 12)

57. d.
(Objective 10)

58. b. A patient with this mechanism and symptoms of hypoxia clearly needs the highest percentage of oxygen available.
(Objective 10)

59. c. Ideally this should be done 3 minutes before intubation.
(Objective 12)

60. b. If the tube passes into tissue outside of the trachea, ventilation will not be possible. Aspiration, vocal cord injury, and perforation of great vessels also are complications but still may allow delivery of ventilation.
(Objective 12)

WRAP IT UP

1. External respiration is interrupted because the substance aspirated and resulting inflammation of the alveoli impair the passage of oxygen to the pulmonary capillaries.
   (Objective 1)

2. b. The drugs the patient ingested are central nervous system depressants that will inhibit the respiratory center in the brain and also impair the protective airway reflexes.
   (Objective 6)

3. Suctioning secretions from the airway, nasogastric tube insertion with suction of gastric contents, and endotracheal intubation will help to prevent further aspiration.
   (Objective 8)

4. c. Air trapping occurs from chronic obstructive pulmonary disease; bradypnea is a slow regular respiratory pattern; Kussmaul's respirations are rapid and deep and occur in diabetic ketoacidosis.
   (Objective 9)

5. A nonrebreather mask delivers the highest amount of oxygen.
   (Objective 10)

6. c. Respiratory acidosis occurs when ventilation is impaired, resulting in decreased oxygen and increased CO_2.
   (Objectives 9 and 15)

7. Hyperventilation helps to reverse respiratory acidosis.
   (Objective 15)

8. Measure the oropharyngeal airway from the tragus of the ear to the corner of the mouth or the angle of the jaw.
   (Objective 12)

9. a. Suctioning vomit from the oropharynx before intubation reduces the risk of aspiration and improves visualization of the vocal cords.
   b. After intubation suctioning with a soft whistle-tipped catheter would help to eliminate vomit that previously was aspirated.
   (Objectives 8 and 12)

10. a. No sounds heard over epigastrium
    b. Breath sounds clearly audible bilaterally
    c. Syringe fills freely with air and no stomach contents aspirated
    d. Bulb fills with air within 2 seconds and no stomach contents are aspirated
    e. Yellow color
    f. CO_2 reads 35 to 45 mm Hg
    g. Oxygen saturation increases or reads from 93% to 100%
    h. Tube directly observed to be passing through vocal cords
    (Objective 13)

11. Rate, 11-12; volume, 6 to 7 mL/kg
    (Objective 11)

PART SIX

IN THIS PART

Trauma Systems and Mechanism of Injury

READING ASSIGNMENT
Chapter 20, pages 499-519, in *Mosby's Paramedic Textbook,* ed. 3

OBJECTIVES
Upon completion of this chapter, the paramedic student will be able to:
1. Describe the incidence and scope of traumatic injuries and deaths.
2. Identify the role of each component of the trauma system.
3. Predict injury patterns based on knowledge of the laws of physics related to forces involved in trauma.
4. Describe injury patterns that should be suspected when injury occurs related to a specific type of blunt trauma.
5. Describe the role of restraints in injury prevention and injury patterns.
6. Discuss how organ motion can contribute to injury in each body region depending on the forces applied.
7. Identify selected injury patterns associated with motorcycle and all-terrain vehicle collisions.
8. Describe injury patterns associated with pedestrian collisions.
9. Identify injury patterns associated with sports injuries, blast injuries, and vertical falls.
10. Describe factors that influence tissue damage related to penetrating injury.

SUMMARY
- Trauma is the leading cause of death among persons 1 to 34 years of age and is the fifth leading cause of death among all Americans.
- Trauma care is divided into three phases: preincident, incident, and postincident.
- Components of the trauma system include injury prevention, prehospital care, emergency department care, interfacility transportation (if needed), definitive care, trauma critical care, rehabilitation, data collection, and trauma registry.
- Injuries are caused by a transfer of energy from some external source to the human body. The extent of injury is determined by the type of energy applied, by how quickly it is applied, and by the part of the body to which the energy is applied.
- Blunt trauma is an injury produced by the wounding forces of compression and change of speed, which can disrupt tissues.
- Four restraining systems are available in the United States. These are lap belts, diagonal shoulder straps, child safety seats, and air bags. All of these significantly reduce injuries. However, if they are used inappropriately, these protective devices also can produce injuries.

- Organ injuries can result from sudden movement caused by deceleration and compression forces. The recognition of these injuries requires a high degree of suspicion. The paramedic must use the principles of kinematics.
- Small motorized vehicles such as motorcycles, all-terrain vehicles, snowmobiles, motorboats, water bikes, and farm machinery are considered to be more dangerous than other motor vehicles. They are more dangerous because they offer little protection to the rider. They offer minimal protection from the transfer of energy associated with collisions.
- All auto-pedestrian collisions can produce serious injuries. They require a high degree of suspicion for multiple-system trauma.
- Sports provide a variety of health benefits. However, they also can produce severe injury.
- Blast injury is damage to a patient exposed to a pressure field that is produced by an explosion of volatile substances. Blasts release large amounts of energy in the form of pressure and heat.
- Falls from greater than 3 times the height of a person (15 to 20 feet) are associated with an increased incidence of severe injuries. In predicting injuries associated with falls, the paramedic should evaluate three things: the distance fallen, the body position of the patient on impact, and the type of landing surface struck.
- All penetrating objects, regardless of velocity, cause tissue disruption. The character of the penetrating object, its speed of penetration, and the type of body tissue it passes through or into determine whether crushing or stretching forces will cause injury.

REVIEW QUESTIONS

Match the appropriate energy law listed in Column II with its description in Column I.

Column I		Column II
1. _B_ Force is equal to mass times acceleration or deceleration.		a. Newton's first law of motion
2. _E_ Equal to ½ mass × velocity².		b. Newton's second law of motion
3. _A_ An object at rest or in motion remains in that state unless force is applied.		c. Conservation of energy law
		d. Joule's law
4. _C_ Energy can neither be created nor destroyed; it can only change form.		e. Kinetic energy law

5. Identify three causes of death for each of the periods of the trimodal distribution of traumatic death; for each period, identify prehospital interventions that may increase patient survival.
   a. Immediate:

   _____

   b. Early:

   _____

   c. Late:

   _____

6. A 17-year-old female falls asleep at the wheel, rides the median for 50 feet, and then strikes a concrete bridge abutment head-on.
   a. Identify the three collisions that occur in this situation.

   Vehicle strikes structure, Body strikes inside of Vehicle,

   Organs strike the bony structures

   _____

   b. Assuming that this driver took the down-and-under pathway during the collision, what injuries should you anticipate?

   Dislocated knees, Patellar fractures, fractured femurs, vascular injury or

   hemmorage

7. Aside from speed and size, what factor affects the injury pattern found in a lateral impact collision?

Whether car remains stationary, or moves from point of impact

8. In which of the following rear-end collisions will damage be greater, assuming that mass and other factors are equal? Why?
   a. A vehicle traveling 50 mph is struck by a vehicle traveling 70 mph.
   b. A vehicle traveling 5 mph is struck by a vehicle traveling 40 mph.

B. Because the difference in speed between vehicles is greater

9. For each of the body regions, list the injury or injuries that may occur during sudden, rapid deceleration.
   a. Head and neck injuries:

   b. Thoracic injuries:

   c. Abdominal injuries:

10. You are called to the scene of a high-speed frontal crash caused by a crossover accident. The driver of one of the vehicles complains of severe dyspnea and has a large circular bruise on her chest. You note greatly decreased lung sounds on the right side of the chest and suspect a pneumothorax.
    a. What traumatic mechanism can cause a pneumothorax in this example?

fx rib could puncture a lung - or - paper bag injury when gas is inhaled against a closed glottis

    b. The driver of the other vehicle has severe abdominal pain and is exhibiting signs of hypovolemic shock. Which abdominal organs or structures can be injured from sudden compression of the abdomen?

Lacerated spleen, liver or kidney, Rupture of bladder, Diaphragm, Duodenum colon, stomach + bowels

11. Identify the type of motorcycle collision most frequently associated with the pattern of injuries listed.
    a. A seasoned biker has a severely angulated fracture of the right forearm and extensive abrasions to the right side of the body.

laying bike down (skid)

    b. A 47-year-old executive has bilateral fractured femurs and facial injuries.

Head on crash, up and over handle bars.

    c. A traffic officer has a severe crush injury to the left lower leg.

Angular

12. Identify the injuries to be anticipated in the following situations:
    a. A motorist swerves across the highway and is struck by an oncoming vehicle.

fx of lower legs, femur, pelvis, thorax + spine, injuries to intra abdominal face and neck

    b. As a young child hurries to avoid being late to school, he is struck by a full-size automobile.

13. When evaluating a sports injury, what principles of kinematics must be considered to determine probable areas of injury?

Energy forces involved, Body part in which energy is transferred, speed of acceleration and deceleration, forces involved, protective gear

14. A suitcase filled with plastic explosives detonates in a locker at a busy urban airport. Describe the type of injuries the paramedic should anticipate in each of the following categories:

    a. Primary blast injuries:

    Hearing loss, Pulmonary Hemorage, Cerebral Air Embolism, thermal injurys Abdominal Hemmorage, Bowel Perfacation

    b. Secondary blast injuries:

    Lacerations, Contusions, fractures and impaled objects.

    c. Tertiary blast injuries:

    Fractures, head, spine, abdomind pelvic

15. You are called to a home to care for a person who has fallen.

    a. List three things you must determine to predict injuries associated with this fall.

    Height of fall, How pt landed, type of landing surface.

    b. What age of patient is most likely to fall?

    Children and Elderly

    c. If the person who fell is an adult, how is she likely to land?

    Adults are more likely to land on their feet.

16. Briefly describe the way each of the following ballistic properties influences injury patterns in penetrating trauma.

    a. Character of the penetrating object:

    b. Speed of penetration:

    c. Distance from patient that a bullet is fired:

STUDENT SELF-ASSESSMENT

17. Trauma is the leading cause of death in persons of which of the following ages?
    a. Less than 1 year
    b. 1 to 34 years
    c. 35 to 65 years
    d. More than 65 years

18. What actions can a paramedic take to intervene at the incident phase of trauma?
    a. Educate the community
    b. Decrease scene time
    c. Promote safety legislation
    d. Wear personal restraint systems

19. Which of the following is a component of a trauma system as defined in the National Standard Paramedic Curriculum?
    a. Emergency medical services education
    b. Fire suppression
    c. Pain management
    d. Rehabilitation
20. What factor influences trauma triage guidelines?
    a. Mechanism of injury
    b. Patient's ability to pay
    c. Paramedic preference
    d. Patient preference
21. What is the process of predicting injury patterns that may result from the forces and motions of energy known as?
    a. Force of energy applied
    b. Index of suspicion
    c. Kinematics
    d. Mechanism of injury
22. Injury resulting from blunt trauma most often is caused by which of the following forces?
    a. Compression
    b. Deceleration
    c. Distraction
    d. Torsion
23. Your patient was restrained when her car was struck on the right side on her door at a high rate of speed. What injuries do you predict?
    a. Aortic injury
    b. Liver injury
    c. Pancreatic injury
    d. Splenic injury
24. Which injuries are more likely if the lap belt is applied improperly?
    a. Duodenal injuries
    b. Maxillofacial injuries
    c. Pelvic fractures
    d. Sternal fractures *All possible*
25. Which of the following is true regarding ejection from a vehicle?
    a. It will not happen if the person is restrained.
    b. It usually happens before impact.
    c. Spinal injuries are common.
    d. There is little risk of death.
26. Steering wheel/dash air bags are designed to reduce injuries in which of the following collisions?
    a. Frontal collisions
    b. Lateral collisions
    c. Rollover collisions
    d. All of the above
27. Which of the following are predictable injuries from all-terrain vehicle crashes?
    a. Abdominal injuries
    b. Kidney injuries
    c. Thoracic injuries
    d. Upper extremity injuries
28. Which of the following is more likely to occur when a child is struck by a car, compared with an adult?
    a. The child may strike the hood of the vehicle.
    b. The child may be dragged under the vehicle.
    c. The child may land on the ground.
    d. The child may strike the bumper of the vehicle.
29. A roofer falls from the top of a two-story residence. What type of injuries do you anticipate?
    a. Minor injuries to the feet and spine
    b. Severe injuries to the feet and spine
    c. Minor injuries to the head and neck
    d. Major injuries to the head and neck
30. A 2-year-old child falls from a second-story window. What area of the body is most likely to be injured?
    a. Head and neck
    b. Arm
    c. Leg
    d. Pelvis
31. Which of the following is a high-energy weapon with the potential to cause the greatest injury to tissues?
    a. M-16
    b. .357 magnum
    c. 12-gauge shotgun
    d. Knife
32. Which organ is likely to experience the most severe injury from tissue crushing caused by cavitation after a gunshot wound?
    a. Bowel
    b. Liver
    c. Lung
    d. Muscle

WRAP IT UP

You are checking your ambulance at shift change on a foggy September morning when you are dispatched to the interstate highway for a chain reaction collision involving multiple vehicles. You and your supervisor arrive on the scene simultaneously, and she sends you to begin triage. As you move from vehicle to vehicle, you note the following. The first two cars appear to have struck each other head on—there is major damage. In vehicle #1 there are two front seat passengers, both restrained with air bags that now are deflated. They are conscious, but the passenger has abdominal and low back pain and lifts his shirt to show you the abrasion over his abdomen. In vehicle #2 the passengers were not restrained. The driver was thrown up and over the steering wheel and into the now starred windshield. He is dyspneic, pale, and anxious. His passenger was ejected and lies motionless at the side of the road; there is no breathing, even after you open his airway, so you move on. Vehicle #3, a small sedan, struck vehicle #2 on the right rear fender in a glancing blow and then swerved into the ditch and rolled several times. The front seat passenger, who is belted with her lap and shoulder belt, and her child, appropriately secured in a child seat in the middle rear seat, are crying, are alert, and have normal skin color. As vehicle #3 swerved, it struck a sport utility vehicle (vehicle #4) that spun and came to rest sideways in the highway. The SUV was then struck laterally on the driver door by a national express delivery truck (vehicle #5). There were no side air bags, and the restrained SUV driver has chest pain and severe arm and hip pain. The truck driver was restrained and is ambulatory with no complaints. A motorcyclist (vehicle #6), seeing an imminent collision with vehicle #5, laid his bike down and slid on his side 30 feet before striking the rear dual wheels of the truck. The protective coating on his helmet has been worn away on the lateral side, as has his jacket, and he is conscious, alert and complaining of severe pain from his deep skin abrasions. A police officer, struck by a car as he set up traffic cones, is unconscious on the ground. You report to command a brief synopsis of patient condition so that appropriate transport decisions can be made; the closest level I or II trauma center is 75 miles away.

1. Which phase of trauma care will you be involved with on this scene?
   a. Preincident
   b. Incident
   c. Postincident
   d. Preventive

2. Place a check mark beside the components of a sophisticated trauma system that could (or did) benefit any of the patients on this call.
   a. _____ Injury prevention
   b. ___✓___ Prehospital care
   c. ___✓___ Emergency department care
   d. ___✓___ Interfacility transportation if needed
   e. ___✓___ Definitive care
   f. ___✓___ Trauma critical care
   g. ___✓___ Rehabilitation
   h. ___✓___ Data collection and trauma registry

3. List injuries that you would anticipate based on the mechanism of injury for each of the following patients.

   Patient   **Injuries Predicted**
   a. Passenger vehicle #1 (restrained with air bag)

   _____

   b. Driver vehicle #2 (up and over)

   _____

   c. Passenger car #2 (ejected)

   _____

   d. Passenger vehicle #3 (child in car seat)

   _____

   e. Driver vehicle #4 (SUV)

   _____

   f. Rider vehicle #6 (motorcycle)

   _____

   g. Police officer

   _____

CHAPTER 20 ANSWERS

REVIEW QUESTIONS

1. b
(Objective 3)

2. e
(Objective 3)

3. a
(Objective 3)

4. c
(Objective 3)

5. a. Lacerations of the brain, brainstem, upper spinal cord, heart, aorta, and other large vessels; injury prevention programs
b. Subdural or epidural hematoma, hemopneumothorax, ruptured spleen, lacerated liver, pelvic fracture, and numerous injuries associated with significant blood loss; decreasing time from injury to definitive care, which must be brief
c. Sepsis, infection, and multiple organ failure; early recognition and treatment of life-threatening injury in the field, with adequate fluid resuscitation and aseptic technique
(Objective 1)

6. a. The vehicle strikes the abutment, the passenger strikes the inside of the vehicle, and the internal organs pull forward rapidly and strike the bony structures inside the body.
b. Dislocated knees, patellar fractures, fractured femurs, posterior fracture or dislocation of the acetabulum, vascular injury, and hemorrhage
(Objective 1)

7. Whether the car struck remains stationary (injuries likely on the side of the impact) or moves away from the point of impact (injuries likely on the side opposite the impact)
(Objective 4)

8. b. The velocity that produces damage is determined by calculating the difference between the speed of the two vehicles. In example a it is $70 - 50 = 20$, and in example b it is $40 - 5 = 35$.
(Objective 3)

9. a. Intracerebral hemorrhage and cervical fracture; b. ruptured aorta; c. kidney, liver, and spleen lacerations
(Objective 4)

10. a. Pneumothorax could be caused by displaced rib fractures that puncture a lung or by a paper bag injury, in which impact occurs after the patient has inhaled against a closed glottis.
b. Lacerated spleen, liver, or kidney; rupture of the bladder, diaphragm, gallbladder, duodenum, colon, stomach, and small bowel
(Objective 4)

11. a. Laying the bike down; b. head-on (up and over the handle bars); c. angular
(Objective 7)

12. a. Fractures of the lower legs, femur, pelvis, thorax, and spine; injuries to the intraabdominal or intrathoracic contents; and head and spinal injuries
    b. Fractures of the femur and pelvis; abdominopelvic and thoracic trauma; and head and neck injuries
    (Objective 8)

13. Energy forces involved, body part to which energy is transferred, speed of acceleration and deceleration, forces involved (compression, twisting, hyperextension, hyperflexion), protective gear
    (Objective 9)

14. a. Hearing loss, pulmonary hemorrhage, cerebral air embolism, thermal injuries, abdominal hemorrhage, and bowel perforation
    b. Lacerations, contusions, fractures, and impaled objects
    c. Fractures and abdominopelvic, thoracic, head, and spine injuries
    (Objective 9)

15. a. The paramedic should evaluate: the distance fallen; the body position of the patient on impact; and the type of landing surface.
    b. Children and elderly are more likely to fall.
    c. An adult is more likely to land on her feet.
    (Objective 9)

16. a. Length and width of knives determine the depth and extent of the injury. With bullets, missile damage increases if the bullet is designed to rotate, flatten, or fragment during or after impact.
    b. Kinetic injury increases with increased speed, and tissue damage increases with increased energy applied.
    c. As the range increases, the damage decreases because of decreased velocity. Close-range injuries produce more damage because of the direct injury of gases from combustion and the explosion of powder.
    (Objective 10)

17. b. Trauma is the fifth leading cause of death overall.
    (Objective 1)

18. d. Community education and legislation are preincident interventions, and decreasing scene time is a postinjury intervention.
    (Objective 1)

19. d. The other components are injury prevention, prehospital care, emergency department care, interfacility transportation, definitive care, trauma critical care, data collection, and trauma registry.
    (Objective 2)

20. a. Other factors include patient condition, injury severity indices, and available patient care resources.
    (Objective 2)

21. c. Kinematics is based on mechanism of injury and force of energy applied. Index of suspicion for certain types of injuries is related to kinematics, the age of the patient, and preexisting illness.
    (Objective 3)

22. a. Direct compression or pressure on a structure is the most common type of force applied in blunt trauma.
    (Objective 4)

23. b. Because she was struck on the right side, injury to the liver is more likely than injury to the spleen.
    (Objective 4)

24. a. All the other injuries can occur in high-speed crashes in which the lap belt is applied properly.
    (Objective 5)

25. c. A small number of restrained persons are ejected. Risk of death is 6 times greater than the risk for those who are not ejected. Ejection typically happens after impact.
(Objective 5)

26. a. The air bag inflates and then rapidly deflates after the first frontal collision.
(Objective 5)

27. d. Head and neck injuries also are common.
(Objective 7)

28. b. This may compound other injuries and cause traumatic amputation.
(Objective 8)

29. b. Falls from more than 3 times the height of the individual are likely to produce serious injury. Adults who fall from a height greater than 15 feet usually land on their feet.
(Objective 9)

30. a. Children tend to fall head first because their heads are proportionately larger.
(Objective 9)

31. a.
(Objective 10)

32. b. Nonelastic organs do not stretch.
(Objective 10)

WRAP IT UP

1. b.
(Objective 1)

2. a. Injury prevention (seat belt education, passive restraint [air bags] systems; prehospital care (triage, treatment, transport); emergency department care (examination, diagnostics, interventions); interfacility transport if needed (to higher-level trauma centers); definitive care (surgery for intraabdominal injuries); trauma critical care (early postresuscitation care); rehabilitation (physical, head injury); data collection and trauma registry (to monitor trauma quality, track demographics)
(Objective 2)

3. a. If lap belt was improperly worn too high, injury to T12, L1, and L2 could occur. If compressed, injury could be provided to the liver, spleen, duodenum, or pancreas could be present.
(Objectives 3, 4, and 5)

b. Rib fractures, ruptured diaphragm, hemopneumothorax, pulmonary contusion, cardiac contusion, myocardial rupture, or aortic rupture are possible if thorax absorbed impact. If abdomen absorbed impact, tears to liver, spleen, or blood vessels are possible. Head and neck injuries are also common.
(Objectives 3 and 4)

c. Spinal fracture, death
(Objectives 3 and 4)

d. Rollover: difficult to categorize injuries—None may be present if proper restraints were used.
(Objectives 3 and 4)

e. Lateral impact: fractured ribs, pulmonary contusion, ruptured liver or spleen, fractured clavicle, fractured pelvis, and head and neck injury
(Objectives 3 and 4)

f. Motorcyclist laying the bike down: abrasions, fractures to the affected side
(Objective 7)

g. Pedestrian struck: lower extremity fractures; femur, pelvis, spine fractures; head injuries, internal hemorrhage
(Objective 8)

Hemorrhage and Shock

READING ASSIGNMENT
Chapter 21, pages 520-537, in *Mosby's Paramedic Textbook,* ed. 3

OBJECTIVES
Upon completion of this chapter, the paramedic student will be able to:
1. Describe how to recognize signs and symptoms of internal or external hemorrhage.
2. Define shock.
3. Outline the factors necessary to achieve adequate tissue oxygenation.
4. Describe how the diameter of resistance vessels influences preload.
5. Describe the function of the components of blood.
6. Outline the changes in the microcirculation during the progression of shock.
7. List the causes of hypovolemic, cardiogenic, neurogenic, anaphylactic, and septic shock.
8. Describe pathophysiology as a basis for signs and symptoms associated with the progression through the stages of shock.
9. Describe key assessment findings to distinguish the etiology of the shock state.
10. Outline the prehospital management of the patient in shock based on knowledge of the pathophysiology associated with each type of shock.
11. Discuss how to integrate the assessment and management of the patient in shock.

SUMMARY
- The seriousness of external hemorrhage depends on the anatomical source of the hemorrhage, the degree of vascular disruption, and the amount of blood loss that can be tolerated by the patient. Internal bleeding that causes the patient to be unstable usually occurs in one of three body cavities: the chest, abdomen, or retroperitoneum.
- Shock is not a single entity. Shock does not have one specific cause and treatment. Rather, shock is a complex group of physiological abnormalities. Moreover, shock can result from a variety of disease states and injuries.
- To achieve adequate oxygenation of tissue cells (perfusion), three distinct components of the cardiovascular system must function properly: the heart, vasculature, and lungs.
- The healthy body is a smooth-flowing fluid delivery system inside a container. The volume of the container is related directly to the diameter of the resistance vessels. This diameter can change rapidly.
- Normal adult blood volume is 4.5 to 5 L.

- The progression of shock affects the microcirculation. This progression follows a sequence of stages related to changes in capillary perfusion and cellular necrosis. These stages include vasoconstriction, capillary and venule opening, disseminated intravascular coagulation, and multiple organ failure.
- In emergency care, shock commonly is classified based on the cause. (For example, the cause may be hypovolemic, cardiogenic, neurogenic, anaphylactic, or septic.)
- The response of the body to the shock syndrome (hypoperfusion and its associated anaerobic metabolism) can be categorized into stages: compensated shock, uncompensated (or decompensated) shock, and irreversible shock.
- Variations in the physiological response to shock can occur based on a number of factors. The patient's age and health are factors. The patient's ability to activate compensatory mechanisms plays a role. The specific organ affected is a factor as well.
- The management and treatment plan for the patient in shock focuses on assessment. The paramedic must assess oxygenation and perfusion of the body organs. The goals of the treatment plan are to ensure a patent airway, to provide adequate oxygenation and ventilation, and to restore perfusion. The initial survey can help to identify the adequacy of cellular perfusion.

REVIEW QUESTIONS

Match the blood component in Column II with its definition in Column I. Use each answer only once.

Column I

1. __b__ Provides oxygen to and removes carbon dioxide from cells
2. __g__ Forms sticky plugs and initiates clotting
3. __e__ Destroys red blood cells and bacteria
4. __A__ Large protein that moves water from tissues into the blood
5. __D__ Important in human immune response
6. __f__ Solvent of blood through which salts, minerals, and fats travel

Column II

a. Albumin
b. Erythrocytes
c. Fibrinogen
d. Gamma globulin
e. Leukocyte
f. Plasma
g. Platelet

7. You are called to evaluate a 20-year-old butcher who sustained a stab wound to the femoral artery. Evaluation of the patient reveals a large amount of blood loss from an inguinal wound that is spurting bright red blood. The patient is anxious and confused. Vital signs are as follows: blood pressure, 86/70 mm Hg; pulse, 136; respirations, 28; and lungs, clear. The patient's lips and nail beds are pale and cyanotic, and capillary refill is greater than 2 seconds. List the three physiological components necessary for normal cellular oxygenation as measured by the Fick principle and determine whether each has been met.

   a.

   b.

   c.

8. Describe the structural elements of the vascular system that enable it to adjust its size and adapt to pressure changes.

_____

_____

9. Complete the following sentences: The pressure that blood exerts against the vessel walls is known as

   (a) _Systemic_____ pressure. Pressure that results from contraction of the ventricles is

   (b) _Systolic_____ pressure, whereas the residual pressure

   between contractions is (c) _Diastolic_____ pressure. The pulse felt in an artery resulting from the difference in (b) and (c) pressure is known as (d) _Pulse_____ pressure.

Pressure in the vessels is greatest at the (e) _Heart (or Aorta)_____ and least at the

(f) _Vena Cava_____.

10. State the effect that each of the following patient situations has on the size of the patient's vascular container and on preload.
    a. A patient with a cervical spine injury from a motor vehicle collision has the following vital signs: blood pressure, 80/60 mm Hg; pulse, 60; and respirations, 28. His skin is cool and pale above the level of the injury and warm and dry below it.

_____

    b. A 55-year-old woman with heavy vaginal bleeding has been dizzy. Vital signs are as follows: blood pressure, 106/92 mm Hg; pulse, 116; and respirations, 20.

_____

11. For each of the following intravenous fluids, indicate whether the solution is isotonic, hypotonic, or hypertonic. Indicate whether there will be immediate net movement of fluid into or out of the intravascular space if this fluid is given, or whether no movement is observed.

Intravenous Fluid **Isotonic, Hypotonic, or Hypertonic** **Fluid Movement**

D50W

Lactated Ringer's

Normal saline

0.45% normal saline

D_5W

12. A 65-year-old complains of severe abdominal pain that radiates to the back. A large pulsatile mass is evident in the abdomen. Vital signs are as follows: blood pressure, 80/70 mm Hg; pulse, 128; and respirations, 28. Predict the pathophysiological changes and associated signs and symptoms that will occur during the stages of shock for this patient.
    a. Stage 1: Vasoconstriction

_____

    b. Stage 2: Capillary and venule opening

_____

    c. Stage 3: Disseminated intravascular coagulation

_____

_____

    d. Stage 4: Multiple organ failure

_____

_____

13. For each of the following situations, list the type of shock and briefly describe interventions necessary for patient management.

a. You are called to evaluate a 72-year-old man whose wife states that he had chest pain all day yesterday and earlier today. He has no pain when you arrive, but he is confused, pale, and diaphoretic. No bleeding is evident. Lung sounds reveal crackles in the bases. Vital signs are as follows: blood pressure, 86/76 mm Hg; pulse, 128 and irregular; and respirations, 28.

Classification:

Interventions:

---

b. Your 17-year-old patient was unrestrained in a motor vehicle collision. He has no sensation below the nipple line and is confused. He has a large laceration on the parietal area and complains of neck pain. No other injuries are evident. His skin is pale and cool above the nipple line and warm and dry below. Vital signs are as follows: blood pressure, 84 mm Hg by palpation; pulse, 56; and respirations, 28 and very shallow.

Classification:

Interventions:

---

c. A 26-year-old woman who states that her last menstrual period was 8 weeks ago is complaining of severe right lower quadrant abdominal pain. She is pale, cool, and diaphoretic. Vital signs are as follows: blood pressure, 106/78 mm Hg; pulse, 120; and respirations, 20 while supine; blood pressure, 88/76 mm Hg; pulse, 136; and respirations, 28 while standing.

Classification:

Interventions:

---

d. A 42-year-old woman experiences acute shortness of breath, urticaria, nausea, and dizziness after ingesting a penicillin tablet prescribed by her dentist. Vital signs are as follows: blood pressure, 80 mm Hg by palpation; pulse, 140; and respirations, 40 and labored.

Classification:

Interventions:

---

e. A 72-year-old resident of a nursing home has a fever and is restless and agitated. The urine in the indwelling catheter collection bag is milky and green. Vital signs are as follows: blood pressure, 94/60 mm Hg; pulse, 132; and respirations, 30.

Classification:

Interventions:

_____

_____

f. A 55-year-old office worker has complained of a pounding sensation in his chest and has fallen from his chair, striking his head on the desk. You note a 5-cm laceration on the frontal area that is freely oozing dark red blood (about 20 mL on the floor). The patient is unconscious, and vital signs are as follows: blood pressure, 60 mm Hg by palpation; pulse, 180; and respirations, 28.

Classification:

Interventions:

_____

_____

14. For each of the following situations, identify whether the patient is in compensated or uncompensated shock and explain why.
   a. A 48-year-old has sustained second- and third-degree burns to 70% of his body. He is pale, cool, and diaphoretic. His nail beds are cyanotic, and his vital signs are as follows: blood pressure, 84/76 mm Hg; pulse, 136; and respirations, 32.

_____

_____

   b. A 22-year-old passenger in a high-speed motor vehicle crash was restrained with a lap belt. She complains of severe abdominal pain. Her skin is cool and pale. Vital signs are as follows: blood pressure, 110/86 mm Hg; pulse, 128; and respirations, 28.

_____

_____

15. Describe the characteristics of irreversible shock.

_____

16. List three conditions, situations, or characteristics that decrease a patient's ability to compensate in shock.

_____

17. For each of the following scenarios, select the appropriate intervention(s) from the following list. Briefly justify your answer.

Pneumatic antishock garment   Drug therapy
Rapid fluid replacement   Blood transfusions
Intraosseous infusion

   a. A 72-year-old after experiencing a myocardial infarction with pulmonary edema and vital signs as follows: blood pressure, 86/60 mm Hg; pulse, 124; and respirations, 28.

   _____

   _____

   b. A 2-year-old was struck by an automobile, and you suspect that he has numerous pelvic and abdominal injuries. Vital signs are as follows: blood pressure, unobtainable; pulse, 170 carotid and weak; and respirations, 40 and shallow.

   _____

   _____

   c. A 44-year-old with a sudden onset of dizziness followed by syncope and vital signs as follows: blood pressure, 86/68 mm Hg; pulse, 44; and respirations, 20.

   _____

   _____

   d. An 18-year-old stung by a bee at a park has generalized redness and hives and is acutely short of breath. Vital signs are as follows: blood pressure, 70 mm Hg by palpation; pulse, 132; and respirations, 36.

   _____

   _____

   e. A 53-year-old woman with heavy vaginal bleeding for 1 week became lethargic and confused. Vital signs are as follows: blood pressure, 66 mm Hg by palpation; pulse, 136; and respirations, 32.

   _____

   _____

   f. A 19-year-old sustained a gunshot wound to the chest. Vital signs are as follows: blood pressure, 106/88 mm Hg; pulse, 128; and respirations, 24. ETA to the hospital is 40 minutes.

   _____

   _____

STUDENT SELF-ASSESSMENT

18. Your patient is passing bright red blood through the rectum. What is this called?
   a. Coffee-ground emesis   c. Hematochezia
   b. Epistaxis   d. Melena
19. Which of the following is the best definition of shock?
   a. Systolic blood pressure less than 90 mm Hg
   b. Greater than 25% loss of circulating blood
   c. Inadequate perfusion of the capillaries
   d. Blood flow deficit to the myocardium

20. Which of the following is true according to the Fick principle?
    a. Glucose must be available for cellular oxygenation.
    b. Precapillary and postcapillary sphincters must be open for adequate flow.
    c. Red blood cells must be able to load and unload oxygen.
    d. The pH should be at least 6.5 for adequate perfusion to occur.
21. Which of the following blood characteristics is the greatest determinant of afterload (peripheral vascular resistance)?
    a. Vessel diameter   c. Viscosity
    b. Vessel length   d. Volume
22. A decrease in peripheral vascular resistance will cause the container size of the body to _____ and the blood pressure to _____.
    a. decrease, decrease   c. increase, increase
    b. decrease, increase   d. increase, decrease
23. Which blood vessels act as collecting channels and storage (capacitance) vessels?
    a. Arterioles   c. Capillaries
    b. Arteries   d. Venules/veins
24. Which of the following blood cells are responsible for transporting about 99% of the oxygen carried to body tissues?
    a. Erythrocytes   c. Plasma proteins
    b. Leukocytes   d. Platelets
25. In what phase of shock does the microcirculation develop the leaky capillary syndrome?
    a. Capillary and venule opening
    b. Disseminated intravascular coagulation
    c. Multiple organ failure
    d. Vasoconstriction
26. What happens to fluid in stage 2 of the progression of shock?
    a. It is pulled into the intravascular space because of vasoconstriction.
    b. It leaks out of the intravascular space because of vasoconstriction.
    c. It is pulled into the intravascular space because of increased hydrostatic pressure.
    d. It leaks out of the intravascular space because of decreased hydrostatic pressure.
27. What occurs when there is dilation of the precapillary sphincter while the postcapillary sphincter remains constricted during lactic acidosis?
    a. No net movement of fluid between the fluid compartments
    b. Loss of vascular fluid into the interstitial spaces
    c. Movement of fluid from the interstitial spaces to the intravascular spaces
    d. Fluid shunting around the capillaries through the arterioles
28. What is shock caused by heart (pump) failure known as?
    a. Anaphylactic shock   c. Hypovolemic shock
    b. Cardiogenic shock   d. Neurogenic shock
29. Which of the following shock states does not produce vasodilation?
    a. Anaphylactic   c. Neurogenic
    b. Cardiogenic   d. Septic
30. Your patient was stabbed in the abdomen 20 minutes ago. Vital signs are as follows: blood pressure, 80/50 mm Hg; pulse, 136; and respirations, 26. He is anxious and pale. He is probably in which stage of shock?
    a. Compensated   c. Transitional
    b. Irreversible   d. Uncompensated
31. Increases in peripheral vascular resistance can be measured indirectly by noting which of the following?
    a. Diastolic blood pressure   c. Pulse rate
    b. Jugular distention   d. Systolic blood pressure
32. For which of the following conditions is the pneumatic antishock garment considered helpful?
    a. Cardiogenic shock   c. Penetrating chest injuries
    b. Pelvic fractures   d. Pulmonary edema
33. Which of the following fluids is a colloid solution?
    a. Dextran   c. Lactated Ringer's solution
    b. 0.45% sodium chloride d. Normal saline

34. Which of the following blood products has the greatest oxygen-carrying capacity per volume?
   a. Fibrinogen
   b. Packed red blood cells
   c. Plasma
   d. Whole blood

35. You arrive at the emergency department with a patient who has been vomiting bright red blood and is exhibiting signs and symptoms of shock. Which fluid is most beneficial to him at this time?
   a. Blood plasma
   b. Dextran
   c. Packed red blood cells
   d. Plasmanate

36. Your patient has fallen 30 feet from scaffolding and is anxious, confused, and in obvious shock. Which of the following is your priority of care, in the proper order?
   a. Rapid transport, oxygen, intravenous therapy
   b. Oxygen, intravenous therapy, rapid transport
   c. Intravenous therapy, rapid transport, oxygen
   d. Oxygen, rapid transport, intravenous therapy

37. In the absence of spinal or head injury, in what position should the hypovolemic patient in shock be placed?
   a. Lateral recumbent
   b. Modified Trendelenberg's
   c. Supine hypotension
   d. Trendelenberg's

38. Which of the following is not an appropriate initial prehospital management technique for the patient in hypovolemic shock?
   a. Crystalloid fluid replacement
   b. External hemorrhage control
   c. Pneumatic antishock garment
   d. Treatment with dopamine

39. Fluid therapy in cardiogenic shock should be slowed to the keep-open rate in which of the following cases?
   a. If lung crackles (rales) increase.
   b. If jugular vein distention decreases.
   c. If heart rate decreases.
   d. If peripheral edema increases.

40. Which of the following is the treatment of choice for the patient in severe anaphylactic shock?
   a. Antihistamines
   b. Epinephrine
   c. Fluid challenge
   d. Pneumatic antishock garments

41. You suspect that your patient has a ruptured ectopic pregnancy. She is in profound shock. Which intravenous catheter will you select?
   a. 14 gauge, 1½ inch
   b. 14 gauge, 3 inch
   c. 18 gauge, 1½ inch
   d. 18 gauge, 3 inch

42. A 200-mL fluid challenge is to be infused over 20 minutes. The drop factor is 10 drops/mL. How fast will you run it?
   a. 1 drop/min
   b. 33 drops/min
   c. 100 drops/min
   d. 400 drops/min

43. Which of the following is not a goal of prehospital care for the patient with severe hemorrhage and shock?
   a. Definitive care for internal hemorrhage
   b. Initiation of treatment
   c. Rapid recognition of the event
   d. Rapid transport to the appropriate hospital

WRAP IT UP

You are dispatched to a construction site for a fall. When you arrive, you are directed to the rear of an apartment building under construction. A 35-year-old worker has fallen about 30 feet onto a pile of dirt and rock. She is conscious but confused and is bleeding from a large head laceration. You immediately apply direct pressure to the laceration with a 5 × 9 inch dressing as you hold in-line immobilization of her head and continue your assessment. Her airway is patent, breathing is rapid, skin is pale and cool, and heart rate is rapid. The bleeding from her head laceration appears to have been controlled from direct pressure, so your partner wraps it with a gauze roller bandage as you continue your assessments. Her trachea is midline, neck veins are flat, and breath sounds are clear and equal bilaterally. A large reddened area begins on her lateral chest and extends down across her upper abdomen. There is tenderness to palpation over the left lateral ribs and diffuse tenderness over her abdomen. Both lower legs are swollen, tender, and deformed, with weak pedal pulses noted. She is rolled onto the backboard with spinal precautions and support of her legs and is moved to the ambulance. Vital signs are BP 84/66 mm Hg, P 136, R 28, SaO$_2$ not obtainable. Oxygen is delivered by non-rebreather mask at 15 L/min, transport is initiated, and the trauma center is notified that you are en route with an unstable patient who has fallen. En route to the hospital, an IV of normal saline is initiated in the left antecubital space and administered wide open; ECG monitoring is performed, and serial blood pressures obtained by an automatic BP cuff show a slight improvement in blood pressure, although her heart rate does not come down. Her head bandage is reinforced when blood soaks through the first one. The trauma team is awaiting you in the resuscitation room. Immediately, cross-table cervical spine, and chest radiographs are performed. Uncrossmatched blood is transfused, and as the patient's condition rapidly deteriorates, she is rushed to the surgical suite where her severely injured spleen is removed.

1. Were this patient's signs and symptoms of shock a result of external or internal hemorrhage? Explain your answer.

_____

2. Which of the following factors needed for adequate tissue perfusion was impaired in this patient?
   a. Adequate oxygen must be available in the lungs.
   b. Oxygen must be able to move freely across the alveolar walls.
   c. Normal hemoglobin levels must exist to carry oxygen.
   d. Tissue cells must close to capillaries so oxygen can off-load.
3. Circle the appropriate answer. The pale color of the patient's skin reflected a narrowing/widening of the blood vessels, which would cause a(n) decrease/increase in cardiac preload.
4. Which blood component most urgently needs replacement in this patient?
   a. Erythrocytes
   b. Fibrinogen
   c. Leukocytes
   d. Plasma
5. Your initial assessment of this patient reveals that she is in what stage of shock?
   a. Compensated
   b. Irreversible
   c. Multiple organ dysfunction syndrome
   d. Uncompensated
6. What sites (injuries) were possible causes for her shock?

_____

7. Pick the compensatory responses in shock that would be responsible for the following signs or symptoms present in this patient.
   a. Sympathetic response   b. Hormonal response   c. Adrenal response

   Sign or Symptom   **Compensatory Mechanism**
   Narrowed pulse pressure
   Pale, cool skin
   Tachycardia

8. Which of the following represents definitive care for this patient?
   a. Isotonic fluid administration
   b. High-concentration oxygen delivery
   c. Surgical intervention
   d. Uncrossmatched blood transfusion

REVIEW QUESTIONS

1. b
(Objective 5)

2. g
(Objective 5)

3. e
(Objective 5)

4. a
(Objective 5)

5. d
(Objective 5)

6. f
(Objective 5)

7. a. An adequate amount of oxygen is available to red blood cells. There is a sufficient F_{IO_2}, his airway is patent, and his lungs are clear.
b. Red blood cells must be circulated to all tissue cells. Based on the history of significant blood loss and the physical findings that indicate decreased cerebral perfusion (anxiety and confusion) and peripheral perfusion (pale, cyanotic lips and nail beds), it is evident that red blood cell transport is inadequate.
c. Red blood cells must be able to off-load oxygen adequately. This seems to be occurring in this situation, although acid-base abnormalities can impair this ability, and insufficient information is available to determine this accurately.
(Objective 3)

8. All blood vessels larger than capillaries are surrounded by layers of connective tissue that counter the pressure of blood in the vascular system, have elastic properties to dampen pressure pulsations and minimize flow variations throughout the cardiac cycle, and contain muscle fibers to control vessel diameter.
(Objective 4)

9. a. systemic; b. systolic; c. diastolic; d. pulse; e. heart (or aorta); f. vena cava
(Objective 4)

10. a. Spinal cord injury results in a loss of sympathetic tone and therefore impairs the ability of the blood vessels to constrict below the level of the injury. This increases the container size, decreasing the effective circulating volume and preload.
b. When blood loss occurs, a situation potentially exists in which the container is the same size but the volume has decreased, reducing the preload. Body compensatory mechanisms attempt to decrease the size of the container by vasoconstriction in an effort to match the container to the volume.
(Objective 4)

11.

Intravenous Fluid	Isotonic, Hypotonic, or Hypertonic	Fluid Movement
D50W	Hypertonic	Into intravascular space
Lactated Ringer's	Isotonic	No net movement
Normal saline	Isotonic	No net movement
0.45% normal saline	Hypotonic	Out of intravascular space
D_5W	Isotonic initially but rapidly hypotonic because of glucose metabolism	Out of intravascular space

(Objective 10)

12. a. Oxygen to cells in vasoconstricted areas decreases. Anaerobic metabolism occurs. Leaky capillary syndrome evolves. Pale, sweaty skin; rapid, thready pulse; elevation in blood glucose; and dilation of coronary, cerebral, and skeletal muscle arterioles occur.

b. Precapillary sphincters open. Blood pools and vascular space is expanded greatly, resulting in increased container size. Decreased preload and congestion of the viscera occur. Increased anaerobic metabolism results in increased respiratory rate. Rouleaux formation inhibits perfusion in visceral capillaries and impedes flow. Hypercoagulability develops.

c. Blood coagulates in microcirculation, clogging capillaries and causing congestion; fibrinolytic mechanisms then are overstimulated, causing pulmonary edema and hemorrhage. Cell membrane function is lost, and anaerobic metabolism increases. Water and sodium leak into cells and potassium leaks out. Cells swell and die. Oxygen absorption and carbon dioxide elimination are impaired in the lungs, and acute respiratory distress syndrome may result.

d. After 1 to 2 hours a dramatic decrease in blood pressure occurs. Cellular metabolism stops. Organ failure occurs and may include liver, kidney, and heart failure; gastrointestinal bleeding; pancreatitis; and pulmonary thrombosis.
(Objective 6)

13. a. Cardiogenic shock: Administer high-flow oxygen, continue assessment, initiate intravenous normal saline to keep the vein open, consider a fluid challenge of 100 to 200 mL of lactated Ringer's solution or normal saline, monitor lung sounds and patient response carefully, and consider vasopressor drug therapy.

b. Neurogenic shock: Apply cervical spine immobilization, assess the need to assist ventilations, administer high-flow oxygen, initiate intravenous lactated Ringer's solution or normal saline (avoiding excessive amounts), monitor lung sounds frequently, apply and inflate pneumatic antishock garments if local protocol advises, continue assessment, and consider vasopressor drug therapy.

c. Hypovolemic shock: Administer high-flow oxygen, place patient in modified Trendelenberg's position, transport rapidly, initiate two large-bore (14- or 16-gauge) intravenous lines with lactated Ringer's solution or normal saline and infuse rapidly, apply pneumatic antishock garment if local protocol advises, and prepare to inflate it if patient's condition deteriorates.

d. Anaphylactic shock: Ensure a patent airway, administer high-flow oxygen (administer subcutaneous epinephrine), initiate intravenous lactated Ringer's solution or normal saline with a 14- or 16-gauge catheter, consider administration of diphenhydramine (Benadryl).

e. Septic shock: Administer high-flow oxygen, determine whether the patient has preexisting obstructive pulmonary disease, initiate intravenous therapy with a 14- or 16-gauge catheter, and obtain an accurate patient history.

f. Cardiogenic shock: Assess for a patent airway, administer high-flow oxygen, initiate a 16- or 18-gauge intravenous line with normal saline to keep the vein open, institute electrocardiographic monitoring, initiate maneuvers to decrease heart rate based on the electrocardiographic tracing and patient symptoms (drugs, cardioversion), and apply dressing to head wound.
(Objectives 7 and 10)

14. a. Uncompensated shock: The compensatory mechanisms can no longer sustain a normal systolic blood pressure. The pulse pressure is narrowed. Blood oxygenation is decreased as evidenced by cyanosis.

b. Compensated shock: Systolic blood pressure is adequate, but other signs of shock are evident (cool, pale skin and increased pulse and respiratory rate).
(Objective 8)

15. Irreversible shock may occur suddenly or 1 to 3 weeks after the event. Clinical signs include bradycardia; pale, cold, clammy skin; and cardiac arrest.
(Objective 8)

16. Preexisting disease, medication, older or young age
(Objective 8)

17. a. Drug therapy: Neither pneumatic antishock garments nor rapid fluid infusion is considered because this patient is already in heart failure. Therapy should be directed at improving the function of the heart with drugs.
b. Pediatric pneumatic antishock garments (if indicated by local medical direction), rapid fluid replacement, blood transfusions, and intraosseous infusion: The patient has a mechanism of injury for significant blood loss and is exhibiting signs of uncompensated shock. Pneumatic antishock garments may decrease the container size and maximize flow to the vital organs. Rapid fluid infusion may restore circulating volume. Blood transfusion may be necessary on arrival to emergency department to enhance oxygen-carrying capability and restore the vascular volume. Rapid peripheral intravenous therapy may be impossible in this situation, making intraosseous infusion the vascular access method of choice. Rapid transport is essential.
c. Drug therapy: The heart rate is slow and is likely the reason why this person is exhibiting signs of shock. None of the other interventions increases heart rate.
d. Drug therapy and rapid fluid replacement: The primary cause of the shock state in this patient is probably histamine release. Drug therapy is the only intervention that can arrest and reverse these symptoms. Rapid fluid replacement also may help restore circulating volume until drug therapy is effective.
e. Pneumatic antishock garments, rapid fluid replacement, and blood transfusions: The primary cause of the shock symptoms according to the patient history is loss of blood. Rapid fluid replacement can restore circulating volume. At the emergency department the blood transfusion helps restore oxygen-carrying capacity and circulating volume.
f. Rapid fluid replacement is not indicated. At this time the patient is maintaining a normal blood pressure. The pulse and respiratory rate are elevated somewhat, so assessment should be frequent. Rapid fluid replacement may be necessary if the patient's blood pressure drops below 90 mmHg.
(Objective 10)

18. c. Coffee-ground emesis indicates gastrointestinal bleeding. Epistaxis is bleeding from the nose. Melena is dark, black, tarry stools.
(Objective 1)

19. c. A systolic blood pressure less than 90 mm Hg may be normal in certain individuals. Loss of blood volume may lead to shock but does not define it. Shock leads to decreased myocardial blood flow.
(Objective 2)

20. c. The Fick principle states that adequate oxygen must be available to red blood cells through the alveolar cells of the lungs. So that hemoglobin can be oxygenated, red blood cells must be circulated to the tissue cells, and red blood cells must be able to load oxygen at the lungs and unload oxygen at the peripheral cells.
(Objective 3)

21. a. Vessel length and viscosity are relatively constant. Blood volume may influence pressure but not resistance.
(Objective 4)

22. d. As peripheral vascular resistance decreases, vessel capacitance increases and the container size increases. This makes the existing blood volume insufficient to maintain an adequate preload.
(Objective 4)

23. d
(Objective 4)

24. a
(Objective 5)

25. d. Leaky capillary syndrome develops after lactate and hydrogen ions build up in the capillaries and their linings lose their ability to retain large molecular structures within their walls.
(Objective 6)

26. b. This fluid loss is caused by the increased hydrostatic pressure created in this situation.
(Objective 6)

27. b. The precapillary sphincter opens, whereas the postcapillary sphincter remains closed, increasing the pressure inside the capillary and forcing fluid out through the already compromised capillary walls.
(Objective 6)

28. b. Anaphylactic shock is caused by the release of chemicals after an antigen-antibody reaction. Hypovolemic shock results from a loss of body fluid (water, plasma, blood). Neurogenic shock is a loss of vasomotor tone.
(Objective 7)

29. b. Loss of vasomotor tone is a contributing factor to shock in each of the other types of shock.
(Objective 9)

30. d. The compensatory mechanisms of vasoconstriction, increased heart rate, and increased contractility are no longer sufficient to maintain adequate blood pressure.
(Objective 8)

31. a. As peripheral vascular resistance increases, diastolic blood pressure also increases.
(Objective 8)

32. b. Use of pneumatic antishock garments generally is not recommended for any of the other situations.
(Objective 10)

33. a. All the others are crystalloid solutions.
(Objective 10)

34. b. Whole blood and packed red blood cells have red cells and therefore the greatest ability to carry oxygen. Packed cells do not contain plasma and therefore have a greater concentration of red blood cells per unit volume. Only a small amount of oxygen is carried dissolved in plasma.
(Objective 10)

35. c. This is the only fluid that contains red blood cells.
(Objective 10)

36. d. Priorities of care always follow the ABCs; therefore oxygen should be first and intravenous therapy should be initiated en route unless a transportation delay exists; in this case, definitive care may be expedited.
(Objective 10)

37. b. This position permits better perfusion without compromising respiratory status.
(Objective 10)

38. d. Vasoactive drugs are not indicated for use in the patient with hypovolemic shock until adequate fluid volume has been replaced at the hospital. Pneumatic antishock garments occasionally may be used to treat hypovolemic shock associated with pelvic fractures.
(Objective 10)

39. a. Increased lung congestion indicates that the failing heart cannot deal with the existing fluid volume. Jugular venous distention should increase with fluid overload. Peripheral edema has a slow onset and is not an acute sign evident in the prehospital phase of care. A moderate decrease in heart rate indicates patient improvement. (Objective 10)

40. b. Epinephrine is the only treatment that rapidly improves all the life-threatening effects of anaphylaxis. Other adjunct therapy may be used after epinephrine has been given. (Objective 10)

41. a. The shortest catheter with the widest diameter should be selected. (Objective 10)

42. c. Drops/minute $= \dfrac{200 \times 10}{20} = 100$ (Objective 10)

43. a. Control of internal hemorrhage often requires surgical intervention or other definitive care measures available only in the hospital. (Objective 11)

WRAP IT UP

1. This patient had internal bleeding and external bleeding. The internal bleeding was most likely responsible for her shock. (Objective 1)

2. c. Most of the oxygen in the body is carried on hemoglobin. This patient's blood loss has caused a decrease in hemoglobin. (Objective 2)

3. The blood vessels narrow in an attempt to increase the preload. (Objective 4)

4. a. The red blood cells contain hemoglobin, which carry oxygen and are critical for normal tissue oxygenation. (Objective 5)

5. d. Because the blood pressure has decreased, the patient is no longer compensating adequately for the shock. (Objective 6)

6. Bleeding from head, concealed intraabdominal bleeding, or long bone fractures of lower legs (Objective 7)

7. Narrow pulse pressure: a, b, c
   Pale, cool, skin: a, b, c
   Tachycardia: a, b, c
   (Objective 8)

8. c. If the patient had uncontrolled bleeding from the spleen, the only definitive intervention would be surgical. Prehospital care includes oxygenation, monitoring, fluid replacement, and transport to the closest appropriate hospital (trauma center preferred). (Objective 10)

Soft Tissue Trauma

READING ASSIGNMENT

Chapter 22, pages 538-557, in *Mosby's Paramedic Textbook*, ed. 3

OBJECTIVES

Upon completion of this chapter, the paramedic student will be able to:
1. Describe the normal structure and function of the skin.
2. Describe the pathophysiological responses to soft tissue injury.
3. Discuss pathophysiology as a basis for key signs and symptoms, and describe the mechanism of injury and signs and symptoms of specific soft tissue injuries.
4. Outline management principles for prehospital care of soft tissue injuries.
5. Describe, in the correct sequence, patient management techniques for control of hemorrhage.
6. Identify the characteristics of general categories of dressings and bandages.
7. Describe prehospital management of specific soft tissue injuries not requiring closure.
8. Discuss factors that increase the potential for wound infection.
9. Describe the prehospital management of selected soft tissue injuries.

SUMMARY

- The skin and its accessory organs are the main cosmetic structures of the body. These structures perform many functions that are critical to survival. The skin is composed of two distinct layers of tissue: the outer layer (epidermis) and the inner layer (dermis).
- Surface trauma can disrupt the normal distribution of body fluids and electrolytes. Surface trauma also can interfere with the maintenance of body temperature. The two physiological responses to surface trauma are vascular and inflammatory reactions. These can lead to healing, scar formation, or both. Many factors can affect or alter wound healing.
- Soft tissue injuries are classified as closed or open. Classification is determined by the absence or presence of a break in the continuity of the epidermis. Closed wounds include contusions, hematoma, and crush injury. Open wounds are classified as abrasions, lacerations, punctures, avulsions, amputations, and bites.
- Assessment of life-threatening injuries and resuscitation precedes evaluation and intervention of non–life-threatening soft tissue injuries. General wound assessment should include a history of the event that caused the wound and a careful examination of the injury.
- Methods of hemorrhage control include direct pressure, elevation, pressure point, immobilization by splinting, and pneumatic pressure devices.
- The general categories of dressings used in trauma care are sterile, nonsterile, occlusive, nonocclusive, adherent, and nonadherent. The general categories of bandages are absorbent, nonabsorbent, adherent, and nonadherent.
- Depending on the nature and location of the patient's injury, cleansing, dressings, bandages, and immobilization may be indicated to care for a wound properly.

- The goals of wound care are to prevent infection and protect from infection. Factors that influence the likelihood of infection include unclean wounds and wound mechanisms and a patient's poor state of health.
- Special considerations for specific wounds include penetrating chest or abdominal injury, avulsion, amputation, and crush syndrome.

REVIEW QUESTIONS

Match the type of dressing listed in Column II with its description in Column I. Use each answer only once.

Column I

1. _E_   Air does not pass through this dressing.
2. _f_   Bacteria have been eliminated from this dressing.
3. _D_   This dressing can be used when infection is not a concern.
4. _A_   This dressing sticks to the wound surface.
5. _C_   This dressing allows air to pass through to the wound.
6. _b_   This dressing does not stick to the wound.

Column II

a. Adherent dressing
b. Nonadherent
c. Nonocclusive dressing
d. Nonsterile dressing
e. Occlusive dressing
f. Sterile dressing

7. List at least six structures or tissues located in the dermis.

a. CONNECTIVE tissue

b. ELAStic Fibers

c. Blood vessels

d. lymphatic vessels

e. motor + SENSORY FiBERS

f. HAIR, NAILS AND glANDS

8. Identify at least three functions of the integumentary system.

a. PROTECTION From infection

b. TEMPERATURE REGULATION

c. CUSHIONING OF INJURY - PRESERVATION of BODY FluiDs

9. Identify the three crucial steps in the clotting mechanism.

a. RELEASE OF PlAtelet fACtors At iNJURY SITE

b. FORMATION OF thromBiN

c. TRApping of RED Blood cells in fiBRIN to form A clot

10. Why are redness, swelling, warmth, and pain found at the site of an inflammatory response?

WARMth AND REDNESS iS CAUSED By VASODIAhAtion AND ENHANCED Blood supply to Affected AREA. Swelling is CAUSED By iNCREASED CAPILLARY PERMEABility which allows things to leak into EXtRACELLULAR SPACE, PAIN is CAUSED By CHEMICALS AND iNCREASED PRESSURE RESULTING From Fluid BuilDup.

11. List six types of drugs that can impair normal wound healing.

a. CORticO StEROIDS

b. NSAIDS

c. PCN

d. Cholchicine

e. ANti COAgulANts

f. ANtiNEOplastic AgENts .

295

12. List six types of wounds that are likely to require closure.

a. WOUNDS to COSMETIC REGIONS

b. GAPING WOUNDS

c. WOUNDS OVER TENSION AREAS

d. DEGLOVING INJURIES

e. RING FINGER INJURIES

f. SKIN TEARING

13. For each of the following scenarios, list the soft tissue injury described and key prehospital interventions to manage the trauma.

a. A 45-year-old woman is being transported for care after her husband repeatedly struck her head and face with his fist. You note numerous swollen, ecchymotic areas on the face and head.

Injury:

Interventions:

CONTUSIONS OR HEMATOMA —

APPLY ICE PACKS

b. Rescuers have just removed a victim who had been trapped in a concrete structure for 2 days. The patient's lower torso had been pinned under a concrete piling. During the rescue phase, the patient was alert but somewhat confused. Vital signs were within normal limits. Shortly after extrication the patient's physiological status begins to deteriorate.

Injury:

Interventions:

CRUSH SYNDROME

AIRWAY MAINTENANCE — SODIUM BICARBONATE.

c. A wallpaper hanger has sustained a deep linear wound after cutting himself with an Exacto knife. The wound is oozing dark red blood, and fatty tissue is visible at the edges of the injury.

Injury:

Interventions:

LACERATIONS — CONTROL BLEEDING, MONITOR FOR SIGNS OF SHOCK.

d. A motorcyclist wearing only her swimsuit had to lay the bike down to avoid a collision. The patient states that the bike slid about 100 feet along the asphalt road. She has huge scrape-type injuries on her entire left side. She denies pain or tenderness anywhere else.

Injury:

Interventions:

ABRASIONS. CLEAN WOUNDS, lightly cover with sterile Dressing.

e. Neighbors direct you to a yard where a young child has been attacked by a large dog. No one is sure of the dog's present location. The child is screaming, and his left arm has many puncture wounds and lacerations.

Injury:

Interventions:

Rinse contaminates, splint extremity

f. A hunter has been impaled with an arrow. The arrow has penetrated the right upper quadrant of the abdomen. She is pale and cool.

Injury:

Interventions:

Stabilize arrow with bulky dressing. Treat for shock if present.

g. A mechanic reports an injury to her right hand while working with a high-pressure grease gun. You note a small puncture wound with a drop of grease on it at the distal end of the left thumb.

Injury:

Interventions:

h. A butcher slices off the distal tip of his index finger.

Injury:

Interventions:

i. A factory employee catches his hair in some large machinery and avulses a large portion of the posterior aspect of his scalp.

Injury:

Interventions:

j. A weekend handyman severs his right index finger with a skill saw. He drives himself to a nearby firehouse but does not have the digit with him.

Injury:

Interventions:

Questions 14 and 15 pertain to the following case study:

Your patient was treated and released from the emergency department with a diagnosis of tibial fracture after a fall. He has a plaster splint that was applied there and is complaining of pain so severe, "I just can't take it anymore."

14. What further assessments should you perform on this patient's leg to look for compartment syndrome?

15. If he has compartment syndrome, what could a delay in treatment cause?

_____

Questions 16 and 17 pertain to the following case study:

    You are called to the scene of a construction site, where a 57-year-old workman has lacerated his left hand.

16. What questions should you ask to obtain the wound history on this patient?

_____

_____

17. Outline the physical examination of the wound and hand.

_____

_____

18. You are called to a rural farm, where a 17-year-old has sustained a partial amputation of his left lower arm after tangling it in a corn picker. There is extensive soft tissue damage and deformity of the extremity, which is squirting bright red blood. Your estimated time of arrival to the nearest hospital is 30 minutes. Describe in the proper sequence six measures you can use to control the bleeding in this patient and briefly describe the proper technique for using each skill.

    a. _____

_____

    b. _____

_____

    c. _____

_____

    d. _____

_____

    e. _____

_____

    f. _____

_____

    For questions 19 to 23, circle (a) or (b) to indicate the wound that is at _greater risk_ for infection. Explain why you chose your answer in (c).

19. a. A farmer lacerates his hand on a combine.
     b. A chef cuts his hand on a butcher knife.
     c.

20. a. A 25-year-old athlete is stabbed.
     b. A 79-year-old nursing home resident is stabbed.
     c.

21. a. The patient cut his abdomen.
   b. The patient's laceration is on his hand.
   c.

22. a. Your patient reports to the emergency department for sutures 18 hours after the injury.
   b. The patient drives to the emergency department 2 hours after injury.
   c.

23. a. His finger was split open after he jammed it in a door.
   b. He sliced his finger on a piece of metal on the door.
   c.

STUDENT SELF-ASSESSMENT

24. What is the avascular layer of the skin called?
   a. Dermis
   b. Epidermis
   c. Sebaceous
   d. Subcutaneous tissue

25. Which of the following does *not* play a role in normal hemostasis?
   a. Activation of platelets
   b. Aldosterone synthesis
   c. Thrombin formation
   d. Vasoconstriction

26. Which medications can interfere with hemostasis?
   a. Acetaminophen
   b. Aspirin
   c. Decongestants
   d. Insulin

27. Which of the following medical conditions is associated with delayed healing?
   a. Alcoholism
   b. Asthma
   c. Cardiac dysrhythmias
   d. Stroke

28. Which of the following wound forces is least likely to be associated with a high risk for infection?
   a. Foreign bodies
   b. Human and animal bites
   c. Injection injuries
   d. Paring knife wounds

29. Which of the following is considered a closed injury?
   a. Avulsion
   b. Bite
   c. Hematoma
   d. Puncture

30. High-pressure injection injuries can be limb-threatening. Why is the severity of this wound difficult to assess in the prehospital environment?
   a. The light is too poor to evaluate the wound adequately.
   b. The location of the wound is difficult to visualize.
   c. The equipment needed for assessment is not available.
   d. The wound is small with minimal external signs.

31. What is the appropriate prehospital care for avulsed body tissue?
   a. Placing it directly on ice
   b. Sealing it in a plastic bag
   c. Soaking it in a cup of lactated Ringer's solution
   d. Débriding it of all dirt

32. Which type of soft tissue injury may result in abscesses, lymphangitis, cellulitis, osteomyelitis, tenosynovitis, tuberculosis, hepatitis B, and tetanus?
   a. Amputation
   b. Avulsion
   c. Bites
   d. Crush injury

33. Which of the following is an early finding in crush injury?
   a. Paralysis
   b. Paresis
   c. Paresthesia
   d. Pulselessness

34. Where is compartment syndrome most likely to be found?
   a. Abdomen
   b. Upper arm
   c. Head
   d. Thorax

35. What causes life-threatening symptoms in patients with crush syndrome after being released from entrapment?
    a. Circulatory overload when blood rushes back to the central circulation
    b. Hypokalemia, hypouricemia, hypercalcemia, and hypophosphatemia
    c. Myoglobin is released and filtered through the liver, causing liver failure.
    d. Toxic substances from anaerobic metabolism are released into the blood.
36. Blast injuries can cause rupture in air-filled organs such as which of the following?
    a. Bladder   **c.** Lungs
    b. Heart   d. Pancreas
37. Which wound is least likely to require physician evaluation if tetanus immunization is up to date?
    a. A needle fragment imbedded in the wound.
    b. Weakness in the finger distal to the laceration.
    c. Laceration extending over the border of the lip.
    d. A painful abrasion on the leg that is oozing slightly.
38. Who would *not* be a candidate for tetanus toxoid if the person reports not having had a booster in more than 10 years?
    a. A patient who takes insulin for diabetes
    b. A patient whose baby is due in 3 weeks
    c. A patient whose arm was sore the last time he had one
    d. A patient whose home medicines include digoxin (Lanoxin)

WRAP IT UP

You are dispatched to a ranger's cabin deep in a rugged national park for "traumatic injuries." A 20-year-old climber initially injured when he fell about 12 feet, sliding down a steep rock face a day ago, lost his way, was bitten by a wild dog, and then cut his forearm in a desperate attempt to enter the cabin when there was no response to his initial knocks at the door. He has numerous swollen, painful blunt injuries because of small collections of blood under the skin; several puncture wounds to the left forearm from the bite around which the skin is now tender, red, warm, and swollen; several areas on his hands, arms, and legs where the skin was scraped off and is oozing clear liquid; and a deep wound on the right forearm from the glass injury that is bleeding freely and in which fatty tissue is visible. You easily control the bleeding and complete your assessment of this patient, finding no additional injuries, and assess his vital signs, which are BP 126/72 mm Hg, P 98, R 16, SaO$_2$ 98%. You transport him to the local hospital where he is treated and released 8 hours later.

1. Which of the skin layers were injured?

_____

2. What signs and symptoms of inflammation are present from his wounds?

_____

3. Place a check mark beside the soft tissue injuries present in this patient.
    a. _____ Closed wounds   f. _____ Laceration
    b. _____ Contusions   g. _____ Puncture
    c. _____ Crush injury   h. _____ Avulsion
    d. _____ Open wounds   i. _____ Amputation
    e. _____ Abrasion   j. _____ Bites

4. Describe appropriate steps in management of this patient's bleeding.

_____

5. How will you treat his other wounds? _____

6. What risk factors are present in this patient for the development of infection?

_____

REVIEW QUESTIONS

1. e
(Objective 6)

2. f
(Objective 6)

3. d
(Objective 6)

4. a
(Objective 6)

5. c
(Objective 6)

6. b
(Objective 6)

7. Connective tissue, elastic fibers, blood vessels, lymphatic vessels, motor and sensory fibers, hair, nails, and glands
(Objective 1)

8. Protection and cushioning against injury, barrier against infection, temperature regulation, and preservation of body fluids
(Objective 1)

9. a. Release of platelet factors at injury site
b. Formation of thrombin
c. Trapping of red blood cells in fibrin to form a clot
(Objective 2)

10. The warmth and redness are caused by vasodilation and enhanced blood supply to the affected area. Swelling is caused by increased capillary permeability, which allows plasma, plasma proteins, and electrolytes to leak into extracellular space. Pain is caused by chemicals and increased pressure resulting from fluid buildup.
(Objective 2)

11. a. Corticosteroids; b. nonsteroidal antiinflammatory drugs; c. penicillin; d. colchicine; e. anticoagulants; f. antineoplastic agents
(Objective 2)

12. a. Wounds to cosmetic regions; b. gaping wounds; c. wounds over tension areas; d. degloving injuries; e. ring finger injuries; f. skin tearing
(Objective 2)

13. a. Contusion or hematoma: Apply ice or cold packs and compression with manual pressure or compression bandage. Assess for underlying injury.
b. Crush syndrome: Provide airway and ventilation support, administer high-flow oxygen, maintain body temperature, rehydrate with expanding intravenous fluids (1 to 1.5 L initial bolus), and administer pharmacological agents such as sodium bicarbonate (to help control hyperkalemia and acidosis), glucose and insulin (to decrease serum potassium), and mannitol (to promote diuresis).

c. Laceration: Control hemorrhage and monitor for signs of hypovolemic shock.

d. Abrasions: Clean gross contaminants from injured surface and lightly cover with sterile dressing.

e. Dog bite: Ensure that animal is contained, control bleeding, rinse off gross contaminants, splint extremity, and obtain a medical history from the pet owner.

f. Penetrating or impaled object: Leave object in place, do not manipulate object unless it is necessary for patient extrication or transport, control bleeding with direct pressure around the impaling object, stabilize the object with bulky dressings, and immobilize the patient. Treat shock if present.

g. Puncture wound: Evaluate wound, elevate affected extremity, immobilize, and transport.

h. Avulsion: Control bleeding, retrieve the avulsed tissue, wrap tissue in gauze that is dry or moistened with lactated Ringer's or saline solution (per local protocol), seal in plastic bag, and place sealed bag on crushed ice.

i. Degloving: Control bleeding, evaluate for hypovolemia, elevate head of stretcher after you rule out mechanism for cervical spine injury.

j. Amputation: Control bleeding, retrieve amputated tissue, and treat as for avulsion.

(Objectives 3 and 9)

14. Assess for pain, paresis, paresthesia, pallor, and pulselessness in the affected extremity. Determine whether there is swelling or tightness of the compartment, tenderness to palpation, weakness in the leg, or pain on passive stretch (early sign).
(Objective 3)

15. A delay in treatment of compartment syndrome can cause nerve death, muscle necrosis, and crush syndrome.
(Objective 3)

16. When did you cut yourself? Was it a dirty place where you got the cut? How did the injury happen? Does anything else hurt? How much blood did you lose? Rate your pain on a scale of 1 to 10 with 1 being no pain and 10 the worst pain you have ever had. Do you take any medicines? Do you have any major illnesses? When was your last tetanus shot?
(Objective 4)

17. Inspect the wound for bleeding, size, depth, presence of foreign bodies, amount of tissue lost, edema, and deformity. Inspect the surrounding area for damage to arteries, nerves, tendons, and muscle. Assess the sensory and motor function of his hand. Evaluate the perfusion of the wound and of the tissues of the hand distal to the wound. Assess capillary refill, distal pulse, tenderness, temperature, edema, and crepitus (if underlying bone injury is suspected).
(Objective 4)

18. a. Apply direct pressure to the wound with a gloved hand or handheld dressing (4 to 6 minutes), and then secure a pressure dressing firmly with an elastic bandage. Reinforce the dressing if bleeding continues.

b. Elevate the affected area above the level of the heart.

c. Apply pressure point control if other measures have failed. Select the appropriate pressure point proximal to the wound and compress the artery against the underlying bone for at least 10 minutes.

d. Immobilize by splinting if movement increases the bleeding. (Immobilization is used as an adjunct to other control devices.) Select the appropriate splint for the body area and apply it to minimize blood flow.

e. Use pneumatic pressure devices. (Devices such as air splints or pneumatic antishock garments serve as adjuncts for pressure control after the bleeding is controlled by other methods.)

f. Use a tourniquet only when other methods are unsuccessful in controlling bleeding and when preservation of life is selected over preservation of the limb. Notify medical control and select a site 2 inches proximal to the wound over the brachial or femoral artery. Place a tourniquet over the artery and a pad over the artery to be compressed. Wind tourniquet twice around the extremity and tie it in a half knot over the pad. Place a windlass on the half knot and secure it with a square knot. Tighten the windlass until the hemorrhage stops and secure it. Note the time of application and mark "TK" on the patient's forehead and notify the receiving hospital. Carefully monitor the time the tourniquet is on.

(Objective 5)

19. a. This wound is likely much more contaminated than one that occurred in a clean indoor setting.
(Objective 8)

20. b. The risk of infection increases in older patients and in those who have preexisting medical conditions.
(Objective 8)

21. b. Injuries of the hand, foot, lower extremity, scalp, and face have a higher than normal risk of infection.
(Objective 8)

22. a. The risk of infection is greater in wounds that are not cleaned and repaired for longer than 8 to 12 hours after the injury.
(Objective 8)

23. a. Injuries associated with a crushing mechanism are more susceptible to infection than those caused by fine cutting forces.
(Objective 8)

24. b. The dermis provides the vascular supply to the epidermis. The sebaceous glands are in the dermis. The subcutaneous tissue lies under the dermis.
(Objective 1)

25. b. Aldosterone aids in body fluid regulation.
(Objective 2)

26. b. Aspirin decreases platelet activity.
(Objective 2)

27. a. Other conditions associated with impaired healing are advanced age, uremia, diabetes, hypoxia, peripheral vascular disease, malnutrition, advanced cancer, hepatic failure, and cardiovascular disease.
(Objective 2)

28. d. A knife wound would be considered high risk if it were contaminated with organic material or if the patient were immunocompromised or had poor circulation.
(Objective 2)

29. c. All the others are open wounds.
(Objective 3)

30. d. The wound site may only have minimal bleeding, numbness, and blanching. Surgical intervention is often necessary.
(Objective 3)

31. b. All other interventions could cause further damage.
(Objective 9)

32. c. Bites may be a combination of puncture, laceration, avulsion, and crush injuries heavily laden with infectious organisms.
(Objective 3)

33. c. All others are late findings.
(Objective 3)

34. b. The most common sites are below the knee and above the elbow.
(Objective 3)

35. d. Blood pools in the injured extremity, causing hypovolemia. Elevated blood potassium, phosphate and uric acid levels, and low blood calcium levels occur. Myoglobin is filtered in the kidneys, resulting in acute renal failure.
(Objective 3)

36. c. Other air-filled structures that may be affected are the eardrum, sinuses, stomach, and intestines.
(Objective 3)

37. d. All the other injuries have a high potential for impaired wound healing or infection if not treated by a physician.
(Objective 7)

38. b. Tetanus toxoid should not be given to pregnant patients or children younger than 6 weeks.
(Objective 7)

WRAP IT UP

1. Epidermis and dermis (puncture wounds may be deeper)
(Objective 1)

2. Pain, warmth, redness, swelling
(Objective 2)

3. Closed wounds, contusions, crush injury is possible (from dog bite), open wounds, abrasions, lacerations, punctures (bites), bites
(Objective 3)

4. Direct pressure may be all that is necessary to control bleeding. If not, elevation of the extremity and reinforcement of the bandage may be helpful. For severe and persistent bleeding, arterial pressure point control. If medical control approves, when life is threatened, a tourniquet may be applied for a brief period.
(Objective 5)

5. The wounds should be cleansed with clean, running water until no debris is seen. If transport time will be prolonged, wounds may be covered with nonadherent dressings to prevent further contamination. Antibiotic ointment can be applied to superficial wounds.
(Objectives 7 and 9)

6. Wounds were sustained in a dirty environment; bite wounds are highly susceptible to infection; no wound care was provided for a prolonged period of time.
(Objective 8)

READING ASSIGNMENT
Chapter 23, pages 558-579, in *Mosby's Paramedic Textbook,* ed. 3

OBJECTIVES
Upon completion of this chapter, the paramedic student will be able to:
1. Describe the incidence, patterns, and sources of burn injury.
2. Describe the pathophysiology of local and systemic responses to burn injury.
3. Classify burn injury according to depth, extent, and severity based on established standards.
4. Discuss the pathophysiology of burn shock as a basis for key signs and symptoms.
5. Outline the physical examination of the burned patient.
6. Describe the prehospital management of the patient who has sustained a burn injury.
7. Discuss pathophysiology as a basis for key signs, symptoms, and management of the patient with an inhalation injury.
8. Outline the general assessment and management of the patient who has a chemical injury.
9. Describe specific complications and management techniques for selected chemical injuries.
10. Describe the physiological effects of electrical injuries as they relate to each body system based on an understanding of key principles of electricity.
11. Outline assessment and management of the patient with electrical injury.
12. Describe the distinguishing features of radiation injury and considerations in the prehospital management of these patients.

SUMMARY
- Each year more than 2 million Americans seek medical attention for burns. Morbidity and mortality rates from burn injury follow significant patterns regarding gender, age, and socioeconomic status. A burn injury is caused by an interaction between thermal, chemical, electrical, or radiation energy and biological matter.
- Tissue damage from burns depends on the degree of the heat and on the duration of exposure to the thermal source. As local events occur at the injury site, other organ systems become involved in a general response to the stress caused by the burn.
- Burns are classified in terms of depth as superficial, partial-thickness, and full-thickness. The rule of nines provides a rough estimate of burn injury size (extent) and is most accurate for adults and for children older than age 10. The Lund and Browder chart is a more accurate method of determining the area of burn injury. Severity of burn injury and burn center referral guidelines are based on standards that take into account the depth, extent, and severity of the burn wound; the source of injury; patient age; presence of concurrent medical or surgical problems; and the body region that is burned.
- Shock after thermal injury results from edema and accumulation of vascular fluid. These tissue changes occur in the area of injury and can produce systemic hypovolemia if the burn area is large.

- Emergency care for a burn patient begins with the initial assessment. The goal is to recognize and treat life-threatening injuries.
- Goals for prehospital management of the severely burned patient include preventing further tissue injury, maintaining the airway, administering oxygen and ventilatory support, providing fluid resuscitation, providing rapid transport to an appropriate medical facility, using aseptic (clean) technique to minimize the patient's exposure to infectious agents, managing pain, and providing psychological and emotional support.
- Prehospital considerations in caring for patients with inhalation injury include recognition of the dangers inherent in the fire environment, pathophysiology of inhalation injury, and early detection and treatment of impending airway or respiratory problems.
- The severity of chemical injury is related to three things: the chemical agent, the concentration and volume of the chemical, and the duration of contact. Treatment is directed at stopping the burning process by using copious irrigation.
- Three types of injury may occur as a result of contact with electrical current: direct contact burns, arc injuries, and flash burns. Once the scene is safe, patient intervention may begin. Internal damage from electrical current may be much more significant than external wounds.
- Persons who are injured by radiation rarely require emergency care. Radioactive particles are classified into three types: alpha, beta, and gamma. The Federal Emergency Management Agency recommends that basic radiation protection for the rescuer and the patient include four factors: minimize time in the radiation field; maintain a safe distance from the source; place shielding between the rescuers and the source; and limit the amount of radioactive material in a specific area.

REVIEW QUESTIONS

Match the chemicals listed in Column II with the appropriate description in Column I.

Column I	Column II
1. _____ Chemical used to clean fabric and metal, can cause hypocalcemia and severe burns	a. Alkali
2. _____ Noxious gas that, when in solution, can cause blindness if it contaminates the eye	b. Ammonia
	c. Hydrofluoric acid
3. _____ Chemical that causes burns after prolonged exposure and also may result in lead poisoning	d. Petroleum
4. _____ Chemical that produces heat if exposed to water and should be removed or covered with oil	e. Phenol
5. _____ Exposure to this chemical may be painless and result in dysrhythmias and central nervous system depression	

6. Identify the four major sources of burn injury.

   a.

   b.

   c.

   d.

7. Label the three zones of burn injury on Fig. 23-1 and briefly describe the characteristics of the tissue in each.

   A. _____

   _____

   B. _____

   _____

C. _____

_____

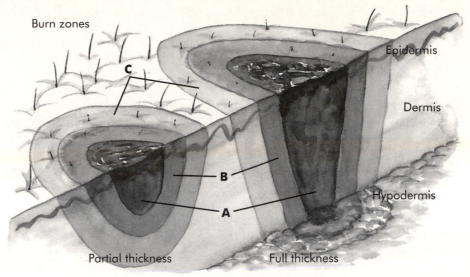

Figure 23-1

8. Explain two mechanisms that cause swelling in the burned tissue.

  a.

  b.

9. Describe the response in each of the following body systems to a major burn injury:

  a. Cardiovascular:

_____

  b. Pulmonary:

_____

  c. Gastrointestinal:

_____

  d. Musculoskeletal:

_____

  e. Neuroendocrine:

_____

  f. Metabolic:

_____

  g. Immune:

_____

  h. Emotional:

_____

10. For each of the following situations, classify the burn according to depth (first-, second-, or third-degree), extent (body surface area), and severity (according to the American Burn Association). Identify those patients who meet the American Burn Association criteria for referral to a burn center.

   a. A chef at a local restaurant has spilled hot grease down the anterior surface of his body. The wound is extremely painful, moist, and red, with many blisters. The burns cover the anterior surface of his chest, abdomen, arms, and left leg.

   Depth:
   Extent:
   Severity:
   Referral:

   b. On a hot summer day a young motorist opens his radiator cap and sprays hot steam and fluid over the upper half of his torso. The wounds are painful, moist, and red, with some blistering, and they blanch to the touch. The burns cover his face, anterior chest, and abdomen.

   Depth:
   Extent:
   Severity:
   Referral:

   c. An 80-year-old woman steps into a tub of extremely hot water. Because of her severe arthritis, she takes a long time to get out. She has circumferential burns around the right lower extremity up to the knee. The burn wound appears white and leathery and has no capillary refill.

   Depth:
   Extent:
   Severity:
   Referral:

11. As you arrive at the scene of a residential fire, rescue workers carry out an approximately 40-year-old, 80-kg man who is unconscious and has white, leathery burns. The burns cover the entire body surface except the posterior surface of both legs. He has shallow respirations at a rate of 24/min, and his blood pressure is 106/70 mm Hg. Patchy pieces of his smoldering clothing remain.

   a. Describe your initial assessment of this patient, including depth, extent, and severity of burns.

   _____

   _____

   b. Describe the prehospital care, including airway and fluid resuscitation, with type of fluid and rate.

   _____

   _____

12. Describe the specific interventions to be used when the following third-degree burns are present:

   a. Burns to the face:

   _____

   b. Extremity burns:

   _____

   c. Circumferential burns:

   _____

Questions 13 to 16 pertain to the following case study:

A 13-year-old boy uses gasoline to start a bonfire and ignites his clothing. As he attempts to pull his flaming jacket over his head, it gets stuck while continuing to burn. On your arrival, he is alert after an initial brief loss of consciousness. He has extensive burns on his face, neck, and chest. The burns are white and dry, with charred patches. They do not blanch when touched. His nasal hair is singed, and he is coughing up black, sooty sputum.

13. What aspects of the mechanism of injury and history of the event lead you to believe that this patient may have an inhalation injury?

_____

14. What physical findings suggest inhalation injury?

_____

15. At what point would you consider intubation?

_____

16. Do you suspect an inhalation injury above or below the glottis, and why?

_____

17. You are responding to a call for a person who has a chemical burn. En route to the industrial complex, you review the questions you will ask to determine the potential seriousness of the burn.

　a. Provide two examples of these questions.

_____

_____

　b. You find your patient covered with a powder known to cause chemical burns to the skin. Describe patient decontamination techniques.

_____

_____

18. Identify two examples of chemicals that can cause burn injury in each of the following categories:

　a. Acids:

_____

　b. Alkalis:

_____

　c. Organic compounds:

_____

19. The amount of tissue damage caused by an electrical current depends on six factors: (a) _____,

_____, _____, _____ _____, and _____. Amperage is

the measure of current (b) _____ per unit time. Voltage is a continuous (c) _____ applied to any electrical circuit causing a flow of electricity. High-voltage electrical injuries result from contact with an

electrical source of (d) _____ or greater. Resistance to electricity depends on four factors:

(e) _____ _____, _____, _____, and _____. Resistance to

electrical flow in the body is greatest in the (f) _____ tissue. The two types of current commonly used

are (g) _____ and _____. Direct current flows in (h) _____ direction. It is used

in (i) _____. Alternating current periodically reverses (j) _____ of flow. This reversal may

cause muscle contractions that may (k) _____ the patient to the source. In general, the current

pathway in low-voltage current follows the path of (l) _____ _____, and high-voltage

current follows the (m) _____ path. As the duration of contact with the patient increases, tissue

damage (n) _____.

20. Name the three burn patterns that can result from electrical current.

   a.

   b.

   c.

21. Briefly describe the potential effects of electrical injury on each of the following body regions.

   a. Cutaneous:

   _____

   b. Cardiovascular:

   _____

   c. Neurological:

   _____

   d. Vascular:

   _____

   e. Muscular:

   _____

   f. Renal:

   _____

   g. Pulmonary:

   _____

   h. Orthopedic:

   _____

   i. Ocular and otic:

   _____

22. A home owner was trimming his trees when he came into contact with overhead electrical wires. On your arrival, he is still in contact with the electrical source.

    a. What must be done before treatment commences?

_____

    The patient falls 10 feet from the tree to the ground. The scene is now safe. He is conscious and alert. You note multiple small, round, white burns on his right hand. When his clothing is removed, you discover significant burns and tissue injury to both feet.

    b. Describe your history and physical examination of this patient.

_____

_____

_____

    c. Describe treatment, including fluid resuscitation (rate and type).

_____

_____

23. Describe the appearance of wounds characteristically associated with lightning burns.

_____

24. For each of the following classes of lightning injury, list two physical signs:

    a. Minor:

_____

    b. Moderate:

_____

    c. Severe:

_____

25. Describe the characteristics of the following three types of radiation particles:

    a. Alpha:

_____

    b. Beta:

_____

    c. Gamma:

_____

26. Describe the physical effects that can be expected at the following levels of radiation exposure:

    a. Less than 100 rem:

_____

b. 100 to 200 rem:

_____

c. Greater than 450 rem:

_____

Questions 27 to 29 pertain to the following case study:

You arrive at a clinical laboratory, where a significant amount of radioactive material reportedly was released when a worker fell 1 foot from a platform.

27. Describe your approach to the emergency scene.

_____

_____

28. The victim must be accessed. Describe how the crew members designated to perform the rescue can minimize their radiation exposure.

_____

_____

_____

29. Describe any special measures that you should use to care for this patient after you reach him or her.

_____

_____

STUDENT SELF-ASSESSMENT

30. Which is an example of a thermal mechanism of injury?
  a. Arcing
  b. Alkali agents
  c. Ionizing agents
  d. Scalding

31. Which of the following risk factors is associated with a high incidence of burn fatality?
  a. Female gender
  b. Child
  c. Industrial setting
  d. High-income family

32. The most common source of burn injury is
  a. Chemical
  b. Electrical
  c. Radiation
  d. Thermal

33. Which of the following is a systemic response to burn injury?
  a. Hypoventilation
  b. Hyperactive gastrointestinal tract
  c. Decreased metabolic rate
  d. Depressed inflammatory response

34. A burn characterized by a moist, red appearance with blisters is probably what degree?
  a. First
  b. Second
  c. Third
  d. Fourth

35. A 5-year-old patient with third-degree burns of the anterior and posterior surfaces of both legs would be estimated to have a(n) _____ burn.
  a. 18%
  b. 24%
  c. 28%
  d. 36%

36. Hypovolemia in burn injury occurs because of which of the following?
    a. Blood loss
    b. Condensation of tissue fluid
    c. Increased capillary permeability
    d. Decrease in fluid intake
37. When calculating the extent of burn injury to ensure accurate fluid resuscitation, the paramedic should do which of the following?
    a. Calculate the burn size after arriving at the hospital.
    b. Estimate size before cooling the burn.
    c. Not include first-degree burns.
    d. Use the Lund and Browder chart.
38. To cool the burn of a patient burned on 50% of the body surface area, the paramedic should do which of the following?
    a. Apply ice intermittently in 15-minute cycles.
    b. Leave the patient exposed to air and apply a fan.
    c. Apply cool water and then cover the patient with sheets and blankets.
    d. Continuously apply cool water while en route to the hospital.
39. Using the consensus burn formula, calculate the minimum fluid requirement during the first hour for a 100-kg patient who has 60% third-degree burns covering his body.
    a. 250 mL
    b. 500 mL
    c. 750 mL
    d. 6000 mL
40. Which of the following is *not* a reason to suspect inhalation injury?
    a. Burns involving petroleum products
    b. Documented loss of consciousness
    c. Hoarseness or stridor
    d. Burns in an enclosed space
41. Which of the following statements is true regarding carbon monoxide poisoning?
    a. Oxygen saturation on the pulse oximeter is 80 or less.
    b. Skin color is cyanotic and often mottled.
    c. Respiratory rate is depressed in the early stages.
    d. Oxygen administration reduces the half-life of carbon monoxide.
42. What is the treatment of choice for almost all chemical injuries?
    a. Vigorous drying of the chemical
    b. Application of a chemical antidote
    c. Copious irrigation with water
    d. Delayed treatment until arrival at the hospital
43. Severity of chemical injury is related to all of the following except which one?
    a. Chemical concentration
    b. Duration of contact
    c. Environmental temperature
    d. Type of chemical agent
44. Calcium gluconate gel and solution are used to treat which of the following chemical injuries?
    a. Ammonia
    b. Hydrofluoric acid
    c. Petroleum
    d. Phenol
45. Electrical burns that result when the heat of the electrical current ignites the patient's clothing are what type of burns?
    a. Alternating
    b. Arc
    c. Direct
    d. Flame
46. Which tissue does electrical current flow through most easily?
    a. Bone
    b. Blood
    c. Muscle
    d. Nerve
47. Death in lightning injury most frequently results from which of the following?
    a. Cardiac or respiratory arrest
    b. Central nervous system injury
    c. Coagulation of the blood
    d. Severe burn shock
48. Which type of radiation requires a lead shield to stop penetration?
    a. Alpha
    b. Beta
    c. Gamma
    d. Nonionizing

WRAP IT UP

You are dispatched to a refinery for an explosion. When you arrive, you are directed into a dock area where you find a 37-year-old worker who was touching a forklift when it contacted a high-voltage electrical line, breaking it. He was thrown into some packing material that ignited because of the arcing. It took several minutes for the power to be interrupted so the fire could be extinguished. When you arrive, he is conscious, alert, and complaining of severe pain of his right arm. You provide cervical spine immobilization and continue your assessment as your partner applies high-concentration oxygen. You note a brown leathery wound on his left hand, and a charred wound on his right foot. He has moist, painful, partially blistered burns on his abdomen, and waxy, pale, tan-colored burns on his back from his shoulders to his buttocks. His vital signs are BP 170/100 mm Hg, P 124 irregular, R 20, SaO_2 on room air of 95%. You cool the burns with sterile saline, apply a clean sheet over the long spine board, secure him, cover his burns with clean sheets and warm blankets, and move him into the ambulance where you initiate an IV of LR at a rate prescribed by medical direction. An ECG monitor is applied, and morphine is administered for his increasing pain. Medical direction advises you to transport him to the burn center. En route, you monitor vital signs, peripheral pulses, which are diminished in the right foot, and continue to administer pain medication. When the urinary catheter is inserted in the ED, you note that it is a dark red wine color. The patient is hospitalized for 3 months, has his right lower leg amputated, and requires numerous skin grafts.

1. What source(s) caused this patient's burns?
   a. Chemical
   b. Electrical
   c. Thermal
   d. Electrical and thermal

2. Why did this patient have no signs of burn shock? _____

   _____

3. What was the burn depth? _____ Extent? _____ Severity? _____

4. Why was it necessary to monitor peripheral pulses? _____

   _____

5. Explain the following treatment decisions.

   a. Application of cool saline to the wound _____

   b. Administration of oxygen despite normal SaO_2_____

   _____

   c. Initiating the IV in the left arm_____

   d. Giving morphine intravenously instead of intramuscularly_____

   _____

6. What should you specifically assess to determine whether this patient has any indication of inhalation injury?

   _____

   _____

7. His electrical wounds were on the hand and on the foot. Explain why you did not find electrical burns in other places.

   _____

8. Place a check mark beside each of the signs or symptoms this patient had that indicate electrical injury.

a. _____ Hypertension

b. _____ Tachycardia

c. _____ Dysrhythmias

d. _____ Seizures

e. _____ Coma

f. _____ Motor/sensory deficits

g. _____ Respiratory depression

h. _____ Peripheral circulation impaired

i. _____ Myoglobinuria

REVIEW QUESTIONS

1. c
(Objective 8)

2. b
(Objective 8)

3. d
(Objective 8)

4. a
(Objective 8)

5. e
(Objective 8)

6. a. Thermal
b. Electrical
c. Chemical
d. Radiation
(Objective 1)

7. A. Zone of coagulation: nonviable tissue
B. Zone of stasis: seriously injured but potentially viable (Cells will die if no supportive measures are taken within 24 hours.)
C. Zone of hyperemia: increased blood flow caused by inflammatory response (Cells will recover in 7 to 10 days if no shock or infection develops.)
(Objective 2)

8. a. Chemical mediators cause increased capillary permeability and a fluid shift from the intravascular space to burned tissues.
b. The sodium pump in cell walls is damaged, and sodium moves into injured cells and increases swelling.
(Objective 2)

9. a. Decreased venous return, decreased cardiac output, increased vascular resistance (except in zone of hyperemia), hemolysis, and rhabdomyolysis that may lead to renal failure
b. Increased respiratory rate to meet increased metabolic demands
c. Adynamic ileus, vomiting, and stress ulcer
d. Decreased range of motion resulting from edema and immobilization; osteoporosis and demineralization later
e. Increased circulating levels of epinephrine, norepinephrine, and aldosterone
f. Increased basal metabolic rate
g. Increased susceptibility to infection and depressed inflammatory response
h. Pain, isolation, and fear of disfigurement
(Objectives 2 and 4)

10.

Depth	Extent	Severity	Referral
a. Second degree (partial thickness)	36%	Major	Yes
b. Second degree (partial thickness)	22.5%	Moderate	Yes
c. Third degree (full thickness)	9%	Major	Yes (involves feet)

(Objective 3)

11. a. Simultaneously put out the fire and cool the burn with clean water while performing initial assessment; monitor vital signs; assess burn depth (third degree), extent (82%), and severity (major); perform a head-to-toe survey; assess lung sounds and distal pulse, movement, sensation, and capillary refill in all extremities.
b. Cool the burn with clean water for ≤ 10 minutes; open the airway; intubate as necessary; ventilate with 100% oxygen; prepare to intubate; remove remaining clothing and jewelry; cover the patient to maintain warmth; initiate lactated Ringer's solution intravenously at 820 mL/hr (2 mL/kg per percent body surface area burned 24 hours [half of daily fluid to be given in first 8 hours]) up to 1640 mL/hr (4 mL/kg per percent body surface area burned, over 24 hours) in an unburned extremity; and rapidly transport patient.
(Objectives 5 and 6)

12. a. Realize that the burns may swell and be associated with airway problems. Raise the head of the stretcher 30 degrees if spinal injury is not suspected. If the ears are burned, do not use a pillow.
b. Remove jewelry, assess neurovascular status frequently, and elevate extremities.
c. Monitor distal pulse, movement, sensation, and respirations and rapidly transport the patient to the nearest appropriate facility.
(Objective 6)

13. His jacket created an enclosed space, and he experienced a loss of consciousness.
(Objective 7)

14. Facial burns, singed nasal hair, and carbonaceous sputum suggest inhalation injury.
(Objective 7)

15. Increased dyspnea, decreased level of consciousness, hoarseness, and stridor indicate the need for intubation.
(Objective 7)

16. Above the glottis is the most likely area of injury. The mechanism of injury does not suggest injury below the glottis.
(Objective 7)

17. a. What type, concentration, and volume of chemical was involved? How did the injury occur? When did the injury occur? Was any first aid given? Does the patient feel any pain?
b. With appropriate protective clothing, brush most of the powder off and then irrigate profusely (using a shower if available).
(Objective 7)

18. a. Rust removers, bathroom cleaners, and swimming pool acidifiers
b. Drain cleaners, fertilizers, heavy industrial cleaners, and cement and concrete
c. Phenols, creosote, and gasoline
(Objective 8)

19. a. Amperage, voltage, resistance, type of current, current pathway, duration of current flow
b. Flow (intensity)
c. Force (tension)
d. 1000 volts
e. Resistivity, size of object pathway, length of object pathway, and temperature
f. Bone
g. Alternating, direct
h. One
i. Industry
j. Direction
k. Freeze
l. Least resistance
m. Shortest
n. Increases
(Objective 10)

20. a. Direct contact
b. Arc
c. Flash
(Objective 10)

21. a. Direct contact can create large areas of coagulation necrosis. The entry wound is often a characteristic bull's-eye (dry and leathery), and the exit is ulcerated and explosive.
b. Dysrhythmias and damage to the myocardium may occur. Cardiac arrest is the most common cause of death after electrical injury. Hypertension caused by increased catecholamine levels is common.
c. Central nervous system injury may result in coma, seizures, and peripheral nerve injury and may lead to sensory or motor deficits. Brainstem injury may cause respiratory depression or arrest or cerebral edema or hemorrhage, which can lead to death.
d. Blood vessel necrosis may cause immediate or delayed hemorrhage or thrombosis.
e. Muscle injury may result in release of myoglobin, which can cause renal failure.
f. Acute renal failure occurs in 10% of significant electrical injuries.
g. The patient may have decreased ventilation or respiratory arrest because of central nervous system injury or chest wall dysfunction.
h. Fractures and dislocations can result from direct electrical injury or from injury caused by fall or electrocution.
i. Burns to conjunctiva or cornea and ruptured tympanic membrane are common.
(Objective 10)

22. a. The electrical source must be removed safely from the patient, preferably by interruption of power by the electric company.
b. Perform cervical spine immobilization and ABCDEs. Determine the patient's chief complaint, source of electricity, duration of exposure, level of consciousness before and after injury, and medical history. Perform a head-to-toe survey, looking for entry and exit burn wounds or trauma associated with the fall. Assess distal pulse, movement, sensation, and capillary refill in all extremities and document them. Monitor electrocardiographic rhythm.
c. Immobilize the cervical spine, open the airway, apply 100% oxygen, assess the need to assist ventilations, remove all jewelry, initiate lactated Ringer's solution intravenously at 20 to 40 mL/kg, monitor the vital signs and electrocardiogram, and maintain body warmth.
(Objective 11)

23. Linear, feathery, pinpoint appearance
(Objective 10)

24. a. The patient is usually conscious and may be confused and amnesic, with stable vital signs.
b. The patient may be combative or comatose, with associated injuries from lightning strike, first- and second-degree burns, tympanic membrane rupture (common), and possible internal injuries.
c. The patient may have immediate brain damage, seizures, respiratory paralysis, and cardiac arrest.
(Objective 10)

25. a. Alpha particles are positively charged atoms with minimal penetrability; however, they are dangerous when internal exposure occurs.
b. Beta particles are positively or negatively charged electrons that have more penetrating power than alpha particles and can permeate subcutaneous tissue.
c. Gamma particles have a much higher penetrating power than alpha or beta rays and require lead shielding to stop penetration. (Protective clothing does not stop these rays.) Exposure may produce local skin burns and extensive internal damage.
(Objective 12)

26. a. Less than 100 rem usually causes no significant acute problems.
b. A total of 100 to 200 rem can cause symptoms such as nausea and vomiting but is not life threatening.
c. Exposure of greater than 450 rem has a 50% mortality rate within 30 days.
(Objective 12)

27. The rescuers and emergency vehicle initially should be positioned 200 to 300 feet upwind of the site. No eating, smoking, or drinking should be permitted at the site. The appropriate local authorities and medical control should be notified of the situation.
(Objective 12)

28. Protective clothing should be worn, if available. The victim should be approached quickly by trained rescue teams. Rescue personnel should trade off frequently until the victim is stabilized sufficiently to remove him or her a safe distance from the contaminated area. If possible, the crew members should position themselves behind any protective barrier available.
(Objective 12)

29. If ventilation is required for the radiation-contaminated victim, an airway adjunct should be used. The patient should be moved away from the radiation source as soon as possible, but lifesaving care should not be delayed if the patient cannot be moved immediately. Intravenous lines should be initiated only if absolutely necessary, and good aseptic technique should be used to minimize the risk of introducing contaminants into the patient's body.
(Objective 12)

30. d. Alkali agents cause chemical burns, ionizing agents cause radiation burns, and arcing is caused by electrical energy.
(Objective 1)

31. b. Men die more frequently than women from burns. Three fourths of burn fatalities occur in the home. Deaths are also common in low-income homes.
(Objective 1)

32. d. This source includes flames, scalds, or contact with hot substances.
(Objective 1)

33. d. The patient hyperventilates to adapt to the increased metabolic rate. The gastrointestinal tract slows and, with large burns, adynamic ileus is a frequent complication.
(Objective 2)

34. b. First-degree burns are usually red, dry, and painful without blisters. Third-degree burns are white, yellow, tan, brown, or black; leathery; and often painless.
(Objective 3)

35. c. Each leg is between 13.5% and 14% body surface area.
(Objective 3)

36. c. Evaporation of fluid from the injured area also accounts for significant fluid loss.
(Objective 4)

37. c. The presence of first-degree burns should be noted in the narrative; however, these burns should not be included in the estimate of percent body surface area burned.
(Objective 3)

38. c. The burn should be cooled rapidly, and then body temperature should be maintained with sheets and blankets.
(Objective 6)

39. c. 2 mL × 60 × 100 = 12,000 mL in the first 24 hours
One half in the first 8 hours = 6,000 mL
6,000 mL ÷ 8 = 750 mL
The formula states that 2 to 4 mL/kg per percent body surface area burned is given in 24 hours, so the range would be 750 to 1500 mL.
(Objective 6)

40. a. Petroleum products are not associated with inhalation burns unless they occur in an enclosed space or meet one of the other criteria.
(Objective 6)

41. d. Oxygen saturation levels may be normal because the hemoglobin still is saturated (with carbon monoxide, not oxygen), and the oximeter may not differentiate between the two. Intravenous fluid therapy is not helpful in these patients.
(Objective 7)

42. c. Drying the chemical or delaying treatment only prolongs contact with the skin and increases the burn injury. Application of a chemical antidote is recommended only for a few chemicals.
(Objective 8)

43. c. Each other factor has a direct effect on the severity of the injury.
(Objective 7)

44. b. Subcutaneous injection of the calcium gluconate gel under the burn eschar is the most effective method.
(Objective 9)

45. d. An arc occurs when electrical energy "jumps" from its source through the air to another conductive medium. Direct burns result when the current passes through a person. *Alternating* is a description of a type of electrical current.
(Objective 10)

46. d. Bone provides the most resistance to electrical energy.
(Objective 10)

47. a. All the other pathological conditions can occur following lightning injury but cause death less frequently than cardiac or respiratory arrest.
(Objective 10)

48. c. Gamma rays have 10,000 times the penetrating power of alpha particles and 100 times the penetrating power of beta particles.
(Objective 12)

WRAP IT UP

1. d. Direct contact electrical and flame burns.
(Objective 1)

2. Burn shock evolves over 8 to 24 hours after injury and often is not seen immediately after injury.
(Objective 2)

3. Depth: Second- and third-degree (partial and full thickness)
Extent: ~24% (rule of nines); ~28% (Lund and Browder chart)
Severity: Major burn (>25%; electrical injury; significant involvement of hands/feet)
(Objective 3)

4. Damage from direct electrical current is often greatest in the tissues between the entrance and exit wounds. If the swelling occurs in the tissue compartments, severe circulatory compromise to the extremities can occur, causing progressive loss of pulses.
(Objective 5)

5. a. Cools the wound to minimize tissue damage.

b. Progressive burn shock should be anticipated, and oxygen should be delivered despite an initially normal SaO_2. Additionally, if the possibility of carbon monoxide exposure exists, SaO_2 will be normal despite tissue hypoxia.

c. Electrical burns were present in the right hand and right foot. The current had to travel through the right arm to reach the foot so that arm should be avoided because of the potential for impaired circulation.

d. As burn shock progresses, blood flow to the muscles will decline, resulting in ineffective management of pain.

(Objective 6)

6. Did the burns occur in an enclosed space? Does the patient have any stridor, facial burns, soot in the nose or mouth, facial burns, singed facial or nasal hair, edema of the lips or oral cavity, coughing, difficulty swallowing, hoarse voice, or circumferential neck burns?
(Objective 7)

7. Electrical current usually follows the path of least resistance to ground. Body tissues with the least resistance include the nerves and the blood vessels, not external skin structures.
(Objective 10)

8. a, b, c, h, i
(Objective 10)

Head and Facial Trauma

READING ASSIGNMENT

Chapter 24, pages 580-605, in *Mosby's Paramedic Textbook,* ed. 3

OBJECTIVES

Upon completion of this chapter, the paramedic student will be able to:

1. Describe the mechanisms of injury, assessment, and management of maxillofacial injuries.
2. Describe the mechanisms of injury, assessment, and management of ear, eye, and dental injuries.
3. Describe the mechanisms of injury, assessment, and management of anterior neck trauma.
4. Describe the mechanisms of injury, assessment, and management of injuries to the scalp, cranial vault, or cranial nerves.
5. Distinguish between types of traumatic brain injury based on an understanding of pathophysiology and assessment findings.
6. Outline the prehospital management of the patient with cerebral injury.
7. Calculate a Glasgow Coma Scale, trauma score, Revised Trauma Score, and pediatric trauma score when given appropriate patient information.

SUMMARY

- Major causes of maxillofacial trauma are motor vehicle crashes, home accidents, athletic injuries, animal bites, intentional violent acts, and industrial injuries.
- With the exception of compromised airway and the potential for significant bleeding, damage to the tissues of the maxillofacial area is seldom life threatening. Blunt trauma injuries may be classified as fractures to the mandible, midface, zygoma, orbit, and nose.
- Injury to the ears, eyes, or teeth may be minor or may result in permanent sensory function loss and disfigurement. Trauma to the ear may include lacerations and contusions, thermal injuries, chemical injuries, traumatic perforation, and barotitis. Evaluation of the eye should include a thorough history. Assessment also should include measurement of visual acuity, pupillary reaction, and extraocular movements.
- Anterior neck injuries may result in damage to the skeletal structures, vascular structures, nerves, muscles, and glands of the neck.
- Injuries to the skull may be classified as soft tissue injuries to the scalp and skull fractures. Skull fractures may be classified as linear fractures, basilar fractures, depressed fractures, and open vault fractures.

- The categories of brain injury include DAI and focal injury. Diffuse axonal injury may be mild (concussion), moderate, or severe. Focal injuries are specific, grossly observable brain lesions. Included in this category are lesions that result from skull fracture, contusion, edema with associated increased ICP, ischemia, and hemorrhage.
- The prehospital management of a patient with head injuries is determined by a number of factors. One factor is the mechanism of injury. A second factor is the severity of injury. A third factor is the patient's level of consciousness. Associated injuries affect the priorities of care.
- Several injury rating systems are used to triage, guide patient care, predict patient outcome, identify changes in patient status, and evaluate trauma care. Rating systems commonly used in emergency care include the Glasgow Coma Scale, trauma score/Revised Trauma Score, and pediatric trauma score.

REVIEW QUESTIONS

Match the type of skull fracture listed in Column II with the appropriate description in Column I. Use each answer only once.

Column I

1. _____ Associated with Battle's sign and raccoon's eyes
2. _____ Most common skull fracture; has low complication rate
3. _____ Direct communication between scalp laceration and brain tissue
4. _____ Fracture when bone is pushed downward; often associated with scalp laceration

Column II

a. Basilar
b. Depressed
c. Linear
d. Open vault

Match the cranial nerve in Column II with the abnormal sign or symptom associated with it in Column I. Use each cranial nerve only once.

Column I

5. _____ Hearing loss
6. _____ Loss of vision in one eye
7. _____ Weakness of one side of the face
8. _____ Double vision
9. _____ Loss of sense of smell

Column II

a. Olfactory
b. Optic
c. Oculomotor
d. Facial
e. Acoustic
f. Glossopharyngeal

10. A 6-year-old unrestrained child strikes his face on the stick shift of a truck in a head-on collision. On arrival, you find him seated in the cab of the truck, alert, crying, and complaining of pain in his face. Blood is oozing from his mouth.

    a. Describe your focused assessment of his head and face.

    _____

    _____

    b. On physical examination, you note the child's difficulty closing his mouth and an apparent space between the two lower front teeth, as well as a laceration that extends down through the gums. The bleeding continues, and you note excessive oral secretions. Vital signs are stable. Describe how you would transport and manage this child.

    _____

    _____

11. Briefly describe the evaluation of a suspected eye injury on a patient with no life threats.

_____

_____

12. For each of the following patients, identify the injury you suspect and list prehospital management techniques:

a. A 10-year-old complains of severe pain in the right eye after he was struck in the face with a handful of sand. The right eye is reddened and tearing.

_____

b. A 35-year-old has sustained a partially avulsed right upper lid.

_____

_____

c. A fish hook is embedded in the eye of a 42-year-old woman.

_____

_____

d. A handball player is struck directly in the eye by the ball. He is having difficulty seeing from the injured eye. You note blood in the anterior chamber of the eye.

_____

_____

e. During hockey playoffs, a high stick strikes a player in the eye. You note an irregular pupil on the affected side. A jellylike substance extrudes from an apparent laceration to the globe.

_____

_____

Questions 13 and 14 pertain to the following case study:

You are en route to a domestic disturbance in which a 45-year-old man reportedly has been stabbed in the neck with an ice pick.

13. Identify possible signs and symptoms of penetrating neck trauma that you should anticipate.

_____

On arrival, you note an ashen-colored unconscious patient who is breathing and has a weak pulse. A large pool of blood surrounds him, and a large amount of blood is coming from his neck.

14. List the steps in management of this patient with respect to the neck wound.

_____

_____

15. Briefly list the signs and symptoms associated with the following brain injuries, and state whether the injury is a diffuse axonal injury or focal brain injury:

a. Concussion:

_____

b. Contusion:

_____

c. Subdural hematoma:

_____

d. Epidural hematoma:

_____

e. Severe diffuse axonal injury:

_____

16. A man has been struck on the head with a baseball bat during a barroom brawl. He is alert and oriented, with an obvious depression and laceration at the right temporal area. Describe the signs and symptoms you will see if his intracranial pressure progressively rises en route to the hospital.

_____

17. You are transporting by air a patient who has sustained an isolated head injury in a motorcycle accident. Initially, he was awake and talking, but over the past 10 minutes, his condition has deteriorated rapidly. He now has a fixed, dilated right pupil; irregular respirations; a blood pressure of 170/100 mm Hg; and a pulse of 64. Identify treatment modalities you would provide for this patient.

_____

_____

18. Calculate the score indicated (Glasgow Coma scale [GCS], Revised Trauma Score [RTS], pediatric trauma score [PTS]) for each of the following patient examples:

a. Your patient opens her eyes to voice, is confused, and pulls her hand away when you start intravenous therapy. Her vital signs are blood pressure, 90/70 mm Hg; pulse, 120; and respirations, 24 and unlabored. Capillary refill is 1 second. GCS_____ RTS_____

b. Your patient opens his eyes to deep pain, moans some unrecognizable sounds, and withdraws slightly from pain. His vital signs are blood pressure, 70 mm Hg by palpation; pulse, 136; and respirations, 30 and shallow. His capillary refill is 4 seconds.
GCS_____ RTS _____

c. Your 10-day-old, 4-kg patient fell to the floor. She is crying vigorously. You note a small abrasion on her head, with a slight amount of swelling but no palpable crepitus. No other injuries are noted. Her blood pressure is 80 mm Hg. PTS _____

STUDENT SELF-ASSESSMENT

19. Which of the following is a sign of midface fracture?
    a. Diplopia
    b. Lengthening of the face
    c. Mastoid ecchymosis
    d. Numbness of the forehead

20. Your patient has signs and symptoms of midface fractures with a Glasgow Coma Scale score of 6. Which of the following is an appropriate prehospital intervention?
    a. Elevation of the head of the cot
    b. Nasogastric intubation
    c. Orotracheal intubation
    d. Pressure dressing over the nares

21. What is the name of the bone that, when fractured, often is associated with signs and symptoms similar to orbital fractures?
    a. Frontal
    b. Mandible
    c. Maxilla
    d. Zygoma

22. Your patient has been struck in the eye with a ball. She has diplopia, subconjunctival ecchymosis, enophthalmos, and numbness in the cheek. Which of the following bone fractures is consistent with these findings?
    a. Mandible
    b. Maxilla
    c. Orbit
    d. Zygoma

23. Displaced nasal fractures are most significant when they
    a. Are displaced to one side.
    b. Are associated with bleeding.
    c. Depress the dorsum of the nose.
    d. Occur in children.

24. The upper segment of the patient's pinna was avulsed in a motor vehicle collision. Which of the following treatments is appropriate for this patient?
    a. Approximate the edges of the avulsed tissue to the ear and apply a pressure dressing.
    b. Care for the remaining ear only. No chance exists to reimplant avulsed ear tissue.
    c. Scrub the avulsed tissue before wrapping it for transport to prevent infection.
    d. Wrap the avulsed tissue in moist gauze, seal it in a plastic bag, and place the bag on ice.

25. Prehospital management of ear pain following barotrauma may include which of the following?
    a. Administration of nitrous oxide by inhalation
    b. A request that the patient perform the Valsalva maneuver
    c. Oxygen delivery to increase the absorption of trapped air
    d. Placement of the patient in the lateral recumbent position

26. Which of the following is an acceptable way to transport an avulsed tooth?
    a. In a mild soap solution
    b. In sterile water
    c. In a dry gauze dressing
    d. In fresh whole milk

27. Why are zone I neck injuries associated with the highest mortality? It contains which of the following?
    a. Brainstem, carotid artery, and nasopharynx
    b. Carotid artery, jugular vein, trachea, larynx, esophagus, and cervical spine
    c. Distal carotid arteries, salivary glands, and pharynx
    d. Subclavian and jugular vessels, lung, esophagus, trachea, cervical spine, cervical nerve roots

28. Which sign or symptom may indicate compromise of the upper airway associated with a hematoma in the neck?
    a. Cough
    b. Dysphagia
    c. Stridor
    d. Wheezing

29. Intubation of the patient with laryngeal or tracheal trauma may be difficult because of which of the following?
    a. Absence of spontaneous respirations
    b. Collapse of the trachea and bronchial tubes
    c. The presence of acute hypoxia
    d. Distorted and invisible vocal cords

30. Which of the following is an injury associated with focal brain injury?
    a. Concussion
    b. Contusion
    c. Minute petechial bruising of brain tissue in several areas
    d. Mechanical disruption of axons in both cerebral hemispheres

31. Which of the following is the most reliable indicator of increasing intracranial pressure?
    a. Deteriorating level of consciousness
    b. Nausea and vomiting
    c. Increased blood pressure and decreased pulse
    d. Unilateral dilated pupil
32. Which of the following breathing patterns is *not* likely to be exhibited by the patient with a brain injury?
    a. Ataxic breathing
    b. Cheyne-Stokes respirations
    c. Hypoventilation
    d. Kussmaul's respirations
33. Characteristic signs and symptoms of subarachnoid hemorrhage include which of the following?
    a. Clinical signs of unexplained hypovolemia
    b. Gradual onset of unilateral weakness of the arms
    c. Intermittent pain and double vision in both eyes
    d. Sudden onset of "the worst headache I've ever had"
34. Which is the most rapid and effective intervention to decrease intracranial pressure in a patient with a severe head injury and a Glasgow Coma Scale score of 6?
    a. Elevation of the head of the bed
    b. Intravenous administration of mannitol
    c. Intubation and adequate ventilation
    d. Massive doses of steroids
35. You wish to give 40 g of mannitol to a patient who has a head injury. You have a 20% solution of the drug. How many milliliters do you give?
    a. 8
    b. 50
    c. 80
    d. 200
36. Which drug may be administered before intubation to prevent a sudden increase in intracranial pressure?
    a. Atropine
    b. Lidocaine
    c. Mannitol
    d. Midazolam

WRAP IT UP

You are working at an amusement park, when a call comes over your walkie-talkie for a person who has fallen off a ride. You respond in a motorized golf cart and find a 17-year-old who has fallen about 20 feet from a ride onto the concrete. Bystanders found her prone and rolled her onto her back. Your direct a security officer to maintain spinal immobilization while you assess that her only response to painful stimulation is flexion of her arms. She is making no sounds and her eyes remain closed; pupils are midline, 5 mm, and reactive. She has multiple contusions and lacerations to her face, her nose is flattened, and there is thin bloody drainage from it. You insert an oral airway, and because her respirations are shallow and only about eight per minute, you begin to ventilate her with a bag-valve-mask resuscitator and oxygen as the local ambulance crew arrives. Her radial pulse is 60 per minute, her skin is pale and cool, and her blood pressure is 80/50 mm Hg. She is logrolled with spinal precautions, her back is examined quickly, and after she is secured to the long spine board and stretcher, she is moved into the ambulance where the paramedic crew leader intubates her trachea. An ECG and noninvasive blood pressure monitor are attached, and an IV of normal saline is initiated. After a bolus of 200 mL is given, her pressure rises to 100/70 mm Hg. Physical exam shows no crepitus or deformity anywhere except her face. Moments before arrival at the ED, her right pupil dilates to 7 mm and becomes nonreactive, BP is 130/50 mm Hg, P 50, and she has no motor response to painful stimulus and no spontaneous respirations when bagging is paused. You begin hyperventilation at 20 per minute. She is diagnosed with a severe diffuse axonal injury and dies during the flight to the regional trauma center.

1. If this patient had a gag reflex, should you have considered nasal instead of oral intubation?
    a. No, there is a possibility of midface fracture and penetration of the cranial vault.
    b. No, there would not have been a need to intubate if that patient had a gag reflex.
    c. Yes, nasal intubation would have been less likely to raise intracranial pressure.
    d. Yes, nasal intubation would have tamponaded the nasal bleeding when in place.
2. Based on the information given, which type of skull fractures would you anticipate?
    a. Basilar
    b. Depressed
    c. Linear

d. a and b

e. a and c

3. What type of brain hemorrhage is present in diffuse axonal injury?

   a. Cerebral hematoma

   b. Epidural hematoma

   c. Subarachnoid hemorrhage

   d. Subdural hematoma

   e. None of the above

4. Explain your rationale for providing the following treatment:

   a. Tracheal intubation:_____

   b. Fluid bolus with normal saline:_____

   c. Hyperventilation after the pupil dilated_____

_____

5. Calculate the following scores for this patient:

<table>
<tr><td></td><td align="center">Glasgow Coma Scale</td><td align="center">Revised Trauma Score</td></tr>
<tr><td>Initial</td><td></td><td></td></tr>
<tr><td>During transport</td><td></td><td></td></tr>
</table>

6. Place a check mark beside the indicators of increasing intracranial pressure that were present in this patient.

   a. _____ Headache

   b. _____ Nausea/vomiting

   c. _____ Altered level of consciousness

   d. _____ Blood pressure rises

   e. _____ Pulse slows

   f. _____ Cheyne-Stokes respirations

   g. _____ Widening pulse pressure

   h. _____ Fixed, dilated pupil

   i. _____ Central neurogenic hyperventilation

   j. _____ Abnormal posturing

   k. _____ Ataxic respirations

   l. _____ Irregular pulse rate

CHAPTER 24 ANSWERS

REVIEW QUESTIONS

1. a
   (Objective 4)

2. c
   (Objective 4)

3. d
   (Objective 4)

4. b
   (Objective 4)

5. e. This nerve is associated with basilar skull fracture.
   (Objective 4)

6. b. Injury to the brain affecting the optic nerve may cause blindness in one or both eyes or visual field defects.
   (Objective 4)

7. d. Damage involving the facial nerve may cause immediate or delayed facial paralysis and is associated with basilar skull fracture.
   (Objective 4)

8. c. Injury affecting the oculomotor nerve can result in double vision because of the inability of the eye to move medially and down and out. Ptosis and pupil dilation or unresponsiveness to light also may occur.
   (Objective 4)

9. a. Loss or alteration of sense of smell associated with injury affecting the olfactory nerve is a common finding associated with basilar skull fracture.
   (Objective 4)

10. a. Inspect and palpate the head for lacerations, contusions, and deformities. Inspect the face for asymmetry and soft tissue injury. Evaluate the child's vision by holding up fingers and assessing pupil response. Assess for EOMs by asking the child to look up and down and side to side. Look for deformity of the nose and any drainage of blood or cerebrospinal fluid. Inspect the oral cavity for bleeding, soft tissue injury, and missing teeth. Palpate the face for crepitus, and question the child about tenderness or numbness. Ask the child to open and close the mouth and move the lower jaw from side to side. Gently palpate for loose teeth.
    b. Immobilize the cervical spine, and secure the child to the backboard while frequently suctioning the oral cavity. Tilt the backboard to the side and secure it firmly with straps. Suction the oral cavity frequently, and instruct the child to signal when he needs additional suctioning or if he has difficulty breathing. Continually reevaluate for life threats.
    (Objective 1)

11. Obtain a history to include the exact mode of injury; previous ocular, medical, and drug history, including cataracts, glaucoma, and presence of hepatitis or human immunodeficiency virus; use of eye medications; use of corrective glasses or contact lenses; presence of ocular prostheses; and symptoms and treatment interventions that may have been attempted before emergency medical services arrival. Observe the patient for signs of external trauma, discoloration, injury to the lid, fluid or jelly extruding from the eye, bleeding, blood in the anterior chamber, and the presence of contact lenses. Measure visual acuity with a handheld acuity chart or any printed material with small, medium, and large point sizes. Record the distance at which the visual material was held. Measure each eye separately and assess vision with and without corrective lenses. Evaluate pupil reaction

to ensure that they constrict in concert when light is applied and dilate in response to darkness. Assess extraocular muscles by asking the patient to track an object with the eyes (without head movement) up, down, right, and left.
(Objective 2)

12. a. Injury: foreign body (or corneal abrasion); management: irrigate with normal saline.
    b. Injury: lid avulsion; management: assess for underlying injury to the eye; control bleeding with gentle pressure; for transport, cover with a dressing moistened with normal saline and an eye shield.
    c. Injury: embedded foreign body; management: patch uninjured eye; stabilize hook and cover with cardboard cup secured with tape.
    d. Injury: traumatic hyphema; management: elevate head of ambulance cot or spine board 40 to 45 degrees; instruct patient to avoid straining.
    e. Injury: ruptured globe; management: cover affected eye with damp, sterile dressings and an eye shield.
    (Objective 2)

13. Bleeding, shock, hematoma, pulse deficit, neurological deficit, dyspnea, hoarseness, stridor, subcutaneous emphysema, hemoptysis, dysphagia, and hematemesis
    (Objective 3)

14. Secure airway and breathing. Maintain spinal immobilization. Apply firm, direct pressure to the affected vessels, and tamponade the vessel by direct pressure with a gloved finger only to the affected vessel(s). If venous injury is suspected, keep the patient supine or in Trendelenberg's position to prevent an air embolism. If air embolism is suspected, turn the immobilized patient on the left side, head lower than feet, to attempt to trap the air embolus in the right ventricle.
    (Objective 3)

15. a. Diffuse axonal injury; loss of consciousness (usually less than 5 minutes), retrograde or antegrade amnesia, vomiting, combativeness, transient visual disturbances, and problems with coordination; should all improve, not deteriorate
    b. Focal injury; seizures, hemiparesis, aphasia, personality changes, and loss of consciousness (lasting hours, days, or longer)
    c. Focal injury; headache, nausea, vomiting, decreasing level of consciousness, coma, abnormal posturing, paralysis, and bulging fontanelles in infants
    d. Focal injury; transient loss of consciousness followed by a lucid interval (6 to 18 hours) and a subsequent decreasing level of consciousness, headache, and contralateral hemiparesis (opposite the side of the bleeding); 50% unconscious without improvement
    e. Diffuse axonal injury; patients being usually unconscious for prolonged periods; may have posturing and signs of increased intracranial pressure
    (Objective 5)

16. Headache, nausea, vomiting, altered level of consciousness, increased systolic blood pressure, widened pulse pressure, decreased pulse rate, abnormally slow respiratory pattern, unilateral dilated pupil, and abnormal posturing
    (Objective 5)

17. Intubate tracheally (possibly nasally if signs of basilar skull fracture are not present) using spinal precautions. Hyperventilate the lungs with 100% oxygen at a rate of 24 per minute. Consider gastric tube insertion if available. Maintain fluids to keep the vein open unless signs of shock develop. Consider pharmacological agents, such as mannitol and furosemide, in consultation with medical direction. Notify medical direction, and transport the patient to the closest appropriate trauma center.
    (Objective 6)

18. a. GCS is 12, and RTS is 11.
    b. GCS is 8, and RTS is 7.
    c. PTS is 7.
    (Objective 7)

19. b. "Donkey face" is associated with this injury. Edema, unstable maxilla, epistaxis, numb upper teeth, nasal flattening, and cerebrospinal fluid rhinorrhea are also signs of midface fracture.
(Objective 1)

20. c. Neither an endotracheal tube nor a gastric tube should be placed nasally in the patient with midface fracture because they may pass into the cranial vault. Elevation of the head of the cot would be appropriate only after the cervical spine is cleared by radiographs in the emergency department. Cerebrospinal fluid drainage often accompanies these injuries and should be allowed to drain freely.
(Objective 1)

21. d. The zygoma commonly is called the *cheek bone*.
(Objective 1)

22. c. Orbital fractures often are associated with other fractures, such as Le Fort II and III and zygomatic fractures.
(Objective 1)

23. d. In children, minimal displacement may result in growth changes and ultimate deformity.
(Objective 1)

24. d. A chance to reimplant does exist, so if possible, the ear should be transported as described. However, ear injuries that involve cartilage often heal poorly and are infected easily.
(Objective 2)

25. b. Nitrous oxide is contraindicated and may increase the pain. Other measures that may help include requests that the patient yawn, swallow, and move the lower jaw.
(Objective 2)

26. d. Milk may be used if a commercial tooth solution, such as Hank's solution, is not available.
(Objective 2)

27. d. Zone II injuries (b) occur more often but are associated with lower mortality.
(Objective 3)

28. c. Stridor indicates that the upper airway is compromised significantly.
(Objective 3)

29. d. Attempting intubation actually may increase the damage associated with the injury and, if unsuccessful, cause partial airway obstruction to become complete.
(Objective 3)

30. b. Contusion is bruising of a specific area of the brain. All other answers reflect injuries that represent diffuse axonal injury.
(Objective 5)

31. a. This is the earliest sign and is consistent with all patients who have increased intracranial pressure.
(Objective 5)

32. d. The patient in diabetic ketoacidosis demonstrates Kussmaul's respirations in an attempt to correct acidosis.
(Objective 5)

33. d. Other common signs and symptoms include dizziness, neck stiffness, unequal pupils, vomiting, seizures, and loss of consciousness.
(Objective 5)

34. c. All other interventions are indicated (depending on medical control) to decrease intracranial pressure; however, ventilation at a rate not to exceed 24 per minute is the fastest method with the least risk to the patient. (Objective 6)

35. d. $\dfrac{40\,\text{g} \times 100\,\text{mL}}{20\,\text{g}} = 200\,\text{mL}$

or 20 g:100 mL = 40 g:x mL

4000 = 20x

200 mL = x

36. b. Atropine may be given to children before intubation to counteract the vagal stimulation. Mannitol is an osmotic diuretic given to decrease intracranial pressure but usually is not given for this purpose. Midazolam (Versed) is often given during rapid sequence induction procedures to sedate the patient. (Objective 6)

WRAP IT UP

1. a. The nasal bleeding, massive facial trauma, and flattened nose are indicators of midface fractures. Nasal intubation of this patient is associated with the risk of perforation of the cranial vault. (Objective 1)

2. e. Midface fractures are associated with basilar skull fractures. There is no indication of depression of the skull bones. (Objective 1)

3. e. Diffuse axonal injury is associated with severe shearing, stretching, or tearing of the nerve fibers of the brain rather than a large collection of blood in an area of the brain. (Objective 4)

4. a. Intubation will protect the airway of a patient with a severe head injury with altered level of consciousness as evidenced by a Glasgow Coma Scale score of less than 8. (Objective 6)

b. Fluid bolus is given to raise the blood pressure. Because the cerebral perfusion pressure (pressure needed to deliver oxygenated blood to the brain tissue) is equal to the mean arterial pressure less the intracranial pressure, if the blood pressure falls too low, the blood delivery to the brain is severely compromised. Fluid bolus may be needed to increase the blood pressure. (Objective 6)

c. Hyperventilation is indicated when the pupil dilates and the Glasgow Coma Scale score is less than 9. This will cause constriction of the blood vessels in the brain and a resulting decrease in the intracranial pressure, which will decrease the risk of brain herniation. (Objective 6)

5. Initial Glasgow Coma Scale score: 5; initial Revised Trauma Score: 6
Transport Glasgow Coma Scale score: 3; transport Revised Trauma Score: 4
(Objective 7)

6. c, d, e, g, h, j. There is insufficient information given to determine whether the patient had ataxic or Cheyne-Stokes respirations. (Objective 5)

CHAPTER
25
Spinal Trauma

READING ASSIGNMENT
Chapter 25, pages 606-629, in *Mosby's Paramedic Textbook,* ed. 3

OBJECTIVES
Upon completion of this chapter, the paramedic student will be able to:
1. Describe the incidence, morbidity, and mortality related to spinal injury.
2. Predict mechanisms of injury that are likely to cause spinal injury.
3. Describe the anatomy and physiology of the spine and spinal cord.
4. Outline the general assessment of a patient with suspected spinal injury.
5. Distinguish between types of spinal injury.
6. Describe prehospital evaluation and assessment of spinal cord injury.
7. Identify prehospital management of the patient with spinal injuries.
8. Distinguish between spinal shock, neurogenic shock, and autonomic hyperreflexia syndrome.
9. Describe selected nontraumatic spinal conditions and the prehospital assessment and treatment of them.

SUMMARY
- Most SCIs are the result of motor vehicle crashes. Other causes are falls, penetrating injuries from acts of human violence, and sport injuries.
- The paramedic can classify the MOI as positive, negative, or uncertain. This classification is combined with the clinical guidelines for evaluating SCI, which include the following signs and symptoms: pain, tenderness, painful movement, deformity, cuts/bruises over spinal area, paralysis, paresthesias, and weakness. This system can help to identify cases in which spinal immobilization is appropriate.
- The spinal column is composed of 33 vertebrae. These are divided into five sections. The sections are 7 cervical, 12 thoracic, 5 lumbar, 5 sacral (fused), and 4 coccygeal (fused).
- The specific mechanisms of injury that frequently cause spinal trauma are axial loading; extremes of flexion, hyperextension, or hyperrotation; excessive lateral bending; and distraction.
- Spinal injuries may be classified as sprains and strains, fractures and dislocations, sacral and coccygeal fractures, and cord injuries. The spinal cord may sustain a primary or a secondary injury. Lesions (transections) of the spinal cord are classified as complete or incomplete.
- With spinal injuries, the first priority is to evaluate and manage any threats to life. The second priority is to preserve spinal cord function. This includes avoiding secondary injury to the spinal cord. These goals are best met by maintaining a high degree of suspicion for the presence of spinal trauma, by providing early spinal immobilization, by rapidly correcting any volume deficit, and by administering oxygen.
- General principles of spinal immobilization include prevention of further injury; treating the spine as a long bone with a joint at either end (the head and pelvis); always using complete spinal immobilization; beginning spinal

immobilization in the initial assessment and maintaining it until the spine is immobilized completely on the long spine board; and placing the patient's head in a neutral, in-line position, unless contraindicated.
- Spinal shock refers to a temporary loss of all types of spinal cord function distal to the injury.
- Neurogenic shock produces a loss of sympathetic tone to the vessels. This causes relative hypotension; warm, dry, and pink skin; and relative bradycardia.
- Autonomic hyperreflexia syndrome results from a massive, uncompensated cardiovascular response that stimulates the sympathetic nervous system. This response in turn causes an increase in blood pressure and other symptoms.
- Some nontraumatic spinal conditions include low back pain, degenerative disk disease, spondylolysis, herniated intervertebral disk, and spinal cord tumors. The management of patients with nontraumatic back pain in the prehospital setting is mainly supportive. The goal is to help patients decrease their pain and discomfort.

REVIEW QUESTIONS

Match the spinal illness/injury in Column II with the description in Column I. Use each term only once.

Column I		**Column II**
1. _____ A tear in the capsule that encloses the center of the disk		**a.** Anterior cord syndrome
2. _____ Nontraumatic structural defect that involves the lamina or vertebral joint		**b.** Autonomic hyperreflexia syndrome
3. _____ Paralysis and decreased pain and temperature sensation below a flexion injury		**c.** Brown-Séquard syndrome **d.** Central cord syndrome
4. _____ Sprain causing partial dislocation of intervertebral joints		**e.** Herniated nucleus pulposus **f.** Hyperextension strain
5. _____ Hemitransection of cord with weakness on the injured side		**g.** Neurogenic hypotension **h.** Spinal cord tumors
6. _____ Whiplash from a low-speed, rear-end collision		**i.** Spinal shock **j.** Spondylosis
7. _____ Sudden rapid increase in blood pressure, relieved by emptying of the bladder		**k.** Subluxation
8. _____ Bradycardia, warm skin, and low blood pressure		
9. _____ Abnormal tissue growth in the spine that may cause spasticity		
10. _____ Injury characterized by paralysis of the arms with sacral sparing		

11. In each of the following situations, state whether the mechanism of injury is negative, positive, or uncertain related to your assessment of the spine.

   a. A soccer player falls and twists her knee._____

   b. A patient is ejected during a rollover crash._____

   c. A patient has a gunshot wound lateral to the spine._____

   d. A young man falls 3 feet off a porch._____

   e. A patient is the restrained driver in a motor vehicle crash, and the rear hood is buckled.

   _____

   f. A child dives off the high board and strikes the bottom of the pool with his head.

   _____

   g. A woman who was running slips and falls, striking her head on a ceramic tile floor.

   _____

12. List five preexisting conditions that can increase the risk of spine injury or complicate the injury.

a.

b.

c.

d.

e.

13. Spinal sprains and strains usually result from (a) _____ and (b) _____ forces. A hyperflexion sprain occurs when a tear is present in the posterior (c) _____ and _____, which allows partial (d) _____ of the intervertebral joints. Hyperextension strains are common with low-velocity, rear-end automobile collisions and are known commonly as (e) _____. The most frequently injured spinal regions, in descending order, are (f) _____ to _____, (g) _____ to _____, and (h) _____ to _____. The most common are wedge-shaped (i) _____ fractures. (j) _____ and (k) _____ are extremely unstable injuries caused by a combination of severe hyperflexion and compression forces.

14. A cyclist was thrown from his bike and has severe pain in the back between his scapulae. List signs and symptoms that can indicate a complete cord lesion as a result of this injury.

_____

_____

Questions 15 to 17 pertain to the following case study:

A 35-year-old was involved in a motor vehicle crash with moderate damage, which you classify as an uncertain mechanism for spine injury. She says she is fine and just wants to be "checked out" at the hospital.

15. Which conditions or situations would make her unreliable to perform spinal examination for clinical criteria?

_____

_____

16. Describe your examination for motor findings suggestive of spine injury.

_____

_____

17. Describe how to perform the sensory exam to evaluate for spine injury on this patient.

_____

18. Identify five situations involving suspected cervical spine injury when the head should *not* be moved to a neutral inline position with manual immobilization.

a.

b.

c.

d.

e.

19. Identify the steps involved in rolling of a supine patient (Fig. 25-1), including positioning of rescuers.

A.

B.

C.

D.

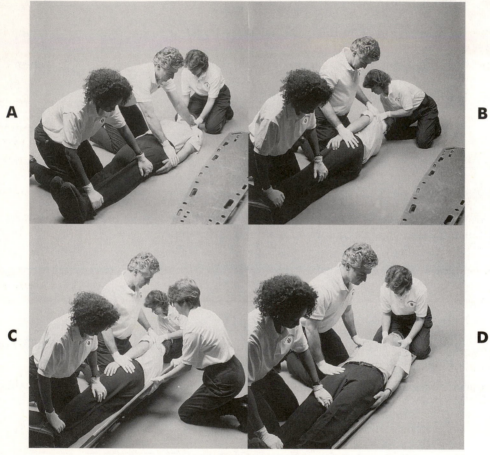

Figure 25-1

20. Identify drugs that may be used for each of the following spinal cord emergencies:

a. Spinal cord injury with paralysis:

_____

b. Spinal cord injury with hypotension and bradycardia:

_____

STUDENT SELF-ASSESSMENT

21. Most spinal injuries occur as a result of which of the following?
    a. Falls
    b. Motor vehicle crashes
    c. Sports-related injuries
    d. Penetrating injuries from acts of violence

22. Which of the following classifications of mechanism of injury would be given to a fall from the roof of a single-story residence?
    a. Alternative mechanism of injury
    b. Negative mechanism of injury
    c. Positive mechanism of injury
    d. Uncertain mechanism of injury

23. Which of the following patients would be considered reliable to assess for spinal cord injury?
    a. A patient who witnessed the death of his or her child in crash.
    b. A patient with a severely angulated, partially amputated foot.
    c. A patient who cannot communicate in a language you understand.
    d. A patient who is complaining of knee and hip pain with no deformity.

24. Which is the most flexible area of the spine?
    a. Cervical spine
    b. Lumbar spine
    c. Sacral spine
    d. Thoracic spine

25. A side-impact motor vehicle collision is most likely to produce spinal injury from extremes in which motion?
    a. Axial loading
    b. Distraction
    c. Flexion
    d. Lateral bending

26. Which finding on a patient with uncertain mechanism of injury should cause you to suspect spine trauma and to immobilize the spine?
    a. High blood pressure
    b. History of Parkinson's disease
    c. Laceration on the scalp
    d. Pain or tenderness of the neck

27. Hyperflexion sprains can cause partial dislocation of the intervertebral joints. This condition is known as which of the following?
    a. Axial loading
    b. Herniated disks
    c. Subluxation
    d. Whiplash

28. Fractures at the level of S1 and S2 may lead to which of the following?
    a. Loss of bowel and bladder function
    b. Neurogenic shock
    c. Paralysis of the legs
    d. Transection of the spinal cord

29. Paralysis and loss of sensation below the umbilicus indicate an injury at the level of which of the following?
    a. C4
    b. T4
    c. T10
    d. S1

30. Which of the following is a sign of autonomic dysfunction resulting from spinal cord injury?
    a. Bradycardia
    b. Hypertension
    c. Profuse sweating
    d. Polyuria

31. Which of the following signs or symptoms is associated with central cord syndrome?
    a. Intact light touch and position sensation
    b. Greater motor weakness or paralysis in the arms than legs
    c. Loss of pain and temperature sensation on the side of injury
    d. Weakness in the upper and lower extremities on the side opposite the injury

32. Respiratory distress should be anticipated in the patient with which of the following?
    a. Brown-Séquard syndrome
    b. Herniated thoracic disk
    c. Hyperextension strain
    d. Spinal cord transection above C5 to C6

33. The purpose of immobilizing the patient suspected to have spinal injury in the prehospital setting is which of the following?
    a. To apply traction to pull apart injured bones
    b. To minimize neurogenic shock
    c. To prevent primary injury
    d. To prevent additional cord hypoxia or edema
34. When a patient on a long spine board is immobilized, which of the following body regions should be secured first?
    a. Arms
    b. Head
    c. Legs
    d. Torso
35. Which of the following cord injury presentations involves flaccid paralysis that usually resolves within 24 hours?
    a. Autonomic hyperreflexia syndrome
    b. Neurogenic hypotension
    c. Spinal shock
    d. Spondylosis
36. Which of the following medical conditions of the spine can increase the risk of spinal fractures?
    a. Degenerative disk disease
    b. Herniated intervertebral disk
    c. Spinal cord tumors
    d. Spondylolysis

WRAP IT UP

You are dispatched to a call to "assist the invalid." As per protocol, you respond "on the quiet" with no lights or sirens. When you arrive at the home of the 87-year-old patient, his wife tells you that he tripped over a videotape in the living room and fell forward, striking his forehead on the coffee table. As you approach him, he apologizes profusely for calling you to help him up off the floor. He is conscious, alert, and oriented, and you can see a small abrasion on his mid-forehead. When you ask him if anything hurts, he reaches around to his neck, rubs it vigorously, and says that his neck is sore. You palpate his neck, and he says the cervical spine area is tender, but you feel no crepitus and note no deformity. Your partner begins cervical-spine immobilization as you continue your exam. You can see that his breathing is normal, and palpation of his radial pulse reveals a normal, regular rate with warm, dry skin. A quick head-to-toe exam is unremarkable except for his persistent complaint of an "electric shock" sensation in his extremities. You explain to the patient your concern that he may have a spine injury, and he consents to transport. After application of the cervical collar, you logroll him and secure him to the long backboard. Vital signs are BP 134/78 mm Hg, P 60, R 20, SaO$_2$ 96%. You initiate an IV and contact medical direction, who advises no further. The patient's condition remains stable, and you give report to the charge nurse in the ED. Later, the charge nurse calls you to let you know that the patient has an unstable fracture of C2 and C3. A halo vest has been applied, and his condition remains stable.

1. Which is the most common mechanism of injury for spinal injuries?
    a. Falls
    b. Motor vehicle crashes
    c. Penetrating injuries
    d. Sport injuries
2. Which mechanism of injury occurred in this case?
    a. Negative
    b. Positive
    c. Uncertain
3. Place a check mark beside the signs or symptoms that made you determine that spinal immobilization was indicated for this patient.
    a. _____ Trauma with use of intoxicating substances
    b. _____ Seizure activity
    c. _____ Complaints of pain in neck or arms
    d. _____ Tender neck on examination
    e. _____ Unconscious after head injury
    f. _____ Significant injury above clavicle
    g. _____ Fall greater than 3 times patient's height
    h. _____ Fall and bilateral heel fracture
    i. _____ Injury from high-speed motor vehicle collision

4. Which forces likely injured the spine in this case?
   a. Axial loading
   b. Distraction
   c. Lateral bending
   d. Hyperextension and/or hyperflexion

5. If you had merely assisted the patient to his feet without performing a history or examination on him, what could have happened to his spinal cord?

_____

6. List some signs or symptoms that would indicate that this patient had a spinal cord injury.

_____

7. Place a check mark beside the signs or symptoms you would anticipate if the spinal cord were injured and the patient were developing neurogenic shock.
   a. _____ Bradycardia
   b. _____ Cool skin
   c. _____ Dry skin
   d. _____ Hypertension
   e. _____ Hypotension
   f. _____ Moist skin
   g. _____ Tachycardia
   h. _____ Warm skin

CHAPTER 25 ANSWERS

REVIEW QUESTIONS

1. e
   (Objective 9)

2. j
   (Objective 9)

3. a
   (Objective 5)

4. k
   (Objective 5)

5. c
   (Objective 5)

6. f
   (Objective 5)

7. b
   (Objective 8)

8. g
   (Objective 8)

9. h
   (Objective 9)

10. d
    (Objective 5)

11. a. Negative
    b. Positive
    c. Positive
    d. Uncertain
    e. Uncertain
    f. Positive
    g. Uncertain
    (Objective 2)

12. Damage from spinal injury can occur more easily or be complicated by one or more of the following:
    a. Increased age
    b. Osteoporosis
    c. Spondylosis
    d. Rheumatoid arthritis
    e. Paget's disease
    f. Congenital cord anomalies (fusion, narrow spinal canal)
    (Objective 4)

13. a. Hyperflexion
    b. Hyperextension
    c. Ligamentous complex and joint capsule
    d. Dislocation (subluxation)
    e. Whiplash
    f. C5 to C7
    g. C1 to C2
    h. T12 to L2
    i. Compression
    j. Teardrop fractures
    k. Dislocations
    (Objective 5)

14. Absence of motor and sensory function below the nipple, relative bradycardia, hypotension, priapism, unstable body temperature, loss of bowel and bladder control, and decreased depth of respiration (loss of inervation of most intercostal muscles)
    (Objective 6)

15. To be reliable, she must be calm, cooperative, sober, alert, and oriented. If she exhibits any of the following, she should be considered unreliable: acute stress reaction, brain injury, intoxication, abnormal mental status, distracting injuries, or problems in communication.
    (Objective 4)

16. Motor evaluation: Ask the patient to move her arms and legs. Ask her to flex her elbow, grab and squeeze your fingers, and extend her elbows. Have the patient spread the fingers of both hands and keep them apart while you squeeze the second and fourth fingers. A normal exam produces springlike resistance. Support the patient's lower arm and ask her to hold her wrists or fingers out straight while you press down on her fingers. Moderate resistance should be felt. Place your hands at the sole of each foot and ask the patient to push against your hands. Both sides should feel equal and strong. Then, hold the patient's feet (with fingers on her toes) and instruct her to pull them back to her nose. Both sides should feel equal and strong.
    (Objectives 4 and 6)

17. Sensory evaluation: Question the patient about pain in the neck or back and any feelings of numbness or tingling in the body. Assess light touch on each hand and each foot (with the patient's eyes closed) and then, if necessary, prick the hands and feet with a sharp object (without breaking the skin).
    (Objectives 4 and 6)

18. a. Increasing pain or neurological deficits during movement
    b. Resistance to movement
    c. Muscle spasm
    d. Airway compromise caused by repositioning
    e. Severe misalignment of head from midline
    (Objective 7)

19. a. Rescuer 1 is positioned at the patient's head, providing in-line manual stabilization. Rescuers 2 and 3 are positioned at the patient's midthorax and knees.
    b. While maintaining immobilization, the rescuers, in one organized move, slowly logroll the patient onto his or her side, perpendicular to the ground.
    c. Rescuer 4 positions the long spine board by placing the device flat on the ground or at a 30- to 40-degree angle against the patient's back.
    d. In one organized move, the rescuers slowly logroll and center the patient onto the long spine board.
    (Objective 7)

20. a. Methylprednisolone 30 mg/kg bolus, followed by 5.4 mg/kg/hr for 23 hours
    Other experimental treatments include naloxone and calcium channel blockers (consult medical direction).
    b. Dopamine

21. b. In order of frequency of occurrence, they are motor vehicle crashes, falls, penetrating injuries, and sports injuries.
(Objective 1)

22. c. Most single-story homes are more than 3 times a person's height, which is classified as positive mechanism of injury.

23. d. The patient in (a) may be experiencing a stress reaction. The patient in (b) has a distracting injury. You cannot examine the patient in (c) well enough to rule out spinal injury by clinical criteria because of the language barrier.
(Objective 2)

24. a. The cervical spine allows the head to rotate with an almost 180-degree range of motion, 60 degrees of flexion, and 70 degrees of extension.
(Objective 3)

25. d. Axial loading occurs when the spine is compressed vertically. Distraction results from excessive "pulling" on the spinal cord. Flexion is a bending motion that decreases the angle between two joints, which more often results from anterior/posterior-type motion.
(Objective 2)

26. d. Pain or tenderness of the neck with or without palpation always should indicate immobilization of the spine.
(Objective 4)

27. c. Axial loading is a vertical loading mechanism of injury. A herniated disk occurs when the cartilage surrounding an intervertebral disk ruptures and releases the pulpy elastic substance that cushions the vertebrae above and below, causing pain and damage to nerve roots.[1]
(Objective 5)

28. a. The spinal cord terminates at L2.
(Objective 5)

29. c. C3 and C4 would involve sensory loss at the top of the shoulder; T4 at the nipple; and S1 on the lateral foot.
(Objectives 4 and 6)

30. a. Hypotension, priapism, loss of sweating and shivering, poikilothermy, and loss of bowel and bladder control are also signs.
(Objective 6)

31. b. This weakness usually results from hyperextension or hyperflexion injuries.
(Objective 5)

32. d. Transection of the cord above C3 usually results in respiratory arrest. Lesions that occur at C4 may result in diaphragmatic paralysis. Lesions at C5-C6 spare the diaphragm but result in loss of significant intercostal muscle function.
(Objective 6)

33. d. Traction should not be applied on the spine in the field. Primary injury occurs at the time the initial forces are applied.
(Objective 7)

34. d. Immobilize the torso first to prevent angulation of the cervical spine.
(Objective 7)

---

[1] Anderson KN, Anderson LE: *Mosby's medical, nursing, & allied health dictionary,* ed 3, St Louis, 1990, Mosby.

35. c. Spinal shock results from a temporary loss of all spinal cord function distal to the injury.
(Objective 8)

36. d. Rotational stress fractures are common at the affected site of spondylosis.
(Objective 9)

WRAP IT UP

1. b. Motor vehicle collisions, falls, and then penetrating trauma and sports injuries.
(Objective 1)

2. c. This was a single-level fall.
(Objective 2)

3. c, d. Neck pain is the most important predictor of cervical spine injury.
(Objective 4)

4. d. The mechanism of injury and abrasion to his forehead lead us to believe that his head was flexed or extended forcefully.
(Objective 2)

5. It could have caused a partial or complete cord injury (causing paralysis) if the unstable cervical spine impinged on the delicate spinal cord.
(Objective 2)

6. The patient was complaining of radicular (electrical shock) pain, a symptom of cord injury. Additional signs or symptoms could include paralysis, paresthesias, weakness, neurological deficit, priapism, loss of sweating/shivering, poikilothermy, and loss of bowel and bladder control.
(Objective 6)

7. a, c, e, h
(Objective 8)

Thoracic Trauma

READING ASSIGNMENT
Chapter 26, pages 630-643, in *Mosby's Paramedic Textbook,* ed. 3

OBJECTIVES
Upon completion of this chapter, the paramedic student will be able to:
1. Discuss the factor and mechanism of injury associated with thoracic trauma.
2. Describe the mechanism of injury, signs and symptoms, and management of skeletal injuries to the chest.
3. Describe the mechanism of injury, signs and symptoms, and prehospital management of pulmonary trauma.
4. Describe the mechanism of injury, signs and symptoms, and prehospital management of injuries to the heart and great vessels.
5. Outline the mechanism of injury, signs and symptoms, and prehospital care of the patient with esophageal and tracheobronchial injury and diaphragmatic rupture.

SUMMARY
- Thoracic trauma injuries are caused by blunt or penetrating trauma. Such trauma often results from motor vehicle crashes, falls from heights, blast injuries, blows to the chest, chest compression, gunshot wounds, and stab wounds.
- Fractures of the clavicle, ribs, or sternum, and as well as flail chest, may be caused by blunt or penetrating trauma. Complications of skeletal trauma of the chest may include cardiac, vascular, or pulmonary injuries.
- Closed pneumothorax may be life-threatening if (1) it is a tension pneumothorax, (2) it occupies more than 40% of the hemithorax, or (3) it occurs in a patient in shock or a preexisting pulmonary or cardiovascular disease. Open pneumothorax may result in severe ventilatory dysfunction, hypoxemia, and death unless it is quickly recognized and corrected. Tension pneumothorax is a true emergency. It results in profound hypoventilation. It may result in death if it is not quickly recognized and managed. Hemothorax may result in massive blood loss. These patients often have hypovolemia and hypoxemia. Pulmonary contusion results when trauma to the lung causes alveolar and capillary damage. Severe hypoxemia may develop. The degree of hypoxemia is directly related to the size of the contused area. Traumatic asphyxia results from forces that cause an increase in intrathoracic pressure. When it occurs alone, it is often not lethal. However, brain hemorrhages, seizures, coma, and death have been reported after these injuries.
- The extent of injury from myocardial contusion may vary. The injury may be only a localized bruise. However, it also may be a full-thickness injury to the wall of the heart. The full-thickness injury may result in cardiac rupture, ventricular aneurysm, or a traumatic myocardial infarction. Pericardial tamponade occurs if 150 to 200 mL of blood enters the pericardial space suddenly. This results in a decrease in stroke volume and cardiac output. *Myocardial rupture* refers to an acute traumatic perforation of the ventricles or atria. It is nearly always immediately fatal. However, death may be delayed for several weeks after blunt trauma. Aortic rupture is a severe injury. There is

an 80% to 90% mortality rate in the first hour. The paramedic should consider the possibility of aortic rupture in any trauma patient who has unexplained shock after a rapid deceleration injury.

- Esophageal injuries most frequently often are caused by penetrating trauma (e.g., missile projectile and knife wounds). Tracheobronchial injuries are rare. (They occur in fewer than 3% of victims of blunt or penetrating chest trauma, but the mortality rate is over 30%.) A tension pneumothorax that does not improve following needle decompression or the absence of a continuous flow of air from the needle following decompression should alert the paramedic to the possibility of a tracheobronchial injury.
- Diaphragmatic ruptures may allow abdominal organs to enter the thoracic cavity. There they may cause compression of the lung, resulting in a reduction in ventilation, a decrease in venous return, a decrease in cardiac output, and shock.

REVIEW QUESTIONS

Questions 1 to 3 pertain to the following case study:

> You are transferring a 26-year-old woman who was a passenger in a car struck laterally on her door. She has a fractured right humerus and multiple fractures of ribs 3 to 8. En route to the trauma center, you note paradoxical movement of her chest.

1. What chest injury do you suspect?

   flail chest

2. Why is the patient likely to become hypoxic following this injury?

   The injury causes lungs difficulty in

3. What patient care measures should you use to improve ventilation?

4. Identify three symptoms common to all types of pneumothorax.

   a.

   b.

   c.

5. A deer hunter is shot accidentally with a 30-30 caliber rifle. The hunter has an open wound inferior to the right nipple, and you cannot find an exit wound.

   a. Why is this patient likely to become hypoxic?

   b. What interventions must be taken immediately to correct the hypoxia?

6. A patient from a motor vehicle crash has sustained severe blunt chest trauma. He has diminished breath sounds on the right side of the chest. He is anxious and dyspneic.

   a. What additional signs and symptoms would indicate that he has developed a tension pneumothorax?

b. Describe the prehospital intervention for tension pneumothorax.

INSERT 14G catheter midclavicular line of 2nd or 3rd intercostal space on the side of the pneumothorax. Listen for a rush of air, consider a flutter valve. Re-evaluate and repeat steps if needle clots

7. What two life-threatening conditions may be caused by hemothorax?

a. *Hypoxia*

b. *Hypovolemic shock*

8. You are called to care for a worker who was crushed momentarily between a truck and a loading dock. His face and head are a bright, reddish purple, and his jugular veins are greatly distended.

a. What injury do you suspect?

Traumatic Asphyxia

b. What treatment would you provide?

Oxygenate, Maintain Airway

9. A 28-year-old woman was involved in a frontal collision, during which her chest struck the steering wheel. She complains of crushing substernal chest pain and palpitations. Her blood pressure is normal, her pulse is 110 and irregular, and her lungs are clear.

a. What injury do you suspect?

Myocardial Contusion

b. What treatment measures should be instituted for this patient?

O^2, EKG, treatment of Dysrhythmia per protocol

10. A 27-year-old was splitting wood when a metal splinter flew off the ax and penetrated his chest. On your arrival, he is confused, with a systolic blood pressure of 80 mm Hg, a narrow pulse pressure, muffled heart sounds, and distended neck veins. You notice bulging veins on his forearm when you prepare to start an IV.

a. What chest injury do you suspect?

Pericardial Tamponade

b. What prehospital care should be rendered?

O^2, fluid replacement, rapid transport

11. What signs should be anticipated in a patient with an aortic rupture caused by a rapid deceleration injury?

Upper extremity or generalized hypertension, systolic murmur, severe shock (paraplegia

STUDENT SELF-ASSESSMENT

12. Which of the following is true regarding chest trauma?
    a. It is associated with a small number of deaths each year.
    b. It only occurs with motor vehicle crashes and penetrating injury.
    c. It only includes soft tissue injuries to the chest.
    d. The use of seat belts decreases the mortality associated with it.

13. Which of the following is true regarding clavicle fractures?
    a. Clavicle fractures are unusual injuries.
    b. They are never serious injuries.
    c. They usually occur when the arm is twisted.
    d. They can be treated with a sling and swath.
14. Which of the following is true regarding rib fractures?
    a. They are more common in children.
    b. The first rib frequently is fractured.
    c. They are associated with pancreatic injury.
    d. Ribs 3 to 8 are most commonly fractured.
15. Respiratory distress in a patient with flail chest most often is associated with which of the following?
    a. Impaired mechanics of respiration
    b. Open chest wounds
    c. Severe pain that increases with respiration
    d. Underlying pulmonary contusion
16. Sternal injuries frequently are associated with which of the following?
    a. Airway compromise
    b. Flail chest
    c. Myocardial injury
    d. Spleen injury
17. Which is the most common cause of pneumothorax?
    a. Excessive pressure on the chest wall
    b. Penetration from a gun or knife
    c. Penetration from a rib fracture
    d. Spontaneous pneumothorax
18. When is a pneumothorax least likely to cause a life threat?
    a. It is closed.
    b. It is a tension pneumothorax.
    c. It occupies more than 40% of the hemithorax.
    d. It occurs in a patient with shock.
19. Your patient has a pneumothorax and may be developing a hemothorax. What signs or symptoms will you anticipate?
    a. Bradypnea
    b. Hypotension
    c. Tracheal deviation away from the affected side
    d. Widened pulse pressure
20. Injury to the lung tissue may occur when overexpansion of air in the lungs occurs after the primary energy wave has passed. This is known as which of the following?
    a. Implosion effect
    b. Inertial effect
    c. Paper-bag effect
    d. Spalding effect
21. What often occurs as a result of pulmonary contusion?
    a. Hypovolemia
    b. Hypoxia
    c. Pericardial tamponade
    d. Pneumothorax
22. Which of the following is *not* a sign associated with Beck's triad (found in pericardial tamponade)?
    a. Jugular vein distention
    b. Muffled heart sounds
    c. Narrowing pulse pressure
    d. Tracheal deviation
23. Which of the following is a complication of pericardiocentesis?
    a. Cardiac dysrhythmias
    b. Increased tamponade
    c. Laceration of a coronary artery
    d. Laceration of the ventricle
    e. All of the above
24. Your patient was involved in a high-speed motor vehicle crash. Which of the following signs may signal aortic rupture?
    a. Congestive heart failure
    b. Decreased breath sounds
    c. Hypertension
    d. Jugular venous distention
25. Your patient was in a motorcycle crash and has dyspnea and bowel sounds at the nipple line on the left side of the chest. You suspect which of the following?
    a. Pericardial tamponade
    b. Liver rupture
    c. Diaphragmatic rupture
    d. Kidney injury

WRAP IT UP

You respond to a "vehicle accident" with possible rescue. When you arrive, you see a single car that has struck a light standard, knocking it to the ground. The safety officer verifies that you can approach the vehicle after he determines that it is not in contact with the pole, and he ensures that the scene is blocked from oncoming traffic. You are able to open the driver door to access your only patient, an 18-year-old man who was not restrained and was driving an older car with no air bags. He is conscious and alert, with a laceration on his forehead. He is moaning loudly and complaining of pain in his legs. Your partner takes spinal precautions while you quickly assess his condition. He has a weak, rapid radial and carotid pulse with pale, cool skin and rapid respirations, and you think that his breath sounds are diminished slightly on the left. He has tenderness and redness over his anterior chest and both lower legs. You and the fire crew on the scene apply oxygen and a cervical collar and perform a rapid extrication, moving him quickly to the ambulance after he is secured onto the stretcher. In the ambulance your team moves quickly to assess vital signs: BP 130/80 mm Hg, P 128, R 24, and SaO_2 on non-rebreather mask is 95%. His breath sounds are difficult to hear, but it seems they are still decreased on the left. The rest of your exam shows bilateral tenderness, deformity, and swelling in the lower legs with weak pedal pulses palpable. You ask your partner to get en route to the trauma center quickly and initiate two IVs and call a report en route. Repeat vital signs remain unchanged during transport. Your medical officer calls back an hour later and is told that the patient was diagnosed with concussion, left pneumothorax, fractured second left rib, and bilateral closed fractures of the tibia and fibula and that they are monitoring the patient for an aortic tear because the initial films show some widening in the mediastinum. He is presently stable with a chest tube in the left side of his chest.

1. Circle the classifications of chest trauma with which the patient has been diagnosed or for which he is being evaluated.
   a. Diaphragmatic injury
   b. Heart and great vessel injury
   c. Pulmonary injury
   d. Skeletal injury

2. What signs or symptoms were present that indicated possible bony chest injury?

_____

3. i. Place a check mark beside the signs or symptoms of pneumothorax that this patient displayed.
   ii. Place a *t* beside additional signs or symptoms that would have indicated this patient was developing a tension pneumothorax.

   a. _____ Chest pain
   b. _____ Cyanosis
   c. _____ Decreased breath sounds on affected side
   d. _____ Distended neck veins
   e. _____ Dyspnea

   f. _____ Hypotension
   g. _____ Subcutaneous emphysema
   h. _____ Tachycardia
   i. _____ Tachypnea
   j. _____ Tracheal deviation

4. How did you treat the pneumothorax in the field?

_____

_____

5. Which of the following is true regarding aortic rupture?
   a. Fracture of the second rib is associated with this injury.
   b. Hypotension will always be seen.
   c. Immediate death rarely is seen with aortic tears.
   d. Quadriplegia can be associated with this injury.

CHAPTER 26 ANSWERS

REVIEW QUESTIONS

1. Flail chest
   (Objective 2)

2. The pulmonary contusion and injured segment of the chest will not expand; therefore insufficient negative pressure is generated in the chest to draw in a normal amount of air.
   (Objective 2)

3. Intubate if the Glasgow Coma Scale score is less than 8 or if the patient has severe hypoxia and assist ventilations with positive pressure (demand valve, bag-valve) with 100% oxygen. Monitor vital signs, electrocardiogram, and oxygen saturation.
   (Objective 2)

4. Dyspnea, tachypnea, diminished breath sounds on the affected side, and chest pain on inspiration
   (Objective 3)

5. a. During inspiration, some air will enter the wound instead of the trachea, which decreases air entering the lung for ventilation
   b. Seal wound on three sides with occlusive dressing. Administer high-flow oxygen by non-rebreather mask.
   (Objective 3)

6. a. Cyanosis, tracheal deviation, tachycardia, hypotension, and distended neck veins
   b. Insert a 14-gauge catheter in the midclavicular line of the second or third intercostal space on the side of the pneumothorax. Listen for a rush of air, consider a flutter valve, reevaluate the patient, and repeat these steps en route if the needle clots.
   (Objective 3)

7. Hypoxia and hypovolemic shock
   (Objective 3)

8. a. Traumatic asphyxia
   b. Oxygenate and maintain airway and ventilation and evaluate for associated injuries.
   (Objective 3)

9. a. Myocardial contusion
   b. Oxygen administration, electrocardiographic monitoring, and treatment of dysrhythmias per protocol
   (Objective 4)

10. a. Pericardial tamponade
    b. Oxygen administration, fluid replacement, rapid transport, consideration of pericardiocentesis (only with authorization and specialized training)
    (Objective 4)

11. Upper extremity or generalized hypertension, systolic murmur, paraplegia (rare), and severe shock
    (Objective 4)

12. d. At least 25% of trauma deaths are associated with chest trauma. Falls, crush injuries, blast injuries, and blows to the chest also can cause significant thoracic trauma.
    (Objective 1)

13. d. The clavicle is one of the most commonly fractured bones. Rarely, clavicle fracture can be complicated by injury to the subclavian vein or artery from bony fragment penetration. The mechanism typically involves a fall on outstretched arms or the shoulder.
(Objective 2)

14. d. Children have more elastic chests and are less likely to have rib fractures. The first rib is rarely fractured. The pancreas lies protected behind other abdominal organs and is unlikely to be affected by rib fractures.
(Objective 2)

15. d. The damaged tissue often results in significant hypoxia.
(Objective 2)

16. c. The heart lies under the sternum and may be compressed if it is injured.
(Objective 2)

17. c. Excessive pressure on the chest wall can cause pneumothorax (paper-bag effect). Spontaneous pneumothorax occurs when a rupture or tear develops in the lung parenchyma for no apparent reason.
(Objective 3)

18. a. Pneumothorax in a patient with preexisting lung or heart disease also can be lethal.
(Objective 3)

19. b. Hypotension will develop as a result of hypovolemic shock. Tachypnea, deviation to the affected side (rare), and narrowed pulse pressure also may occur.
(Objective 3)

20. c. Inertial effect is a stretching and shearing of alveoli and intravascular structures. When the kinetic wave of energy is reflected partially at the alveolar membrane surface and the remainder causes a localized release of energy, it is referred to as the *Spalding effect*.
(Objective 3)

21. b. Profound hypoxia can result from abnormal lung function.
(Objective 3)

22. d. Tracheal deviation may be found in some patients with tension pneumothorax.
(Objective 4)

23. e. Laceration of the liver also may occur.
(Objective 4)

24. c. Pulses may be decreased in the lower extremities.
(Objective 5)

25. c. When the bowel moves into the chest, severe respiratory compromise occurs.
(Objective 5)

WRAP IT UP

1. b, c, d
(Objective 1)

2. Pain, redness of the skin over the area, tenderness on palpation
(Objective 2)

3. i. a, c, e, h, i
ii. b, d, f, g, j
(Objective 3)

4. High-concentration oxygen
(Objective 3)

5. a. Hypertension can be seen initially if vessel tamponade has occurred. There is an 80% to 90% chance of immediate death. Paraplegia is possible.
(Objective 4)

CHAPTER

27

Abdominal Trauma

READING ASSIGNMENT

Chapter 27, pages 644-651, in *Mosby's Paramedic Textbook*, ed. 3

OBJECTIVES

Upon completion of this chapter, the paramedic student will be able to:
1. Identify mechanisms of injury associated with abdominal trauma.
2. Describe mechanisms of injury, signs and symptoms, and complications associated with abdominal solid organ, hollow organ, retroperitoneal organ, and pelvic organ injuries.
3. Outline the significance of injury to intraabdominal vascular structures.
4. Describe the prehospital assessment priorities for the patient suspected of having an abdominal injury.
5. Outline the prehospital care of the patient with abdominal trauma.

SUMMARY

- Blunt trauma to abdominal organs usually results from compression or shearing forces.
- Penetrating injury may result from stab wounds, gunshot wounds, or impaled objects.
- The two solid organs most commonly injured are the liver and the spleen. Both of these organs are primary sources of death from hemorrhage. Injuries to the hollow abdominal organs may result in sepsis, wound infection, and abscess formation.
- Injury to the retroperitoneal organs (kidneys, ureters, pancreas, duodenum) may cause massive hemorrhage.
- Injury to the pelvic organs (bladder, urethra) usually results from motor vehicle crashes that produce pelvic fractures.
- Injuries to abdominal vascular structures may be life threatening. This is due to their potential for massive hemorrhage.
- The most significant sign of severe abdominal trauma is the presence of unexplained shock.
- Emergency care of patients with abdominal trauma usually is limited to two courses of action. One is to stabilize the patient. The other is to rapidly transport the patient to a hospital for surgery to repair the injury.

REVIEW QUESTIONS

1. A 12-year-old boy recovering from mononucleosis has been hit on the left side by another child. He complains of severe left upper quadrant abdominal pain and left shoulder pain. He has signs of shock.

   a. What solid organ has most likely been injured in this situation?

b. Why would the boy complain of shoulder pain?

_____

c. What care should you provide for him?

_____

2. Describe complications that may result when hollow organs of the abdomen are injured.

_____

_____

3. List nine signs or symptoms associated with abdominal trauma.

a.

b.

c.

d.

e.

f.

g.

h.

i.

STUDENT SELF-ASSESSMENT

4. Which of the following is true of abdominal trauma?
   a. Blunt injuries do not occur when personal restraints are used.
   b. Complications of penetrating abdominal trauma appear immediately.
   c. Penetrating injury is associated with higher mortality than blunt trauma.
   d. Shearing forces may produce a tear or rupture of solid organs or blood vessels.
5. Which one of the following is the most commonly injured solid organ?
   a. Adrenal gland   c. Liver
   b. Kidney   d. Pancreas
6. After injury to the liver, patients often experience which of the following?
   a. Bowel obstruction   c. Peritoneal irritation
   b. Gastrointestinal bleeding   d. Renal failure
7. Which of the following is true about renal trauma?
   a. Bleeding is usually minimal.
   b. Fractures often need surgical repair.
   c. It occurs only as a result of posterior trauma.
   d. Urine output stops.
8. Which of the following mechanisms of blunt trauma is most often associated with pancreatic injury?
   a. Bicycle handlebar impalement
   b. Falls from higher than 20 feet
   c. Punch injuries from abuse
   d. Restrained passenger in head-on crash
9. What sign or symptom is a contraindication to insertion of an indwelling Foley catheter?
   a. Blood at the urinary meatus   c. Burning during urination
   b. Bruising over the flank   d. Microscopic hematuria

10. Intraabdominal arterial and venous injuries
    a. Always present with a palpable mass
    b. Have the potential for massive hemorrhage
    c. Involve only the aorta or vena cava
    d. Occur only with penetrating trauma
11. The patient was involved in a high-speed motor vehicle crash. He refuses care. When he stands to leave, he becomes pale and states that he feels nauseated and dizzy. For which condition should you first assess as a possible cause of these signs and symptoms?
    a. Hyperventilation
    b. Preexisting medical problem
    c. Severe abdominal injury
    d. Vagal reaction to pain
12. Scene care of the patient who has signs of shock from abdominal injury should include which of the following?
    a. Comprehensive physical examination
    b. Initiation of IV fluid therapy
    c. Ongoing assessment
    d. Oxygen administration

    Questions 13 to 15 pertain to the following case study:

    Your patient is a 30-year-old woman who was shot in the right upper quadrant of the abdomen. She is pale and restless and has cool, clammy skin. Vital signs are blood pressure, 76/58 mm Hg; pulse, 128/min; and respirations, 28/min.

13. You would suspect injury to the (1) chest, (2) liver, (3) spleen, (4) urinary bladder?
    a. (1) and (2)
    b. (1) and (3)
    c. (2) and (4)
    d. (3) and (4)
14. Interventions for this patient include which of the following?
    a. Oxygen (4 L/min via nasal cannula) and intravenous lactated Ringer solution to keep the vein open
    b. Oxygen (10 L/min via mask) and intravenous lactated Ringer solution to keep the vein open
    c. Oxygen (4 L/min via nasal cannula) and intravenous lactated Ringer solution via rapid infusion
    d. Oxygen (10 L/min via mask) and intravenous lactated Ringer solution via rapid infusion
15. Your *first* priority on arrival at this call would be
    a. Airway maintenance
    b. Administration of oxygen
    c. Scene safety
    d. Stopping the bleeding

WRAP IT UP

Dispatch radios you to respond to a call for a "cutting," stating that the scene is not safe and police are en route. You stage in the area and notify dispatch, waiting to proceed in when police notify you that the scene has been secured. Your patient is a 55-year-old obese male who was stabbed in the abdomen with a 6-inch kitchen knife by an "unknown" assailant. He is awake and alert but very anxious, and he wants to get up and walk around despite his blood-soaked shirt. You note his pale, cool skin; feel a thready, rapid, radial pulse; and then quickly pull off his shirt and pants. One stab wound is visible in the right upper quadrant on his abdomen, just below his rib cage. He denies being short of breath when you question him, and you hear clear and equal breath sounds bilaterally, but his abdomen is rigid and very tender to palpation. No other wounds are visible on your quick head to toe assessment. You quickly administer oxygen and move him to the ambulance, where you assess his vital signs: BP, 78/50 mm Hg; P, 136/min; R, 28/min; Sao$_2$ is unobtainable. You realize that the patient is a critical trauma case, but your rural location is too far from the trauma center, and no helicopter is available. You tell your partner to head for the nearest hospital. Then you continue care; you insert one IV of normal saline, wide open on blood tubing, and another in the other arm of lactated Ringer solution. By the time you have established the second line, you have arrived at the hospital, where the patient is transfused with uncrossmatched blood. Luckily the surgeon is available in-house; she determines that immediate surgery is indicated. The patient is rushed to the operating room, where his lacerated liver is repaired. He is discharged home in 10 days.

1. What other mechanisms can cause injuries to the abdominal organs?

2. Which of the following is true regarding his injury?
  a. Liver contents spilling into the peritoneal cavity cause no signs or symptoms.
  b. The liver is a solid organ, therefore the chief concern after injury is bleeding.
  c. The liver is very vascular and can be removed to prevent death from uncontrolled hemorrhage.
  d. Retroperitoneal bleeding can be severe and is hard to control after liver injury.
3. Place a ✔ beside the signs or symptoms of peritoneal irritation that this patient displayed.
  a. _____ Distention   **d.** _____ Pain
  b. _____ Fever   **e.** _____ Tenderness to palpation
  c. _____ Guarding/rigidity
4. What major artery that supplies the liver could have been injured by this penetrating wound?
  a. Celiac artery
  b. Iliac artery
  c. Inferior mesenteric artery
  d. Hepatic artery
5. What three critical interventions needed to enhance the chance of survival for patients with abdominal trauma were performed on this patient?

  a.

  b.

  c.
6. How would your care change if his initial vital signs were BP 108/78 P 120 R 24/min SaO$_2$ 96%?

_____

CHAPTER 27 ANSWERS

REVIEW QUESTIONS

1. a. Spleen; b. referred pain caused by irritation of the diaphragm by a splenic hematoma or blood in the peritoneum (Kehr sign); c. This child should have a rapid assessment. Oxygen should be administered, and rapid transport to the closest appropriate trauma center should begin immediately. Intravenous therapy using an isotonic solution should be administered at 20 mL/kg during transport. Repeat IV bolus may be indicated based on the reevaluation.
(Objective 2)

2. Sepsis, infection, abscess formation, and peritonitis (resulting from leakage of the contents of hollow organs).
(Objective 2)

3. a. Unexplained shock; b. bruising and discoloration of the abdomen; c. abrasions; d. obvious bleeding; e. pain, abdominal tenderness, or guarding; f. abdominal rigidity, distention; g. evisceration; h. rib fractures; i. pelvic fractures.
(Objective 4)

STUDENT SELF-ASSESSMENT

4. d. This injury is caused by stretching of organs and blood vessels.
(Objective 1)

5. c. The other organ most often injured is the spleen.
(Objective 2)

6. c. Shock also occurs often.
(Objective 2)

7. b. Bleeding can be severe and difficult to detect. Injury can result from anterior or posterior trauma. Urine output may contain blood.
(Objective 2)

8. a. Steering wheel trauma and penetrating trauma are also associated with pancreatic injury.
(Objective 2)

9. a. This may indicate urethral injury, which could be complicated by insertion of a catheter.
(Objective 2)

10. b. The patient often presents with signs and symptoms of shock.
(Objective 3)

11. c. With unexplained shock in a trauma patient, abdominal injury should always be at the top of your "rule out" list.
(Objective 4)

12. d. The initial exam can be done on the scene. Further examination and IV therapy may be performed en route to the hospital.
(Objective 5)

13. a. The liver is located in the right upper quadrant. The diaphragm extends low, therefore the chest cavity is easily penetrated in these types of injuries.
(Objective 1)

14. d. Administration of high-concentration oxygen and fluid resuscitation are indicated.
   (Objective 5)

15. c. Scene safety should always be the first priority on every call, especially when a crime has been committed.
   (Objective 5)

WRAP IT UP

1. Blunt: assault, motor vehicle collisions, falls, industrial injuries, pedestrian injuries, blast injuries. Penetrating: impaled objects, gunshot wounds.
   (Objective 1)

2. b. When bile and blood spill into the peritoneal cavity after liver injury, signs and symptoms of peritoneal irritation occur. The liver is necessary for life; it can be partially removed, but complete removal results in death.
   (Objective 2)

3. c, d, e
   (Objective 2)

4. a. The iliac and inferior mesenteric arteries are lower in the abdomen. The portal vessel is a vein, not an artery.
   (Objective 3)

5. a. Rapid transport for definitive care (surgery)
   b. Oxygenation
   c. Fluid resuscitation
   (Objective 5)

6. Venous access would be obtained with a large bore catheter, but fluids would be run at a keep-open rate unless his systolic BP dropped below 100 mmHg
   (Objective 5)

Musculoskeletal Trauma

READING ASSIGNMENT

Chapter 28, pages 652-672, in *Mosby's Paramedic Textbook,* ed. 3

OBJECTIVES

Upon completion of this chapter, the paramedic student will be able to do the following:

1. Describe the features of each class of musculoskeletal injury.
2. Describe the features of bursitis, tendonitis, and arthritis.
3. Given a specific patient scenario, outline the prehospital assessment of the musculoskeletal system.
4. Outline general principles of splinting.
5. Describe the significance and prehospital management principles for selected upper extremity injuries.
6. Describe the significance and prehospital management principles for selected lower extremity injuries.
7. Identify prehospital management priorities for open fractures.
8. Describe the principles of realignment of angular fractures and dislocations.
9. Outline the process for referral of patients with a minor musculoskeletal injury.

SUMMARY

- Injuries that can result from traumatic force on the musculoskeletal system include fractures, sprains, strains, and joint dislocations. Problems associated with musculoskeletal injuries include hemorrhage, instability, loss of tissue, simple laceration and contamination, interruption of blood supply, and long-term disability.
- Several inflammatory and degenerative conditions may manifest as or may be complicated by extremity injury. These include bursitis, tendonitis, and arthritis.
- Common signs and symptoms of extremity trauma include pain on palpation or movement, swelling or deformity, crepitus, decreased range of motion, false movement, and decreased or absent sensory perception or circulation distal to the injury.
- Once the paramedic has assessed for life-threatening conditions, the extremity injury should be examined for pain, pallor, paresthesia, pulses, paralysis, and pressure. In addition, DCAP-BTLS should be evaluated for the injured extremity.
- Immobilization by splinting helps alleviate pain; reduces tissue injury, bleeding, and contamination of an open wound; and simplifies and facilitates transport of the patient. Splints can be categorized as rigid, soft or formable, and traction splints.
- Upper extremity injuries can be classified as fractures or dislocations of the shoulder, humerus, elbow, radius and ulna, wrist, hand, and finger. Most upper extremity injuries can be adequately immobilized by application of a sling and swathe.

- Lower extremity injuries include fractures of the pelvis and fractures or dislocations of the hip, femur, knee and patella, tibia and fibula, ankle and foot, and toes.
- Most open fractures are obvious because of associated hemorrhage. However, a small puncture wound may not be initially apparent. In addition, bleeding may be minimal. Therefore the paramedic must consider any soft tissue wound in the area of a suspected fracture to be evidence of an open fracture. Open fractures are considered a true surgical emergency. This is due to the potential for infection.
- Only *one* attempt at realignment should be made. This should be done *only* if severe neurovascular compromise is present (e.g., extremely weak or absent distal pulses). Moreover, it should be done *only* after consultation with medical direction.
- The paramedic should evaluate the need for emergency department assessment versus having the patient see his or her private physician. This need is determined by the patient's condition and the mechanism of injury.

REVIEW QUESTIONS

Match the type of fracture in column II with the description in column I. Use each answer only once.

Column I

1. _____ A cancer patient sustains a fracture despite no apparent trauma.
2. _____ A fracture is incomplete, and the bone is bent.
3. _____ Bone is sticking out of a laceration.
4. _____ A runner feels increased pain in the foot and is found to have a fracture.
5. _____ A patient's arm is broken after having been twisted in an auger.
6. _____ The skin over a deformed ankle is intact.
7. _____ The fracture extends through the growth plate.
8. _____ The x-ray reveals a shattered bone.
9. _____ The fracture appears to be at a 45-degree angle across the bone.

Column II

a. Closed
b. Comminuted
c. Epiphyseal
d. Greenstick
e. Oblique
f. Open
g. Pathological
h. Spiral
i. Stress
j. Transverse

Select *all* the appropriate immobilization devices from column II that would be used to treat the fractures in column I. You may use each term *more* than once.

Column I

10. _____ Shoulder
11. _____ Humerus
12. _____ Elbow
13. _____ Forearm
14. _____ Wrist
15. _____ Hand
16. _____ Finger
17. _____ Pelvis
18. _____ Hip
19. _____ Femur
20. _____ Knee or patella
21. _____ Tibia or fibula
22. _____ Ankle or foot
23. _____ Toes

Column II

a. Buddy splint
b. Formable splint
c. Long spine board
d. Rigid splint
e. Pneumatic antishock garment
f. Sling
g. Swathe
h. Traction splint

Questions 24 to 26 pertain to the following case study:

A 16-year-old injured his wrist after falling during a hockey game.

24. What is your primary objective when performing the initial assessment on this patient?

_____

25. What are the six *P*s of assessment for this injury?

P

P

P

P

P

P

26. As you examine this patient, you inspect and palpate the extremity to identify

D

C

A

P

B

T

L

S

27. Identify at least 11 general principles of splinting.

a.

b.

c.

d.

e.

f.

g.

h.

i.

j.

k.

Questions 28 and 29 pertain to the following case study:

A 55-year-old patient has a shortened and externally rotated hip with no pedal pulse distal to the injury. You antici-pate a 45-minute transport to the nearest medical center.

28. Why is it appropriate to attempt to realign this dislocation?

_____

29. Explain the procedure for attempting to realign the hip in this situation.

_____

STUDENT SELF-ASSESSMENT

30. Which of the following is true about a sprain?
   a. It means injury to a tendon.
   b. No tissue disruption occurs, but bruising does occur.
   c. Severe hemorrhage can occur.
   d. Joint instability and dislocation may result.

31. A _subluxation_ is another name for which of the following?
   a. Complete dislocation
   b. Incomplete dislocation
   c. Open fracture
   d. Strain

32. What is the cause of the pain associated with bursitis, tendonitis, and arthritis?
   a. Aging
   b. Degeneration
   c. Infection
   d. Inflammation

33. What group of drugs is often used to treat arthritis?
   a. Antibiotics
   b. Antipyretics
   c. Muscle relaxants
   d. NSAIDs

34. Signs or symptoms of extremity trauma that have a high urgency include which of the following?
   a. Absent distal pulses
   b. Crepitus
   c. Decreased range of motion
   d. Swelling and deformity

35. Your patient has been intubated and has signs of severe shock. His right wrist is swollen and deformed, and crepitus is present. How will you manage this extremity injury during your 7-minute transport time to the hospital?
   a. Elevation and application of ice
   b. Forearm splint
   c. Long spine board
   d. Sling and swathe

36. Boxer's fracture is the most common fracture of which bone(s)?
   a. Carpals
   b. Metacarpal
   c. Phalanges
   d. Radius

37. When a patient has a dislocation of the hip, the affected leg is usually which of the following?
   a. Lengthened and externally rotated
   b. Lengthened and internally rotated
   c. Shortened and externally rotated
   d. Shortened and internally rotated

38. A traction splint may be helpful for a patient with which of the following fractures?
   a. Femoral fracture
   b. Humeral fracture
   c. Tibial fracture
   d. Pelvic fracture

39. Your patient has severe deformity of the knee and a diminished pulse in the foot on the affected leg. This may be an indication of injury to which of the following?
   a. Femoral artery
   b. Dorsalis pedis artery
   c. Popliteal artery
   d. Posterior tibial artery

40. A bone is protruding through a wound on the lower leg. When you immobilize the fracture, the bone end slips back into the wound. What action should you take?
   a. Cover the wound with a dry sterile dressing.
   b. Irrigate the wound with sterile normal saline.
   c. Move the leg gently until the bone reappears.
   d. Soak the wound with Betadine solution.

41. Your patient fell and has a grossly deformed shoulder. Which of the following is a contraindication to realignment?
   a. Absent radial pulse
   b. Paresthesias
   c. Severe pain
   d. Thoracic spine injury

42. A woman injured her ankle during a skating activity. She has refused care and transport by EMS. What should you do before leaving the scene?
   a. Administer morphine intramuscularly for the pain.
   b. Instruct her to elevate the leg and apply ice.
   c. Have her try to bear weight and walk.
   d. Tell her to see a physician if pain persists for 2 days.

WRAP IT UP

At 0230 your pager beeps you to respond to a vehicle collision in your township. You know that you are the closest volunteer, so you respond in your truck, knowing that the ambulance will be about 10 minutes behind you. Your patient is a 45-year-old nurse whom you recognize from the ED. She was heading home from her shift when she apparently dozed off and her car ran off the road, striking a tree. Major damage was done to the front of her car, and her airbags deployed. She is conscious and crying. She says the only thing she remembers is looking up, seeing the tree, and holding on to the steering wheel. As you speak with her, you unbuckle her belt. Her skin is pink and warm, and her heart rate is increased. She tells you she thinks she has broken her arms and legs. She denies any other pain or difficulty breathing. She has bilaterally equal breath sounds and no obvious chest or abdominal trauma. Her wrists are both tender and deformed but have good pulses. Her right femur is swollen and very tender; her left lower leg is deformed, and a laceration is slowly oozing blood over the painful area. She has good sensation and movement distal to all her extremity injuries. You and another volunteer administer oxygen, assess her vital signs (BP, 110/70 mm Hg; P, 124/min; R, 20/min), initiate an IV of normal saline in the left antecubital space, and splint her left lower leg. As the ambulance arrives, she vomits and says she is feeling faint. A repeat set of vital signs shows BP, 106/70 mm Hg; P, 128/min; and R, 20/min. Even though the patient denies neck pain or tenderness, a collar is applied and she is rapidly extricated to the long spine board. A traction splint is applied to her right leg, and she is secured to the stretcher and moved to the ambulance. Under the guidance of medical direction, IV morphine is given in 2 mg doses to relieve her pain. Her forearms are splinted and elevated on pillows, and ice is applied to all injured extremities. Continuous monitoring of vital signs and extremity pulses, movement, and sensation shows no change during transport. After a total of 6 mg of morphine, the patient reports that the pain has dulled from a "10" to a "7," so you give an additional 2 mg, knowing that the movement on arrival at the ED will be painful. You apply a sterile 4 × 4 gauze to the wound on her left lower leg. You note fat globules in the oozing dark blood.

On your next trip to the hospital, you visit the patient. She will miss at least 3 months of work because of her multiple fractures. She thanks you repeatedly for giving her the pain medicine; she says her attitude toward patients who are in pain has been changed forever.

1. List six things you should assess each time you think a patient has fractured an extremity.

_____

2. Describe how you would have changed your treatment if you suspected a fracture in her lower right leg as well.

_____

3. Identify which splint (or splints) would be appropriate for each of the patient's injuries on this call.
   a. Sling and swathe   **d.** Traction splint
   b. Rigid splint   **e.** Pillow splint
   c. Formable splint
   _____ Right and left upper extremity injuries
   _____ Right upper leg injury
   _____ Left lower leg injury

4. Explain the principles that should be followed in applying the splints to both arms and the left lower leg.

_____

5. What was the significance of the wound over the patient's painful leg deformity?
   a. It could greatly increase the risk of blood loss.
   b. It could signify an open fracture, which poses a high risk of infection.
   c. Unless bone can be seen sticking out, it is not significant.
   d. Unless the bleeding is uncontrolled, the wound should not be covered.

6. Explain the rationale for administering oxygen and initiating an IV in this patient.

CHAPTER 28 ANSWERS

REVIEW QUESTIONS

1. g
2. d
3. f
4. i
5. h
6. a
7. c
8. b
9. e
   (Questions 1-9: Objective 1)

10. f and g
11. b, d, f, and g
12. b, d, f, and g
13. b, d, and f
14. b, d, and f
15. b and d
16. a, b, and d
    (Questions 10-16: Objective 5)

17. c and e
18. c
19. c and h
20. b and d
21. b and d
22. b
23. a
    (Questions 17-23: Objective 6)

24. With every patient you must assess for the presence of life threats in the initial assessment.
    (Objective 3)

25. The six *P*s are pain, pallor, paresthesia, pulses, paralysis, and pressure.
    (Objective 3)

26. The initials *DCAP-BTLS* refer to deformity, contusions, abrasions, penetrations or punctures, burns, tenderness, lacerations, and swelling.
    (Objective 3)

27. The general principles of splinting are: splint joints above and below, as well as bone ends; immobilize open and closed fractures in the same manner; cover open fractures to minimize contamination; check pulses, sensation, and motor function before and after splinting; stabilize the extremity with gentle, in-line traction to the position of normal alignment; immobilize a long bone extremity in a straight position that can easily be splinted; immobilize dislocations in a position of comfort; ensure good vascular supply; immobilize joints as found; joint injuries are aligned only if no distal pulse is detected; apply cold to reduce swelling and pain; apply compression to reduce swelling; and elevate the extremity if possible.
    (Objective 4)

28. No pulse is present distal to the injury; this is an indication to attempt realignment in the prehospital setting.
    (Objective 8)

29. Administer an analgesic and/or benzodiazepine (with appropriate monitoring) if not contraindicated by other injuries. Apply in-line traction along the shaft of the femur with the hip and knee flexed at 90 degrees. Apply slow and steady traction to relax the muscle spasm. Listen for a "pop," with accompanying sudden relief of pain and easy manipulation of the leg to full extension. Immobilize the leg in full extension with the patient supine on a long spine board; reevaluate pulses and neurovascular status. If attempt is unsuccessful, place the patient supine and use pillows or blankets to immobilize the leg at a flexion not exceeding 90 degrees.
(Objective 8)

STUDENT SELF-ASSESSMENT

30. d. Sprains represent injuries to ligaments.
(Objective 1)

31. b. A complete dislocation is a *luxation*.
(Objective 1)

32. d. Bursitis involves inflammation of the bursa; tendonitis is inflammation of a tendon caused by injury; and arthritis is inflammation of the joint.
(Objective 2)

33. d. The traditional drugs in this group cause gastrointestinal complications and are being replaced by newer agents with fewer side effects.
(Objective 2)

34. a. Treatment is needed for all the other signs; however, emergent interventions are needed to preserve the limb when distal pulses are absent.
(Objective 3)

35. c. Because of the life threats present in this patient, time would not be taken to treat this isolated injury except to provide full-body immobilization on a spine board.
(Objective 3)

36. b. The fifth metacarpal is broken in a boxer's fracture.
(Objective 5)

37. d. After a hip fracture, the extremity is usually shortened and externally rotated.
(Objective 6)

38. a. It is not indicated for other types of fractures.
(Objective 6)

39. c. Injury to the popliteal artery is associated with knee trauma.
(Objective 6)

40. a. Make sure that this is reported to the receiving medical personnel and documented in the patient care report. Assess distal pulse and sensation.
(Objective 7)

41. d. The movement necessary to realign the arm could cause further injury to the back.
(Objective 8)

42. b. Instructions about care of the injury should be given to the patient (preferably in writing) before you depart.
(Objective 9)

WRAP IT UP

1. Assess for pain, tenderness, deformity, swelling, crepitus, any soft tissue wounds in the area of a suspected fracture, as well as distal pulses, sensation, and movement before and after splinting
(Objective 3)

2. A traction splint would not have been appropriate if the lower leg also had been fractured. The patient could have been splinted on the spine board, using blankets or pillows to stabilize the extremity or perhaps long board splints.
(Objective 4)

3. Upper extremity injuries: b or c. Although a sling may be helpful for immobilizing and elevating the splinted isolated upper extremity, in this case, because the patient was supine on the spine board, it wouldn't have been indicated.
(Objectives 4, 5)

   Right upper leg injury: d
   (Objectives 4, 6)

   Left lower leg injury: b or c
   (Objectives 4, 6)

4. The distal pulse, movement, and sensation should be assessed before and after splinting. The splint should be applied to include the joints above and below the injury and should be secured firmly. The extremity should be elevated if possible and ice applied.
(Objective 4)

5. b. Although significant open fractures pose an increased risk of bleeding, the chief concern is infection of the bone, which is very difficult and time-consuming to treat.
(Objective 7)

6. Aside from the potential for chest and abdominal injuries based on the mechanism of injury, there is significant risk of internal bleeding from long bone fractures. This is particularly true for the femur and secondarily for the tibia and fibula.
(Objective 3)

PART SEVEN

IN THIS PART

CHAPTER

29

Cardiology

READING ASSIGNMENT

Chapter 29, pages 673-815, in *Mosby's Paramedic Textbook,* ed. 3

OBJECTIVES

Upon completion of this chapter, the paramedic student will be able to do the following:
1. Identify risk factors and prevention strategies associated with cardiovascular disease.
2. Describe the normal physiology of the heart.
3. Discuss electrophysiology as it relates to the normal electrical and mechanical events in the cardiac cycle.
4. Outline the activity of each component of the electrical conduction system of the heart.
5. Outline the appropriate assessment of a patient who may be experiencing a cardiovascular disorder.
6. Describe basic monitoring techniques that permit electrocardiogram interpretation.
7. Explain the relationship of the electrocardiogram tracing to the electrical activity of the heart.
8. Describe in sequence the steps in electrocardiogram interpretation.
9. Identify the characteristics of normal sinus rhythm.
10. When shown an electrocardiogram tracing, identify the rhythm, site of origin, possible causes, clinical significance, and prehospital management that is indicated.
11. Describe prehospital assessment and management of patients with selected cardiovascular disorders based on knowledge of the pathophysiology of the illness.
12. List indications, contraindications, and prehospital considerations when using selected cardiac interventions, including basic life support, monitor-defibrillators, defibrillation, implantable cardioverter defibrillators, synchronized cardioversion, and transcutaneous cardiac pacing.
13. List indications, contraindications, dose, and mechanism of action for pharmacological agents used to manage cardiovascular disorders.
14. Identify appropriate actions to take in the prehospital setting to terminate resuscitation.

SUMMARY

- Persons at high risk for cardiovascular disease include those with diabetes, a family history of premature cardiovascular disease, and prior myocardial infarction. Prevention strategies include community educational programs in nutrition, cessation of smoking (smoking prevention for children), and screening for hypertension and high cholesterol.
- The left coronary artery carries about 85% of the blood supply to the myocardium. The right coronary artery carries the rest. The pumping action of the heart is a product of rhythmic, alternate contraction and relaxation of the atria and ventricles. The stroke volume is the amount of blood ejected from each ventricle with one contraction. Stroke volume depends on preload, afterload, and myocardial contractility. Cardiac output is the amount of blood pumped by each ventricle per minute.

- In addition to the intrinsic control of the body in regulating the heart, extrinsic control by the parasympathetic and sympathetic nerves of the autonomic nervous system is a major factor influencing the heart rate, conductivity, and contractility. Sympathetic impulses cause the adrenal medulla to secrete epinephrine and norepinephrine into the blood.
- The major electrolytes that influence cardiac function are calcium, potassium, sodium, and magnesium. The electrical charge (potential difference) between the inside and outside of cells is expressed in millivolts. When the cell is in a resting state, the electrical charge difference is referred to as a resting membrane potential. The specialized sodium-potassium exchange pump actively pumps sodium ions out of the cell. It also pumps potassium ions into the cell. The cell membrane appears to have individual protein-lined channels. These channels allow for passage of a specific ion or group of ions.
- Nerve and muscle cells are capable of producing action potentials. This property is known as *excitability*. An action potential at any point on the cell membrane stimulates an excitation process. This process is spread down the length of the cell and is conducted across synapses from cell to cell.
- The contraction of cardiac and skeletal muscle is believed to be activated by calcium ions. This results in a binding between myosin and actin myofilaments.
- The conduction system of the heart is composed of two nodes and a conducting bundle. One of the nodes is the sinoatrial node. The other is the atrioventricular node.
- Common chief complaints of the patient with cardiovascular disease include chest pain or discomfort, including shoulder, arm, neck, or jaw pain or discomfort; dyspnea; syncope; and abnormal heartbeat or palpitations. Paramedics should ask patients suspected of having a cardiovascular disorder whether they take prescription medications, especially cardiac drugs. Paramedics should ask whether patients are being treated for any serious illness as well. They also should ask whether patients have a history of myocardial infarction, angina, heart failure, hypertension, diabetes, or chronic lung disease. In addition, paramedics should ask whether patients have any allergies or have other risk factors for heart disease.
- After performing the initial assessment of the patient with cardiovascular disease, the paramedic should look for skin color, jugular venous distention, and the presence of edema or other signs of heart disease. The paramedic should listen for lung sounds, heart sounds, and carotid artery bruit. The paramedic should feel for edema, pulses, skin temperature, and moisture.
- The electrocardiogram represents the electrical activity of the heart. The electrocardiogram is generated by depolarization and repolarization of the atria and ventricles.
- Routine monitoring of cardiac rhythm in the prehospital setting usually is obtained in lead II or MCL_1. These are the best leads to monitor for dysrhythmias because they allow visualization of P waves. A 12-lead electrocardiogram can be used to help identify changes relative to myocardial ischemia, injury, and infarction; distinguish ventricular tachycardia from supraventricular tachycardia; determine the electrical axis and the presence of fascicular blocks; and determine the presence of bundle branch blocks.
- The paper used to record electrocardiograms is standardized. This allows comparative analysis of an electrocardiogram wave.
- The normal electrocardiogram consists of a P wave, QRS complex, and T wave. The P wave is the first positive deflection on the electrocardiogram. The P wave represents atrial depolarization. The P-R interval is the time it takes for an electrical impulse to be conducted through the atria and the atrioventricular node up to the instant of ventricular depolarization. The QRS complex represents ventricular depolarization. The ST segment represents the early part of repolarization of the right and left ventricles. The T wave represents repolarization of the ventricular myocardial cells. Repolarization occurs during the last part of ventricular systole. The Q-T interval is the period from the beginning of ventricular depolarization (onset of the QRS complex) until the end of ventricular repolarization or the end of the T wave.
- The steps in electrocardiogram analysis include analyzing the QRS complex, P waves, rate, rhythm, and P-R interval.
- Dysrhythmias originating in the sinoatrial node include sinus bradycardia, sinus tachycardia, sinus dysrhythmia, and sinus arrest. Most sinus dysrhythmias are the result of increases or decreases in vagal tone.
- Dysrhythmias originating in the atria include wandering pacemaker, premature atrial complexes, paroxysmal supraventricular tachycardia, atrial flutter, and atrial fibrillation. Common causes of atrial dysrhythmias are ischemia, hypoxia, and atrial dilation caused by congestive heart failure or mitral valve abnormalities.
- When the sinoatrial node and the atria cannot generate the electrical impulses needed to begin depolarization because of factors such as hypoxia, ischemia, myocardial infarction, and drug toxicity, the atrioventricular node or the area surrounding the atrioventricular node may assume the role of the secondary pacemaker. Dysrhythmias

originating in the atrioventricular junction include premature junctional contractions, junctional escape complexes or rhythms, and accelerated junctional rhythm.

- Ventricular dysrhythmias pose a threat to life. Ventricular rhythm disturbances generally result from failure of the atria, atrioventricular junction, or both to initiate an electrical impulse. They also may result from enhanced automaticity or reentry phenomena in the ventricles. Dysrhythmias originating in the ventricles include ventricular escape complexes or rhythms, premature ventricular complexes, ventricular tachycardia, ventricular fibrillation, asystole, and artificial pacemaker rhythm.
- Partial delays or full interruptions in cardiac electrical conduction are called *heart blocks*. Causes of heart blocks include atrioventricular junctional ischemia, atrioventricular junctional necrosis, degenerative disease of the conduction system, and drug toxicity. Dysrhythmias that are disorders of conduction are first-degree atrioventricular block, type I second-degree atrioventricular block (Wenckebach), type II second-degree atrioventricular block, third-degree atrioventricular block, disturbances of ventricular conduction, pulseless electrical activity, and preexcitation (Wolff-Parkinson-White) syndrome.
- Atherosclerosis is a disease process characterized by progressive narrowing of the lumen of medium and large arteries. Atherosclerosis has two major effects on blood vessels. First, the disease disrupts the intimal surface. This causes a loss of vessel elasticity and an increase in thrombogenesis. Second, the atheroma reduces the diameter of the vessel lumen. Thus this decreases the blood supply to tissues.
- Angina pectoris is a symptom of myocardial ischemia. Angina is caused by an imbalance between myocardial oxygen supply and demand. Prehospital management includes placing the patient at rest, administering oxygen, initiating intravenous therapy, administering nitroglycerin and possibly morphine, monitoring the patient for dysrhythmias, and transporting the patient for physician evaluation.
- Acute myocardial infarction occurs when a coronary artery is blocked and blood does not reach an area of heart muscle. This results in ischemia, injury, and necrosis to the area of myocardium supplied by the affected artery. Death caused by myocardial infarction usually results from lethal dysrhythmias (ventricular tachycardia, ventricular fibrillation, and cardiac standstill), pump failure (cardiogenic shock and congestive heart failure), or myocardial tissue rupture (rupture of the ventricle, septum, or papillary muscle). Some patients with acute myocardial infarction, particularly those in the older age groups, have only symptoms of dyspnea, syncope, or confusion. However, substernal chest pain is usually present in patients with acute myocardial infarction (70% to 90% of patients). ST segment elevation greater than or equal to 1 mV in at least two side-by-side electrocardiogram leads indicates an acute myocardial infarction. However, some patients infarct without ST segment elevation changes. Other conditions also can produce ST segment elevation. Prehospital management of the patient with a suspected myocardial infarction should include placing the patient at rest; administering oxygen at 4 L per minute via nasal cannula; frequently assessing vital signs and breath sounds; initiating an intravenous line with normal saline or lactated Ringer's solution to keep the vein open; monitoring for dysrhythmias; administering medications such as nitroglycerin, morphine, and aspirin; and screening for risk factors for fibrinolytic therapy.
- Left ventricular failure occurs when the left ventricle fails to function as an effective forward pump. This causes a back-pressure of blood into the pulmonary circulation. This in turn may lead to pulmonary edema. Emergency management is directed at decreasing the venous return to the heart, improving myocardial contractility, decreasing myocardial oxygen demand, improving ventilation and oxygenation, and rapidly transporting the patient to a medical facility.
- Right ventricular failure occurs when the right ventricle fails as a pump. This causes back-pressure of blood into the systemic venous circulation. Right ventricular failure is not usually a medical emergency in itself; that is, unless it is associated with pulmonary edema or hypotension.
- Cardiogenic shock is the most extreme form of pump failure. It usually is caused by extensive myocardial infarction. Even with aggressive therapy, cardiogenic shock has a mortality rate of 70% or higher. Patients in cardiogenic shock need rapid transport to a medical facility.
- *Cardiac tamponade* is defined as impaired filling of the heart caused by increased pressure in the pericardial sac.
- Abdominal aortic aneurysms are usually asymptomatic. However, signs and symptoms will signal impending or active rupture. If the vessel tears, bleeding initially may be stopped by the retroperitoneal tissues. The patient may be normotensive on the arrival of emergency medical services. If the rupture opens into the peritoneal cavity, however, massive fatal hemorrhage may follow.
- Acute dissection is the most common aortic catastrophe. Any area of the aorta may be involved. However, in 60% to 70% of cases the site of a dissecting aneurysm is in the ascending aorta, just beyond the takeoff of the left subclavian artery. The signs and symptoms depend on the site of the intimal tear. They also depend on the extent of

dissection. The goals of managing suspected aortic dissection in the prehospital setting are relief of pain and immediate transport to a medical facility.

- Acute arterial occlusion is a sudden blockage of arterial flow. Occlusion most commonly is caused by trauma, an embolus, or thrombosis. The most common sites of embolic occlusion are the abdominal aorta, common femoral artery, popliteal artery, carotid artery, brachial artery, and mesenteric artery. The location of ischemic pain is related to the site of occlusion.
- Noncritical peripheral vascular conditions include varicose veins, superficial thrombophlebitis, and acute deep vein thrombosis. Of these conditions, deep vein thrombosis is the only one that can cause a life-threatening problem. This problem is pulmonary embolus.
- Hypertension often is defined by a resting blood pressure that is consistently greater than 140/90 mm Hg. Chronic hypertension has an adverse effect on the heart and blood vessels. It requires the heart to perform more work than normal. This leads to hypertrophy of the cardiac muscle and left ventricular failure. Conditions associated with chronic, uncontrolled hypertension are cerebral hemorrhage and stroke, myocardial infarction, and renal failure.
- Hypertensive emergencies are conditions in which a blood pressure increase leads to significant, irreversible end-organ damage within hours if not treated. The organs most likely to be at risk are the brain, heart, and kidneys. As a rule, the diagnosis is based on altered end-organ function and the rate of the rise in blood pressure, not on the level of blood pressure.
- Basic cardiac life support helps to maintain the circulation and respiration of a victim of cardiac arrest. Basic life support is continued until advanced cardiac life support is available. Two mechanisms are thought to be responsible for blood flow during cardiopulmonary resuscitation. One is direct compression of the heart between the sternum and the spine. This increases pressure within the ventricles to provide a small, but critical amount of blood flow to the lungs and body organs. The second one is increased intrathoracic pressure transmitted to all intrathoracic vascular structures. This creates an intrathoracic-to-extrathoracic pressure gradient. This gradient causes blood to flow out of the thorax. A number of mechanical devices provide external chest compression. Others provide chest compression with ventilation in the cardiac arrest patient.
- Cardiac monitor-defibrillators are classified as manual or automated external defibrillators. Defibrillation is the delivery of electrical current through the chest wall. Its purpose is to terminate ventricular fibrillation and certain other nonperfusing rhythms.
- Implantable cardioverter defibrillators work by monitoring the patient's cardiac rhythm. When a monitored ventricular rate exceeds the preprogrammed rate, the implantable cardioverter defibrillator delivers a shock of about 6 to 30 J through the patches. This is an attempt to restore a normal sinus rhythm.
- Synchronized cardioversion is designed to deliver a shock about 10 milliseconds after the peak of the R wave of the cardiac cycle. (Thus the device avoids the relative refractory period.) Synchronization may reduce the amount of energy needed to end the dysrhythmia. It also may decrease the chances of causing another dysrhythmia.
- Transcutaneous cardiac pacing is an effective emergency therapy for bradycardia, complete heart block, and suppression of some malignant ventricular dysrhythmias. Proper electrode placement is important for effective external pacing.
- What is becoming more and more evident is that patients who cannot be resuscitated in the prehospital setting rarely survive. This is the case even if they are resuscitated temporarily in the emergency department. Cessation of resuscitative efforts in the prehospital setting should follow system-specific criteria established by medical direction

REVIEW QUESTIONS

Match each term in Column II with its definition in Column I. Use each answer only once.

Column I

1. _c_ Heart rate × stroke volume
2. _f_ Volume available for ventricles to pump each contraction
3. _a_ Peripheral vascular resistance produces this pressure
4. _e_ Ventricular relaxation
5. _b_ Cardiac output × peripheral vascular resistance
6. _g_ Increased myocardial contractility in response to increased preload
7. _h_ Ventricular ejection per heartbeat

Column II

a. Afterload
b. Blood pressure
c. Cardiac output
d. Contractility
e. Diastole
f. Preload
g. Starling's law
h. Stroke volume
i. Systole

8. Identify a prevention strategy for each of the following risk factors for cardiovascular disease and a community resource where you can refer the patient to assist with modification of this risk factor.

Risk Factor	Prevention Strategy	Resource
a. Smoking		
b. Hypercholesterolemia		
c. Obesity		
d. Sedentary lifestyle		

9. Explain how the sympathetic and parasympathetic divisions of the autonomic nervous system influence cardiac function in the following areas.

	Sympathetic	Parasympathetic
a. Heart rate		
b. Myocardial contractility		
c. Lungs		
d. Blood vessels (peripheral)		

10. Name the two adrenal hormones and describe the effects of each on the cardiovascular system.

	Name	Function
a.		
b.		

11. Fill in the blanks in the following sentences about electrophysiology: Within the body, separated charged particles with opposite charges have a (a) _____ force of attraction that gives them (b) _____ energy. This energy is released when the cell membrane becomes (c) _____ to the charged particles and allows the charges to come together. The electrical charge between the inside and outside of cells is the (d) _____ difference and is measured in (e) _____. Although there is a relatively equal number of positively and negatively charged ions inside and outside the cell, the intracellular area has a (f) _____ charge because of the (g) _____ charged proteins that cannot move outside the cell. The electrical charge difference in the resting state has the potential to do work and is known as the resting membrane (h) _____ (RMP). During this phase, the inside of the cell is electrically (i) _____ relative to the outside of the cell (approximately [j] _____mV). The RMP results primarily from the difference between the intracellular and extracellular (k) _____ion level.

Because of the chemical gradient (more of these ions inside than outside of the cell), the (l) _____ would move out of the cell in an attempt to achieve equilibrium. However, these ions remain in the cell because of the negtive intracellular charge generated by the (m). _____ In the RMP, sodium will not rush into the cell because the cell membrane is not (n) _____ to sodium. The ability of nerve and muscle cells to produce action potentials is known as (o) _____. If this action potential results in a decreased charge difference across the cell membrane, the RMP becomes less negative, and this is called (p) _____. If a stimulus is strong enough to cause depolarization of a cell membrane to a level called the (q) _____, a chain reaction of permeability changes cause an (r) _____ to spread over the entire cell membrane. Action potentials have two phases: a (s) _____ phase and a

(t) _____ phase. During an action potential, the sodium ions rush into the cell, and RMP becomes

(u) _____ on the inside and (v) _____ on the outside of the cell membrane. This occurs

during the (w) _____ phase. The repolarization phase results from potassium leakage outside the

cell and the return of the cell membrane to its normal resting (x) _____ state.

12. Answer the following questions regarding the five phases of the cardiac action potential:

a. During phase 0 (rapid depolarization), what causes the inside of the cell to become positive?

_____

b. What is the membrane potential during phase 1 (early rapid repolarization)?

_____

c. How is the membrane potential held at 0 during phase 2 (plateau phase)?

_____

d. What happens to the membrane potential of the cell during phase 3 (terminal phase of rapid repolarization)?

_____

e. How is the balance of sodium and potassium restored during phase 4?

_____

f. Why can cardiac pacemaker cells depolarize without an external stimulus to initiate an action potential?

INTRODUCTION TO ELECTROCARDIOGRAM MONITORING

13. Circle the correct response in each of the following statements:

The electrocardiogram tracing represents an amplified view of the myocardial (a) action potentials/contractions. If the voltage displayed is positive, the electrocardiogram tracing will display a(n) (b) upward/downward/isoelectric deflection. Cardiac pacemaker cells spontaneously can generate impulses, a property known as (c) automaticity/conductivity. This rhythmic activity occurs because these cells do not have a stable (d) action potential/resting membrane potential.

14. Label Fig. 29-1 illustrating the cardiac conduction system.

A.

B.

C.

D.

E.

F.

G.

H.

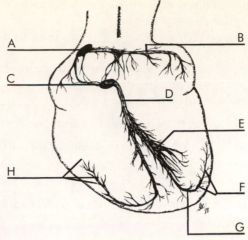

Figure 29-1

15. The sinoatrial node is the dominant pacemaker. If it fails to fire, what will happen?

_____

16. Briefly describe the mechanism for ectopic impulse formation by each of the following mechanisms:

a. Enhanced automaticity:

_____

b. Reentry:

_____

ASSESSMENT OF THE PATIENT WITH CARDIAC DISEASE

17. A 62-year-old woman complains of chest pain. What questions should you ask using the OPQRST mnemonic to determine the nature and severity of her pain?

O

P

Q

R

S

T

18. List three chief complaints that may lead you to believe a patient has a cardiovascular problem.

a.

b.

c.

19. An older man experiences a syncopal episode at a local gym. List at least two questions you should ask in an attempt to determine the nature of his syncopal episode.

a.

b.

20. A 34-year-old woman walks into your ambulance base complaining of a fluttering sensation in her chest. What will your history and physical examination include to determine the cause of this sensation?

_____

_____

Questions 21 to 23 pertain to the following case study:

An 87-year-old woman calls you to her home and complains of weakness and nausea. On arrival, you find her seated on the commode. She is pale, cool, and diaphoretic. Her blood pressure is 70 mm Hg by palpation, and her electrocardiogram is shown in Fig. 29-2.

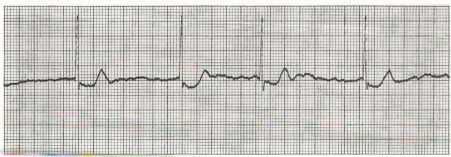

Figure 29-2

21. What information from this patient's medical history will be important to elicit at this time?

_____

22. What is your interpretation of her electrocardiogram?

_____

23. She tells you that she is taking digoxin, diltiazem, potassium, and furosemide. Could any of her home medicines be playing a role in her problem? If yes, which ones and why?

_____

_____

24. An older man is found unresponsive and bradycardic in a local park. A caretaker states that he complained of chest pain before collapsing. No one is available to give you any information regarding his history. Briefly outline specific findings you may encounter in your patient assessment if he has a history of cardiac problems.

_____

_____

ELECTROCARDIOGRAM MONITORING

25. Place the positive (+) and negative (−) and electrodes for the four leads shown in Fig. 29-3.

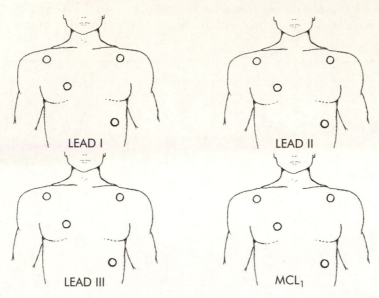

Figure 29-3

26. Describe the location of each of the 10 electrodes needed to record a 12-lead electrocardiogram.

a.   f.

b.   g.

c.   h.

d.   i.

e.   j.

27. List six problems that may interfere with a clear electrocardiogram recording. For each problem, discuss a possible solution.

a.   d.

b.   e.

c.   f.

28. Label Fig. 29-4 with the appropriate measurement intervals

a. _____ mm

b. _____ second

c. _____ second

d. _____ second

e. _____ second

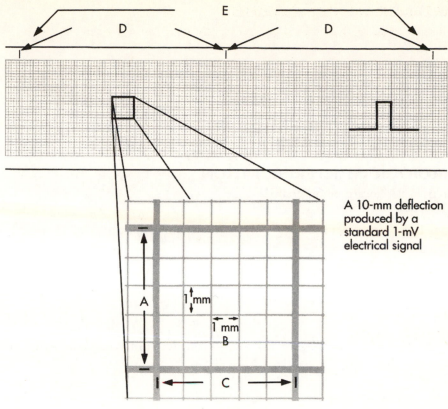

Figure 29-4

29. Label the sample electrocardiogram tracing in Fig. 29-5.

a. P WAVE

b. QRS

c.

d.

e.

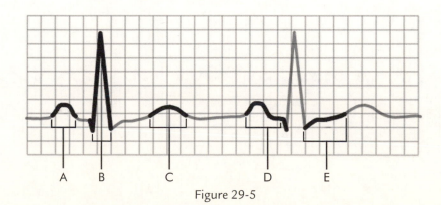

Figure 29-5

30. List five causes of artifact.

a.

b.

c.

d.

e.

ELECTROCARDIOGRAM INTERPRETATION

31. List the five steps in electrocardiogram analysis.

a.

b.

c.

d.

e.

32. Calculate the rate of the electrocardiogram in Fig. 29-6 using four different methods, describing the steps you use in each method.

a. _____

_____

b. _____

_____

c. _____

_____

d. _____

_____

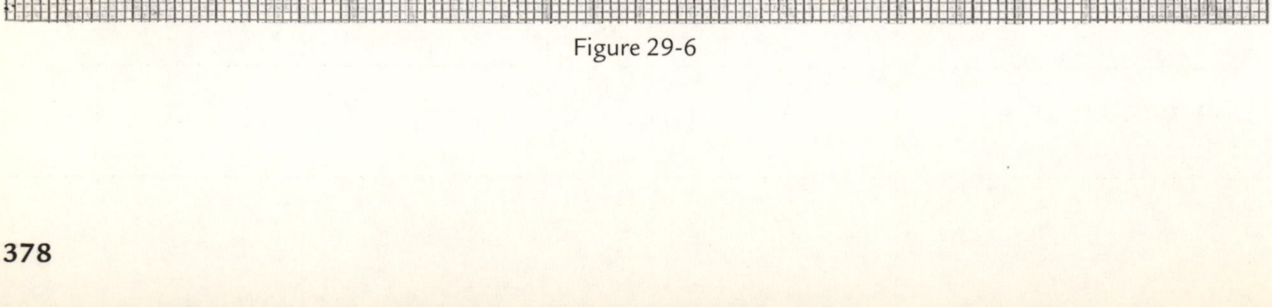

Figure 29-6

33. If the rate in question 32 is within normal limits, can we assume the patient is stable in this situation?

_____

34. Which method of calculation would be *most* accurate if the rhythm in question 32 was

   a. Regular?

_____

   b. Irregularly irregular?

_____

35. What criterion must be met when analyzing the electrocardiogram rhythm to determine that the rhythm is regular?

_____

36. What analysis can be made about conduction in each of the following examples?

   a. The QRS complex width is less than or equal to 0.12 second.

_____

   b. The QRS complex width is greater than 0.12 second.

_____

37. List the four criteria that must be evaluated when analyzing the P waves.

   a.

   b.

   c.

   d.

38. Briefly describe the significance of each of the following P-R interval findings.

   a. P-R interval 0.08 second:

_____

   b. P-R interval 0.16 second:

_____

_____

   c. P-R interval 0.24 second:

_____

39. Analyze the electrocardiogram rhythm strip in Fig. 29-7 using the five steps described in question 31, and give your interpretation.

   a. Step 1:

_____

   b. Step 2:

_____

c. Step 3:

_____

d. Step 4:

_____

e. Step 5:

_____

Interpretation:

_____

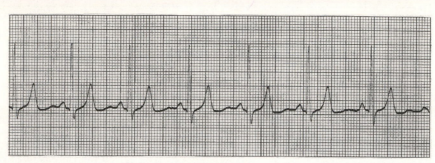

Figure 29-7

INTRODUCTION TO DYSRHYTHMIAS

40. When a dysrhythmia is noted on the monitor, what factors must be considered to determine whether any intervention is necessary?

_____

41. Dysrhythmias originating in the sinoatrial node frequently result from increases or decreases in

a. _____. Electrocardiogram features common to all sinoatrial node dysrhythmias are

b. QRS complex.

_____

c. P waves (lead II).

_____

d. P-R interval.

_____

42. List two causes of each bradycardic and tachycardic dysrhythmia that originates in the sinus node.

a. Sinus bradycardia:

_____

b. Sinus tachycardia:

_____

Complete the missing information on Flashcards 1 to 4 at the end of the text.

43. Complete Flashcard 1 (Fig. 29-8): sinus bradycardia.

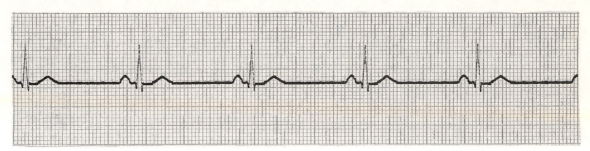

Figure 29-8

44. Complete Flashcard 2 (Fig. 29-9): sinus tachycardia.

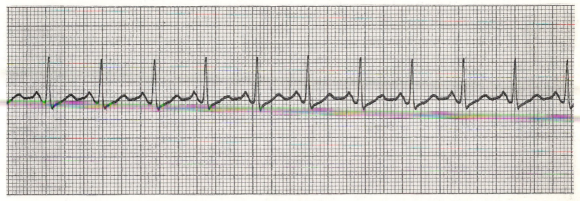

Figure 29-9

45. Complete Flashcard 3 (Fig. 29-10): sinus dysrhythmia.

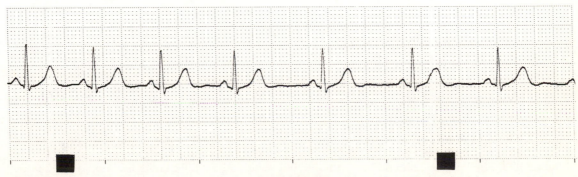

Figure 29-10

46. Complete Flashcard 4 (Fig. 29-11): sinus arrest.

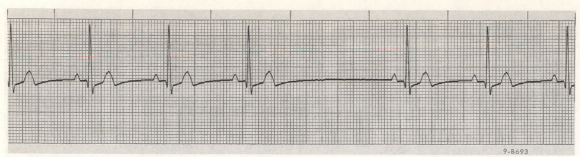

Figure 29-11

47. Atrial dysrhythmias originate in the (a) _____ of the (b) _____ or in the (c) _____ pathways.

48. Common features of atrial dysrhythmias are

    a. QRS complex.

_____

    b. P waves (if present).

_____

    c. P-R intervals.

_____

49. List four causes of dysrhythmias that originate in the atria.

    a.

    b.

    c.

    d.

Complete the missing information on Flashcards 5 to 9 showing dysrhythmias originating in the atria.

50. Complete Flashcard 5 (Fig. 29-12): wandering atrial pacemaker.

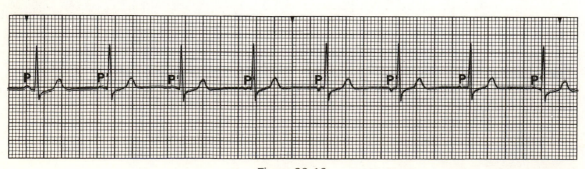

Figure 29-12

51. Complete Flashcard 6 (Fig. 29-13): premature atrial contraction.

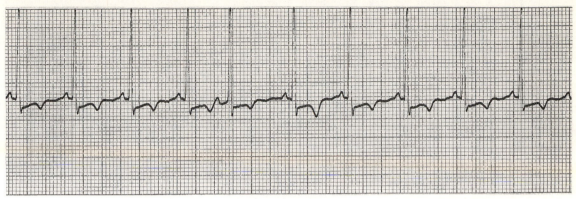

Figure 29-13

52. Complete Flashcard 7 (Fig. 29-14): supraventricular tachycardia.

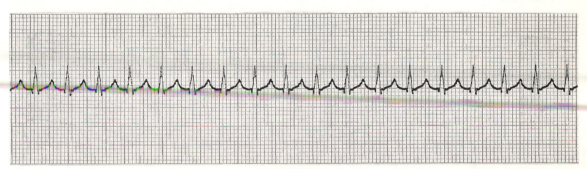

Figure 29-14

53. Complete Flashcard 8 (Fig. 29-15): atrial flutter with 3:1 conduction.

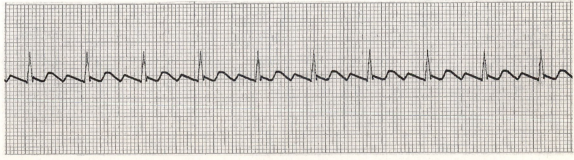

Figure 29-15

54. Complete Flashcard 9 (Fig. 29-16): atrial fibrillation.

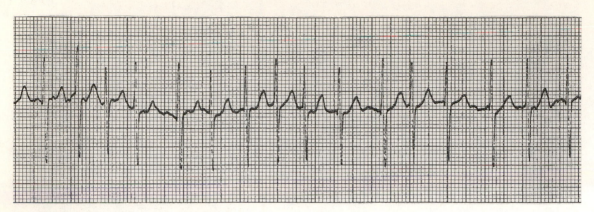

Figure 29-16

55. Rhythms that start in the atrioventricular node or junction are called (a) _____ rhythms. These rhythms share the following common features:

b. QRS complex:

_____

c. P waves:

_____

d. P-R interval:

_____

56. List four causes of dysrhythmias that start in the atrioventricular junction.

a.

b.

c.

d.

Complete the missing information on Flashcards 10 to 12 showing dysrhythmias originating in the atrioventricular junction.

57. Complete Flashcard 10 (Fig. 29-17): sinus rhythm (borderline bradycardia) with two premature junctional contractions.

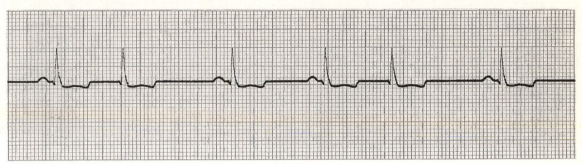

Figure 29-17

58. Complete Flashcard 11 (Fig. 29-18): junctional escape rhythm.

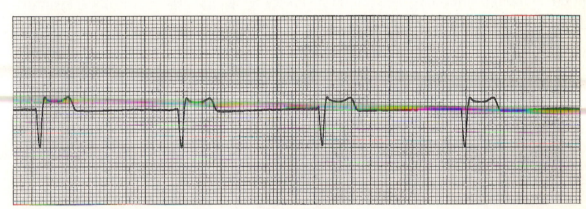

Figure 29-18

59. Complete Flashcard 12 (Fig. 29-19): accelerated junctional rhythm.

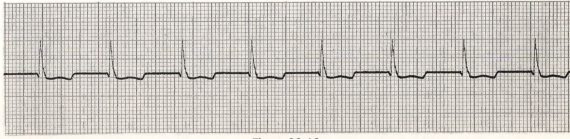

Figure 29-19

60. Rhythms originating from the ventricle have an intrinsic rate of (a) _____ to _____ but can be accelerated at rates up to (b) _____ or tachycardic at rates greater than (c)_____.

61. List five causes of dysrhythmias that originate in the ventricles.

a.

b.

c.

d.

e.

62. Identify five steps that can be used when evaluating a 12-lead electrocardiogram to distinguish between wide-complex tachycardias of ventricular versus supraventricular origin.

a.

b.

c.

d.

e.

Complete the missing information on Flashcards 13 to 18 showing dysrhythmias originating in the ventricles.

63. Complete Flashcard 13 (Fig. 29-20): ventricular escape rhythm.

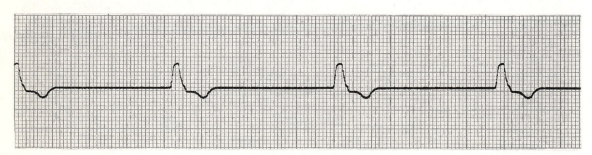

Figure 29-20

64. Complete Flashcard 14 (Fig. 29-21): normal sinus rhythm with one premature ventricular contraction.

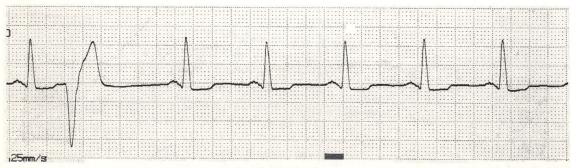

Figure 29-21

65. Complete Flashcard 15 (Fig. 29-22): monomorphic ventricular tachycardia.

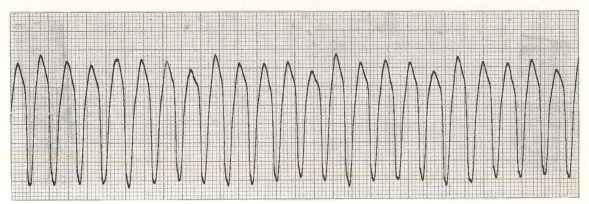

Figure 29-22

66. Complete Flashcard 16 (Fig. 29-23): ventricular fibrillation.

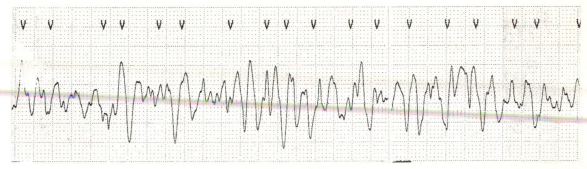

Figure 29-23

67. Complete Flashcard 17 (Fig. 29-24): asystole.

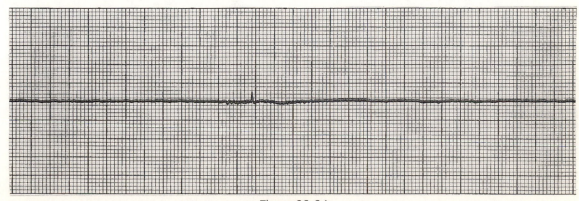

Figure 29-24

68. Complete Flashcard 18 (Fig. 29-25): ventricular paced rhythm.

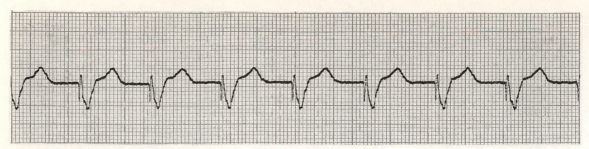

Figure 29-25

69. Delays or interruptions in cardiac electrical conduction are called (a) _____. They may be caused by disease of the (b) _____.

70. List five causes of dysrhythmias caused by delays in cardiac electrical conduction.

a.

b.

c.

d.

e.

Complete the missing information on Flashcards 19 to 22 showing dysrhythmias originating from conduction disorders.

71. Complete Flashcard 19 (Fig. 29-26): sinus rhythm with first-degree atrioventricular block.

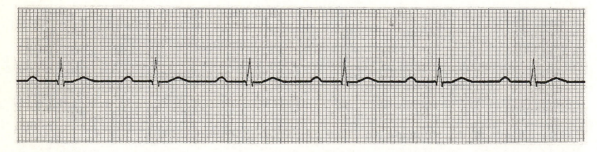

Figure 29-26

72. Complete Flashcard 20 (Fig. 29-27): second-degree atrioventricular block (Mobitz type I or Wenckebach).

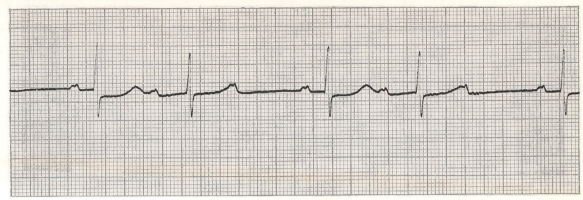

Figure 29-27

73. Complete Flashcard 21 (Fig. 29-28): second-degree atrioventricular block (Mobitz type II).

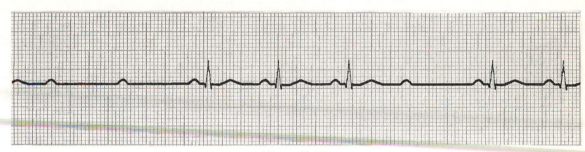

Figure 29-28

74. Complete Flashcard 22 (Fig. 29-29): third-degree (complete) atrioventricular block.

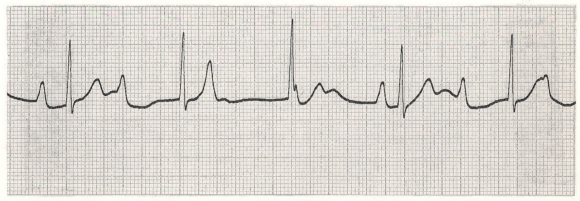

Figure 29-29

75. List the characteristics to identify the following:

  a. Right bundle branch block _____

  b. Left bundle branch block _____

  c. Anterior hemiblock _____

  d. Posterior hemiblock _____

76. Identify patients at risk for developing complete heart block if they are given procainamide, digoxin, verapamil, or diltiazem:

  a.

  b.

  c.

77. An approximately 50-year-old man is found unconscious in a parking lot downtown. He is pulseless and apneic. The attendant is certain he has been there less than 5 minutes but does not know what happened. The patient's electrocardiogram is shown in Fig. 29-30.

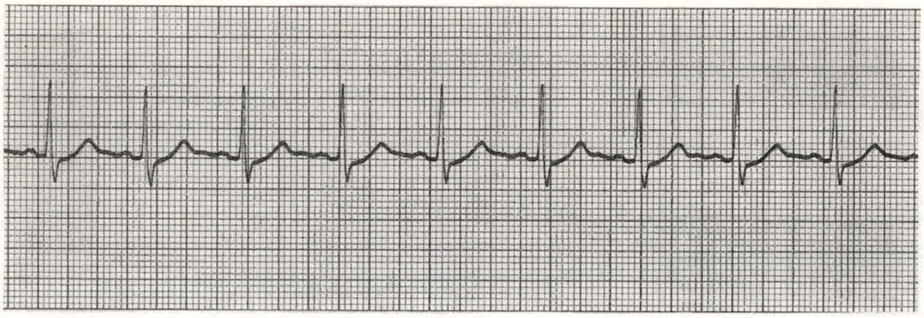

Figure 29-30

  a. You identify the rhythm as

_____

  b. Outline the appropriate interventions for this patient based on current treatment guidelines by the American Heart Association.

_____

78. Outline the electrocardiogram features that may allow detection of a patient with Wolff-Parkinson-White syndrome.

  a. QRS complex:

_____

  b. P-R interval:

_____

79. Why is it clinically important to recognize a patient with a history of Wolff-Parkinson-White syndrome?

_____

_____

SPECIFIC CARDIOVASCULAR DISEASES

80. Explain the pathophysiology of atherosclerotic effects on blood vessels.

_____

_____

81. List two triggers that may initiate an anginal attack in a susceptible patient:

a.

b.

82. Describe the following features of angina:

a. Duration:

_____

b. Relieved by:

_____

83. How can a paramedic distinguish between unstable angina and myocardial infarction in the prehospital environment?

_____

84. Briefly outline the sequence of pathophysiological events that occur from the time that a clot forms until cardiac tissue dies in acute myocardial infarction.

_____

_____

85. Complete the information regarding myocardial infarction that is missing in the following table:

Area of Heart Injured or Infarcted	Coronary Vessel Involved Most Often	Leads with Visible ST Segment Changes
Anterior		
Lateral		
Septal		
Inferior		

86. How much ST segment elevation must be present to be clinically significant?

_____

87. List six conditions other than myocardial infarction that can cause ST segment elevation.

a.

b.

c.

d.

e.

f.

88. List the five-step analysis described in this text for infarct recognition.

    a.

    b.

    c.

    d.

    e.

89. Identify four complications resulting from myocardial infarction.

    a.

    b.

    c.

    d.

Questions 90 to 94 pertain to the following case study:

A 57-year-old, 80-kg man with a history of untreated hypertension complains of crushing midsternal chest pain that began 2 hours ago. He takes no medicines but admits to smoking two packs of cigarettes per day. His blood pressure is 162/102 mm Hg. His electrocardiogram strip is shown in Fig. 29-31.

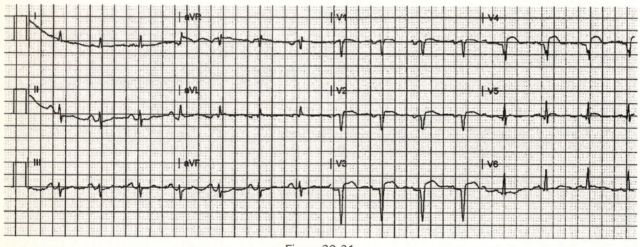

Figure 29-31

90. What other associated signs or symptoms may be present if the patient is experiencing a myocardial infarction?

_____

91. What is your interpretation of his electrocardiogram?

_____

92. Describe general treatment measures you will use for this patient.

_____

93. List three drugs (excluding oxygen) with the appropriate dosage to administer to this patient.

   a.

   b.

   c.

94. You transmit the 12-lead to the hospital and are asked to determine whether the patient meets inclusion or exclusion criteria for fibrinolytic therapy.

   a. List 4 inclusion criteria:

_____

   b. List 10 contraindications to fibrinolytic administration.

_____

_____

   c. Aside from the contraindications above, what three high-risk criteria suggest that this patient would benefit from PCI?

95. Interpret each of the following 12-lead electrocardiograms.

   a. Fig. 29-32:

_____

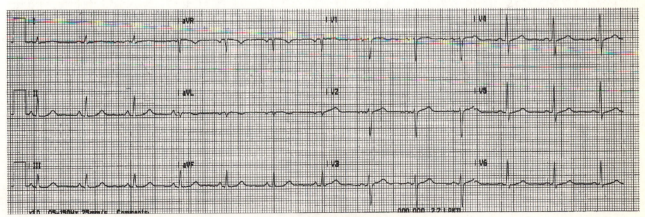

Figure 29-32

b. Fig. 29-33:

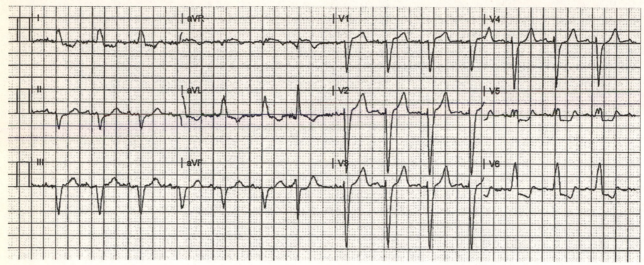

Figure 29-33

c. Fig. 29-34:

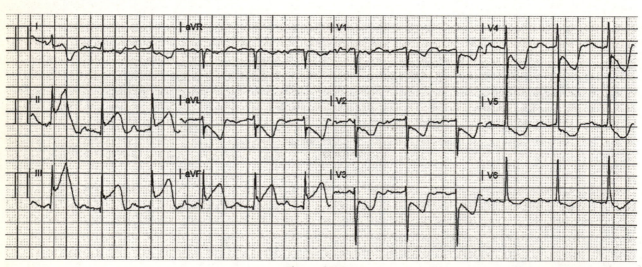

Figure 29-34

d. Fig. 29-35:

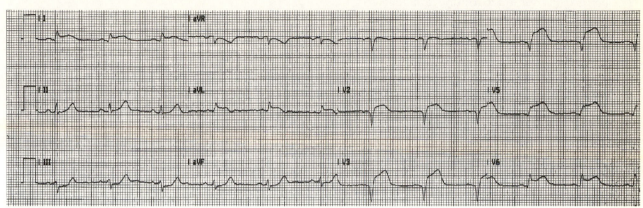

Figure 29-35

Questions 96 to 100 pertain to the following case study:

An 80-kg patient who had a syncopal episode and chest pain has the following electrocardiogram (Fig. 29-36).

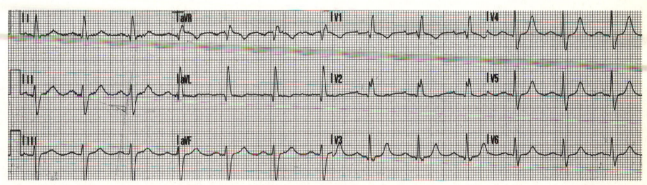

Figure 29-36

96. What is the axis of this electrocardiogram? _____

97. The QRS complex duration is 0.134 second. Draw a triangle that begins at the J point in lead V_1 and, working backward, ends at the first QRS deflection that is encountered. Does the triangle point up or down?

_____

98. Based on your determination of axis, the QRS duration, and the triangle you drew, identify the two blocks that are present in this electrocardiogram.

_____

99. What is the significance of these blocks?

_____

100. Based on the patient's chief complaint and your electrocardiogram findings, what interventions would you perform in addition to routine cardiac care?

_____

Questions 101 to 105 pertain to the following case study:

A 72-year-old, 70-kg woman calls you to her home and complains of a sudden onset of severe dyspnea without chest pain. You find her anxious, sitting upright, with diaphoretic skin and circumoral cyanosis. Her only home medicine is a diuretic. Vital signs are blood pressure, 170/106 mm Hg; pulse, 124; and respirations, 28 and labored. Rales are audible to the level of the scapulae. SaO_2 is 86%. Her electrocardiogram is shown in Fig. 29-37.

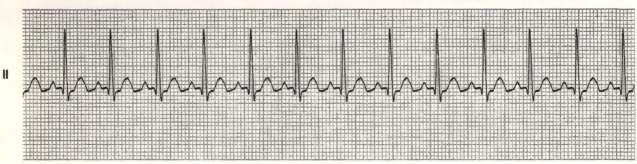

Figure 29-37

101. What medical condition or conditions do you suspect?

_____

102. What other physical findings would help confirm this diagnosis?

_____

103. What is your interpretation of her electrocardiogram?

_____

104. You have placed the patient on oxygen and wish to administer other pharmacological agents to improve her oxygenation. List three drugs that you would consider, and give the correct dose and desired effect of each.

    a._____

    b._____

    c._____

105. You decide to administer furosemide 0.5 mg/kg. It is supplied in a 4-mL ampule that contains 40 mg of the drug. How many milliliters will you give? _____ mL

106. List causes and signs and symptoms of right ventricular failure.

    a. Causes:

_____

b. Signs and symptoms:

_____

Questions 107 to 110 pertain to the following case study:

You are evaluating a 67-year-old man who has a history of two myocardial infarctions. His wife states he had chest pain that began 4 hours ago but that he refused to let her call emergency medical services and then passed out. He is conscious but confused and is pale and diaphoretic. His blood pressure is 80/50 mm Hg, his respiratory rate is 20, his SaO_2 is 90%, and his breath sounds are clear. His only home medicine is nitroglycerin paste, which he has on his left chest. This patient's electrocardiogram is shown in Fig. 29-38.

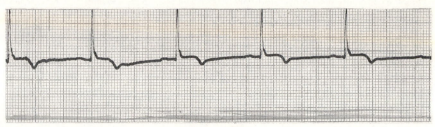

Figure 29-38

107. What is your interpretation of his electrocardiogram?

_____

108. What drug and dosage will you administer in consultation with medical direction to correct this dysrhythmia?

_____

After administering the first dose of this drug, the heart rate accelerates to 70 beats/min; however, the patient's other physical findings remain unchanged.

109. What do you suspect this patient is suffering from?

_____

110. List critical interventions, including drug therapy, that you should use, assuming that your estimated time of arrival to the hospital is 30 minutes.

_____

_____

Questions 111 to 114 pertain to the following case study:

A 70-year-old man experiences a sudden onset of a "tearing" abdominal pain at the area of the umbilicus that radiates to his back. He is pale and complains of the urge to defecate. His only history is hypertension, for which he takes captopril. Vital signs are blood pressure, 106/70 mm Hg; pulse, 100; and respirations, 20. On physical examination, you auscultate a bruit over the periumbilical area.

111. What illness do you suspect?

_____

112. Should you palpate this patient's abdomen?

_____

113. Should you allow this patient to go to the toilet and defecate?

_____

114. Briefly outline your management of this patient.

_____

_____

Questions 115 to 117 pertain to the following case study:

An older man complains of a severe "ripping" pain between his scapulae that extends down to his legs. He is pale and diaphoretic and has the following vital signs: blood pressure 170/110 mm Hg in the right arm and 130/80 mm Hg in the left arm.

115. What medical emergency do you suspect?

_____

116. Describe other physical findings that may confirm your suspicions.

_____

117. Outline your management of this patient in the prehospital phase.

_____

_____

118. Differentiate between the following characteristics of embolic arterial occlusion and thrombotic arterial occlusion.

	Embolic	**Thrombotic**
Causes:		
Onset:		
Signs and symptoms:		

119. An older woman calls you to her home because she bumped her leg and a varicose vein is bleeding. What care should be rendered to this patient?

_____

120. List three signs or symptoms of acute deep vein thrombosis.

a.

b.

c.

Questions 121 to 124 pertain to the following case study:

A 60-year-old man complains of a severe headache, blurred vision, and vomiting. He states that he has a history of hypertension but has not been taking his medicine because the cost is too high. His vital signs are blood pressure, 190/128 mm Hg; pulse, 88; and respirations, 20.

121. What medical emergency do you suspect?

_____

122. If this man is not treated promptly, what other signs and/or symptoms may result?

_____

123. Outline general management principles for this patient.

_____

124. If your transport time is delayed, list one drug (with the appropriate dose) that medical direction may order to lower this patient's blood pressure.

_____

TECHNIQUES OF MANAGING CARDIAC EMERGENCIES

125. You are at a friend's home playing tennis. After retrieving the ball, you turn around see that your friend has collapsed on the court. Outline the steps you must take from this moment until emergency medical services arrives if he has had a cardiac arrest. (Assume that no one else is nearby to help.)

_____

_____

_____

126. A basic life support unit is caring for a patient who is in cardiac arrest when your advanced life support unit arrives on the scene. An automated external defibrillator without a display is attached to the patient, and five shocks already have been delivered.

    a. When should you defibrillate this patient if you determine that ventricular fibrillation is present?

_____

    b. If a rescuer is in contact with the patient when the automated external defibrillator fires, will an injury occur?

_____

Questions 127 to 129 pertain to the following case study:

    You arrive on the scene to care for a patient who is pulseless and apneic. A bystander is performing CPR when you arrive. The monitor displays the rhythm shown in Fig. 29-39.

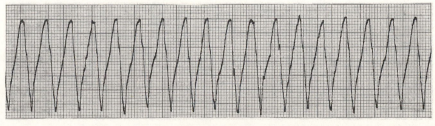

Figure 29-39

127. What is your interpretation of the electrocardiogram?

_____

128. What is your first intervention after rhythm determination and verification of pulselessness?

_____

129. List two factors that will improve the success rate of this treatment.

a.

b.

130. List the steps in performing this intervention.

_____

_____

_____

131. You are at the home of a patient whose wife states that he was experiencing severe chest pain. Moments after you hook up the patient to your monitor, he loses consciousness, and the rhythm shown in Fig. 29-40 is displayed. Blood pressure is 60 mm Hg by palpation, and ventilations are adequate. Another paramedic applies oxygen by non-rebreather mask at 12 L/min. State the appropriate therapy for this patient up to and including administration of the first drug.

_____

_____

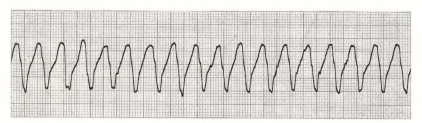

Figure 29-40

132. What is the advantage of synchronized cardioversion?

_____

133. Briefly outline the steps in synchronized cardioversion that are different from unsynchronized cardioversion.

_____

_____

134. An unresponsive 69-year-old patient has a blood pressure of 76/50 mm Hg. The ECG is shown in Fig. 29-41.

a. What is your interpretation of the electrocardiogram?

_____

b. Assuming that IV access is not obtainable, and no drugs are readily available, list the steps you would take to initiate transcutaneous pacing on this patient.

_____

_____

_____

_____

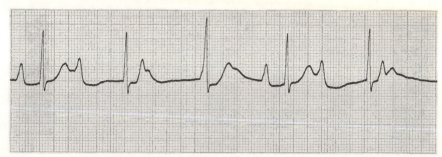

Figure 29-41

135. An older man is found unresponsive, apneic, and pulseless in the busy bathroom of a shopping mall. A quick examination reveals the monitor pattern shown in Fig. 29-42.

    a. What is your interpretation of the rhythm?

_____

    b. What drugs (with appropriate doses) should be administered?

_____

    c. What causes for this arrest should you consider?

_____

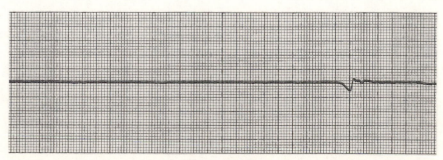

Figure 29-42

136. You are en route to the hospital with a 55-year-old man whom you suspect is having an acute myocardial infarction. Suddenly, the patient gasps and becomes pulseless and apneic. As you look at the monitor, you note the electrocardiogram shown in Fig. 29-43.

    a. What is the rhythm?

_____

    b. What single treatment modality is most likely to restore circulation in this patient?

_____

    c. List the appropriate drugs (in the proper order) with correct doses that may be given to this patient if the answer in (b) is unsuccessful.

_____

_____

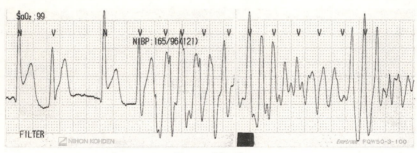

Figure 29-43

137. For each of the following situations, state whether criteria to stop resuscitation have been met. Explain your decision. Assume the patient is now in asystole.

    a. The patient is 94 years old and was found in asystolic arrest, having last been seen 30 minutes previously. You have intubated the patient, given epinephrine and atropine twice.

_____

_____

    b. A 65-year-old patient collapses outside a mall. You have been resuscitating for 20 minutes, although you have not been able to intubate. You have administered epinephrine (three doses), and administered atropine sulfate (two doses). It is a snowy day.

_____

c. A 16-year-old is in full arrest after falling from a fourth-floor balcony. You initially got back a sinus rhythm with a pulse, but now asystole is on the monitor. The patient was intubated en route, and you have two large-bore intravenous lines infusing wide open and have given three doses of epinephrine, and given two doses of atropine.

_____

_____

d. A 70-year-old is in asystole. You have intubated and given epinephrine (three doses) and administered the maximum dose of atropine with no success. You elect to terminate resuscitation, but the family is objecting strongly.

_____

_____

STUDENT SELF-ASSESSMENT

138. Your patient is experiencing chest pain. He is 75 years of age, says his last cholesterol test result was 300 mg/dL, and takes Glucophage (metformin), Accupril, and indapamide. How many risk factors for cardiovascular disease did you identify in this patient?
    a. Two   **c.** Four
    b. Three   **d.** Five

139. Blood pressure is equal to which of the following?
    a. Heart rate × Stroke volume × Cardiac output
    b. Stroke volume × Peripheral vascular resistance
    c. Heart rate × Stroke volume × Peripheral vascular resistance
    d. Heart rate × Contractility × Stroke volume

140. Your patient is experiencing signs of a large infarct affecting the anterior portion of the left ventricle. Which coronary vessel most likely is involved?
    a. Circumflex artery   **c.** Left anterior descending
    b. Coronary sinus   **d.** Right coronary artery

141. Which valve separates the left atrium from the left ventricle?
    a. Aortic   **c.** Pulmonic
    b. Mitral   **d.** Tricuspid

142. The magnetic force that occurs when particles with opposite charges are separated across the cell membrane is known as which of the following?
    a. Action potential   **c.** Millivolts
    b. Depolarization   **d.** Potential energy

143. Which ions are critical to maintain the normal resting membrane potential?
    a. Chloride   **c.** Sodium
    b. Phosphate   **d.** Sulfate

144. Which drugs may affect the threshold level of cardiac conduction cells?
    a. Atropine   **c.** Nitroglycerin
    b. Morphine   **d.** Verapamil

145. Which phase of the cardiac action potential represents depolarization?
    a. Phase 1   **c.** Phase 3
    b. Phase 2   **d.** Phase 4

146. What is the purpose of the absolute refractory period in the heart?
    a. To allow electrolyte balance to be restored
    b. To initiate the next action potential
    c. To permit the muscle to relax so the heart can fill
    d. To stretch the cardiac fibers for more forceful contraction

147. Which are the smallest divisions of the His bundles?
  a. Anterior-superior fascicles
  b. Posterior-inferior fascicles
  c. Right and left bundle branches
  d. Purkinje fibers

148. Why do pacemaker cells fire repeatedly without external stimulation?
  a. Cerebral biorhythms cause intrinsic stimulation.
  b. Epinephrine initiates the action potential in regular cycles.
  c. Sympathetic nervous system causes hormonal stimulation.
  d. They have an unstable resting membrane potential.

149. Why is there a conduction delay in the atrioventricular node of the normal cardiac cycle?
  a. So ectopic rhythms do not have a chance to enter the cycle
  b. So simultaneous contraction of the atria can occur
  c. To allow for contraction of the atria before ventricular contraction
  d. To permit refilling of the coronary arteries before atrial systole

150. Which of the following may cause a decrease in sinoatrial node discharge, resulting in decreased heart rate?
  a. Acetylcholine
  b. Epinephrine
  c. Norepinephrine
  d. Parasympatholytic effects

151. Mechanisms that produce dysrhythmias following reentry include which of the following?
  a. Atropine administration
  b. Digitalis toxicity
  c. Hypercapnia
  d. Hyperkalemia

152. Which of the following signs or symptoms would be atypical for a coronary event?
  a. Abdominal discomfort
  b. Dyspnea
  c. Jaw pain
  d. Syncope

153. Dyspnea associated with myocardial infarction usually is related to which of the following?
  a. Chronic obstructive pulmonary disease
  b. Drug administration
  c. Hypercarbia
  d. Pulmonary congestion

154. Syncope should be assumed to be caused by a dysrhythmia if which of the following is associated with it?
  a. Nausea preceded the event.
  b. The patient is older.
  c. The patient has a history of diabetes.
  d. It occurred when the patient was standing.

155. When evaluating a patient for jugular venous distention, the paramedic should do which of the following?
  a. Raise the head of the bed 90 degrees.
  b. Raise the head of the bed 45 degrees.
  c. Lay the patient in the supine position.
  d. Have the patient stand with assistance.

156. Why may it be helpful to find the point of maximum impulse on the patient's chest?
  a. For appropriate defibrillation or pacing patch placement
  b. For assessment of strength of myocardial contractions
  c. To identify a point to auscultate the mitral valve
  d. To place electrodes for monitoring a 12-lead electrocardiogram

157. What does the electrocardiogram tracing assess?
  a. Cardiac output
  b. Electrical conduction
  c. Myocardial contractility
  d. Stroke volume

158. Which of the following represents a bipolar lead?
  a. aV_F
  b. aV_R
  c. Lead II
  d. V_1

159. In lead II the positive electrode is located on the left lower extremity. During normal conduction, which way should the QRS complex deflect?
  a. Biphasic
  b. Downward
  c. Isoelectric
  d. Upward

160. You are looking at leads II, III, and aV$_F$. What part of the heart can you "view" in those leads?

    a. Anterior   **c.** Lateral

    b. Inferior   **d.** Septum

161. Modified chest leads mimic the view that can be obtained by looking at which of the following?

    a. Augmented leads   **c.** Posterior leads

    b. Limb leads   **d.** V leads

162. Where should the positive electrode be placed for MCL$_1$?

    a. Below the lateral end of the left clavicle

    b. Below the lateral end of the right clavicle

    c. Fourth intercostal space to the right of the sternum

    d. Left axillary line at the level of the fifth intercostal space

163. Why are leads II and MCL$_1$ preferred for routine monitoring for dysrhythmias?

    a. P waves can be visualized easily.

    b. The tallest QRS complex can be seen.

    c. Rates are calculated more easily.

    d. ST segment elevation or depression can be viewed.

164. Which precordial leads are septal leads?

    a. aV$_L$ **c.** V$_3$ and V$_4$

    b. V$_1$ and V$_2$ **d.** V$_5$ and V$_6$

165. What represents the absence of electrical activity in the heart on the electrocardiogram strip?

    a. Isoelectric line   **c.** QRS complex

    b. P wave   **d.** ST segment

166. What is the normal duration of the QRS complex?

    a. 0.04 to 0.08 second   **c.** 0.12 to 0.14 second

    b. 0.08 to 0.10 second   **d.** 0.14 to 0.16 second

167. During what point does the absolute refractory period occur in the heart?

    a. P wave   **c.** Q-T interval

    b. P-R interval   **d.** T wave

168. To assess abnormal QRS width accurately, the paramedic should do which of the following?

    a. Determine the J point and measure back from it.

    b. Identify the lead with the widest QRS complex and then measure it.

    c. Measure from the end of the P wave to the end of the S wave.

    d. Measure from R-R wave from left to right.

169. There are 10 small boxes between the R waves on the electrocardiogram tracing. What is the heart rate?

    a. 6 beats/min   **c.** 60 beats/min

    b. 30 beats/min   **d.** 150 beats/min

170. Identify the electrocardiogram tracing in Fig. 29-44.

    a. Normal sinus rhythm

    b. Sinus rhythm with first-degree atrioventricular block

    c. Second-degree heart block type II

    d. Ventricular demand pacer with capture

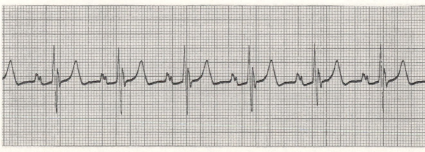

Figure 29-44

171. Identify the electrocardiogram tracing in Fig. 29-45.
  a. Accelerated idioventricular rhythm
  b. Junctional tachycardia
  c. Ventricular pacemaker
  d. Ventricular tachycardia

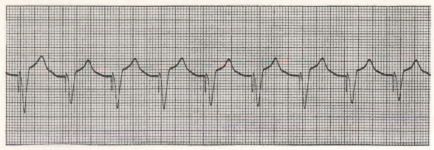

Figure 29-45

172. Identify the electrocardiogram tracing in Fig. 29-46.
  a. Multifocal premature ventricular contractions
  b. Couplet of premature ventricular contractions
  c. Ventricular bigeminy
  d. Ventricular escape rhythm

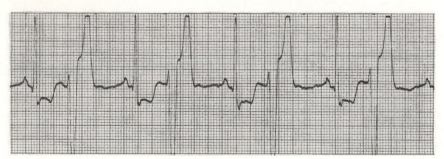

Figure 29-46

173. Identify the electrocardiogram tracing in Fig. 29-47.
  a. Second-degree atrioventricular block type I
  b. Second-degree atrioventricular block type II
  c. Sinus arrest
  d. Sinus arrhythmia

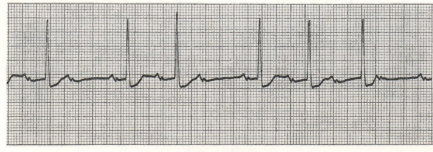

Figure 29-47

174. Identify the electrocardiogram tracing in Fig. 29-48.
  a. Atrial fibrillation
  b. Atrial flutter
  c. Junctional tachycardia
  d. Third-degree atrioventricular block

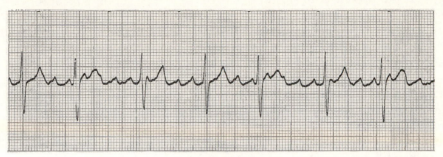

Figure 29-48

175. Identify the electrocardiogram tracing in Fig. 29-49.
  a. Atrial fibrillation   **c.** Atrial tachycardia
  b. Atrial flutter   **d.** Sinus tachycardia

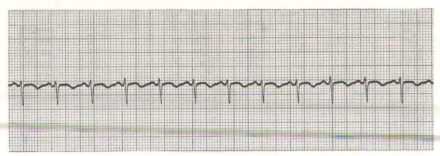

Figure 29-49

176. Identify the electrocardiogram tracing in Fig. 29-50.
  a. Accelerated junctional rhythm followed by pacemaker
  b. Junctional rhythm followed by pacemaker
  c. Junctional rhythm followed by idioventricular
  d. Second-degree atrioventricular block type II followed by idioventricular

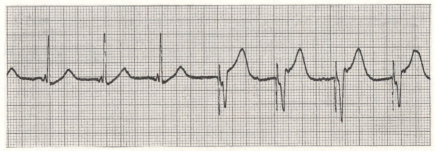

Figure 29-50

177. You are treating a 60-year-old woman with atrial fibrillation at a rate of 168 beats/min. Her blood pressure is 80 mm Hg by palpation, and she feels faint. Which of the following interventions is appropriate?
   a. Adenosine 6 mg via rapid intravenous administration
   b. Verapamil 2.5 mg intravenously over 2 minutes
   c. Procainamide 30 mg/min intravenously
   d. Synchronized cardioversion at 100 J

178. Which of the following is an ectopic rhythm?
   a. Atrial tachycardia   **c.** Normal sinus rhythm
   b. Junctional tachycardia   **d.** Sinus bradycardia

179. Which of the following will *not* cause sinus bradycardia?
   a. Digoxin   **c.** Isoproterenol
   b. Increased vagal tone   **d.** Sleep

180. What is the most common cause of decreased cardiac output in atrial fibrillation or atrial flutter?
   a. Decreased ventricular contractility
   b. Development of blood clots
   c. Inadequate atrial filling
   d. Loss of atrial kick

181. What can result from atrial fibrillation?
   a. Congestive heart failure   **c.** Rheumatic heart disease
   b. Pericarditis   **d.** Vagal stimulation

182. If your patient has accelerated junctional rhythm, what medical history should you inquire about that is associated specifically with this rhythm?
   a. Chronic obstructive pulmonary disease
   b. Diabetes
   c. Marijuana use
   d. Treatment with digoxin

183. Which of the following mechanisms may cause ventricular dysrhythmias?
   a. Enhanced automaticity
   b. Reentry phenomena
   c. Enhanced automaticity and reentry phenomena
   d. Neither enhanced automaticity nor reentry phenomena

184. Premature ventricular contractions that occur every second complex are known as which of the following?
   a. Bigeminy   **c.** Idioventricular
   b. Couplets   **d.** Multifocal

185. Your patient has a wide-complex tachycardia. Which of the following electrocardiogram findings would indicate ventricular tachycardia?
   a. All precordial leads (V leads) have a positive deflection.
   b. Negative QRS deflection with a single peak in MCL_1 and MCL_6.
   c. Positive QRS complex in leads I, II, and III.
   d. RS interval is less than 0.10 second in any V lead.

186. What type of pacemaker fires only when the patient's own heart rate drops below a predetermined rate?
   a. Asynchronous   **c.** Dual chamber
   b. Demand   **d.** Fixed rate

187. What rhythm occurs when a complete block develops at or below the atrioventricular node?
   a. Bundle branch block
   b. Fascicular block
   c. Second-degree atrioventricular block type II
   d. Third-degree atrioventricular block

188. Which of the following is true regarding left bundle branch block?
   a. It produces an initial R wave in V_1 instead of the normal small Q wave.
   b. There is a shallow, narrow QS pattern, and the QRS complex is less than 0.12 second.
   c. There is an RSR prime pattern seen in V_1 with a QRS complex greater than 0.12 second.
   d. The fibers that usually fire the interventricular septum are blocked.

189. Which of the following has the greatest potential to deteriorate into complete heart block?
   a. Anterior hemiblock
   c. Posterior hemiblock
   b. Bifascicular block
   d. Right bundle branch block

190. Your patient has a history of Wolff-Parkinson-White syndrome. You note a rapid wide-complex atrial fibrillation. Which drug is appropriate for this patient?
   a. Adenosine
   c. Diltiazem
   b. Amiodarone
   d. Magnesium

191. What distinguishes unstable angina from stable angina?
   a. It is caused by atherosclerotic disease of the coronary arteries.
   b. The pain lasts 1 to 5 minutes and is relieved by oxygen or nitroglycerin.
   c. The pain changes in its onset, frequency, duration, or quality.
   d. It is precipitated by physical exertion or emotional stress.

192. Death from myocardial infarction is *most commonly* the result of which of the following?
   a. Dysrhythmias
   c. Pulmonary embolism
   b. Low blood pressure
   d. Cardiac rupture

193. Appropriate care for a stable patient with acute ST segment elevation myocardial infarction would include all of the following except which one?
   a. Placing the patient in a semi-Fowler position
   b. Administering lactated Ringer's solution at 500 mL/hr intravenously
   c. Administering oxygen by nasal cannula
   d. Documenting and reporting all intravenous sticks

194. Which of the following is *not* diagnostic of an acute myocardial infarction?
   a. Pathological Q waves
   c. ST segment depression
   b. Peaked tented T waves
   d. ST segment elevation

195. Medications that may help in the management of a patient with cardiac pulmonary edema include all of the following *except* which one?
   a. Epinephrine
   c. Morphine
   b. Furosemide
   d. Nitroglycerin

196. When a patient suffers from right ventricular heart failure, blood backs up into which of the following?
   a. Aorta
   c. Pulmonary veins
   b. Pulmonary arteries
   d. Venae cavae

197. Cardiogenic shock is
   a. Fatal in only 10% to 15% of patients.
   b. Caused by extensive myocardial damage.
   c. The result of an intravascular electrolyte imbalance.
   d. Caused by obstruction of the renal vessels.

198. Your patient has a history of cancer and is having chest pain and tachycardia. What is an early sign that may indicate the development of cardiac tamponade?
   a. Decreased systolic pressure
   c. Pericardial friction rub
   b. Jugular venous distention
   d. Tracheal deviation

199. Which is the most common presentation of dissection of the thoracic aorta?
   a. Chest heaviness of slow onset
   b. Intense back pain with sudden onset
   c. Neck pain that began suddenly
   d. Substernal dull pain that increased gradually

200. Acute arterial occlusion may result in which of the following?
   a. Absent distal pulses
   c. Pulmonary congestion
   b. Hypertension
   d. Torsades de pointes

201. You suspect that your patient has an arterial occlusion affecting the lower leg. Which of the following treatment measures would be appropriate?
   a. Initiate intravenous fluid therapy and administer a fluid challenge.
   b. Massage the affected extremity to encourage circulation.
   c. Immobilize the affected extremity and protect it from injury.
   d. Administer furosemide 40 mg intravenously to flush out the embolus.

202. Chronic, uncontrolled hypertension puts a patient at risk for all *except* which of the following?
    a. Cerebral hemorrhage
    c. Myocardial infarction
    b. Diabetes mellitus
    d. Renal failure
203. According to the American Heart Association, what ratio of compressions and ventilations should be performed in the patient in cardiac arrest?
    a. 2:15
    c. 2:30
    b. 15:2
    d. 30:2
204. You work at a service that uses biphasic defibrillation. Which of the following is true regarding this device?
    a. Higher defibrillation doses are needed.
    b. It compensates for chest impedence.
    c. The batteries are larger.
    d. The energy flows in one direction.
205. What principle should be followed when placing paddles or patches on the chest for defibrillation?
    a. Anterior-posterior placement may be used for patches.
    b. Never reverse the polarity, or defibrillation will not occur.
    c. Place one paddle over the sternum directly over the heart.
    d. Use pediatric paddles for children up to 8 years of age.
206. What should you consider when caring for a patient who has an implantable cardioverter defibrillator?
    a. Apply a magnet to the chest to activate these devices if the patient is unresponsive.
    b. If the first defibrillation attempt is unsuccessful, paddle placement should be changed.
    c. Three shocks should be delivered before CPR.
    d. Touching the patient during implantable cardioverter defibrillator defibrillation is dangerous.
207. Which of the following statements is true regarding synchronized cardioversion?
    a. It is faster than unsynchronized cardioversion.
    b. It is not as safe as unsynchronized cardioversion.
    c. It is indicated for pulseless ventricular tachycardia.
    d. It is indicated for unstable paroxysmal supraventricular tachycardia.
208. When attempting to initiate transcutaneous pacing on a conscious patient, set the current at which of the following?
    a. 70 to 80 per minute and increased until the patient is stable
    b. 50 mA and increase until capture occurs
    c. 70 to 80 per minute and decrease until the patient becomes unstable
    d. Maximum mA and decrease until capture is lost
209. Which of the following drugs is used to treat asystole?
    a. Amiodarone
    c. Lidocaine
    b. Atropine
    d. Magnesium
210. Your patient has ST segment elevation in leads II and aVL. His BP drops to 70 mm Hg after a dose of nitroglycerine. What should you do first?
    a. Administer dopamine 2-20 mcg/kg/min.
    b. Deliver a fluid bolus.
    c. Increase oxygen to 6 lpm.
    d. Perform a right-sided 12-lead ECG.
211. Which of the following is an action of morphine sulfate?
    a. Dilation of peripheral vasculature
    b. Increase in cardiac preload
    c. Causes amnesia
    d. Bronchodilation
212. Which of the following is true of digoxin?
    a. It increases the force of ventricular contraction.
    b. It is used to treat bradycardia.
    c. It causes decreased cardiac output.
    d. It increases impulse conduction through the atrioventricular node.
213. Which of the following drugs stimulates the beta receptors?
    a. Amyl nitrite
    c. Epinephrine
    b. Atropine
    d. Labetolol

214. A 60-year-old, 100-kg woman has a blood pressure of 80/50 mm Hg. The electrocardiogram is shown in Fig. 29-51. Which of the following is *not* appropriate to correct this?
  a. Atropine 0.5 mg intravenously
  b. Dopamine 2 to 20 mcg/kg/min
  c. Epinephrine 2 to 10 mcg/kg/min
  d. Transcutaneous pacing

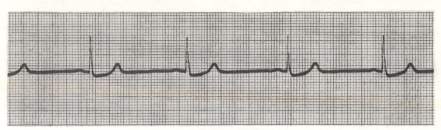

Figure 29-51

215. Which of the following criteria should be considered to determine whether to terminate resuscitation of a patient?
  a. Livor or rigor mortis
  b. Presence of a nonofficial do not resuscitate order
  c. Quality of life judgments
  d. Time of collapse before emergency medical services arrival

WRAP IT UP

"4027 respond to a cardiac arrest, 1425 Humes, 4027 . . .": the dispatcher's familiar voice jolts you awake from a nap. As you respond, you are updated that CPR instructions are in progress. You hear the local fire department announce their arrival at the scene when you are about 10 blocks away, and as you walk into the house you can hear a mechanical voice say, "Deliver shock now." As the firefighter presses the button on the AED, the patient's lifeless body jolts, and then the AED commands, "Assessing rhythm, do not touch the patient," followed what seems like an eternity later by, "No shock advised, check breathing and pulse." You quickly check breathing and pulse and are surprised to feel weak slow pulsations under your fingers at the carotid artery. "Begin ventilations," you instruct the firefighter at the patient's head, and she begins to ventilate the patient with a bag. By now your partner has disconnected the defibrillation pads from the AED and reconnected them to your monitor/defibrillator. You note a bradycardia rhythm that appears to be increasing at a fairly rapid rate. "He's breathing!" the firefighter ventilating the patient exclaims. The patient begins to cough and push away the bag from his face. Vital signs are BP 100/70 mm Hg, P 88, R 18, SaO_2 95%. You calm the patient, apply oxygen, and initiate an IV. The patient's wife says her 55-year-old husband was complaining of indigestion for about an hour before he collapsed. He is normally healthy and takes no medications, and so he would not let her take him to the ER. After the patient is secured in the ambulance, you perform a 12-lead electrocardiogram. You note 4-mm ST segment elevation in leads V_1 to V_4. The patient is awake but slightly confused and rubbing his chest. You give him aspirin and nitroglycerin after obtaining another BP at 116/84 mm Hg. His ER stay is brief; the cardiologist whisks him to the cardiac catheter lab where balloon angiography is performed. As you enter your times in the computer, you note that the initial fire department unit arrived 4 minutes after the 911 call was placed. They delivered the shock 1½ minutes later. You meet the patient a month later at the grocery store with his four children; he is ready to return to work and is emotional as he gives you his thanks.

  1. Place a check mark beside the elements of the chain of survival that were present on this call.
    a. _____ Early recognition of the emergency
    b. _____ Activation of 911
    c. _____ Early cardiopulmonary resuscitation
    d. _____ Early defibrillation
    e. _____ Early advanced care
    f. _____ Rapid interventional cardiology

2. What rhythm(s) was the patient in when the fire department arrived?

_____

3. What antidysrhythmic drug(s) could you administer?

_____

4. What walls of the heart are damaged, based on the 12-lead electrocardiogram findings?

_____

5. What coronary blood vessels are likely occluded?

_____

6. Which element of this patient's situation would be a relative contraindication to fibrinolytic therapy?
   a. Cardiopulmonary resuscitation less than 10 minutes
   b. Suspected aortic dissection
   c. Terminal illness
   d. Uncontrolled hypertension

7. At what rate and volume should the firefighter ventilate after the patient's pulse returns?

   Rate_____   Vol _____

CHAPTER 29 ANSWERS

REVIEW QUESTIONS

1. c
(Objective 2)

2. f
(Objective 2)

3. a
(Objective 2)

4. e
(Objective 2)

5. b
(Objective 2)

6. g
(Objective 2)

7. h
(Objective 2)

8.

Risk Factor	Prevention Strategy	Resource
a. Smoking	Quit smoking with use of medications, hypnosis, behavior modification, health clinic	Private physician, heart association, cancer association, alternative nicotine products
b. Hypercholesterolemia	Diet modification, drugs	Private physician, health clinic, heart association
c. Obesity	Diet, exercise	Private physician, exercise, community health clinic, dietitian, American Heart Association
d. Sedentary lifestyle	Exercise program, leisure activities	Private physician, local hospital

(Objective 1)

9.

	Sympathetic	Parasympathetic
a. Heart rate	Increase	Decrease
b. Myocardial	Increase	No effect contractility
c. Lungs	Beta-bronchiolar dilation	Constriction
d. Blood vessels (peripheral)	Constriction	No effect

(Objective 2)

10. a. Epinephrine: increased heart rate, contractility, bronchiolar dilation, and blood vessel constriction in skin, kidneys, gastrointestinal tract, and viscera
b. Norepinephrine: peripheral vasoconstriction
(Objective 2)

11. a. Magnetic
b. Potential
c. Permeable
d. Potential
e. Millivolts
f. Negative
g. Negatively
h. Potential
i. Negative
j. −70 to −90
k. Potassium
l. Potassium
m. Proteins
n. Permeable
o. Excitability
p. Depolarization
q. Threshold potential
r. Action potential
s. Depolarization
t. Repolarization
u. Positive
v. Negative
w. Depolarization
x. Membrane potential
(Objective 3)

12. a. Sodium rushes into the cell through the fast sodium channels.
b. The membrane potential drops to approximately 0.
c. The slow calcium channels allow calcium to enter the cell while potassium continues to leave, maintaining the membrane potential of 0.
d. The membrane potential returns to −90 mV.
e. The sodium pump allows the exchange of sodium and potassium to their proper compartments.
f. During phase 4, cardiac pacemaker cells slowly depolarize from their most negative membrane potential to a level at which threshold is reached and phase 0 begins. Nonpacemaker cells maintain a stable resting membrane potential and do not depolarize unless stimulated by a sufficiently strong stimulus.
(Objective 3)

13. a. Action potentials; b. upward; c. automaticity; d. resting membrane potential
(Objective 3)

14. a. Sinoatrial node; b. intranodal pathways; c. atrioventricular node; d. common bundle of His; e. left posterior bundle branch; f. Purkinje fibers; g. left anterior bundle branch; h. right bundle branch
(Objective 4)

15. The next pacemaker (atrioventricular node) should take over and fire.
(Objective 4)

16. a. Acceleration of phase 4 depolarization so cells reach their threshold prematurely (may result from digoxin toxicity, increased catecholamine levels, hypoxia, hypercapnia, myocardial ischemia, infarction, increased venous return, hypokalemia, hypocalcemia, heating or cooling of the heart, or atropine administration)
b. Reactivation of tissue by a returning impulse
(Objective 4)

17. O—Onset. What were you doing when the pain began?
    P—Is there anything that makes the pain better or worse?
    Q—What does the pain feel like? (Is it sharp, dull, crushing, squeezing?)
    R—Where is the pain? Does it go anywhere else?
    S—On a scale of 1 to 10, with 1 being no pain and 10 being the worst pain you have ever had, describe your pain.
    T—When did you first feel the pain?
    (Objective 5)

18. Chest pain, dyspnea, syncope, and palpitations
    (Objective 5)

19. How did you feel before you passed out? What were you doing when you passed out? What position were you in before you passed out (i.e., laying down, sitting, or standing)? How long were you unconscious? Do you have a history of heart disease or other significant medical history? What medicines do you take? Do you feel unusual in any other way? How has your health been over the past several days?
    (Objective 5)

20. Pulse rate and regularity, electrocardiogram, vital signs, circumstances of occurrence, duration, associated symptoms, previous history of palpitations, medical history, and daily medicines
    (Objective 5)

21. Major medical illnesses, home medicines, and similar previous episodes
    (Objective 5)

22. Atrial fibrillation with a slow ventricular response
    (Objective 10)

23. Yes. Digoxin (Lanoxin) or calcium channel blocker (Cardizem) toxicity can cause this presentation. Digitalis toxicity is more likely in the patient who also is taking a diuretic (furosemide).
    (Objective 5)

24. Neck: jugular venous distention. Chest: implanted pacemaker generator, median sternotomy scar, lung sounds (crackles), heart sounds (S₃ gallop), and pulse deficit. Abdomen: generator for automatic implantable cardioverter defibrillator visible. Extremities: edema and ulceration. Back: sacral edema. Medical alert tags or medical information in wallet
    (Objective 5)

25.

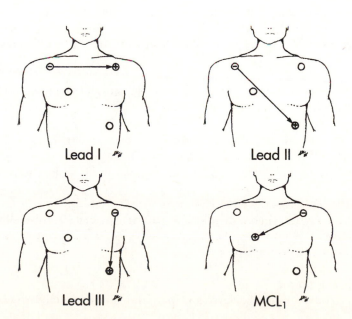

(Objective 6)

26. a. Right arm (right anterior forearm)
b. Left arm (left anterior forearm)
c. Right leg (right lower leg)
d. Left lower leg (left leg)
e. V_1, fourth intercostal space to the right of the sternum
f. V_2, fourth intercostal space to the left of the sternum
g. V_4, fifth intercostal space, midclavicular line
h. V_3, between V_2 and V_4
i. V_5, anterior axillary line in a straight line with V_4
j. V_6, midaxillary line, level with V_4 and V_5 (In women, V_4 to V_6 should be placed under the left breast.)
(Objective 6)

27. a. Excessive body hair: Shave.
b. Diaphoresis: Dry area and apply tincture of benzoin.
c. Poor electrode placement: Reapply correctly.
d. 60-cycle interference: Run monitor on batteries.
e. Poor cable connections: Recheck all connections.
f. Close proximity to electrical motors
(Objective 6)

28. a. 5; b. 0.04; c. 0.20; d. d3; e. 6
(Objective 6)

29. a. P wave; b. QRS complex; c. T wave; d. P-R interval; e. ST segment
(Objective 7)

30. Muscle tremor, AC (60-cycle interference), loose electrodes, patient movement, loss of electrode contact, and external chest compression
(Objective 7)

31. Analyze the QRS complex; analyze the P waves; analyze the rate; analyze the rhythm; analyze the P-R interval.
(Objective 8)

32. a. Triplicate method (120 beats/min.): Find the R wave on the dark line, count 300-150-100-75 for each next dark line until the next R wave. The R wave falls between 100 and 150. Estimate rate to be 120 beats/min.
b. R-R method: 300 ÷ Number of large boxes between R waves = 300 ÷ (almost) 3 = 100 beats/min
c. R-R method: 1500 ÷ Number of small boxes between R waves = 1500 ÷ 13 = 115 beats/min
d. 6-second method: Number of R waves in a 6-second strip × 10 = 12 × 10 = 120 beats/min
(Objective 8)

33. No, this reveals only the rate, not the perfusion status (and the rate is faster than normal for an adult).
(Objective 7)

34. a. R-R method (1500 ÷ Number of small boxes between the R waves) or triplicate method (but only if R waves both fall on dark lines)
b. The 6-second method is the most accurate and quick estimate for irregular rhythm.
(Objective 8)

35. The R-R distance should be equal when measured left to right across an electrocardiogram strip (it can vary no greater than 0.16 second).
(Objective 8)

36. a. Through the ventricles is normal.
b. Conduction through the ventricles is delayed and may follow an abnormal pathway.
(Objective 7)

37. Are they regular? Is there a P wave in front of each QRS complex? Are they upright or inverted? Do they all look the same?
(Objective 8)

38. a. Electrical impulse that progressed from the atria to the ventricles through pathways other than the atrioventricular node of the bundle of His
b. Normal conduction from the sinoatrial node through the atrioventricular node
c. Delay in conduction of impulse through the atrioventricular node or bundle of His
(Objective 7)

39. a. QRS complex: 0.08 sec (normal is less than 0.12 second)
b. P waves: regular, one for each QRS complex, upright, all the same
c. Rate: 75 beats/min (triplicate method)
d. Rhythm: regular (R-R intervals equal)
e. P-R interval: 0.14 second. Interpretation: normal sinus rhythm
(Objectives 8 and 9)

40. Patient history, chief complaint, and physical findings
(Objective 10)

41. a. Parasympathetic stimulation
b. QRS complex less than 0.12 second (unless a conduction delay is present)
c. P waves (regular, preceding each QRS complex, upright, similar)
d. P-R interval: 0.12 to 0.20 second
(Objective 10)

42. a. Sinus node disease, increased parasympathetic vagal tone, hypothermia, hypoxia, and drug effects (digitalis, propranolol, verapamil)
b. Exercise, fever, anxiety, ingestion of stimulants, smoking, hypovolemia, anemia, congestive heart failure, and excessive administration of atropine or vagolytic or sympathomimetic drugs (cocaine, phencyclidine, epinephrine, isoproterenol)
(Objective 10)

43. QRS complex: 0.08 second. P waves: present, upright, similar. Rate: 50 beats/min. Rhythm: regular. P-R interval: 0.16 second. Interpretation: sinus bradycardia. Distinguishing features: all features of normal sinus rhythm except that rate is less than 60 beats/min. Treatment: stable—observe; unstable—atropine 0.5 to 1.0 mg every 3 to 5 minutes to a maximum dose of less than 2.5 mg (0.03 to 0.04 mg/kg), transcutaneous pacing, dopamine 5 to 20 mcg/kg/min, epinephrine 2 to 10 mcg/min, isoproterenol 2 to 10 mcg/min
(Objective 10)

44. QRS complex: 0.06 second. P waves: present, upright, similar. Rate: 110 beats/min. Rhythm: regular. P-R interval: 0.16 second. Interpretation: sinus tachycardia. Distinguishing features: all features of normal sinus rhythm except that rate is greater than 100 beats/min. Treatment: stable—none; unstable—seek and treat underlying cause
(Objective 10)

45. QRS complex: 0.08 second; P waves: present, upright, similar. Rate: 70 beats/min. Rhythm: irregular. P-R interval: 0.12 second. Interpretation: sinus dysrhythmia. Distinguishing features: all features of normal sinus rhythm but irregular rhythm that varies in cycles. Treatment: none
(Objective 10)

46. QRS complex: 0.08 second. P waves: normal, upright. Rate: 50 beats/min. Rhythm: irregular. P-R interval: 0.16 second. Interpretation: sinus arrest. Distinguishing features: normal sinus rhythm until the sinoatrial node fails to fire. Treatment: stable—observe; unstable—atropine and transcutaneous pacing
(Objective 10)

47. a. Tissues; b. atria; c. internodal
(Objective 10)

48. a. QRS complex: normal
b. P waves (if present): different from normal sinus P waves
c. P-R interval: abnormal, shortened, or prolonged
(Objective 10)

49. Stress, overexertion, tobacco, caffeine, Wolff-Parkinson-White syndrome, digoxin toxicity, hypoxia, chronic obstructive pulmonary disease, congestive heart failure, damage to sinoatrial node, rheumatic heart disease, and atherosclerotic heart disease
(Objective 10)

50. QRS complex: 0.06 second. P waves: changes from beat to beat. Rate: 75 beats/min. Rhythm: regular. P-R interval: variable. Interpretation: wandering atrial pacemaker. Distinguishing features: typically slightly irregular P wave shapes and variable P-R interval. Treatment: stable—monitor; unstable following bradycardia—treat as bradycardia
(Objective 10)

51. QRS complex: 0.06 second. P waves: present, upright. Rate: 100 beats/min. Rhythm: regular interrupted by premature beats. P-R interval: 0.10 second (premature atrial contraction 0.16 second). Interpretation: normal sinus rhythm with one premature atrial contraction. Distinguishing features: extra beat occurring earlier than next expected sinus beat; premature atrial contraction has features of sinus beat except that P-R interval may be different. Treatment: none
(Objective 10)

52. QRS complex: 0.06 second. P waves: unable to determine, may be hidden in T wave. Rate: 180 beats/min. Rhythm: regular. P-R interval: unable to determine. Interpretation: supraventricular tachycardia. Distinguishing features: rate greater than 150 beats/min, with complexes originating in atria (QRS complex is <0.12 second unless a conduction defect is present.) Treatment: stable—oxygen, intravenous line, 12-lead electrocardiogram, consideration of vagal maneuvers, adenosine (6 mg, 12 mg, 12 mg rapid intravenous push at 1- to 2-minute intervals), diltiazem or verapamil or beta-blockers, consider digoxin (Class IIb); unstable—synchronized cardioversion at 50, 100, 200, 300, and 360 J
(Objective 10)

53. QRS complex: 0.06 second. P waves: f-R waves. Rate: 100 beats/min. Rhythm: regular. P-R interval: none. F-R interval: may vary. Interpretation: atrial flutter with 3:1 conduction. Distinguishing features: flutter waves. Treatment: stable—(usually no treatment prehospital); with tachycardic rate—diltiazem or verapamil or beta-blockers or digoxin to control rate; if impaired cardiac function is present—diltiazem or amiodarone or digoxin; unstable—synchronized cardioversion at 50, 100, 200, 300, and 360 J
(Objective 10)

54. QRS complex: 0.06 second. P waves: none. Rate: 160 beats/min. Rhythm: irregularly irregular. P-R interval: none. Interpretation: atrial fibrillation. Distinguishing features: irregularly irregular, no P waves, fibrillation waves. Treatment: calcium channel or beta-blocker; impaired cardiac function—diltiazem or amiodarone; acute and associated with serious signs or symptoms—synchronized cardioversion at 100, 200, 300, and 360 J
(Objective 10)

55. a. junctional (nodal); b. normal; c. may occur before, during, or after QRS complex or may be absent; inverted in lead II; d. often less than 0.12 second
(Objective 10)

56. Increased vagal tone on sinoatrial node, pathological slowing of sinoatrial discharge, complete atrioventricular block, digitalis toxicity, damage to the atrioventricular junction, inferior wall myocardial infarction, and rheumatic fever
(Objective 10)

57. QRS complex: 0.08 second. P waves: present, upright, similar in underlying rhythm, absent in premature beats. Rate: 60 beats/min. Rhythm: irregular. P-R interval: 0.16 second (underlying rhythm), none in premature beats. Interpretation: sinus rhythm (borderline bradycardia) with two premature junctional contractions. Distinguishing features: premature beats occurring earlier than next expected sinus beat, lack of P waves, QRS complex within normal limits. Treatment: monitor patient and treat bradycardia if present and symptomatic. (Objective 10)

58. QRS complex: 0.08 second. P waves: absent. Rate: 40 beats/min. Rhythm: regular. P-R interval: none. Interpretation: junctional escape rhythm. Distinguishing features: rate 40 to 60 beats/min, inverted P waves if present (may occur before, during [absent], or after QRS complex). Treatment: stable—monitor; unstable— atropine 0.5 to 1.0 mg every 5 minutes to total dose of 2.5 mg (0.03 to 0.04 mg/kg), transcutaneous pacing, dopamine 5 to 20 mcg/kg/min, epinephrine 2 to 10 mcg/min, and isoproterenol 2 to 10 mcg/min (Objective 10)

59. QRS complex: 0.08 second. P waves: absent. Rate: 80 beats/min. Rhythm: regular. P-R interval: none. Interpretation: accelerated junctional rhythm. Distinguishing features: rate 60 to 100 beats/min, inverted P waves in lead II if present (may be absent or occur before, during, or after QRS complex). Treatment: monitor. (Objective 10)

60. a. 20, 40; b. 100 beats/min; c. 100 beats/min (Objective 10)

61. Failure of higher pacemakers, heart block, myocardial ischemia, hypoxia, acid-base or electrolyte imbalance, congestive heart failure, increased catecholamine levels, use of stimulants, medicine toxicity (digitalis, tricyclic antidepressant overdose), sympathomimetic drugs, cardiac trauma, and electrical injury (Objective 10)

62. If unstable, all rhythms need cardioversion. If stable, the following:
a. Assess leads I, II, III, MCL_1 (V_1), and MCL_6 (V_6) to determine axis deviation. If the QRS complex is negative in leads I, II, and III (extreme right axis or "no-man's land") and positive in MCL_1 (V_1), the rhythm is ventricular tachycardia; if not,
b. Assess the QRS deflection in MCL_1 (V_1) and MCL_6 (V_6). Positive QRS deflections with a single peak, a taller left rabbit ear, or an RS complex with a fat r wave or slurred s wave in MCL_1 (V_1) indicates ventricular tachycardia. A negative QS complex, a negative rS complex, or any wide Q wave in MCL_6 (V_6) also indicates ventricular tachycardia.
c. If right axis deviation is present (negative QRS complex in lead I; positive QRS complex in leads II and III) and the QRS complex is negative in MCL_1 (V_1), it indicates ventricular tachycardia.
d. If all precordial (V) leads are positive or negative (precordial concordance), it indicates ventricular tachycardia.
e. If the RS interval is greater than 0.10 second in any V lead, it indicates ventricular tachycardia.
(Objective 10)

63. QRS complex: 0.16 second. P waves: absent. Rate: 40 beats/min. Rhythm: regular. P-R interval: none. Interpretation: ventricular escape rhythm. Distinguishing features: rate 20 to 40 beats/min, absent P waves, QRS complex greater than 0.12 second. Treatment: oxygen, transcutaneous pacing, dopamine 5 to 20 mcg/kg/min, epinephrine 2 to 10 mcg/min, and isoproterenol 2 to 10 mcg/min (Objective 10)

64. QRS complex: underlying rhythm 0.10 second. Premature beat: 0.16 second. P wave: present, upright (except premature beat). Rate: 75 beats/min. Rhythm: regular interrupted by premature beats. P-R interval: 0.16 second (underlying rhythm). None: premature beat. Interpretation: normal sinus rhythm with one premature ventricular contraction. Distinguishing features: ectopic beat occurs earlier than next expected sinus beat, wide bizarre QRS complex with T wave deflection opposite QRS complex, no P waves, compensatory pause. Treatment: in presence of hemodynamically compromising premature ventricular contractions—oxygen, lidocaine 1.0 to 1.5 mg/kg repeated at 0.5- to 0.75-mg/kg doses to a maximum of 3 mg/kg (Objective 10)

65. QRS complex: 0.20 second. P waves: absent. Rate: 230 beats/min. Rhythm: regular. P-R interval: none. Interpretation: monomorphic ventricular tachycardia. Distinguishing features: rate greater than 100 beats/min (usually greater than 150 beats/min), regular, no P waves, QRS complex equal to or greater than 0.12 second. Treatment: stable—oxygen, procainamide or sotalol or amiodarone or lidocaine; impaired cardiac function—amiodarone or lidocaine; unstable—synchronized cardioversion at 100, 200, 300, and 360 J; or unconsciousness, hypotension, or pulmonary edema—defibrillate at 100, 200, 300, and 360 J or equivalent biphasic energy; pulseless—treat as ventricular fibrillation
(Objective 10)

66. QRS complex: none. P waves: none. Rate: none. Rhythm: none, chaotic. P-R interval: none. Interpretation: ventricular fibrillation. Distinguishing features: no organized rhythm, chaotic fibrillatory waves. Treatment: rapid defibrillation at 200, 300, and 360 J or equivalent biphasic energy, cardiopulmonary resuscitation, intubation, epinephrine or vasopressin, amiodarone or lidocaine, magnesium sulfate, and procainamide; consider sodium bicarbonate
(Objective 10)

67. QRS complex: none. P waves: none. Rate: none. Rhythm: none. P-R interval: none. Interpretation: asystole. Distinguishing features: isoelectric rhythm. Treatment: cardiopulmonary resuscitation, transcutaneous pacing, epinephrine, atropine, and consideration of underlying cause
(Objective 10)

68. QRS complex: 0.16 second. P waves: absent. Rate: 80 beats/min. Rhythm: regular. P-R interval: none. Interpretation: ventricular paced rhythm. Distinguishing features: pacemaker spike followed by wide-complex ventricular beat. Treatment: none
(Objective 10)

69. a. Heart blocks; b. conduction system
(Objective 10)

70. Myocardial ischemia, acute myocardial infarction, increased parasympathetic tone, drug toxicity (digitalis, propranolol, verapamil), and electrolyte imbalance
(Objective 10)

71. QRS complex: 0.06 second. P waves: present, upright. Rate: 60 beats/min. Rhythm: regular. P-R interval: 0.32 second. Interpretation: sinus rhythm with first-degree atrioventricular block. Distinguishing features: P-R interval greater than 0.20 second. Treatment: observe.
(Objective 10)

72. QRS complex: 0.08 second. P waves: present, upright, more P waves than QRS complexes. Rate: 60 beats/min. Rhythm: irregular. P-R interval: progressively longer until one is not conducted. Distinguishing features: more P waves than QRS complexes, progressively lengthens P-R interval until a QRS complex is dropped. Interpretation: second-degree atrioventricular block (Mobitz type I or Wenckebach). Treatment: asymptomatic—observe; if bradycardic with hemodynamic compromise—oxygen, atropine, transcutaneous pacing, dopamine, epinephrine, and isoproterenol
(Objective 10)

73. QRS complex: 0.06 second. P waves: present, upright, more P waves than QRS complexes. Rate: 50 beats/min. Rhythm: irregular. P-R interval: 0.16 second for conducted P waves. Interpretation: second-degree atrioventricular block (Mobitz type II). Treatment: stable—transport for transvenous pacemaker insertion; unstable—oxygen, transcutaneous pacing, dopamine, epinephrine, and isoproterenol
(Objective 10)

74. QRS complex: 0.08 second. P waves: present, upright. Rate: 50 beats/min. Rhythm: regular. P-R interval: no relationship between P waves and QRS complexes. Interpretation: third-degree (complete) atrioventricular block. Distinguishing features: R-R interval usually regular, more P waves than QRS complexes, no relationship

between P waves and QRS complex. Treatment: stable—monitor and transport for transvenous pacemaker insertion; unstable—oxygen, transcutaneous pacing, atropine 0.5 to 1.0 mg (maximum dose 0.04 mg/kg), dopamine 5 to 20 mcg/kg/min, epinephrine 2 to 10 mcg/min, and isoproterenol 2 to 10 mcg/min
(Objective 10)

75. a. QRS complex equal to or greater than 0.12 second. QRS complexes produced by supraventricular activity. RSR prime pattern. In V_1, line drawn backward from the J point into the QRS makes a triangle pointing up.
b. QRS complex less than 0.12 second. QRS complexes produced by supraventricular activity. QS pattern. In V_1, line drawn backward from J point into the QRS makes a triangle pointing down
c. QRS complex less than 0.12 second. QRS complexes produced by supraventricular activity and pathological left axis deviation. A small Q wave followed by a tall R wave in lead I, and a small R wave followed by a deep S wave in lead III
d. Right axis deviation with a normal QRS complex
(Objective 10)

76. a. Any patient with type II atrioventricular block
b. Any patient with evidence of disease of both bundle branches
c. Any patient with two or more blocks of any kind
(Objective 10)

77. a. Pulseless electrical activity (the patient has a rhythm but no perfusing pulse.)
b. Cardiopulmonary resuscitation, intubation, intravenous therapy, epinephrine 1.0 mg every 3 to 5 minutes or one dose of vasopressin 40 u IV/10 to replace first or second dose of epinephrine; consideration of causes (hypovolemia, pulmonary embolus, acidosis, trauma, tension pneumothorax, cardiac tamponade, hypoxia, hypothermia, hypoglycemia, hypokalemia or hyperkalemia, massive myocardial infarction, drug overdose) and treatment if causes are found; if rate is slow, administer atropine 1 mg every 3 to 5 minutes to a maximum dose of 0.04 mg/kg.
(Objective 10)

78. a. QRS normal or wide. Delta wave and onset of QRS complex are slurred or notched
b. P-R interval is usually less than 0.12 second.
(Objective 10)

79. Patients with Wolff-Parkinson-White syndrome are susceptible to paroxysmal supraventricular tachycardias. Verapamil is contraindicated because it may cause rapid atrial to ventricular conduction and lead to ventricular fibrillation and sudden death.
(Objective 10)

80. Atherosclerosis is a process that progressively narrows the lumen of medium and large arteries. Thick, hard atherosclerotic plaques called *atheromata* form especially in areas of turbulent blood flow. The plaques are thought to be an endothelial cell response to chronic mechanical or chemical injury. The response includes platelet adhesion and aggregation and proliferation and migration of smooth muscle cells from the media into the intima. Eventually the atheromata become fibrotic and calcified and partially or totally obstruct the involved arteries. The two major effects are (1) disruption of the intimal surface causing a loss of vessel elasticity and an increase in thrombogenesis and (2) a reduction in the diameter of the vessel lumen with resulting decreased blood supply to tissues.
(Objective 11)

81. a. Physical exertion; b. emotional stress
(Objective 11)

82. a. Angina typically lasts 1 to 5 minutes but may last as long as 15 minutes.
b. Relieved by rest, nitroglycerin, or oxygen
(Objective 11)

83. Unless 12-lead electrocardiogram interpretation is available, it is impossible to distinguish between these two conditions in the field. Even a negative 12-lead electrocardiogram does not exclude acute myocardial infarction. Serial cardiac enzyme tests and electrocardiograms and other tests such as echocardiograms and stress tests may be needed. Both patients should be managed as though they are having a myocardial infarction (excluding thrombolytic therapy).
(Objective 11)

84. Atherosclerotic plaque forms in coronary artery; plaque ruptures; platelets adhere to it, and then thrombus forms on the plaque; as thrombus enlarges, it occludes the coronary artery. (Other causes are coronary vasospasm, coronary embolism, severe hypoxia, hemorrhage into diseased arterial wall, and shock.)
(Objective 11)

85.

Area of Heart Injured or Infarcted	Coronary Vessel Involved Most Often	Leads with Visible ST Segment Changes
Anterior	Left coronary	V_3, V_4
Lateral	Left coronary	V_5, V_6, I, aV_L
Septal	Left coronary	V_1, V_2
Inferior	Right coronary	II, III, aV_F

(Objective 11)

86. a. 0.1 mV in at least two contiguous precordial leads or two or more limb leads.
(Objective 11)

87. Left bundle branch block, some ventricular rhythms, left ventricular hypertrophy, pericarditis, ventricular aneurysm, and early repolarization
(Objective 11)

88. a. Identify rate and rhythm; b. Identify the area of infarct; c. Consider miscellaneous conditions; d. Assess the patient's clinical presentation; e. Recognize the infarction and initiate treatment.
(Objective 11)

89. Lethal dysrhythmias, congestive heart failure, pulmonary edema, cardiogenic shock, and myocardial tissue rupture.
(Objective 11)

90. Nausea; vomiting; diaphoresis; radiation of pain to the neck, jaw, left arm, or back; palpitations; dyspnea; pulmonary edema; hypotension; and a sense of impending doom.
(Objective 11)

91. ST segment elevation in leads V_2, V_3, and V_4. Possible acute anterior myocardial infarction.
(Objective 11)

92. Administer oxygen via nasal cannula, minimize physical activity, monitor electrocardiogram and oxygen saturation (if pulse oximetry is available), assess vital signs frequently (including lung sounds for crackles), and establish an intravenous line to keep the vein open with normal saline or lactated Ringer's solution.
(Objective 11)

93. Aspirin 162 to 325 mg chewed; nitroglycerin 0.4 mg sublingually, repeated 2 times; morphine sulfate 2 to 4 mg intravenously titrated to relieve pain
(Objective 11)

94. a. Patient is alert and able to give informed consent; chest pain or symptoms of acute myocardial infarction for at least 15 minutes and less than 12 hours; electrocardiogram changes consistent with an ST segment elevation myocardial infarction or new LBBB; chest pain and electrocardiogram changes that persist after the administration of sublingual nitroglycerin.

b. SBP >180 mmHg; DBP >110 mm Hg; right vs. left arm systolic BP difference >15 mm Hg; structural CNS disease; CHI within 3 months; major trauma, surgery, GI/GU bleed within <6 weeks; takes blood thinners or has bleeding problems; CPR >10 min; pregnancy; advanced diseases of the liver or kidney or advanced cancer. (Objective 11)

c. HR > 100 bpm and BP < 100 mm Hg; pulmonary edema (rales); or signs of shock (cool, clammy).

95. a. Normal axis; no ST segment elevation, depression. Normal 12-lead electrocardiogram

b. QRS 0.14 second. Pathologic left axis deviation. Left bundle branch block. Cannot detect ST segment elevation in the presence of left bundle branch block

c. Normal axis; ST segment elevation leads II, III, aV_F. ST segment depression in leads aV_L, V_2, V_3, V_4, V_5. Possible inferior myocardial infarction

d. Normal axis; ST segment elevation leads I, aV_L, V_2, V_3, V_4, V_5, V_6. Extensive anterior myocardial infarction

96. There is a pathological left axis deviation. QRS is upright in lead I and down in leads II and III. (Objective 10)

97. The triangle should point upward. (Objective 8)

98. The patient has a left anterior hemiblock (pathological left axis deviation) and a right bundle branch block (QRS >0.12 second and upward triangle). (Objective 10)

99. The presence of more than one block is known as *bifascicular block* and is associated with a high risk of advancement to complete heart block and increased mortality in the presence of myocardial infarction. This patient's symptoms suggest the potential for myocardial infarction. (Objective 10)

100. The potential for serious rhythm deterioration should be anticipated. Prophylactic application of defibrillation or pacing pads in this setting may be indicated based on local protocol. (Objective 10)

101. Left ventricular failure leading to pulmonary edema and possible myocardial infarction (Objective 11)

102. Pulmonary edema: orthopnea and frothy, blood-tinged sputum. Myocardial infarction: chest pain, radiation of pain, nausea, and vomiting (Objective 11)

103. Sinus tachycardia (Objective 10)

104.

Drug	Dose	Desired Effect
a. Furosemide	0.5 to 1.0 mg/kg intravenously	Venodilation and diuresis
b. Morphine	2 to 4 mg intravenously	Venodilation, decreased myocardial work, and decreased anxiety
c. Nitroglycerin	0.4 mg sublingually	Peripheral vasodilation and decreased preload and afterload

(Objectives 11 and 13)

105. 3.5 (Objective 13)

106. a. Left ventricular failure, pulmonary embolism, right ventricle infarct, chronic hypertension, chronic obstructive pulmonary disease, and valvular disease

b. Jugular venous distention, tachycardia, enlarged liver or spleen, peripheral and sacral edema, and ascites

(Objective 11)

107. Sinus bradycardia
(Objective 10)

108. Administer oxygen by non-rebreather mask, and give atropine 0.5 mg intravenously.
(Objectives 10 and 13)

109. Cardiogenic shock
(Objective 11)

110. High-flow oxygen by non-rebreather mask; supine position (if tolerated); intravenous therapy with normal saline—consider fluid challenge (250 to 500 mL); dopamine infusion via intravenous piggyback 5 to 15 mcg/kg/min; (remove nitroglycerin paste and wipe chest with gauze); obtain 12-lead ECG and monitor electrocardiogram for dysrhythmias.
(Objective 11)

111. Expanding or ruptured abdominal aortic aneurysm
(Objective 11)

112. Palpation in this situation could cause a bulging aneurysm to rupture. If medical direction advises palpation, it should be done gently.
(Objective 11)

113. No. Increased intraabdominal pressure could cause rupture of the aneurysm.
(Objective 11)

114. Administer oxygen, transport rapidly, apply pneumatic antishock garments (if available and indicated by protocol) but do not inflate unless the patient's condition deteriorates, initiate two large-bore intravenous lines en route and infuse normal saline or lactated Ringer's solution to keep the vein open unless the patient's condition deteriorates.
(Objective 11)

115. Dissecting thoracic aortic aneurysm
(Objective 11)

116. Unequal peripheral pulses, neurological deficit, or signs of pericardial tamponade
(Objective 11)

117. Minimize movement and anxiety, administer high-concentration oxygen, initiate a 14- or 16-gauge intravenous line in arm with good pulses (higher blood pressure) to keep the vein open, and monitor vital signs and the electrocardiogram frequently.
(Objective 11)

118.

	Embolic	**Thrombotic**
Causes	Clot breaks loose and travels to narrow area in blood vessel	Clot develops at narrow spot in blood vessel
Onset	Rapid	Gradual

	Embolic	**Thrombotic**
Signs and symptoms	Pulseless extremity pain; decreased motor and sensory function; pallor; cool skin temperature distal to the occlusion; decreased capillary refill; possible shock	Pain in hips, lower limbs, buttocks, leg, and abdomen (depends on affected artery); pain; delayed motor and sensory function; pallor; decreased skin temperature distal to the occlusion; decreased CR; possible shock

(Objective 11)

119. Control bleeding with direct pressure and elevation. The bleeding may be persistent and require hospital management.
(Objective 11)

120. Pain, edema, warmth, erythema, tenderness, and a palpable cord
(Objective 11)

121. Hypertensive encephalopathy
(Objective 11)

122. Aphasia, hemiparesis, transient blindness, seizures, stupor, coma, and death
(Objective 11)

123. Calm patient, apply oxygen, and insert intravenous line to keep the vein open; monitor electrocardiogram; and transport rapidly.

124. Nitroglycerin paste. Labetalol 10 to 20 mg intravenously over 1 to 2 minutes
(Objective 13)

125. Determine unresponsiveness; call for help if no one else is available; open the airway; look, listen, and feel for breathing; if there is none, deliver two slow rescue breaths; assess carotid pulse; if there is none, begin cardiopulmonary resuscitation until help arrives (30 compressions: 2 ventilations).
(Objective 12)

126. a. After CPR intubation, intravenous therapy, and the first dose of epinephrine
   b. Yes. Electric shock resulting in injury or death can occur.
   (Objective 12)

127. Ventricular tachycardia (monomorphic)
(Objective 10)

128. Defibrillate (biphasic 120-200J; monophasic 360J) and then reassess the rhythm and pulse.
(Objective 12)

129. Amount of time patient has been in pulseless ventricular tachycardia, quality of bystander CPR, and proper paddle placement
(Objective 12)

130. Apply conductive gel on the patient's chest (or hands-off defibrillation patches); turn on power (there is a separate power source for the defibrillator and monitor with some monitors); select correct energy level; place paddles (or patches) in an appropriate position on the patient's chest; charge the defibrillator; call "clear" and visually check to ensure that no one is in contact with the patient or cot; lean firmly on paddles (if used) with 20 to 25 lb of pressure; discharge both paddle buttons simultaneously (or depress discharge button on monitor for hands-off defibrillator); and resume chest compressions.
(Objective 12)

131. Synchronized cardioversion at 100, 200, 300, and 360 J (or equivalent biphasic).
(Objective 12)

132. It is synchronized with the patient's heartbeat so there is less risk of firing on the relative refractory period and causing ventricular fibrillation.
(Objective 12)

133. Depress the synchronize button before each synchronized shock. If paddles are used, hold the paddles firmly on the chest after activation until they discharge. Ensure monitor is marking QRS complexes.
(Objective 12)

134. a. Third-degree atrioventricular block
b. Apply oxygen and inform the patient that he may feel some discomfort; apply the pacing and monitoring pads; ensure adequate upright R wave on monitor; select pacing mode; select pacing rate (70 to 80 beats/min); set current at 50 mA and slowly increase until capture is observed; reassess patient's vital signs (use right arm for blood pressure); and document and obtain rhythm strips.
(Objective 12)

135. a. Asystole; b. epinephrine 1.0 mg every 3 to 5 minutes and atropine 1 mg every 5 minutes until a maximum dose of 0.04 mg/kg is reached; c. transcutaneous pacing
(Objectives 10 and 12)

136. a. Ventricular fibrillation; b. defibrillation; c. epinephrine 1.0 mg every 3 to 5 minutes or 1 dose vasopressin 40 U (to replace first or second epinephrine dose) intravenous bolus, amiodarone 300 mg intravenous bolus diluted in 20 to 30 mL of NS or D_5W, or lidocaine 1 to 1.5 mg/kg intravenously
(Objectives 10 and 13)

137. a. Stop resuscitation if your protocols allow. Patient is older than 18 years and unresponsive to treatment.
b. Do not stop resuscitation. Patient is older than 18 years. Patient may be hypothermic. Transport and continue resuscitation.
c. Do not stop resuscitation. Patient is younger than 18 years and has sustained trauma, and you were able to get back a perfusing pulse during the resuscitation.
d. Consult with medical direction before you stop resuscitation. The patient has met criteria for resuscitation; however, the family objects strongly, so medical oversight may advise that efforts should continue.
(Objective 14)

138. d. His identified risk factors are male sex, age, hypercholesterolemia, diabetes, and hypertension (Acupril is an angiotensin-converting enzyme inhibitor, and indapamide is a diuretic).
(Objective 1)

139. c. Blood pressure = Cardiac output × Peripheral vascular resistance.
(Objective 1)

140. c. The circumflex supplies the lateral and posterior portions of the left ventricle and part of the right ventricle. The right coronary artery and the left anterior descending supply most of the right atrium and ventricle and the inferior aspect of the left ventricle.
(Objective 2)

141. b. The aortic valve separates the aorta and left ventricle, the pulmonic valve separates the pulmonary arteries and right ventricle, and the tricuspid valve separates the right atrium and right ventricle.
(Objective 2)

142. d. The electrical charge is the potential difference and is measured in millivolts. Depolarization (electrical conduction) occurs when sodium rushes into the cell, altering the electrical balance.
(Objective 3)

143. c. Potassium is also essential.
(Objective 3)

144. d. Calcium channel blockers selectively block the slow channel and alter the threshold level.
(Objective 3)

145. a. Phase 0 is the rapid depolarization phase; phase 1 is the early rapid depolarization phase; phase 2 is the plateau phase; phase 3 is the terminal phase of rapid repolarization; and phase 4 is the period between action potentials.
(Objective 3)

146. c. This allows complete relaxation of the cardiac muscle before another contraction can be initiated.
(Objective 3)

147. d. The His bundle divides into the right and left bundle branches. The left bundle divides into the anterior and posterior fascicles. A third fascicle of the left bundle branch that innervates the interventricular septum and the base of the heart also has been identified. The bundle branches subdivide and become Purkinje fibers.
(Objective 4)

148. d. The resting membrane potential gradually decreases with time until it reaches a critical threshold, at which time depolarization results.
(Objective 4)

149. c. This pause allows the atria to finish contraction and empty before ventricular contraction occurs.
(Objective 4)

150. a. Acetylcholine causes the cell membrane of the sinoatrial node to become hyperpolarized, causing a delay in reaching threshold, and therefore it decreases the heart rate. All other answers increase heart rate.
(Objective 4)

151. d. The other answers represent causes of dysrhythmias that result from enhanced automaticity.
(Objective 4)

152. a. Mental status change, abdominal or gastrointestinal complaints, or vague complaints of ill-being may be presenting symptoms in an older adult patient with a coronary event.
(Objective 5)

153. d. If the heart is unable to pump effectively, blood will back up into the lungs, causing decreased diffusion of gases in the lungs and dyspnea.
(Objective 5)

154. b. Younger patients may experience syncope because of increased vagal tone. Nausea or syncope when standing does not predict the incidence of dysrhythmias.
(Objective 5)

155. b
(Objective 5)

156. c. Peripheral pulses and perfusion would be used to assess strength of myocardial contractions. Placement of patches usually is performed using ribs and gross anatomy.
(Objective 5)

157. b. The electrocardiogram does not measure mechanical events.
(Objective 7)

158. c. The others are unipolar leads (a single positive electrode and a reference point).
(Objective 6)

159. d. If the depolarization moves toward a positive electrode, the tracing should show an upward deflection.
(Objective 6)

160. b. These leads all look up onto the inferior portion of the heart.
(Objective 6)

161. d. These leads may help distinguish between supraventricular tachycardia with aberration and ventricular tachycardia and can help diagnose bundle branch blocks.
(Objective 6)

162. c. The negative lead is placed at the lateral end of the left clavicle. The positive lead for MCL_6 is placed on the left axillary line at the level of the fifth intercostal space.
(Objective 6)

163. a. Many dysrhythmias involve abnormalities of the P wave.
(Objective 6)

164. b. V_3 and V_4 are anterior leads, and V_5 and V_6 are lateral precordial leads.
(Objective 6)

165. a. This is used as the baseline.
(Objective 7)

166. b
(Objective 4)

167. c. The relative refractory period is from the peak of the T wave onward.
(Objective 7)

168. b. In some leads, part of the QRS complex is blended with the baseline and is difficult to measure.
(Objective 8)

169. d. $1500 \div 10 = 150$ beats/min
(Objective 8)

170. b
(Objective 10)

171. c
(Objective 10)

172. c
(Objective 10)

173. a
(Objective 10)

174. b
(Objective 10)

175. d
(Objective 10)

176. a
(Objective 10)

177. d. Adenosine is not indicated for atrial fibrillation, and verapamil is not indicated when a patient is hypotensive. The patient needs electrical cardioversion because her condition is unstable. Procainamide is indicated for ventricular dysrhythmias.
(Objective 10)

178. a. It originates from tissue other than an intrinsic pacemaker.
(Objective 10)

179. c. Isoproterenol is a beta stimulant, so it will increase the heart rate.
(Objective 10)

180. d. The atria cannot contract to empty. This decreases the blood flow to the ventricles and the cardiac output.
(Objective 10)

181. a
(Objective 10)

182. d. It also is associated with excessive catecholamine administration, damage to the atrioventricular junction, inferior wall myocardial infarction, and rheumatic fever.
(Objective 10)

183. c. Other causes include failure of higher pacemakers to initiate impulses.
(Objective 10)

184. a. Couplets are two premature ventricular contractions in a row. An idioventricular rhythm originates in the ventricles and supersedes the underlying rhythm. Multifocal premature ventricular contractions have varied appearance depending on their site of origination.
(Objective 10)

185. a. Precordial concordance with all positive or all negative deflection in the V leads indicates ventricular tachycardia.
(Objective 10)

186. b. Asynchronous (fixed rate) pacemakers stimulate the heart at a set rate regardless of the action of the heart. A dual chamber pacemaker stimulates the atria and the ventricles.
(Objective 10)

187. d. Bundle branch block occurs when one of the bundles of His is blocked. Second-degree atrioventricular block type II is an intermittent block.
(Objective 10)

188. d. It yields an initial Q wave in MCL_1 (V_1) instead of the normal small R wave. There will be a deep QS pattern that is at least 0.12 second.
(Objective 10)

189. b. The blockage of two of the three pathways for ventricular consduction (right bundle branch block with anterior or posterior hemiblock, and left bundle branch block) poses the greatest risk.
(Objective 10)

190. d. Diltiazem may cause rapid atrial to ventricular conduction down the accessory pathway and may lead to ventricular fibrillation and sudden death.
(Objective 10)

191. c. Both have the same cause.
(Objective 11)

192. a. Hypotension caused by pump failure and cardiac rupture can occur but is much less common than lethal dysrhythmias.
(Objective 11)

193. b. A small fluid challenge (250 mL) may be given to a patient with cardiac disease who is hypotensive; however, in the normotensive patient, intravenous fluids should be infused to keep the vein open.
(Objective 11)

194. b. Deep inverted T waves may be present in acute myocardial infarction.
(Objective 11)

195. a. Epinephrine will increase the work, and oxygen demands on the heart precipitate lethal dysrhythmias in this patient.
(Objectives 11 and 13)

196. d. Signs include jugular venous distention and peripheral edema.
(Objective 11)

197. b. Cardiogenic shock is fatal in up to 70% to 80% of patients.
(Objective 11)

198. b. Decreased systolic pressure is a later sign. Muffled heart sounds are associated with this. Tracheal deviation is seen in tension pneumothorax.
(Objective 11)

199. b. The pain often is described as ripping or tearing and is high intensity.
(Objective 11)

200. a
(Objective 11)

201. c
(Objective 11)

202. b. The patient with diabetes is at higher risk for heart disease; however, hypertension does not precipitate diabetes.
(Objective 11)

203. d. The goal is to "push hard and push fast" when performing CPR.
(Objective 12)

204. b. Lower energy levels may be used. Energy flow is bidirectional. Battery size is not affected.
(Objective 12)

205. b. Anterior-posterior placement is not practical for paddle use. Avoid placing the patch or paddle over the sternum because bone is a poor conductor of electricity. Pediatric paddles are indicated for children under 1 year of age.
(Objective 12)

206. b. The implantable cardioverter defibrillator sequence includes up to five shocks in 2 minutes. There is no danger in touching the patients. Strong magnets may inactivate the device.
(Objective 12)

207. d
(Objective 14)

208. b
(Objective 14)

209. b
(Objective 13)

210. b. Inferior wall infarcts often occur with right ventricular infarcts. These make the heart preload dependent. Administer the fluid, then obtain a right-sided ECG.
(Objective 13)

211. a. Morphine will decrease the preload. It is contraindicated in the patient with head injury. It does not cause bronchodilation.
(Objective 13)

212. a
(Objective 13)

213. c
(Objective 13)

214. c. The correct dose is 2 to 10 mcg/min (not mcg/kg/min).
(Objective 13)

215. a. None of the other criteria should be used alone to evaluate whether resuscitation should be stopped.
(Objective 14)

WRAP IT UP

1. a, b, c, d, e, f
(Objective 11)

2. Ventricular fibrillation and ventricular tachycardia are the only two rhythms that will advise a shock on an automated external defibrillator.
(Objective 12)

3. Lidocaine or amiodarone
(Objective 13)

4. ST segment elevation in leads V_1 to V_4 would indicate septal and anterior myocardial infarction.
(Objective 10)

5. Left coronary
(Objective 10)

6. a. The other risk factors mentioned would be absolute contraindications.
(Objective 13)

7. 10-12 breaths/min. 6-7 mL/kg volume.
(Objective 12)

PART EIGHT

IN THIS PART

Pulmonary Emergencies

READING ASSIGNMENT
Chapter 30, pages 816-835, in *Mosby's Paramedic Textbook,* ed. 3

OBJECTIVES
Upon completion of this chapter, the paramedic student will be able to:
1. Distinguish the pathophysiology of respiratory emergencies related to ventilation, diffusion, and perfusion.
2. Describe the causes, complications, signs and symptoms, and prehospital management of patients diagnosed with obstructive airway disease, pneumonia, adult respiratory distress syndrome, pulmonary thromboembolism, upper respiratory infection, spontaneous pneumothorax, hyperventilation syndrome, and lung cancer.

SUMMARY
- Diseases responsible for respiratory emergencies include those related to ventilation, diffusion, and perfusion.
- Obstructive airway disease is a triad of distinct diseases that often coexist. These are chronic bronchitis, emphysema, and asthma. The patient with chronic obstructive pulmonary disease usually has an acute episode of worsening dyspnea that is manifested even at rest, an increase or change in sputum production, or an increase in the malaise that accompanies the disease. The main goal of prehospital care for these patients is the correction of hypoxemia through improved air flow.
- Asthma, or reactive airway disease, is characterized by reversible airflow obstruction caused by bronchial smooth muscle contraction; hypersecretion of mucus, resulting in bronchial plugging; and inflammatory changes in the bronchial walls. The typical patient with asthma is in obvious distress. Respirations are rapid and loud. Initial medications in the prehospital setting probably will have a short onset of action.
- Pneumonia is a group of specific infections (bacterial, viral, or fungal). These infections cause an acute inflammatory process of the respiratory bronchioles and the alveoli. Pneumonia usually manifests with classic signs and symptoms. These include a productive cough and associated fever that produces "shaking chills." Prehospital care of patients with pneumonia includes airway support, oxygen administration, ventilatory assistance as needed, IV fluids, cardiac monitoring, and transport.
- Adult respiratory distress syndrome is a fulminant form of respiratory failure. It is characterized by acute lung inflammation and diffuse alveolar-capillary injury. It develops as a complication of illness or injury. In ARDS, the lungs are wet and heavy, congested, hemorrhagic, and stiff, with decreased perfusion capacity across alveolar membranes and includes airway and ventilatory support.
- Pulmonary thromboembolism is a blockage of a pulmonary artery by a clot or other foreign material. When one or more pulmonary arteries are blocked by an embolism, a section of lung is ventilated but hypoperfused.

Prehospital care is mainly supportive and includes oxygen administration, IV access, and transport for definitive care.

- Upper respiratory infections affect the nose, throat, sinuses, and larynx. Signs and symptoms of a URI include sore throat, fever, chills, headache, cervical adenopathy, and an erythematous pharynx. Prehospital care is based on the patient's symptoms.
- A primary spontaneous pneumothorax usually results when a subpleural bleb ruptures. This allows air to enter the pleural space from within the lung. Signs and symptoms include shortness of breath and chest pain that often are sudden in onset, pallor, diaphoresis, and tachypnea. Prehospital care is based on the patient's symptoms and degree of distress.
- Hyperventilation syndrome is abnormally deep or rapid breathing. This type of breathing results in an excessive loss of carbon dioxide. If the syndrome clearly is caused by anxiety, prehospital care is mainly supportive (i.e., calming measures and reassurance). The paramedic may suspect that the syndrome is a result of illness or drug ingestion. If this is the case, care may include oxygen administration and airway and ventilatory support.
- Lung cancer is an expression of the uncontrolled growth of abnormal cells. As the disease progresses, signs and symptoms may include cough, hemoptysis, dyspnea, hoarseness, and dysphagia. Prehospital management includes airway, ventilatory, and circulatory support.

REVIEW QUESTIONS

Match the description in column I with the correct noninfectious pulmonary disease in column II. Use each answer only once.

Column I

1. _____ Chronic production of excessive mucus, hypoxia, and inflammation of bronchi
2. _____ Pulmonary edema secondary to trauma, inhaled toxins, or metabolic disorders
3. _____ Condition caused by a rupture of a bleb in the lung
4. _____ Impaired oxygenation resulting from blockage of a pulmonary artery by a clot
5. _____ Bronchiolar smooth muscle spasm and excess mucus production caused by allergy
6. _____ Bacterial, viral, or fungal lung infection
7. _____ Uncontrolled abnormal cell growth in the lung
8. _____ Chronic disease that results in a decrease in the alveolar membrane surface area and polycythemia

Column II

a. Adult respiratory distress syndrome
b. Asthma
c. Chronic bronchitis
d. Emphysema
e. Lung cancer
f. Hyperventilation syndrome
g. Pneumonia
h. Pulmonary thromboembolism
i. Spontaneous pneumothorax

9. For each case below, identify whether the respiratory problem is related to ventilation, diffusion, or perfusion or is a combination of two or more of these factors.
   a. Your patient is found unconscious with a plastic bag over her head.
   b. A 26-year-old is found semiconscious with a respiratory rate of 8/min. Track marks are found on the arms, legs, and under the tongue.
   c. An elderly woman with a history of congestive heart failure is acutely dyspneic and cyanotic. She has crackles throughout her lungs and coughs up frothy, bloody sputum.
   d. A woman has experienced vaginal bleeding for 2 weeks. She has profound fatigue and shortness of breath.
   e. A 56-year-old is choking in a restaurant.
   f. Your patient delivered a baby yesterday and has severe chest pain and dyspnea and an Sao_2 of 89% on room air.
   g. An 88-year-old has a large flail segment of the right chest and is hypoxic.

Questions 10 to 12 pertain to the following case study:

You are dispatched to a call for "difficulty breathing." Dispatch tells you en route that the first responders report that the patient is in moderate respiratory distress.

10. What conditions come to mind en route to this call?

_____

11. What findings in your initial assessment would indicate life-threatening respiratory distress?

_____

12. What information should be gathered during the focused history and physical examination of this patient?

_____

_____

13. Differentiate the signs and symptoms of chronic bronchitis and emphysema.
   a. Chronic bronchitis:

_____

   b. Emphysema:

_____

Questions 14 to 16 pertain to the following case study:

> Your 65-year-old patient has a history of chronic bronchitis and emphysema. She states that she has become acutely short of breath today and cannot complete a sentence without gasping for air. Loud wheezing is audible without a stethoscope.

14. How much oxygen should you administer to this patient?_____

15. Name a drug other than oxygen that may be administered to alleviate this patient's dyspnea, if not contraindicated by the history or physical findings.

_____

16. Describe any additional patient care to be given en route to the hospital.

_____

_____

Questions 17 to 22 pertain to the following case study:

> You are called to a junior college to evaluate a 19-year-old who became acutely short of breath during a soccer game. He states that he has a history of asthma. On examination, you note inspiratory and expiratory wheezes throughout the lung fields. Vital signs are: BP, 130/80 mm Hg; pulse, 136/min; and respirations, 30/min. You also note a pulsus paradoxus of 30 mm Hg.

17. Describe the pathophysiological changes in the lungs that cause the patient's signs and symptoms.

_____

18. Why would you perform a peak expiratory flow rate measurement on this patient?

_____

19. Other than oxygen, what drug can be administered to treat this patient? Include the correct dose and route.

_____

20. Describe how you will reassess the patient after the medication has been administered and what you will find if the patient's condition is improving.

_____

21. If therapy is unsuccessful and the patient continues to deteriorate despite aggressive medication therapy, what condition might exist?

_____

22. What additional treatment measures will you use?

_____

23. You respond to a call for difficulty breathing. Your assessment reveals that the patient is wheezing. List one pathological cause of wheezes for each of the following:

  a. Upper airway obstruction:

_____

  b. Lower airway obstruction:

_____

  c. Trauma:

_____

  d. Alveolar pathology:

_____

  e. Interstitial space pathology:

_____

Questions 24 to 26 pertain to the following case study:

A physician calls 9-1-1 to have you transport a patient with a diagnosis of pneumonia from her office to the hospital.

24. List four types of pneumonia.

  a.

  b.

  c.

  d.

25. List the signs and symptoms that may be present if this patient has bacterial pneumonia.

_____

26. Describe the prehospital care of patients with known or suspected pneumonia.

_____

_____

27. You are transporting a 56-year-old man from a small rural hospital to a trauma center 70 miles away. Approximately 24 hours ago, he was involved in a head-on motor vehicle collision. He has been diagnosed with bilateral pulmonary contusions and two fractured ribs. Early in his care, he received a large volume of normal saline intravenously. He has been increasingly short of breath, was intubated before your arrival, and is very difficult to ventilate. Paralytic drugs and sedatives were administered immediately before your departure.

    a. What problem do you suspect?

_____

    b. Describe the measures you will use during transport to assess and care for this patient.

_____

28. List eight factors that increase the risk of pulmonary emboli.

    a.

    b.

    c.

    d.

    e.

    f.

    g.

    h.

29. List the signs and symptoms of pulmonary embolism.

_____

_____

30. List common characteristics of the patient who develops spontaneous pneumothorax.

_____

_____

STUDENT SELF-ASSESSMENT

31. Which of the following is an extrinsic factor associated with the development or exacerbation of respiratory disease?
    a. Cardiac or circulatory pathologies
    b. Smoking
    c. Genetic predisposition
    d. Stress
32. Which of the following is essential for normal ventilation to occur?
    a. Adequate blood volume
    b. Functional diaphragm and intercostal muscles
    c. Interstitial space that is not filled with fluid
    d. Pulmonary capillaries that are not occluded
33. Your patient has a chronic respiratory illness; she called you complaining of difficulty breathing. What is usually the most reliable indicator of the severity of the patient's present condition?
    a. One- or two-word dyspnea   **c.** Patient's description of severity
    b. Pallor and diaphoresis   **d.** Tachycardia
34. Which physical finding indicates chronic hypoxemia?
    a. Accessory muscle use   **c.** Clubbing
    b. Carpopedal spasm   **d.** Pursed-lip breathing

35. Which of the following distinguishes chronic bronchitis from both emphysema and asthma?
    a. Cough
    b. Excessive mucus production
    c. Resistance to air flow
    d. Wheezing
36. Which of the following is evidence of chronic emphysema on physical examination?
    a. Decreased anterior-posterior chest diameter
    b. Decreased capillary refill in the nail beds
    c. Diminished breath sounds throughout the lungs
    d. Decreased diastolic blood pressure
37. Pulmonary hypertension can lead to which of the following?
    a. Pulmonary edema
    b. Pulmonary embolism
    c. Renal failure
    d. Right heart failure
38. Signs and symptoms of an acute asthma attack result from all of the following except which one?
    a. Bronchial muscle contraction
    b. Bronchial inflammation
    c. Mucus hypersecretion
    d. Pulmonary hypertension
39. Which physical finding is the most serious when found in an asthma patient who appears to be having acute respiratory distress?
    a. Expiratory wheezing
    b. Inspiratory wheezing
    c. Silent chest (no wheezing)
    d. Wheezing audible with a stethoscope
40. Pharmacological therapy to treat wheezing in patients with bronchitis or asthma usually includes which of the following?
    a. Albuterol
    b. Aminophylline
    c. Epinephrine
    d. Isoproterenol
41. Which pulmonary function test may be used in the prehospital setting to evaluate the effectiveness of patient ventilation?
    a. Peak expiratory flow rate (PEFR)
    b. Residual capacity
    c. Tidal volume
    d. Vital capacity
42. The most effective preventive measure for bacterial pneumonia is
    a. Antibiotic therapy
    b. Patient positioning
    c. Strict isolation measures
    d. Vaccination
43. What is the most common factor associated with aspiration pneumonia?
    a. Age
    b. Airway pathology
    c. Decreased level of consciousness
    d. Drowning
44. Which of the following is true about adult respiratory distress syndrome regardless of the cause?
    a. Death always occurs as a result of this complication.
    b. Disseminated intravascular coagulation always occurs.
    c. Pneumonia will be a secondary complication.
    d. Pulmonary edema will result.
45. Which ventilation adjunct provides continuous positive airway pressure and may prevent the need for intubation if used successfully?
    a. Venturi mask
    b. BVM
    c. CPAP
    d. PEEP
46. The signs and symptoms of pulmonary embolus vary and are related primarily to
    a. The patient's age
    b. The cause of the embolus
    c. The origin of the embolus
    d. The size of the embolus
47. What is the most important action the paramedic can take to prevent the spread of upper respiratory infections?
    a. Obtain the appropriate immunizations
    b. Place a mask on the patient during transport
    c. Practice good hand washing techniques
    d. Wear a mask and goggles during patient care
48. Which of the following is associated with the development of spontaneous pneumothorax?
    a. Asthma
    b. Free-base cocaine use
    c. IV drug abuse
    d. Thromboembolus

49. Which of the following is *not* a cause of hyperventilation?
  a. Fever
  b. Narcotic overdose
  c. Hyperglycemia
  d. Hypoxia

50. What is the most common risk factor for lung cancer?
  a. Cigarette smoking
  b. Exposure to asbestos
  c. Exposure to coal products
  d. Exposure to ionizing radiation

WRAP IT UP

You know as you respond to a call for "difficulty breathing" that your patient is likely quite ill because the dispatcher has a pumper running the call with you. Your patient is a 74-year-old male with a history of asthma and chronic bronchitis. He is seated leaning forward in a tripod position, using pursed-lip breathing; his neck muscles strain with each breath; and he is able to say only two or three words at a time. His son tells you that his dad hasn't been feeling too good all week, and today he became much worse, developing a fever and coughing up green sputum flecked with blood. His home medicines include ipratropium (Atrovent), beclomethasone (Beclovent), Advair, Singulair, and albuterol.

The patient's skin is gray and wet, the radial pulse is rapid, and an initial oxygen saturation reading is 84% on room air. You pull up his shirt and listen to his lungs; they sound wet and noisy, with wheezes throughout but somewhat diminished in the left base, so you apply a nebulizer mask with albuterol 2.5 mg and set the oxygen at 7 L/min. In the ambulance, the ECG monitor shows sinus tachycardia at 120/min; the Sao_2 is 94% and BP is 164/90 mm Hg; his skin is now dry, and he is speaking a bit more clearly. You start an IV, administer methylprednisolone (125 mg IV), and administer oxygen by nasal cannula at 4 L/min. The patient is admitted with a diagnosis of left lower R lobe pneumonia. He returns home in 4 days.

1. Which of the following was likely the primary problem for this patient's acute hypoxia?
  a. Inadequate diffusion between alveoli and pulmonary capillaries
  b. Inadequate perfusion of blood through the pulmonary capillary bed
  c. Inadequate ventilation in and out of the lungs
  d. a and b
  e. a and c

2. Put a ✔ beside the signs or symptoms of life-threatening respiratory distress that this patient displayed.
  a. _____ Altered mental status
  b. _____ Severe cyanosis
  c. _____ Absent breath sounds
  d. _____ Audible stridor
  e. _____ One- or two-word dyspnea
  f. _____ Tachycardia
  g. _____ Pallor or diaphoresis
  h. _____ Accessory muscle use

3. Based on this patient's reported history, what would you anticipate?
  a. He normally produces very little sputum.
  b. A thin, pink appearance would be normal for him.
  c. Lung tissue is scarred and susceptible to infection.
  d. In the absence of disease, the Po_2 is normal.

4. Explain your rationale for administration of
  a. Albuterol

_____

  b. Methylprednisolone

_____

5. Why might levalbuterol be a better choice for this patient? _____

6. Which is true about pneumonia?
  a. It is always caused by a bacterial infection.
  b. Fever is always present.
  c. Antibiotic treatment always cures it.
  d. Inflammation of the alveoli interferes with gas exchange.

CHAPTER 30 ANSWERS

REVIEW QUESTIONS

1. c
2. a
3. i
4. h
5. b
6. g
7. e
8. d
(Questions 1-8: Objective 3)

9. a. This is a problem with diffusion, because insufficient oxygen is available to diffuse across the alveolar membrane into the capillaries.
b. This represents a problem with ventilation. The drugs may have depressed the central nervous system causing slower, shallower breathing.
c. This is likely to be related to a problem with diffusion from the fluid that has leaked into the interstitial spaces and with perfusion because the left side of the heart is not functioning well.
d. These symptoms are likely related to anemia, which causes a problem with perfusion such that oxygen cannot be carried to the tissues.
e. Airway obstruction creates a problem with ventilation.
f. These signs and symptoms suggest pulmonary embolism, which creates a problem with perfusion.
g. Flail chest is often accompanied by pulmonary contusion. This would create a problem with ventilation because of the mechanical disruption and diffusion related to the fluid in the pulmonary spaces.
(Objective 1)

10. Asthma, chronic obstructive pulmonary disease, heart failure, pulmonary edema, pulmonary embolism, bronchiolitis (infants), foreign body aspiration, toxic inhalation, pneumonia, spontaneous pneumothorax, hyperventilation syndrome, or lung cancer are some of the conditions that may present with this chief complaint.
(Objective 2)

11. Signs and symptoms that indicate a life threat include alterations in mental status, severe cyanosis, absent breath sounds, audible stridor, one- or two-word dyspnea, tachycardia, pallor and diaphoresis, cardiac dysrhythmias, a pulse rate over 130/min, poor, floppy muscle tone, and the presence of retractions and/or the use of accessory muscles.
(Objective 2)

12. You should ask about the patient's chief complaint and determine whether he or she has any chest pain, productive or nonproductive cough, hemoptysis, wheezing, or signs of respiratory infection (e.g., fever or increased sputum production). Inquire about the patient's past history, especially with regard to similar problems and the individual's perceived severity of this episode. Obtain a medication history and ask whether the patient has ever needed intubation to manage this type of illness. The physical examination should begin by noting your general impression of the patient. Note the patient's position, mentation, ability to speak, respiratory effort, and skin color. Observe the heart rate for tachycardia or bradycardia. Note any abnormal respiratory patterns. Assess the face and neck for pursed-lip breathing and use of accessory muscles. Evaluate the neck for jugular venous distention. Inspect the chest for injury, indicators of chronic disease, accessory muscle use, and chest symmetry. Auscultate the lungs for abnormal breath sounds. Assess the extremities for peripheral cyanosis, clubbing of the fingers, and carpopedal spasm.
(Objective 2)

13. a. "Blue bloater," chronic cough with production of a large amount of sputum, hypercapnia, hypoxemia, cyanosis, pulmonary hypertension, and cor pulmonale; b. "pink puffer," hyperexpansion of the lungs, barrel chest, resistance to airflow (especially on expiration), pursed-lip breathing, and thinness.
(Objective 2)

14. Oxygen should be administered initially at 2 L/min if the patient is not in respiratory failure. If rapid improvement does not occur, the flow of oxygen should be increased while the paramedic carefully monitors the patient. If the patient's condition is critical, intubation and assisted ventilation may be necessary. (Objective 2)

15. Albuterol, levalbuterol (Objective 2)

16. Transport the patient in a position of comfort; instruct the patient to use pursed-lip breathing and to minimize physical activity to conserve energy for breathing; calmly reassure and care for the patient and provide a cool environment for transport. (Objective 2)

17. An acute asthma attack is marked by reversible airflow obstruction caused by bronchial smooth muscle contraction; hypersecretion of mucus, causing bronchial plugging; and inflammatory changes in the bronchial walls. (Objective 2)

18. Measurement of the peak expiratory flow rate can aid in the determination of the severity of an asthma attack, as well as the evaluation of the effectiveness of treatment in reversing airway obstruction. (Objective 2)

19. Albuterol, 0.5 mL (2.5 mg) or (levalbuterol 0.63-1.25 mg) in 2.5 mL normal saline by nebulizer at 6 to 7 L/min O_2. (Objective 2)

20. Ask the patient if his breathing is easier. Observe the patient for decreased anxiety, changes in level of consciousness, and ability to converse more easily. Note the degree of respiratory distress by observing the patient's position, use of accessory muscles, and respiratory rate. Monitor vital signs (the pulse and respiratory rate should decrease, and pulsus paradoxus should drop below 20 mm Hg). As the patient improves, the inspiratory and then expiratory wheezes should disappear. (Objective 2)

21. Status asthmaticus (Objective 2)

22. Make sure that oxygen is at 100% and humidified; increase the fluid rate to hydrate the patient; administer other medications (e.g., methylprednisolone, hydrocortisone) as ordered by medical direction; expedite transport; monitor the patient closely for signs of respiratory failure and prepare to intubate if necessary. If intubation is indicated, follow local medical protocols, which may include sedation (ketamine, benzodiazepine, or barbiturates); paralyze the patient; intubate; confirm ET tube placement; and ventilate at 6 to 10 breaths/min and use smaller tidal volumes (6-8 mL/kg); use shorter inspiratory time and longer expiratory time. (Objective 2)

23. a. Upper airway obstruction: foreign body, epiglottitis; b. lower airway obstruction: asthma, airway edema; c. trauma: inhalation injury, adult respiratory distress syndrome (ARDS) secondary to pulmonary contusion; d. alveolar pathology: chronic obstructive pulmonary disease (COPD), lung cancer, inhalation injury; e. interstitial space pathology: pulmonary edema, near drowning. (Objective 2)

24. Viral, bacterial, mycoplasmal, and aspiration (Objective 2)

25. Signs and symptoms of bacterial pneumonia include shaking chills, tachypnea, tachycardia, cough with sputum (rust colored, hemoptysis, yellow, green, or gray), malaise, anorexia, flank or back pain, vomiting, fever, wheezing, fine crackles, dyspnea, and sore throat.
(Objective 2)

26. Care includes airway support, oxygen administration, ventilatory assistance, IV fluids, cardiac and oxygen saturation monitoring, and transportation. If wheezing is present, bronchodilator therapy may be used.
(Objective 2)

27. a. Adult respiratory distress syndrome; b. Monitor the rise and fall of the chest to determine the effectiveness of ventilation; note any difficulty or increasing pressure necessary to ventilate the patient; frequently assess vital signs, observing for an increased heart rate; monitor the electrocardiogram, end-tidal CO_2, and oxygen saturation by pulse oximetry; observe for cyanosis. Ventilate with high-flow oxygen; ventilate with positive end-expiratory pressure, using Boehringer valve if trained and authorized by medical direction; and administer steroids and diuretics if ordered by medical direction.
(Objective 2)

28. Extended travel; prolonged bed rest; obesity; older adulthood; burns; varicose veins; surgery of the thorax, abdomen, pelvis, and legs; pelvic or leg fractures; malignancy; use of birth control pills; congenital or acquired coagulopathies; pregnancy; chronic obstructive pulmonary disease; congestive heart failure; sickle cell anemia; cancer; atrial fibrillation; myocardial infarction; previous pulmonary embolism; deep vein thrombosis; infection; diabetes mellitus; and multiple trauma.
(Objective 2)

29. Dyspnea, cough, hemoptysis, pain, anxiety, syncope, hypotension, diaphoresis, increased respiratory rate, increased heart rate, fever, distended neck veins, chest splinting, pleuritic chest pain, pleural friction rub, crackles, and wheezes (localized).
(Objective 3)

30. This typically occurs in tall, thin males between the ages of 20 and 40. It may also be found in patients with COPD, patients with acquired immunodeficiency syndrome (AIDS) who have pneumonia, and drug abusers who deeply inhale free-base cocaine, marijuana, or inhalants such as glue or solvents.
(Objective 2)

STUDENT SELF-ASSESSMENT

31. b. Cardiac, genetic, and stress factors are all intrinsic factors.
(Objective 1)

32. b. Adequate blood volume and patent pulmonary capillaries are related to perfusion. Normal interstitial space affects diffusion.
(Objective 1)

33. c. All the answers represent findings that indicate respiratory distress; however, in the patient with chronic respiratory illness, the patient's reported level of distress is often the best indication of the severity of the condition.
(Objective 2)

34. c. This sign takes a long time to develop. Acutely hypoxic patients may use accessory muscles or pursed-lip breathing in an attempt to improve ventilation. Carpopedal spasm is seen secondary to hypocapnia.
(Objective 2)

35. b. All will have wheezing and cough when acutely ill. Resistance to airflow is seen in all three conditions, although less so in emphysema.
(Objective 2)

36. c. The patient is more likely to be tachycardic than bradycardic. Capillary refill is an indicator of perfusion (flow) rather than oxygenation.
(Objective 2)

37. d. Right-heart failure can develop secondary to pulmonary hypertension (cor pulmonale). The right side of the heart increasingly is forced to pump harder to overcome the excess pressure in the pulmonary arteries. Eventually it cannot force the blood through, and fluid backs up to the venous side of the system.
(Objective 2)

38. d
(Objective 2)

39. c. Expiratory wheezing indicates narrowing of the smaller airways. As the larger airways become obstructed, inspiratory wheezing becomes audible. When the obstruction becomes so severe that almost no airflow is present, the chest is silent, with diminished breath sounds and no wheezes.
(Objective 2)

40. a. Albuterol is a beta-2 agonist that causes relatively few side effects. Although all the other drugs also cause bronchodilation, they are rarely used because of their high incidence of side effects.
(Objective 2)

41. a. The PEFR is most helpful when the patient's normal baseline peak flow is known.
(Objective 2)

42. d. The vaccine is 80% to 90% effective in the prevention of pneumonia caused by the *pneumococcus* bacillus.
(Objective 2)

43. c. Altered level of consciousness may impair the gag reflex or the patient's ability to handle secretions.
(Objective 2)

44. d. Not all patients die, although the mortality rate is high (over 65%). Disseminated coagulation may occur in some but not all patients.
(Objective 2)

45. a.
(Objective 2)

46. d. The size and location of the embolus determine whether mild signs and symptoms or sudden death occurs.
(Objective 2)

47. c. Most upper respiratory infections have no identifiable cause. Good hand washing is an important action for preventing their spread.
(Objective 2)

48. b. Other risk factors for spontaneous pneumothorax include patients with emphysema, people with AIDS who develop pneumonia, and healthy tall, thin men between the ages of 20 and 40.
(Objective 2)

49. b. Narcotic overdose is associated with respiratory depression.
(Objective 2)

50. a. Heavy smokers have a 25 times greater risk of developing lung cancer than nonsmokers.
(Objective 2)

WRAP IT UP

1. e. Mucus production and inflammation of the alveoli impair ventilation and diffusion.
(Objective 1)

2. b, e, f, g, h
(Objective 2)

3. c. Patients with chronic bronchitis tend to be overweight and have persistent hypoxia and chronic excessive mucus production.
(Objective 2)

4. a. Albuterol is a bronchodilator that relaxes bronchiolar smooth muscle, enlarging the airway passages and allowing better exchange of gases in the lungs.
b. Methylprednisolone is a steroid that reduces swelling and inflammation in the lung tissues, permitting better airflow and diffusion.
(Objective 2)

5. Levalbuterol is less likely to increase the heart rate than albuterol. Since this is an elderly patient who is already tachycardic (HR 120/min), it would be the drug of choice (if available).

6. d. Pneumonia can be caused by bacterial, viral, or fungal infections. Not all these organisms are susceptible to antibiotics. Fever may not be present, especially in immunocompromised patients.
(Objective 2)

31

Neurology

READING ASSIGNMENT
Chapter 31, pages 836-863, in *Mosby's Paramedic Textbook,* ed. 3

OBJECTIVES
Upon completion of this chapter, the paramedic student will be able to do the following:
1. Describe the anatomy and physiology of the nervous system.
2. Outline pathophysiological changes in the nervous system that may alter the cerebral perfusion pressure.
3. Describe the assessment of a patient with a nervous system disorder.
4. Describe the pathophysiology, signs and symptoms, and specific management techniques for each of the following neurological disorders: coma, stroke and intracranial hemorrhage, seizure disorders, headaches, brain neoplasm and brain abscess, and degenerative neurological diseases.

SUMMARY
- The human body's ability to maintain a state of balance, or *homeostasis,* results from the nervous system's regulatory and coordinating activities. The blood supply to the brain comes from the vertebral arteries and the internal carotid arteries.
- Some neurological emergencies are a consequence of structural changes or damage, circulatory changes, or alterations in intracranial pressure that affect cerebral blood flow.
- The initial survey should begin by determining the patient's level of consciousness and by ensuring an open and patent airway. Key elements of the physical examination that may provide clues to the nature of the neurological emergency include the patient history and the history of the event, vital signs, and respiratory patterns.
- *Coma* is an abnormally deep state of unconsciousness. The patient cannot be aroused from this state by external stimuli. In general, two mechanisms produce coma: structural lesions and toxic-metabolic states.
- *Stroke* is a sudden interruption in blood flow to the brain that results in a neurological deficit. Strokes can be classified as ischemic strokes or hemorrhagic strokes.
- A *seizure* is a brief alteration in behavior or consciousness. It is caused by abnormal electrical activity of one or more groups of neurons in the brain. In the prehospital setting, determining the cause of a seizure is not as important as other measures. These include managing the complications and recognizing whether the seizure is reversible with therapy (e.g., it is caused by hypoglycemia).
- The four fairly common types of headaches are tension headaches, migraines, cluster headaches, and sinus headaches.
- A brain tumor, or *neoplasm,* is a mass in the cranial cavity. This mass can be either malignant or benign. Heredity may play a role in the development of brain tumors. They also are associated with several risk factors. These include exposure to radiation, tobacco use, dietary habits, some viruses, and the use of some medications.
- A *brain abscess* is a buildup of purulent material (pus) surrounded by a capsule within the brain. It develops from a bacterial infection. The infection often starts in the nasal cavity, middle ear, or mastoid bone.

- Muscular dystrophy is an inherited muscle disorder. The cause is unknown. The disease is marked by a slow but progressive degeneration of muscle fibers.
- Damage to the white matter of the brain in multiple sclerosis may lead to fatigue, vertigo, clumsiness, unsteady gait, slurred speech, blurred or double vision, and facial numbness or pain.
- The term *dystonia* refers to local or diffuse changes in muscle tone. These may cause painful muscle spasms, unusually fixed postures, and strange movement patterns.
- Parkinson disease usually begins as a slight tremor in one hand, arm, or leg. In the later stages, the disease affects both sides of the body, causing stiffness, weakness, and trembling of the muscles.
- The term *central pain syndrome* refers to infection or disease of the trigeminal nerve.
- *Bell palsy* is paralysis of the facial muscles. It is caused by inflammation of the seventh cranial nerve. The condition is usually one sided and temporary. It often develops suddenly.
- Amyotrophic lateral sclerosis is also called *Lou Gehrig disease*. It is one of a group of rare nervous system disorders. In these disorders, the nerves that control muscular activity degenerate in the brain and spinal cord.
- Peripheral neuropathies usually arise from damage to or irritation of either the axons or their myelin sheaths. This slows or fully blocks the passage of electrical signals.
- The term *myoclonus* refers to rapid and uncontrollable muscle contractions or spasms. These occur at rest or during movement.
- *Spina bifida* is a congenital defect in which part of one or more vertebrae fails to develop completely. This leaves a portion of the spinal cord exposed.
- Polio is caused by a virus. The severity of the disease can range from unapparent infection, to a febrile illness without neurological aftereffects, to aseptic meningitis, and finally to paralytic disease and possibly death.

REVIEW QUESTIONS

For each of the causes in column I, identify the appropriate general cause of coma in column II. Each answer may be used *more* than once.

Column I	Column II
1. _____ The patient's blood pressure rose suddenly to 240/140 mm Hg.	**a.** Cardiovascular system
	b. Drugs
2. _____ The patient's chronic bronchitis is much worse.	**c.** Infectious
3. _____ The patient has missed dialysis for a week.	**d.** Metabolic system
4. _____ The patient's blood alcohol level is 400 mg/dL.	**e.** Respiratory system
5. _____ The patient's glucose level is 30 mg/dL.	**f.** Structural cause
6. _____ The teenage patient has meningitis.	

Match the illness in column II with the description in column I. Use each illness only once.

Column I	Column II
7. _____ Blurred vision and unsteady gait	**a.** Amyotrophic lateral sclerosis
8. _____ Severe muscle spasms because of torticollis	**b.** Bell palsy
9. _____ Burning sensation in the feet because of diabetes	**c.** Central pain syndrome
10. _____ Viral illness causing respiratory paralysis	**d.** Dystonia
11. _____ Muscle trembling because of a decrease in dopamine	**e.** Multiple sclerosis
12. _____ Male genetic disorder that causes muscle wasting	**f.** Muscular dystrophy
13. _____ Intense facial pain activated by a trigger point	**g.** Myoclonus
14. _____ Central nervous system degeneration in patients over age 50 that leads to severe muscle deterioration	**h.** Parkinson disease
	i. Peripheral neuropathy
15. _____ Temporary facial paralysis caused by inflammation	**j.** Polio
16. _____ Genetic defect that leaves the spinal cord exposed	**k.** Spina bifida

17. Complete the following sentences.

The cells of the nervous system that protect the neurons are called **(a)** _____ _____

_____. Each neuron has three main parts. The area that contains the nucleus is the

(b) _____; one or more branching projections that receive impulses are known as

the **(c)** _____; and a single, elongated projection that transmits impulses is called the

(d) _____. In the peripheral nervous system, bundles of axons and their sheaths are called

(e) _____. Neurons are classified by the direction in which they transmit impulses. The neurons that

transmit impulses to the spinal cord and brain from the body are **(f)** _____ neurons. Neurons that

transmit impulses away from the brain to muscle and glandular tissue are **(g)** _____ neurons.

Neurons that conduct impulses from sensory neurons directly to motor neurons are **(h)** _____. In its

resting state the charge inside the neuron is **(i)** _____, and the charge outside the neuron is

(j) _____. When the neuron is stimulated while the outside is positively charged,

(k) _____ ions rush into the cell and begin a wave of **(l)** _____ that travels down the cell.

Myelinated axons have interruptions in the myelin sheaths, called **(m)** _____, _____

that cause the action potential to be conducted more **(n)** _____ than unmyelinated axons. The space

between the nerve endings of two adjacent neurons is known as a **(o)** _____. Impulses are trans-

mitted across these spaces by neurotransmitters such as **(p)** _____, _____, and

_____.

18. List the basic anatomical components of a reflex.

_____

19. Name the two paired arteries that supply blood to the brain.

a.

b.

20. State whether the following factors will *increase, decrease,* or *not change* the cerebral blood flow.
   a. Intracranial pressure of 30 mm Hg:
   b. Mean arterial pressure of 40 mm Hg:
   c. Expanding tumor in the brain:
   d. Hypovolemic shock:

21. List at least two causes of coma for each of the following six general classifications.

   a. Structural:

_____

b. Metabolic:

_____

c. Drug induced:

_____

d. Cardiovascular:

_____

e. Respiratory:

_____

f. Infectious:

_____

22. You have been called to care for a patient who is suspected of suffering from a neurological disorder. He opens his eyes when you call his name but does not know what day it is. He is moving all extremities normally.

   a. List six specific questions you should ask the family to elicit the nature of the neurological problem.

_____

_____

   b. What vital sign findings would suggest increased intracranial pressure?

_____

   c. Using the AVPU assessment, describe the patient's level of consciousness.

_____

   d. What is his score on the Glasgow Coma Scale?

_____

   e. Describe your assessment of this patient's eyes.

_____

23. State whether the following symptoms of coma are most likely to be found in structural or toxic-metabolic coma.
   a. Asymmetrical neurological findings:
   b. Slow onset:
   c. Unilateral fixed and dilated pupil:

24. You arrive at a private residence to evaluate a 65-year-old woman whose neighbors found her unresponsive. She has snoring respirations at a rate of 8/min, and an oral airway is easily placed. Carotid and radial pulses are present and rapid. Blood pressure is 110/70 mm Hg. She flexes to painful stimuli, no history is available, and her blood glucose level is 60 mg/dL. Outline your assessment and management of this patient, including the appropriate dose and route of administration of any drugs you would give.

_____

_____

_____

Questions 25 to 29 refer to the following case study:

You respond to a private residence, where you find an elderly African-American man lying on the sofa. His family states, "He hasn't been acting right." On exam you find him awake and confused, with slurred speech. He follows commands appropriately. When you ask him to smile, he has an apparent facial droop on the right. Ongoing assessment reveals weakness in the left arm and leg. His vital signs are BP, 160/108 mm Hg; P, 72/min; and R, 16/min and regular. His Sao_2 is 95%, and his blood glucose level is 94 mg/dL. History reveals no allergies, and his medications include hydrochlorothiazide, nitroglycerin, and insulin. His family states that a similar incident occurred yesterday and lasted about 5 minutes after he took a walk. He smokes one pack of cigarettes a day.

25. List eight risk factors for stroke that you can identify for this patient and note whether each is modifiable or nonmodifiable.

	Risk Factor	Modifiable (Yes or No)
a.		
b.		
c.		
d.		
e.		
f.		
g.		
h.		

26. List at least six signs or symptoms of cerebrovascular accident that are common to embolic and thrombotic strokes. (Place a star beside the ones experienced by this patient.)

_____

_____

27. List the physical findings that would indicate the probability of stroke for this patient based on

a. The Cincinnati stroke scale_____

_____

b. The Los Angeles Prehospital Stroke Screen_____

_____

28. List the seven Ds of stroke management.

D

D

D

D

D

D

D

450

29. Outline your prehospital care of this patient.

_____

_____

_____

30. Although patients may have diverse presentations, describe the typical progression of signs and symptoms of hemorrhagic stroke.

_____

_____

31. List five causes of seizures:

  a.

  b.

  c.

  d.

  e.

32. State the type of seizure for each of the following signs and symptoms.

  a. Numbness of the body or unusual visual, auditory, or taste symptoms:

  _____

  b. Brief loss of consciousness in a child (without loss of posture) that lasts less than 15 seconds:

  _____

  c. Partial seizure activity that spreads in an orderly fashion to surrounding areas:

  _____

  d. Preceding aura, followed by loss of consciousness and tonic-clonic motor activity, followed by a postictal state:

  _____

  e. Aura followed by automatisms such as lip smacking and chewing, during which time the patient is amnesic:

  _____

33. What history should be obtained from the family of a patient who has had a grand mal seizure?

  _____

34. List two findings that suggest that the seizure is hysterical rather than grand mal.

  a.

  b.

35. State whether each of the following characteristics is more suggestive of seizure or syncope:

  a. It starts in a standing position:

  _____

b. It is preceded by lightheadedness:

_____

c. The patient remains unconscious for minutes to hours:

_____

d. Tachycardia occurs:

_____

36. List two anticonvulsants (with the appropriate doses) that may be given to an adult patient having a seizure.

a.

b.

37. Identify the type of headache (tension, migraine, cluster, or sinus) typically associated with each of the following case presentations.

a. You are dispatched at 0100 to care for a patient who is complaining of a severe headache that woke him. He says the pain is most intense around his left eye, and you note that his eyes are tearing and his nose is

running._____

b. Your partner is recovering from an upper respiratory infection and complaining of a headache that affects her forehead and upper face. She describes an intense pressure sensation that increases when she bends over.

_____

c. Your patient is complaining of a dull, throbbing headache that started a week ago and will not stop.

_____

d. A 24-year-old woman is complaining of a severe headache that began as an intense throbbing on the right side of her head and is now generalized. She has vomited three times. She indicates a history of this and

takes a beta blocker._____

STUDENT SELF-ASSESSMENT

38. Which blood vessel or vessels supply the front lobes of the brain?
   a. Anterior cerebral arteries
   b. Midline basilar artery
   c. Posterior cerebral arteries
   d. Right and left vertebral arteries
39. An important function of the circle of Willis is to maintain blood supply to the brain if which of the following occurs?
   a. The patient becomes hypoxic because of shock.
   b. The patient has a large hemorrhagic stroke.
   c. Intracranial pressure increases suddenly.
   d. The vertebral or internal carotid arteries are blocked.
40. Which of the following will cause a decrease in the cerebral blood flow?
   a. Blood pressure of 70/50 mm Hg
   b. Intracranial pressure of 15 mm Hg
   c. Decreased levels of intraocular fluid
   d. Body temperature of 102° F (38.9° C)
41. Respiratory patterns associated with neurological disorders include all of the following _except_ which symptom?
   a. Ataxic respirations
   b. Cheyne-Stokes respirations
   c. Diaphragmatic breathing
   d. Kussmaul respirations

42. Posturing caused by structural impairment of the subcortical regions of the brain is known as which of the following?
    a. Extension rigidity
    b. Flexion rigidity
    c. Dysconjugate gaze
    d. Flaccidity
43. Your comatose patient's pupils are 2 mm and round and reactive to light. What does this suggest?
    a. Barbiturate overdose
    b. Medullary injury
    c. Opiate overdose
    d. Temporal herniation
44. Management of the postictal patient with a known seizure disorder who initially aroused to pain and then begins to moan and move spontaneously includes which of the following?
    a. Administration of naloxone (2 mg IV)
    b. Administration of diazepam (5 mg IV)
    c. Intravenous fluid therapy with normal saline (100 mL/hr)
    d. Lateral recumbent positioning of the patient
45. Significant findings in the medical history of a patient you suspect is having a stroke include all of the following *except* which characteristic?
    a. Cigarette smoking
    b. Obesity
    c. Oral contraceptive use
    d. Sickle cell disease
46. Which of the following findings would indicate a high probability of stroke based on the Cincinnati prehospital stroke scale?
    a. The patient has the worst headache ever felt.
    b. The patient cannot speak clearly to you.
    c. The patient experiences a new onset of seizures.
    d. The patient complains of double vision.
47. Your patient has continuous, rapid muscle jerking that the family says is related to his neuromuscular disease. What are these movements called?
    a. Dystonia
    b. Inanition
    c. Myoclonus
    d. Palsy

WRAP IT UP

You respond to a call for "seizures." When you arrive, you find a 72-year-old male who opens his eyes to pain, pushes your hand away when you apply nail bed pressure, and calls out cuss words, then quickly appears to sleep again and has snoring respirations. You insert a nasal airway and administer oxygen by mask while you continue your examination. His wife explains that he was in the bathroom having a bowel movement when she heard a noise, and when she got to him, his limbs jerked rhythmically for several minutes and then he "passed out." She says that he had been complaining of a headache this morning. He takes furosemide and enalapril. As you continue your examination, the patient becomes progressively more awake. His vital signs are BP, 192/98 mm Hg; P, 96/min; R, 20/min; Sao_2, 99% (on oxygen); blood glucose, 99 mg/dL; pupils 4 mm, equal, and reactive to light. You initiate an IV of normal saline TKO and, seeing no traumatic injury on your exam, move the patient to your stretcher. In the ambulance you place the patient on an ECG monitor and observe a normal sinus rhythm. You transport him 4 minutes to the closest hospital, continuously monitoring his neurological status and vital signs, which have not changed. As you move him to the ED cot, he experiences another seizure with tonic-clonic movements; his breathing then becomes ataxic, his pupils become fixed and dilated, he is unresponsive to painful stimulus, and his heart rate drops quickly until his ventilations are assisted. CT scan reveals a large hemorrhagic stroke, and the patient dies within 6 hours of arrival at the hospital.

1. What were the patient's Glasgow Coma Scale values
    a. Initially
    b. After his seizure in the ED
2. Were any signs of increased intracranial pressure present
    a. When you arrived
    b. After the patient had his second seizure
3. If the patient had continued to have a seizure, list two drugs (and their appropriate dose) that could have been administered.

    a.

    b.

4. Explain some possible causes of the patient's condition that you tried to rule out as you initially assessed the patient.
5. Identify at least four risk factors for stroke that you have determined this patient had.

_____

_____

6. Place a ✔ beside the signs or symptoms of stroke that this patient showed.
   - **a.** _____ Aphasia
   - **b.** _____ Ataxia
   - **c.** _____ Confusion
   - **d.** _____ Coma
   - **e.** _____ Diplopia
   - **f.** _____ Dizziness
   - **g.** _____ Dysarthria
   - **h.** _____ Headache
   - **i.** _____ Hemiparesis
   - **j.** _____ Incontinence
   - **k.** _____ Monocular blindness
   - **l.** _____ Numbness
   - **m.** _____ Seizure
7. What leads you to believe that this patient had a hemorrhagic rather than an ischemic stroke?

_____

8. Which is true of this patient's Cincinnati or Los Angeles Prehospital Stroke Screen:
   - **a.** Both demonstrate a high probability of stroke.
   - **b.** Both confirm the presence of stoke.
   - **c.** Neither can be performed on this patient.
   - **d.** Only the LAPSS demonstrates stroke in this case.

REVIEW QUESTIONS

1. a
2. e
3. d
4. b
5. d
6. c
7. e
8. d
9. i
10. j
11. h
12. f
13. c
14. a
15. b
16. k
(Questions 1-16: Objective 4)

17. a. Neuroglia; b. cell body; c. dendrites; d. axon; e. white matter; f. sensory; g. motor; h. interneurons; i. negative; j. positive; k. sodium; l. depolarization; m. nodes of Ranvier; n. quickly; o. synapse; p. norepinephrine, epinephrine, and dopamine.
(Objective 1)

18. Sensory receptor, sensory neuron, interneurons, motor neuron, and effector organ.
(Objective 1)

19. Vertebral arteries and internal carotid arteries.
(Objective 1)

20. a. Decrease; b. decrease; c. decrease; d. decrease
(Objective 2)

21. a. Intracranial bleeding, head trauma, brain tumor, or another space-occupying lesion; b. anoxia, hypoglycemia, diabetic ketoacidosis, thiamine deficiency, kidney and liver failure, and postictal phase of a seizure; c. barbiturates, narcotics, hallucinogenics, depressants, and alcohol; d. hypertensive encephalopathy, shock, dysrhythmias, and stroke; e. chronic obstructive pulmonary disease and toxic inhalation; f. meningitis and sepsis.
(Objective 4)

22. a. Why did you call EMS? What happened during the course of this situation? Does the patient have any medical problems, such as heart or lung disease, neurological illness, diabetes, or high blood pressure? Does the patient have a history of drug or alcohol abuse or stroke? Has this ever happened to him before? Do you know if he has had any injuries recently?
b. Increased blood pressure, decreased pulse, widened pulse pressure, slow or irregular respiratory rate.
c. He is responsive to verbal stimuli.
d. GCS = 13
e. Assess the pupils for shape, size, equality, and response to light. Assess the patient's extraocular movements by asking him to follow your finger movements with his eyes (to the extreme left, up and down, to the extreme right, up and down).
(Objective 3)

23. a. Structural; b. toxic-metabolic; c. structural
(Objective 4)

24. Secure the airway and ventilate with 100% oxygen (with in-line immobilization of the spine). Assess the carotid and radial pulses. Assess vital signs, oxygen saturation, breath sounds, ECG, and pupil response. Scan the body for obvious trauma. Draw a blood sample while initiating an IV with 0.9% normal saline. Because the blood glucose level is less than 80 mg/dL, administer thiamine (100 mg IV), reassess, administer 25 g of $D_{50}W$ IV, and reassess. (If the blood glucose level had been normal, you would have administered naloxone [Narcan] [2 mg IV] and reassessed.) If no improvement occurs and patient has no gag reflex, she should be intubated (and tube placement verified). Perform ongoing assessment and transport.
(Objectives 3, 4)

25.

Risk Factor	Modifiable (Yes or No)
a. Age (elderly)	No
b. Race (African-American)	No
c. Gender (male)	No
d. Hypertension	Yes
e. Heart disease (nitroglycerin)	Yes
f. Diabetes (insulin)	Yes
g. Transient ischemic attacks	Yes
h. Cigarette smoking	Yes

(Objective 4)

26. Confusion* or coma, dysarthria*, aphasia, facial droop* or facial numbness, hemiparesis* or hemiplegia, convulsions, incontinence, diplopia, headache, dizziness, ataxia, monocular blindness, or vertigo.
(Objective 4)

27. a. Facial droop, arm drift, and slurred speech; b. Patient is over age 45, has no history of seizures, symptom duration is longer than 24 hours, patient is not wheelchair bound, blood glucose is normal, and patient has obvious asymmetry of smile and arm strength.
(Objective 4)

28. Detection, dispatch, delivery (to a stroke center), door (appropriate hospital for rapid treatment of stroke), data (include CT scan), decision (appropriateness of fibrinolytic therapy), drug.
(Objective 4)

29. Make sure that his airway remains patent, try to determine time of onset, administer supplemental oxygen if his Sao_2 drops below 90% or his condition worsens, monitor vital signs and ECG, elevate head of stretcher 15 degrees, initiate IV LR or NS at 50 mL/hour; protect affected extremities, maintain normal temperature, notify and transport quickly to closest stroke center, control seizures, if present, with benzodiazepines; comfort and reassure the patient and family.
(Objective 4)

30. Hemorrhagic stroke commonly occurs during stress or exertion. It starts abruptly and often begins with a headache, nausea, vomiting, and progressive deterioration of neurological status. The patient may rapidly lose consciousness or have a seizure.
(Objective 4)

31. Stroke, head trauma, toxins, hypoxia, hypoglycemia, infection, metabolic abnormalities, brain tumor, vascular disorders, eclampsia, and drug overdose.
(Objective 4)

32. a. Simple sensory seizure (partial seizure); b. petit mal (generalized seizure); c. jacksonian seizure (partial seizure); d. grand mal seizure (generalized seizure); e. complex partial seizures (partial seizure).
(Objective 4)

33. History of seizures, including frequency and medication compliance; description of seizure (length, features, incontinence, tongue biting); history of head trauma; fever, headache, or nuchal rigidity before seizure; medical history, including diabetes, cardiovascular disease, and stroke.
(Objective 4)

34. With a hysterical seizure, the following do not occur: trauma to the tongue, incontinence, and response to conventional therapy. A hysterical seizure may stop with a sharp command or sternal rub.
(Objective 4)

35. a. Syncope; b. syncope; c. seizure; d. seizure
(Objective 4)

36. Lorazepam (1 to 2 mg IV); or diazepam (5 to 10 mg IV) every 15 minutes as necessary. (Midazolam is sometimes given to treat seizures in children.)
(Objective 4)

37. a. Cluster headache; b. sinus headache; c. tension headache; d. migraine headache.
(Objective 4)

STUDENT SELF-ASSESSMENT

38. a. The internal carotid arteries give rise to the anterior cerebral arteries. The vertebral arteries supply the cerebellum and unite to form the basilar artery.
(Objective 1)

39. d. The circle of Willis would not protect against a large cerebral bleed, systemic hypoxia, or increased ICP. It can help to maintain blood flow if a clot exists in the vertebral or carotid arteries.
(Objective 1)

40. a. This will decrease cerebral perfusion pressure. CPP does not usually decrease until the ICP exceeds 22 mm Hg (the body compensates to that level). Fluid in the eye has no influence on CPP. Metabolic rate will increase, but CPP is not affected by a temperature of 102° F (38.9° C).
(Objective 2)

41. d. Kussmaul respirations occur secondary to the metabolic acidosis that occurs in diabetic ketoacidosis. Each of the other breathing patterns may be encountered in a patient who has a neurological problem.
(Objective 3)

42. a. Flexion posturing occurs with impairment of the cortical regions of the brain. Flaccidity is usually caused by brain stem or cord dysfunction. Dysconjugate gaze is not a posture but an abnormal eye movement.
(Objective 3)

43. c. Barbiturate overdose and medullary injury are more likely to present with dilated pupils. Temporal herniation causes a unilateral dilated pupil.
(Objective 3)

44. d. Airway maintenance is critical. Drug administration would be indicated only if the seizure recurs.
(Objective 4)

45. b. All other choices are risk factors for stroke.
(Objective 4)

46. b. The three components of the stroke scale are facial droop, arm drift, and speech disturbances. All other choices are possible signs or symptoms of stroke but are not included in the stroke scale.
(Objective 4)

47. c. *Dystonia* refers to an alteration in muscle tone that can cause painful spasms, fixed postures, or strange movement patterns. *Inanition* refers to starvation or failure to thrive. *Palsy* is weakness.
(Objective 4)

WRAP IT UP

1. a. 10; b. 3 (no response to pain)
(Objective 3)

2. Altered level of consciousness; hospital: decreasing level of consciousness, bradycardia, fixed and dilated pupils, ataxic breathing
(Objective 3)

3. Lorazepam (Ativan), 1 to 4 mg IV given slowly; or diazepam (Valium), 5 mg over 2 minutes.
(Objective 4)

4. Intracranial bleeding, head trauma, brain tumor, anoxia, hypoglycemia, seizure disorder, drug overdose, poisoning, hypertensive encephalopathy, dysrhythmia, stroke, meningitis
(Objective 3)

5. High blood pressure, age, male gender
(Objective 4)

6. d, h, m
(Objective 4)

7. Symptoms developed abruptly, occurred during exertion (using the toilet), seizure ensued, as did progressive and rapid deterioration
(Objective 4)

8. c. The patient is unconscious and unable to be evaluated using either scale.
(Objective 3)

CHAPTER
32

Endocrinology

READING ASSIGNMENT
Chapter 32, pages 864-881, in *Mosby's Paramedic Textbook*, ed. 3

OBJECTIVES
Upon completion of this chapter, the paramedic student will be able to:
1. Describe how hormones secreted from endocrine glands help the body to maintain homeostasis.
2. Describe the anatomy and physiology of the pancreas and how its hormones work to maintain normal glucose metabolism.
3. Discuss pathophysiology as a basis for key signs and symptoms, patient assessment, and patient management for diabetes and diabetic emergencies of hypoglycemia, diabetic ketoacidosis, and hyperosmolar hyperglycemic nonketotic coma.
4. Discuss pathophysiology as a basis for key signs and symptoms, patient assessment, and patient management for disorders of the thyroid gland.
5. Discuss pathophysiology as a basis for key signs and symptoms, patient assessment, and patient management of Cushing syndrome and Addison disease.

SUMMARY
- The endocrine system consists of ductless glands and tissues. These glands and tissues produce and secrete hormones. Endocrine glands secrete their hormones directly into the bloodstream. They exert a regulatory effect on various metabolic functions. All hormones operate within feedback systems. (These are either positive or negative.) These systems work to maintain an optimal internal environment.
- The pancreatic islets are composed of beta cells, alpha cells, and other cells. The beta cells secrete insulin. The alpha cells secrete glucagon. The other cells are of questionable function. The chief functions of insulin are to increase glucose transport into cells, increase glucose metabolism by cells, increase the liver glycogen level, and decrease the blood glucose concentration toward normal. Glucagon has two major effects: (1) increase blood glucose levels by stimulating the liver to release glucose stores from glycogen and other glucose storage sites (glycogenolysis) and (2) stimulate gluconeogenesis through the breakdown of fats and fatty acids, thereby maintaining a normal blood glucose level.
- Diabetes mellitus is characterized by a deficiency of insulin or an inability of the body to respond to insulin. Diabetes generally is classified as type 1 or type 2. Type 1 is insulin dependent. Type 2 is non-insulin dependent. Type 1 diabetes requires lifelong treatment. This consists of insulin injections, exercise, and diet regulation. Most patients with type 2 diabetes require oral hypoglycemic medications, exercise, and dietary regulation to control the illness.
- Hypoglycemia is a syndrome related to blood glucose levels below 80 mg/dL. Any diabetic patient with behavioral changes or unconsciousness should be treated for hypoglycemia. This condition is a true emergency. It requires immediate administration of glucose to prevent permanent brain damage or death.

- Diabetic ketoacidosis results from an absence of or a resistance to insulin. The signs and symptoms of DKA are related to diuresis and acidosis. They usually are slow in onset.
- Hyperosmolar hyperglycemic nonketotic coma is a life-threatening emergency. It often occurs in older patients with type 2 diabetes. It also frequently occurs in undiagnosed diabetics. The hyperglycemia produces a hyperosmolar state. This is followed by an osmotic diuresis, dehydration, and electrolyte losses.
- Important components of the patient history in the assessment of diabetic patients include the onset of symptoms, food intake, insulin or oral hypoglycemic use, alcohol or other drug consumption, predisposing factors, and any associated symptoms.
- Any patient with a glucose reading below 80 mg/dL and signs and symptoms consistent with hypoglycemia should be given dextrose.
- Thyrotoxicosis is any toxic condition that results from overactivity of the thyroid gland.
- Thyroid storm is a life-threatening condition resulting from an overactive thyroid gland. Thyroid hormones play a key role in controlling body metabolism. They are essential in children for normal physical growth and development.
- Myxedema is a condition that results from a thyroid hormone deficiency. Myxedema coma is a rare illness. In addition to myxedema, it is characterized by hypothermia and mental obtundation. It is a medical emergency.
- Cushing syndrome is caused by an abnormally high circulating level of corticosteroid hormones. These are produced naturally by the adrenal glands.
- Addison disease is a rare but life-threatening disorder. It is caused by a deficiency of the corticosteroid hormones cortisol and aldosterone. These are normally produced by the adrenal cortex.

REVIEW QUESTIONS

Match the signs or symptoms in column II with the appropriate diabetic emergencies in column I. Each answer may be used *more* than once.

Column I	Column II
1. _____ Diabetic ketoacidosis	**a.** Abdominal pain
2. _____ Hyperosmolar hyperglycemic nonketotic coma	**b.** Coma
3. _____ Hypoglycemia	**c.** Cool, clammy skin
	d. Fruity breath odor
	e. Kussmaul respirations
	f. Polyuria
	g. Psychotic behavior
	h. Seizures
	i. Tachycardia
	j. Warm, dry skin
	k. Vomiting

4. Name the hormone secreted from each of these cells in the pancreas.
   a. Alpha cells:
   b. Beta cells:
   c. Delta cells:

5. When food is ingested, it is broken down into smaller units and used or stored. Name the breakdown products and storage sites for the following food types.

Food	Breakdown Products	Storage
a. Carbohydrates		
b. Proteins		
c. Fats		

6. a. How is excess glucose stored in the liver?

_____

   b. How are glucose stores released from the liver?

_____

7. Briefly explain the role of glucagon in the metabolism of food.

_____

8. Why does a patient develop cerebral signs and symptoms of hypoglycemia rapidly?

_____

9. List at least three signs or symptoms that might lead you to suspect that a patient has undetected type 1 diabetes.

_____

_____

_____

10. List at least three medical illnesses associated with long-term diabetes.

_____

_____

_____

11. You arrive on the scene of a suspected diabetic emergency. You find a 35-year-old man whose wife says he took his insulin 2 hours ago and has not eaten. He arouses only to pain and has noisy, snoring respirations. He has no other medical history. Outline the steps in your patient management.

_____

_____

_____

_____

Questions 12 to 16 refer to the following case study:

   A 20-year-old diabetic patient calls you complaining of difficulty breathing. On arrival, the patient states that he has had the flu for 2 days. You note that his respiratory rate is 40/min and his breath has a very sweet odor. You auscultate his lungs, and his breath sounds are clear bilaterally.

12. What do you suspect?

_____

13. What other specific questions will you ask about the history of this patient's illness?

_____

_____

461

14. What specific findings will you be looking for during your physical assessment of the patient?

_____

You perform a blood glucose analysis, and your machine reads "high." The patient appears dehydrated.

15. What interventions should you perform for this patient in the prehospital setting?

_____

16. Should you be concerned about rapid transport for this patient? Why?

_____

17. List six factors that predispose a patient to the development of hyperosmolar hyperglycemic nonketotic coma.

   a.

   b.

   c.

   d.

   e.

   f.

18. Complete the missing information for each endocrine disorder in the table below.

Disorder	Endocrine Gland and Hormone Affected	Hormone Excess or Shortage?	Signs and Symptoms	Life Threat?
Graves disease				
Thyroid storm				
Myxedema				
Cushing syndrome				
Addison disease				

STUDENT SELF-ASSESSMENT

19. How do hormones achieve their desired actions?
   a. They travel by ducts to the specific organ to be stimulated.
   b. They stimulate nerves to send messages to their target tissue.
   c. They trigger cell-specific receptors to initiate specific functions.
   d. They activate the organ adjacent to the gland that produces them.

20. What is the primary action of insulin?
   a. To reduce the glucose needs of the cells
   b. To increase blood glucose levels
   c. To transport glucose into the cells
   d. To manufacture amino acids

21. Oral hypoglycemic agents include all of the following _except_ which drug?
   a. Diabinese   **c.** Insulin
   b. Glucophage   **d.** Orinase

22. Which of the following is often a characteristic of type 2 diabetes?
   a. Requires insulin injections
   b. Develops after age 40
   c. Has a sudden onset of symptoms
   d. Results in life-threatening emergencies
23. What is the breakdown of glucose stores in the liver called?
   a. Glucagon
   b. Glucosuria
   c. Gluconeogenesis
   d. Glycogenolysis
24. Before administration of $D_{50}W$ in a lethargic patient with diabetes, you should do all of the following *except* which procedure?
   a. Initiate intravenous fluids
   b. Administer glucagon
   c. Draw a blood sample
   d. Determine the blood glucose level
25. Before giving $D_{50}W$ to a diabetic who is also a known alcoholic, what should you administer?
   a. Glucagon
   b. Half the usual dose
   c. Insulin
   d. Thiamine
26. An advantage of glucagon over $D_{50}W$ is that it is
   a. Faster acting
   b. Less expensive
   c. Given IM
   d. More effective
27. What is the correct dose of glucagon for an adult?
   a. 0.5 to 1 mg IM
   b. 1 to 2 mg IM
   c. 12.5 g IV
   d. 25 g IV
28. Which of the following signs or symptoms would be *unlikely* in a patient who is in a hyperosmolar hyperglycemic nonketotic coma?
   a. Altered level of consciousness
   b. Dry mucous membranes
   c. Fruity breath odor
   d. Thirst
29. Your patient is very anxious and is complaining of abdominal pain and difficulty breathing. Her vital signs are BP, 80/50 mm Hg; P, 136/min; and R, 24/min. You note basilar rales in her lungs. What endocrine condition may cause this presentation?
   a. Cushing syndrome
   b. Graves disease
   c. Myxedema
   d. Thyroid storm
30. Your patient is a 60-year-old type 2 diabetic who takes glyburide/metformin (Glucovance). He is difficult to arouse and has a blood glucose of 28 mg/dL. Which of the following is true regarding his case?
   a. This may be a rare case of metabolic alkalosis.
   b. Hypoglycemia is common in patients who take oral agents.
   c. If you treat him with $D_{50}W$, his blood glucose will not drop again.
   d. Ask if he has recently started any new medicine and consult medical direction.

WRAP IT UP

At 1400 on a warm summer day, you respond for a "diabetic sick case." When you arrive, you find a 21-year-old patient with type 1 diabetes who is pale, cool, and diaphoretic; she responds to painful stimuli only by telling you to go away. Her husband tells you that she is 8 weeks pregnant, and she hasn't been feeling well for a couple of days because of her "morning sickness." He says her insulin is off schedule, and her sugars have been "all over the place." Her vital signs are BP, 100/70 mm Hg; P, 120/min; and R, 20/min. You start an IV and simultaneously obtain a blood glucose level, which is 34 mg/dL. Minutes after 25 g of $D_{50}W$ has been administered IV, the patient awakens and is embarrassed about the situation. She refuses further treatment and transport; you contact medical direction, which recommends that she call her endocrinologist for an appointment immediately.

1. Which is true about type 1 diabetes?
   a. It results from a pituitary abnormality.
   b. Its symptoms occur when glucagon production decreases.

c. It occurs when the cells lose their ability to absorb glucose.

d. It results from inadequate pancreatic production of insulin.

2. Which hormone is responsible for the initial shakiness, tachycardia, and dry mouth felt by diabetics who are hypoglycemic?

   a. Adrenocorticotrophic hormone

   b. Epinephrine

   c. Glucagon

   d. Vasopressin

3. Put a ✔ beside the signs or symptoms this patient had that could indicate hypoglycemia. Put an 8 beside those that could indicate diabetic ketoacidosis (hyperglycemia).

   a. _____ Altered level of consciousness   **d.** _____ Tachycardia

   b. _____ Cool skin   **e.** _____ Sweaty

   c. _____ Hypotension

4. How would your patient care have changed if

   a. The patient had been alert, and oriented.

_____

_____

   b. Her blood glucose had been 434 mg/dL.

_____

_____

   c. Your blood glucose monitor had not functioned.

_____

_____

CHAPTER 32 ANSWERS

REVIEW QUESTIONS

1. a, b, d, e, f, i, j, k
2. b, f, h, i, j
3. b, c, g, i, j
   (Questions 1-3: Objective 3)

4. a. Glucagon; b. insulin; c. somatostatin
   (Objective 2)

5.

Food	Breakdown Products	Storage
a. Carbohydrates	Glucose	Liver and muscles (excess converted to fat)
b. Proteins	Amino acids	Small amounts in cytoplasm of all cells
c. Fats	Fatty acids, glycerol	Liver and fat cells

   (Objective 2)

6. a. Glucose is stored in the liver as glycogen. b. As the blood sugar begins to drop, glucagon is released from the pancreas and stimulates the breakdown of glycogen to glucose.
   (Objective 2)

7. Glucagon breaks down glycogen and stimulates gluconeogenesis (the formation of glucose from amino acids).
   (Objective 2)

8. Glucose cannot be stored in the brain; therefore when blood sugar drops, no reserves exist. The brain cannot use fats or proteins for energy.
   (Objective 3)

9. New onset of diabetes is associated with increased fluid intake (polydipsia), increased urine output (polyuria), dizziness, blurred vision, and rapid weight loss.
   (Objective 3)

10. Long-term complications of diabetes include blindness, kidney disease, peripheral neuropathy, autonomic neuropathy, peripheral vascular disease, heart disease, and stroke.
    (Objective 3)

11. Assess and protect the airway; place a nasal or oral airway and suction if necessary; evaluate breathing, assist if necessary, and administer oxygen; assess pulse; evaluate vital signs; determine blood glucose level; start an IV in the antecubital space; if the blood glucose is less than 80 mg/dL, administer $D_{50}W$ (25 g IV) and reassess the patient.
    (Objective 3)

12. Diabetic ketoacidosis or a pulmonary problem.
    (Objective 3)

13. Have you had any vomiting or diarrhea? If yes, how much? When did you last eat? What medications do you take and when did you last take them (especially insulin)? How much have you been urinating? Do you feel dizzy when you stand up? Have you lost any weight? Are you thirsty and have you been drinking a lot of fluids? Do you have any abdominal pain?
    (Objective 3)

14. As you perform your total patient assessment, you should check to see if the patient has warm, dry skin; dry mucous membranes; tachycardia; postural hypotension; fruity breath odor; or a decreased level of consciousness. (Objective 3)

15. Oxygen should be administered and the patient monitored for dysrhythmias. An IV of 0.9% normal saline should be initiated. Medical direction likely will advise infusion at a rapid rate, often 250 mL/hour or more. (Objective 3)

16. Transport rapidly because definitive treatment includes administration of insulin, which is not usually available on EMS units. (Objective 3)

17. Type 2 diabetes; advanced age; preexisting cardiac or renal disease; inadequate insulin secretion or action; increased insulin requirements (stress, infection, trauma, burns, myocardial infarction); medications such as thiazide diuretics, glucocorticoids, phenytoin, sympathomimetics, propranolol, and immunosuppressants; and parenteral or enteral feedings. (Objective 17)

18.

Disorder	Endocrine Gland and Hormone Affected	Hormone Excess or Shortage?	Signs and Symptoms	Potentially Life Threatening?
Graves disease	Thyroid hormone	Excess	Enlarged thyroid, swollen neck, protruding eyes	Yes if it progresses to to thyroid storm
Thyroid storm	Thyroid hormone	Excess	Tachycardia, heart failure, dysrhythmias, shock, hyperthermia, restlessness, agitation, abdominal pain, coma	Yes
Myxedema	Thyroid hormone	Shortage	Hoarse voice, fatigue, weight gain, cold intolerance, depression, dry skin, hair loss, infertility, constipation, heavy menses	Not unless it progresses to myxedema coma
Cushing syndrome	Adrenal cortex (corticosteroid hormones)	Excess	Round red face, obese trunk, wasted limbs, acne, purple stretch marks, increased facial and body hair, hump on neck, weight gain, hypertension, psychiatric disturbance, insomnia, diabetes	No
Addison disease	Adrenal cortex (cortisol, aldosterone)	Shortage	Weakness, weight loss, anorexia, hyperpigmented skin, hypotension, hyponatremia, hyperkalemia, gastrointestinal disturbances	Usually not unless a rapid, acute onset occurs

(Objectives 4, 5)

STUDENT SELF-ASSESSMENT

19. c. Hormones travel through the blood and may trigger a receptor site in only one organ or throughout the body, depending on the hormone.
(Objective 1)

20. c. Insulin increases glucose transport into cells, increases glucose metabolism by cells, increases liver glycogen levels, and decreases the blood glucose concentration.
(Objective 2)

21. c. Insulin is administered by parenteral injection.
(Objection 3)

22. b. Most type 2 diabetics can control the disease with diet and oral hypoglycemic agents. This disease has a slow onset and does not often cause life-threatening emergencies.
(Objective 3)

23. d. *Glucagon* is a pancreatic hormone. *Glucosuria* is urine that contains glucose. *Gluconeogenesis* is the formation of glucose from the breakdown of fats and fatty acids.
(Objective 2)

24. b. If IV access can be established, intravenous $D_{50}W$ should be administered.
(Objective 3)

25. d. Thiamine promotes the uptake of glucose in the brain.
(Objective 3)

26. c. When an IV cannot be established in a patient with hypoglycemia, glucagon may be given IM. Glucagon is slower, more expensive, and less effective than $D_{50}W$.
(Objective 3)

27. a. 0.5 to 1 mg IM
(Objective 3)

28. c. No ketogenesis occurs with HHNK, therefore no acetone (fruity) breath odor is noted, as it is in hyperglycemia.
(Objective 3)

29. d. These conditions are caused by adrenergic hyperactivity.
(Objective 4)

30. d. If the patient who takes an oral agent becomes hypoglycemic, use standard treatment for hypoglycemia. Then, try to identify a cause—it may be a recent addition of a new drug (especially antibiotics). Contact medical direction.
(Objective 3)

WRAP IT UP

1. d. Type 1 diabetes is characterized by inadequate production of insulin by the pancreas.
(Objective 3)

2. b. The body releases epinephrine in an attempt to stimulate the release of sugar stored in the liver.
(Objective 3)

3. Hypoglycemia: a, b, c, d, e; hyperglycemia: a, c, d
(Objective 3)

4. a. Oral glucose or foods high in simple sugars (e.g., sweetened orange juice) could have been given.

b. A high blood glucose level would have indicated diabetic ketoacidosis. Oxygenation and rapid administration of lactated Ringers solution would have been indicated, along with careful monitoring of the patient (including ECG). Administration of sodium bicarbonate would usually also be ordered in that situation.

c. If no blood glucose value could be obtained, then based on the patient history and presenting signs and symptoms, $D_{50}W$ would be given and the patient's response monitored. (If the EMS blood glucose monitor is not working, the patient's monitor could be used.)

(Objective 3)

Allergies and Anaphylaxis

READING ASSIGNMENT

Chapter 33, pages 882-891, in *Mosby's Paramedic Textbook,* ed. 3

OBJECTIVES

Upon completion of this chapter, the paramedic student will be able to do the following:

1. Describe the antigen-antibody response.
2. Differentiate between an allergic reaction and a normal immune response.
3. Describe signs and symptoms and management of local allergic reactions based on an understanding of the pathophysiology associated with this condition.
4. Identify allergens associated with anaphylaxis.
5. Describe the pathophysiology, signs and symptoms, and management of anaphylaxis.

SUMMARY

- Antibodies bind to the antigen that produced them. Antibodies aid in neutralizing the antigen and removing it from the body.
- Allergic reaction is an increased physiological response to an antigen after a previous exposure to the same antigen. Localized allergic reactions do not affect the entire body.
- Anaphylaxis is the most extreme form of allergic reaction. Rapid recognition and aggressive therapy are needed for patient survival.
- Almost any substance can cause anaphylaxis. The risk of anaphylaxis increases with the frequency of exposure.
- Symptoms of anaphylaxis may include sneezing and coughing; airway obstruction; wheezing; hypotension or vascular collapse; chest pain; nausea, vomiting, or diarrhea; and weakness, headache, syncope, seizures, or coma.

REVIEW QUESTIONS

1. Complete the following sentences.

   Antigens can enter the body by four routes: **(a)** _____, **(b)** _____,

   (c) _____ or **(d)** _____. The allergic reaction is initiated when a circulating

   (e) _____

combines with a specific antigen, causing a **(f)** _____ reaction or to antibodies bound to

(g) _____ _____ or **(h)** _____.

2. List agents in each of the following groups that can cause anaphylaxis.

   a. Drugs:_____

   b. Insects:_____

   c. Foods:_____

   d. Other:_____

3. List the signs and symptoms associated with each of the following chemical mediators released from basophils and mast cells in an anaphylactic reaction.

   a. Histamines:_____

   _____

   b. Leukotrienes:_____

   _____

   c. Eosinophil chemotactic factor:_____

   _____

4. You are called to a church picnic to care for a 30-year-old woman. Her skin is very red and she has wheezing and dyspnea. After a careful assessment, you determine that she is having an anaphylactic reaction.

   a. What other illness or injury may produce these symptoms?_____

   _____

   b. List two home medicines that may influence your care of this patient._____

   _____

Questions 5 to 7 refer to the following case study:

   You are at a Chinese restaurant caring for a 25-year-old patient experiencing an anaphylactic reaction. His lips are swollen and he is in acute respiratory distress with wheezing and has a blood pressure of 90/70 mm Hg.

5. What are some causative agents that may be found at this restaurant that could trigger this man's anaphylaxis?

6. After a rapid primary survey and vital sign assessment, you determine that immediate pharmacological therapy is indicated. Identify two drugs, with the appropriate dose and route, that may be indicated for this patient.

   a.

   b.

7. Describe other signs or symptoms that this patient may have.

8. You arrive at a dental office, where you find a 35-year-old woman who rapidly developed hives, angioedema, and stridor after an injection of a local anesthetic. She is unconscious and has labored, stridorous respirations, no radial pulse, and a rapid, irregular, barely palpable carotid pulse. No medicines have been administered to treat her. Describe your priorities of care for this patient, including the appropriate drugs, doses, and routes.

_____

_____

9. What is the term used for any substance that causes the formation of antibodies in the body?
   a. Anaphylactic
   c. Basophil
   b. Antigen
   d. Mast cell

10. Which immunoglobulin (antibody) is responsible for anaphylaxis?
    a. IgA
    c. IgG
    b. IgE
    d. IgM

11. Which of the following is a sign or symptom of a type IV (localized) allergic reaction?
    a. Angioedema
    c. Vomiting
    b. Hoarseness
    d. Wheezing

12. Your 20-year-old patient has hives, normal vital signs, and clear breath sounds. He complains of severe itching. Which of the following drugs would be indicated in this situation?
    a. Diphenhydramine (Benadryl), 5 mg IV
    b. Diphenhydramine (Benadryl), 25 mg IM
    c. Epinephrine (Adrenalin), 0.1 mg (1:1000) IV
    d. Epinephrine (Adrenalin), 0.3 mg (1:1000) SQ

13. What term is used for mediators that cause blood vessels to dilate?
    a. Chemotactic substances
    c. Opsonins
    b. Leukotactic substances
    d. Vasoactive substances

14. Which of the following agents is *not* commonly associated with anaphylaxis?
    a. Acetaminophen
    c. Fire ants
    b. Aspirin
    d. Peanuts

15. What is the most likely cause of death in anaphylaxis?
    a. Upper airway obstruction
    b. Hypoxia resulting from bronchospasm
    c. Hypotension resulting from fluid leakage
    d. Vasogenic shock caused by histamines

16. Which of the following signs or symptoms is *not* associated with anaphylaxis?
    a. Abdominal cramps
    c. Rhinorrhea
    b. Cool, pale skin
    d. Urticaria

17. Diphenhydramine is considered which of the following?
    a. Anticholinergic
    c. Bronchodilator
    b. Antihistamine
    d. Sedative-hypnotic

18. Which of the following is a potential complication of IV epinephrine?
    a. Dysrhythmias
    d. Vomiting
    b. Myocardial ischemia
    e. All of the above
    c. Seizures

WRAP IT UP

You are dispatched for a "person down." You find your patient in the cafeteria, lying unconscious. Co-workers tell you that she complained of itching and said, "That bee just stung me." She then complained of difficulty breathing, and after a 9-1-1 call was made, she became unconscious. You ask about any known allergies, and no one seems to know. They tell you she was at her doctor's office this morning for a vaccination, and when the police officer on the scene looks through her purse, he shows you aspirin, ibuprofen, and penicillin tablets. The remnants of her partly eaten lunch are on the table: fried shrimp; deviled eggs; fruit salad with strawberries, mangoes, and a sesame honey dressing; peanut butter crackers; and a glass of milk. Her skin is flushed red, and she has raised welts on her arm; her eyes and lips appear swollen; and her breathing is stridorous. Her vital signs are BP, 76 by palpation; P, 134/min; R, 24/min; and Sao$_2$, 88%. You administer oxygen by nonrebreather mask; at the same time, your partner draws up 0.1 mg of epinephrine and administers it IV over 5 minutes. You start an IV of normal saline and give a fluid bolus; you then administer diphenhydramine (25 mg slow IV), followed by methylprednisolone (125 mg IV). The stridor has now subsided, but you hear some persistent wheezing in the lungs, and the woman's vital signs are now BP, 104/60 mm Hg; P, 120/min; R, 20/min; and Sao$_2$, 98%. You administer an albuterol updraft for the persistent wheezing and continue to monitor her condition, which has improved dramatically by the time you arrive at the hospital. She is discharged with a prescription and instructions for an EpiPen and is told to purchase a bracelet or necklace to alert first responders to her severe allergic condition.

1. Which of the following describes the internal mechanisms responsible for this patient's life-threatening condition?
   a. IgE antibodies react to a foreign antigen, triggering the release of histamines, leukotrienes, and other chemicals
   b. IgM antibodies initiate a type IV allergic reaction, which triggers a life-threatening release of kinins
   c. IgG antibodies trigger the release of antigens, which stimulate the eosinophil chemotactic factor of anaphylaxis
   d. Immunoglobulins begin a process of cellular destruction in the lymphatic system that causes anaphylaxis
2. List the possible causes of anaphylaxis that you observed on this patient call.
3. Put a ✔ beside the signs or symptoms of anaphylaxis that were observed in this patient.

a. _____ Hoarseness	k. _____ Hypotension	u. _____ Weakness
b. _____ Stridor	l. _____ Dysrhythmia	v. _____ Headache
c. _____ Laryngeal edema	m. _____ Chest tightness	w. _____ Seizure
d. _____ Rhinorrhea	n. _____ Nausea	x. _____ Coma
e. _____ Bronchospasm	o. _____ Vomiting	y. _____ Angioedema
f. _____ Increased mucus production	p. _____ Abdominal cramps	z. _____ Urticaria
g. _____ Accessory muscle use	q. _____ Diarrhea	aa. _____ Pruritus
h. _____ Wheezing	r. _____ Anxiety	bb. _____ Erythema
i. _____ Decreased breath sounds	s. _____ Dizziness	cc. _____ Edema
j. _____ Tachycardia	t. _____ Syncope	dd. _____ Tearing of the eyes

4. Explain your rationale for each of the following interventions that were performed for this patient.

   a. Oxygen administration:

   _____

   b. Epinephrine administration:

   _____

   c. Normal saline fluid bolus:

   _____

   d. Diphenhydramine administration:

   _____

   e. Steroid administration:

   _____

   f. Albuterol administration:

   _____

CHAPTER 33 ANSWERS

REVIEW QUESTIONS

1. a. Injection; b. ingestion; c. inhalation; d. absorption; e. antibody; f. hypersensitivity; g. mast cells; h. basophils
(Objective 1)

2. a. Antibiotics (especially penicillin and other beta lactams), local anesthetics, cephalosporins, chemotherapeutics, aspirin, nonsteroidal antiinflammatory agents, opiates, muscle relaxants, IV contrast agents, vaccines, and insulin; b. wasps, bees, and fire ants; c. peanuts, treegrown nuts, soybeans, cod, halibut, shellfish, egg white, strawberries, food additives, wheat and buckwheat, sesame and sunflower seeds, cotton seed, milk, and mango; d. latex.
(Objective 3)

3. a. Histamine release may result in decreased blood pressure, increased gastrointestinal secretions, rhinorrhea, tearing, flushing, urticaria, and angioedema. b. Leukotrienes cause wheezing, which may precipitate chest pain (resulting from coronary vasoconstriction) and enhance the hypotensive effects of histamine. c. Eosinophil chemotactic factor can produce fever, chills, bronchospasm, and pulmonary vasoconstriction.
(Objective 3)

4. a. These same respiratory signs and symptoms could be caused by asthma, upper airway obstruction, pulmonary edema, or toxic inhalation. b. If the patient takes a beta blocker (e.g., atenolol, propranolol), it could interfere with the action of epinephrine. If the patient has already self-administered epinephrine (EpiPen, AnaPen), determine the time it was administered and whether symptoms have improved or worsened since administration.
(Objective 4)

5. Foods such as crab, shrimp, nuts, egg, and food additives are known to cause anaphylaxis.
(Objective 3)

6. a. Epinephrine, 0.3 to 0.5 mg (1:1000) IM; b. diphenhydramine (Benadryl), 25 to 50 mg IM or IV, and then albuterol (Proventil, Ventolin) updraft.
(Objective 4)

7. He may also have stridor, hoarseness, tachypnea, tachycardia, agitation, headache, seizures, decreasing level of consciousness, angioedema, tearing, swelling of the tongue, urticaria, pruritus, sneezing, coughing, tracheal tugging, intercostal retractions, decreased breath sounds, dysrhythmias, chest tightness, nausea, vomiting, and diarrhea.
(Objective 4)

8. Secure the airway, ventilate with 100% oxygen, and intubate. Initiate IV therapy with a large-bore catheter into the antecubital space, infuse fluid rapidly, and administer epinephrine (0.1 mg [1:10,000] IV) over 5 minutes (try to do this simultaneously with airway management if resources permit). If necessary, administer diphenhydramine (25 to 50 mg IM or slow IV) as a second-line drug. Reevaluate the need to administer a second dose of epinephrine if the patient has not responded. Consider giving methylprednisolone. Administer inhaled albuterol if wheezing is present.
(Objective 4)

STUDENT SELF-ASSESSMENT

9. b. An anaphylactic response is a type of life-threatening allergic response. Basophils and mast cells are white blood cells that are involved in the immune response.
(Objective 1)

10. b. IgA immunoglobulins are antibodies found in blood, secretions such as tears, and the respiratory system. IgG antibodies are the most common antibodies involved in the immune response. Production of IgM antibodies precedes IgG production in acute infections.
(Objective 1)

11. a. Angioedema may be found in local or systemic allergic reactions. All of the other signs or symptoms, if present during an allergic reaction, would be most often associated with a systemic (anaphylactic) reaction.
(Objective 2)

12. b. Because no systemic signs or symptoms exist, intramuscular diphenhydramine is indicated. Epinephrine 1:1000 should never be given IVP to treat anaphylaxis.
(Objective 2)

13. d. Chemotactic substances cause the attraction of phagocytic cells toward or away from the antigen; leukotactic substances attract leukocytes to the pathogenic agent; and opsonins bind phagocytes to the invading microorganism.
(Objective 1)

14. a. All the other agents are known to cause anaphylaxis.
(Objective 3)

15. a. Each of the other problems could cause death, but upper airway obstruction is associated with the most deaths from anaphylaxis.
(Objective 4)

16. b. The skin is usually flushed and warm because of the profound vasodilation.
(Objective 4)

17. b
(Objective 2)

18. e
(Objective 4)

WRAP IT UP

1. a. IgE antibodies are the primary mediators in anaphylaxis. Additional chemicals that are triggered include eosinophil chemotactic factor of anaphylaxis, heparin, kinins, prostaglandins, and thromboxanes.
(Objective 1)

2. Antibiotic (penicillin), aspirin, nonsteroidal antiinflammatory agent (ibuprofen), vaccine, possible insect sting, peanuts (peanut butter crackers), shellfish (fried shrimp), egg white (deviled eggs), strawberries, mangoes, sesame seeds (salad), and milk.
(Objective 4)

3. b, c, e, h, j, k, x, y, z, aa, bb, cc
(Objective 5)

4. a. The patient is hypoxic and in shock. Oxygen administration is indicated for both conditions.
b. Epinephrine antagonizes the effects of histamine, and exerts beta-2 effects, which dilate bronchioles; beta-1 effects, which improve myocardial contractility; and alpha effects, which provide vasoconstriction to counteract the effects of anaphylaxis.
c. Normal saline bolus is given as an adjunct to epinephrine in the treatment of the shock associated with anaphylaxis.

d. Diphenhydramine is an antihistamine that can help to reverse some of the symptoms (especially cutaneous) of anaphylaxis.

e. Steroids such as methylprednisolone and dexamethasone suppress acute inflammatory responses that accompany anaphylaxis; they also potentiate smooth muscle relaxation by beta-adrenergic agonists (epinephrine, albuterol) and may alter airway hyperreactivity.

f. Albuterol can aid the management of some of the bronchospasm that is unresolved by epinephrine. However, if signs and symptoms of upper airway edema, severe bronchospasm, or shock persist, an additional dose of epinephrine would be indicated in addition to albuterol.

(Objective 5)

Gastroenterology

READING ASSIGNMENT
Chapter 34, pages 892-907 in *Mosby's Paramedic Textbook,* ed. 3

OBJECTIVES
Upon completion of this chapter, the paramedic student will be able to:
1. Label a diagram of the abdominal organs.
2. Outline prehospital assessment of a patient who has abdominal pain.
3. Describe general prehospital management techniques for the patient with abdominal pain.
4. Describe signs and symptoms, complications, and prehospital management for the following gastrointestinal disorders: gastroenteritis, gastritis, colitis, diverticulosis, appendicitis, peptic ulcer disease, bowel obstruction, Crohn's disease, pancreatitis, esophagogastric varices, hemorrhoids, cholecystitis, and acute hepatitis.

SUMMARY
- The major organs most commonly associated with the gastrointestinal system include the esophagus, stomach, small and large intestine, liver, gallbladder, and pancreas.
- After the initial survey, assessment of abdominal pain should begin with a thorough history. The physical examination may help to determine if the pain is visceral, somatic, or referred.
- The most common treatment for abdominal pain will occur at the hospital. The paramedic should provide supportive treatment, manage life threats, and transport the patient to an appropriate facility.
- Gastroenteritis is inflammation of the stomach and intestines secondary to infectious agents, chemicals, or other conditions.
- Gastritis is acute or chronic inflammation of the gastric mucosa. It commonly results from hyperacidity, alcohol or other drug ingestion, bile reflux, and *Helicobacter pylori* infection.
- Colitis is an inflammatory condition of the large intestine. It is characterized by severe diarrhea and ulceration of the mucosa of the intestine (ulcerative colitis).
- Diverticulosis may result in bright red rectal bleeding if perforation occurs.
- Diverticulitis results when a diverticulum becomes obstructed with fecal matter.
- Appendicitis occurs when the passageway between the appendix and cecum is obstructed by fecal material or by inflammation due to infection.
- Peptic ulcer disease occurs when open wounds or sores develop in the stomach or duodenum.
- Bowel obstruction is an occlusion of the intestinal lumen. It results in blockage of the normal flow of intestinal contents.
- Crohn's disease is a chronic, inflammatory bowel disease. It is of unknown origin.
- Inflammation of the pancreas is called pancreatitis. It causes severe abdominal pain.
- Esophagogastric varices result from obstruction of blood flow to the liver as a result of liver disease.

- Hemorrhoids are distended veins in the rectoanal area.
- Cholecystitis is inflammation of the gallbladder. It most often is associated with the presence of gallstones.
- Hepatitis is characterized by the sudden onset of malaise, weakness, anorexia, intermittent nausea and vomiting, and dull right upper quadrant pain. This is usually followed within 1 week by the onset of jaundice, dark urine, or both.

REVIEW QUESTIONS

Match the gastrointestinal disorder in column II with its description in column I. Use each disorder only once.

Column I	Column II
1. _____ Occlusion of the intestinal lumen	a. Appendicitis
2. _____ Increased pain after ethyl alcohol ingestion; fever and signs of sepsis and shock also possible	b. Arteriovenous malformation
	c. Cholecystitis
3. _____ Protrusion of viscus from normal position through opening in groin or abdominal wall	d. Diverticulitis
	e. Diverticulosis
4. _____ Pain that is most intense at McBurney point	f. Esophageal varices
5. _____ Most common cause of massive rectal bleeding in older adults	g. Esophagitis
	h. Gastritis
6. _____ Open erosion wound in digestive system that may bleed	i. Hemorrhoids
	j. Hernia
7. _____ Characterized by blood dripping into the toilet after a normal bowel movement	k. Intestinal obstruction
	l. Pancreatitis
8. _____ Left lower quadrant abdominal pain resulting from a pouch in the colon wall	m. Peptic ulcer
9. _____ Painless bleeding resulting from a vascular abnormality in the gastrointestinal tract	
10. _____ Bright red hematemesis caused by rupture of vessels distended by portal hypertension	
11. _____ Inflammation of the gallbladder	
12. _____ Inflammation of the gastric mucosa	

13. Label the abdominal organs in Fig. 34-1.

a. _____ f. _____

b. _____ g. _____

c. _____ h. _____

d. _____ i. _____

e. _____

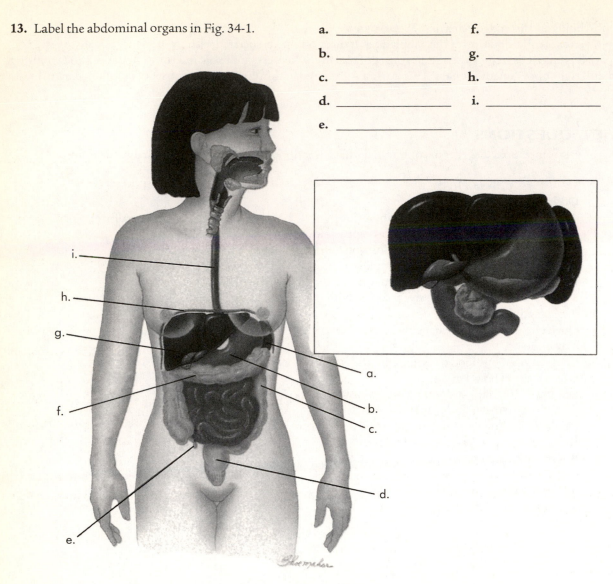

Figure 34-1

14. Your patient is a 72-year-old man complaining of left lower quadrant abdominal pain. State why you would or would not suspect each of the following illnesses as a cause of his pain.

a. Pancreatitis:

_____

b. Cholecystitis:

_____

c. Diverticulitis:

_____

d. Peptic ulcer:

_____

15. A 65-year-old man complains of severe epigastric pain.

   a. List specific questions you must ask this patient to obtain a complete medical history and to determine whether this is a gastrointestinal problem.

   _____

   _____

   _____

   b. What other significant medical problems must you try to rule out by asking these questions?

   _____

   _____

16. Name the type of pain described in each of the following statements.

   a. Your patient is supine with his legs flexed and complains of a constant, sharp, stabbing pain.

   _____

   b. A 40-year-old woman complains of a severe cramping pain at the umbilicus that peaks and then subsides. She is nauseated and has vomited twice.

   _____

   c. An obese 47-year-old female complains of right upper quadrant abdominal pain that travels to her right shoulder blade.

   _____

17. A 17-year-old boy states that he had severe right lower quadrant pain that diminished several hours ago and is now generalized.

   a. What signs and symptoms would indicate that this patient has an acute abdominal condition and may be developing peritonitis?

   _____

   b. Describe the prehospital treatment for this patient.

   _____

   _____

   _____

STUDENT SELF-ASSESSMENT

18. Which of the following abdominal organs is located in the retroperitoneal space?
   a. Liver
   b. Pancreas
   c. Spleen
   d. Stomach

19. A 78-year-old man states that he has been unable to have a bowel movement for a week and has been vomiting profusely. What do you suspect?
   a. Appendicitis
   b. Bowel obstruction
   c. Diverticulosis
   d. Peptic ulcer

20. You are called at 1900 to care for a 40-year-old woman who is complaining of intermittent severe right upper quadrant abdominal pain. She is vomiting and has a low-grade fever. What do you suspect?
- **a.** Colitis
- **b.** Cholecystitis
- **c.** Esophagitis
- **d.** Hepatitis

21. Which of the following is most likely to cause life-threatening hemorrhage?
- **a.** Arteriovenous malformations
- **b.** Diverticulitis
- **c.** Esophagogastric varices
- **d.** Hemorrhoids

22. The cause of acute abdominal pain is most accurately assessed in the prehospital setting by which of the following?
- **a.** Abdominal examination
- **b.** Patient history
- **c.** Secondary survey
- **d.** Vital sign assessment

23. Which of the following is most suggestive of a hemorrhagic gastrointestinal problem?
- **a.** Anorexia
- **b.** Fever
- **c.** Melena
- **d.** Tachycardia

Questions 24 and 25 refer to the following case study:

A pale, elderly man has had severe vomiting and diarrhea for 3 days. His only history is high blood pressure controlled by an ACE inhibitor and a diuretic. He has severe lower abdominal cramping and is in a fetal position. His wife has a similar illness, but it is not as severe. His blood pressure is 92/50 mm Hg; P, 128/min; and R, 20/min.

24. What is a likely cause of the man's pain?
- **a.** Appendicitis
- **b.** Cholecystitis
- **c.** Diverticulosis
- **d.** Gastroenteritis

25. Which is a priority in your care of this patient at this time?
- **a.** Administer pain medicine to relieve his pain.
- **b.** Give him some medicine to relieve his nausea.
- **c.** Position him to allow for maximum comfort.
- **d.** Start an IV and administer fluids to treat shock.

26. Which of the following conditions may cause jaundice?
- **a.** Colitis
- **b.** Gastritis
- **c.** Hepatitis
- **d.** Peptic ulcer disease

Questions 27 and 28 pertain to the following case study:

A 57-year-old alcoholic male is complaining of nausea and vomiting. He has abdominal pain that starts in the area of the umbilicus and goes to both shoulders. He is hot to the touch. Vital signs are BP, 94/58 mm Hg; P, 132/min; and R, 28/min.

27. Which intervention is indicated first for this man?
- **a.** Morphine (4 mg IV push)
- **b.** Normal saline (200 mL bolus)
- **c.** Oxygen (15 L/min by mask)
- **d.** Promethazine (Phenergan), 25 mg IV

28. What abdominal illness is a probable diagnosis for this man?
- **a.** Crohn disease
- **b.** Esophageal varices
- **c.** Pancreatitis
- **d.** Ulcerative colitis

WRAP IT UP

You have just fallen asleep after your third call of the night when the horn sounds and the speaker blares, "4017, respond to an EMS call, abdominal pains, Haven Golden Rest Home, 222 Main, cross street Elm." Your patient is an 80-year-old man who has a history of dementia. The nurse gives you a medication sheet that lists a number of anti-hypertensives, aspirin, some antiarthritic drugs, and some laxatives and stool softeners. She states that he had a shaking chill, vomited twice, seems agitated, and has been moaning and holding his lower abdomen. She thinks his last bowel movement was 4 days ago, and a note in his record states that it was very dark in color. His skin is very warm, moist, and pale, and he is very restless. Vital signs are BP, 100/70 mm Hg; P, 116/min; R, 20/min; Sao$_2$, 93% on room air; and T (axilla), 100.4° F (38° C). His skin is dry and tents slightly, and his mucous membranes are dry. The rest of his physical examination is unremarkable, except that his abdomen is tender to palpation and he is guarding it. Because of his dementia, it is difficult to communicate well enough with him to have him localize the pain. You administer oxygen by nasal cannula at 6 L/min; you then start an IV of normal saline and infuse a bolus of 100 mL, reassessing his breath sounds and vital signs after it has been infused. Medical direction asks you to hold off on pain medicine administration until he can be assessed more thoroughly.

You transport the patient and later find out that free air was present in his abdomen secondary to a ruptured diverticulum. In consultation with his family, after his status deteriorated, the decision was made not to operate.

1. Which abdominal organs could cause pain in the following regions if they are injured, inflamed, or diseased?

   a. Left upper quadrant:

   _____

   b. Right upper quadrant:

   _____

   c. Left lower quadrant:

   _____

   d. Right lower quadrant:

   _____

2. Which of the following describes the correct procedure for an abdominal examination?
   a. Percuss carefully so that painful stimulus can be evaluated.
   b. Auscultate after palpation so that you can focus on tender areas.
   c. Begin palpation in an area of no reported pain and move to the painful area last.
   d. Inspection can often reveal the source of the abdominal pain.

3. Put a ✔ beside any illnesses that could be responsible for this patient's signs and symptoms.

   a. _____ Appendicitis   **e.** _____ Diverticulosis
   b. _____ Bacterial infection   **f.** _____ Hepatitis B
   c. _____ Cholecystitis   **g.** _____ Intestinal obstruction
   d. _____ Crohn disease   **h.** _____ Pancreatitis

4. What additional interventions could have been provided for this patient?

   _____

CHAPTER 34 ANSWERS

REVIEW QUESTIONS

1. k
2. l
3. j
4. a
5. e
6. m
7. i
(Questions 1-7: Objective 2)

8. d
(Objective 2 or 3)

9. b
(Objective 3)

10. f
(Objective 3)

11. c
(Objective 2)

12. h
(Objective 2)

13. a. Spleen; b. stomach; c. descending colon; d. rectum; e. appendix; f. transverse colon; g. liver; h. diaphragm; i. esophagus
(Objective 1)

14. a. No. The pain of pancreatitis is located in the epigastric region or right or left upper quadrant. b. No. The pain of cholecystitis is located in the epigastric region or right upper quadrant. It is more common in women under age 50. c. Yes. Diverticulitis is one possibility. It is common in older adults, and the pain is often in the left lower quadrant. d. No. Pain from a peptic ulcer would typically be in the epigastric area.
(Objective 2)

15. a. Does anything make the pain better or worse? What does the pain feel like (sharp, stabbing, cramping, dull)? Can you show me where the pain is? Does the pain go anywhere else? On a scale of 0 to 10, with 0 being no pain and 10 being the worst pain you have ever had, rate the pain. When did the pain begin? Associated signs and symptoms—Do you have or have you had any nausea, vomiting, diarrhea, constipation, unusual-colored stools, chills, fever, or shortness of breath? Medical history and medications.
b. Myocardial infarction and abdominal aneurysm.
(Objective 4)

16. a. Somatic; b. visceral; c. referred
(Objective 4)

17. a. Fever, chills, tachycardia, tachypnea, position (lying on side with knees flexed and pulled in toward the chest), reluctance to move, skin pallor, absent bowel sounds, generalized involuntary guarding, and rigidity of the abdomen.
(Objective 4)

b. Oxygen by nonrebreather mask; IV by 16-gauge catheter with normal saline or lactated Ringer solution (rate at least 100 mL/hour, determined by patient's vital signs).
(Objective 4)

STUDENT SELF-ASSESSMENT

18. b. All of the other organs are in the abdominal cavity. (Objective 1)

19. b. Appendicitis would be unusual at this age and typically would not cause the symptoms listed. Diverticulosis and peptic ulcer would not typically produce the symptoms described.
(Objective 2)

20. b. Her age, the time of day, and the description of the pain are characteristics of cholecystitis.
(Objective 2)

21. c. All the disorders listed cause bleeding, but rupture of the esophagogastric varices usually produces rapid, life-threatening bleeding. Bleeding from AV malformations may be minor or severe. Bleeding from diverticulitis may be serious but is not typically an acute life-threatening emergency at onset. Hemorrhoidal bleeding is usually not severe.
(Objective 3)

22. b. The patient's age and gender and the description of the medical history often disclose more about the cause of the abdominal illness than a physical examination. The severity of the patient's present condition is determined by the physical examination.
(Objective 4)

23. c. Melena (black or maroon stool) indicates the presence of bleeding. Tachycardia can be caused by bleeding, fever, pain, or other fluid loss.
(Objective 4)

24. d. The signs and symptoms, as well as the fact that the man's wife had the same illness, point to this as a probable cause.
(Objective 2)

25. d. The most pressing problem is the shock from fluid loss. IV fluid replacement is needed as soon as possible.
(Objective 5)

26. c
(Objective 2)

27. c. A normal saline bolus is given next, as soon as an IV line has been established.
(Objective 5)

28. c. Esophageal varices present with life-threatening bleeding. Crohn disease and ulcerative colitis would be unusual in someone of this age without a prior history.
(Objective 2)

WRAP IT UP

1. Left upper quadrant: Liver, bowel, gallbladder
Right upper quadrant: Stomach, bowel, pancreas, spleen
Left lower quadrant: Bowel
Right lower quadrant: Bowel, appendix
(Objective 1)

2. c. Palpate from an area of no pain (if possible) to the area of greatest pain to facilitate the best exam. The exam should be performed in the following order: inspection, auscultation, palpation, percussion
(Objective 2)

3. a, b, c, e, f, g, h
(Objective 4)

4. If the patient's vomiting had persisted, medical direction might have ordered an antiemetic. It's also possible that some pain medicine could have been ordered (a small dose) to relieve his obvious discomfort. This would have had to be done in consultation with medical direction because of the patient's complex history.
(Objective 3)

Urology/Renal

READING ASSIGNMENT
Chapter 35, pages 908-918, in *Mosby's Paramedic Textbook,* ed. 3

OBJECTIVES
Upon completion of this chapter, the paramedic student will be able to:
1. Label a diagram of the urinary system.
2. Describe pathophysiology, signs and symptoms, assessment, and prehospital management of the patient with urinary retention, urinary tract infection, pyelonephritis, urinary calculus, epididymitis, and testicular torsion.
3. Outline the physical examination for patients with genitourinary disorders.
4. Discuss general prehospital management for the patient with a genitourinary disorder.
5. Distinguish between acute and chronic renal failure.
6. Describe the signs and symptoms of renal failure.
7. Describe dialysis and emergent conditions associated with it, including prehospital management.

SUMMARY
- The urinary system removes waste products from the blood. It helps to maintain a constant body fluid volume and composition as well.
- Urinary retention is the inability to urinate.
- Urinary tract infections can involve the upper or lower urinary tract.
- Pyelonephritis is inflammation of the kidney parenchyma.
- Urinary calculi are stones that originate in the kidney.
- Epididymitis is inflammation of the epididymis. The epididymis is the tube that carries sperm from the testicle to the seminal vesicles.
- Testicular torsion is a true emergency. In this condition a testicle twists on its spermatic cord. This disrupts the blood supply to the testicle.
- The physical examination for a patient with a urinary tract problem is similar to that performed for abdominal pain. Patients with genitourinary pain should be managed as any other patient with acute pain.
- Renal failure may result in uremia, hyperkalemia, acidosis, hypertension, and volume overload with congestive heart failure. Renal failure can be classified as acute or chronic. Classification depends on the duration and on the potential for reversibility.
- Dialysis is a technique used to normalize blood chemistry. Dialysis is used in patients who have acute or chronic renal failure. Dialysis also is used to remove blood toxins. The two dialysis techniques are hemodialysis and peritoneal dialysis. Dialysis emergencies may include problems with vascular access, hemorrhage, hypotension, chest pain, severe hyperkalemia, disequilibrium syndrome, and air embolism.

REVIEW QUESTIONS

Match the genitourinary problem in column II with the description in column I. Use each disorder only once.

Column I

1. _____ Can cause vascular infarction and loss of function
2. _____ Inflammation of part of the male reproductive system
3. _____ Systemic disease linked with diabetes and hypertension
4. _____ Infectious process that causes dysuria and hematuria
5. _____ Causes include enlarged prostate and CNS dysfunction
6. _____ Caused by an excess of insoluble salts in the urine
7. _____ Upper urinary infection treated with IV antibiotics

Column II

a. Acute renal failure
b. Chronic renal failure
c. Epididymitis
d. Pyelonephritis
e. Testicular torsion
f. Urinary calculus
g. Urinary retention
h. Urinary tract infection

8. Label the parts of the urinary system shown in Fig. 35-1.

   a.

   b.

   c.

   d.

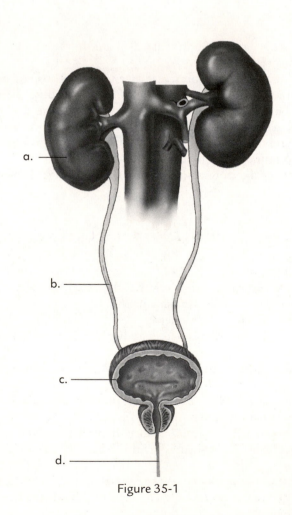

Figure 35-1

9. Identify the genitourinary disorder suspected and the prehospital care needed in each of the following situations.

a. A 35-year-old afebrile man complains of a sudden onset of severe flank pain that radiates into his testicle.

Condition:

_____

Care:

_____

b. Your 21-year-old patient complains of painful swelling in the scrotal sac that is unrelieved by elevation. He is in acute distress and has vomited twice.

Condition:

_____

Care:

_____

c. A 35-year-old woman with a recent history of recurrent urinary infections complains of fever, chills, and severe flank pain.

Condition:

_____

Care:

_____

d. A 27-year-old woman complains of burning on urination and of feeling as if she must urinate every 20 minutes.

Condition:

_____

Care:

_____

10. How can you minimize psychological discomfort for a patient with a urology problem when performing the physical examination?

_____

11. Identify three causes of each of the following disorders.

a. Acute renal failure:

_____

b. Chronic renal failure:

_____

12. You are called to a dialysis center for a person in shock.

a. What types of patient problems should you anticipate en route to this call?

_____

b. If the patient is hypotensive and needs fluid resuscitation, describe how you will initiate fluid therapy and indicate the volume you will infuse.

_____

13. Complete the information in the following table regarding dialysis emergencies.

Disorder	Cause	Effect on Patient	Interventions
Hemorrhage			
Hypotension			
Chest pain			
Hyperkalemia			
Disequilibrium syndrome			
Air embolism			

14. You are dispatched to a private residence for a patient in full arrest. On arrival, you find a 55-year-old man in asystolic cardiac arrest. The family reports that he lost consciousness about 5 minutes before your arrival. The patient's history includes renal failure. He missed hemodialysis this week and was feeling bad before cardiac arrest.

a. You begin CPR. List the first three drugs you should administer to this patient, including dose and route.

_____

b. How will the drug therapy help to correct some of the problems that may have caused the patient's cardiac arrest?

_____

c. What problem may occur if this combination of drugs is administered improperly?

_____

STUDENT SELF-ASSESSMENT

15. Which genitourinary emergency requires treatment within 4 hours to prevent irreversible damage?
   a. Epididymitis
   b. Pyelonephritis
   c. Testicular torsion
   d. Urinary calculus

16. Which of the following is a prerenal cause of acute renal failure?
   a. Kidney infection
   b. Prostatic enlargement
   c. Shock
   d. Ureteral strictures

17. How is prehospital care affected if the patient has a dialysis fistula or shunt?
   a. Blood pressure should be checked in the arm opposite the shunt.
   b. The arm in which the shunt is placed should be elevated.
   c. Vascular access should be initiated in the fistula or shunt.
   d. No special consideration is required.

18. You are caring for a patient with a temperature of 102.5° F (39.2° C) who is on continuous peritoneal dialysis. What is a common cause of fever in patients undergoing this treatment?
   a. Dehydration
   b. Infected fistula
   c. Peritonitis
   d. Pneumonia

19. You are called to the home of an unconscious person in chronic renal failure. The ECG tracing is shown in Fig. 35-2. Which electrolyte imbalance do you suspect?
   a. Hyperkalemia
   b. Hypokalemia
   c. Hypercalcemia
   d. Hypocalcemia

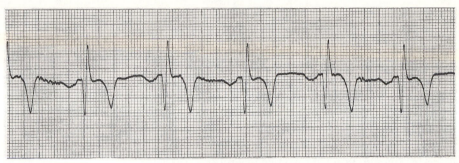

Figure 35-2

20. What drug may be ordered by medical direction to correct the underlying electrolyte imbalance in question 19?
   a. Atropine sulfate (1 mg IV)
   b. Sodium bicarbonate (1 mEq/kg IV)
   c. Magnesium sulfate (1 to 2 g IV)
   d. Verapamil (2.5 mg IV)

21. What physiological problem makes patients in renal failure more susceptible to hypoxia?
   a. Anemia
   b. Glucose intolerance
   c. Pericarditis
   d. Uremia

WRAP IT UP

At 1400 you are dispatched to a dialysis center for a patient who has chest pain. On arrival you find a 59-year-old man who is anxious, pale, and diaphoretic. He missed dialysis for a week because of a severe snowstorm in the area. He came in today fatigued and twitching. About 10 minutes into his dialysis session, he had several episodes of hypotension and then began complaining of chest pain and dyspnea. He has a history of type 1 diabetes, hypertension, and renal failure. He is pale, sweaty, and complains of midsternal chest pain. His oxygen saturation is 94% on room air. You administer oxygen at 4 L/min, which quickly improves his Sao_2 to 98%. The nurse is keeping pressure on the dialysis fistula site in his left arm, so you go to the right arm to assess vital signs. Your findings are BP, 198/106 mm Hg; P, 110/min; R, 20/min; and blood glucose, 170 mg/dL. The patient has generalized edema, and you can hear bibasilar crackles in his lungs. You start an IV in the right forearm, administer one spray (0.4 mg) of nitroglycerin, apply the ECG monitor, and then move him by stretcher into the ambulance. You note tall, tented T waves on his ECG. Just as you are attaching the electrodes to perform a 12-lead ECG, his eyes roll back and his body goes limp, and you note a very wide, slow ventricular complex on the monitor. You immediately determine that he is not breathing and begin to ventilate with a bag-valve-mask; you assess a carotid pulse but find none. Your partner immediately radios for additional help and then takes over CPR. You administer epinephrine IV and set up for intubation. You intubate the patient orally with an 8.0 endotracheal tube and verify its placement by listening to the epigastric area and the lungs and by applying the end-tidal CO_2 monitor, which reads 16.

Because the wide complex rhythm on the monitor is only about 30/min, epinephrine is repeated and atropine is given after absence of a carotid pulse is confirmed. You go en route when the pumper unit arrives; you have one firefighter perform chest compressions while your partner ventilates and another firefighter drives the ambulance. En route, you consider possible causes of arrest in this patient and then administer sodium bicarbonate. As you are giving the bicarbonate, the patient's rhythm changes to asystole; you attempt pacing but can't get capture. The ED staff works for another 10 minutes to resuscitate the patient but are unsuccessful, and the man is pronounced dead.

1. What risk factors does the patient have for chronic renal failure?

_____

_____

2. Put a ✔ beside any of the following signs or symptoms of chronic renal failure that you observed in this patient.

a. ____ Anorexia	**i.** ____ Mental dullness	**q.** ____ Seizures
b. ____ Anemia	**j.** ____ Muscle twitching	**r.** ____ Uremic frost
c. ____ Anxiety	**k.** ____ Nausea	**s.** ____ Vomiting
d. ____ Delirium	**l.** ____ Pericarditis	
e. ____ Electrolyte disturbances	**m.** ____ Peripheral edema	
f. ____ Fatigue	**n.** ____ Progressive obtundation	
g. ____ Glucose intolerance	**o.** ____ Pasty, yellow, skin	
h. ____ Hallucinations	**p.** ____ Pulmonary edema	

3. Which is true regarding the dialysis fistula?
   a. Blood pressures can be obtained in that arm without harm to the fistula.
   b. Patency should be verified by using a Doppler to auscultate pulsation.
   c. Drug administration by this route is contraindicated.
   d. Venous access by this site should be avoided in almost all cases.

4. Explain some possible causes for the following conditions this patient had:
   a. Hypotension:

_____

_____

   b. Chest pain:

_____

_____

   c. Cardiac arrest:

_____

_____

5. Discuss your rationale for the following interventions used in this patient:

   a. Nitroglycerin:

_____

_____

   b. Atropine:

_____

_____

   c. Sodium bicarbonate:

_____

_____

CHAPTER 35 ANSWERS

REVIEW QUESTIONS

1. e
   (Objective 2)

2. c
   (Objective 2)

3. b
   (Objective 5)

4. h
5. g
6. f
7. d
   (Questions 4-7: Objective 2)

8. a. Kidney
   b. Ureter
   c. Bladder
   d. Urethra
   (Objective 1)

9. a. Urinary calculus: Initiate intravenous line; consult with medical direction regarding administration of analgesics such as ketorolac or morphine. b. Testicular torsion: Initiate intravenous line; apply ice pack to scrotum and transport rapidly. c. Pyelonephritis: Initiate intravenous line; transport. d. Urinary tract infection: transport.
   (Objective 2)

10. Protect the patient's privacy with drapes. Have a paramedic who is the same gender as the patient perform the examination if possible. Have a chaperone present during a physical exam of the genitalia (if indicated). Explain all actions to the patient and proceed in a calm, caring manner.
    (Objective 3)

11. a. Trauma, shock, infection, urinary obstruction, and multisystem diseases; b. hypertension, diabetes, congenital condition, and pyelonephritis.
    (Objective 5)

12. a. Too much fluid taken off in dialysis or bleeding at the fistula caused by a pseudoaneurysm (any cause of bleeding is serious because the patient has decreased platelets and is heparinized during dialysis); sepsis; acute myocardial infarction. b. Initiate large-bore intravenous line in the arm without the arteriovenous fistula; infuse a small volume initially (200 to 300 mL) and reevaluate the patient for signs of fluid overload (crackles, engorged neck veins, pulmonary edema).
    (Objective 7)

13.

Disorder	Cause	Effect on Patient	Interventions
Hemorrhage	Decrease in platelet function; anticoagulant use; anemia; bleeding from fistula or graft	Signs and symptoms of shock; dyspnea, angina	Control external bleeding; treat for shock; rapid transport
Hypotension	Hemodialysis because of decreased volume; changes in electrolyte concentration; vascular instability	Decreased blood pressure; signs and symptoms of shock	Small fluid challenge (200 to 300 mL); monitor for signs and symptoms of congestive heart failure
Chest pain	Hypotension and hypoxemia during dialysis	Chest pain, headache, dizziness	Oxygen, fluid replacement, antianginal drugs
Hyperkalemia	Poor diet regulation; missed dialysis	Weakness; may have no symptoms; tall, tented T wave; prolonged PRI (K >6 to 6.5 mmol/L); depressed ST segments and loss of P waves (K >7 mmol/L); wide QRS	Suspect if renal patient in arrest; medical direction may order CaCI and NaHCO3 during arrest
Disequilibrium syndrome	Increased osmolality of the ECF compared with ICF in the brain or with the cerebrospinal fluid	HA, nausea, fatigue; confusion, seizures, coma	Transport; treat seizures with diazepam or lorazepam
Air embolism	Negative pressure in dialysis tubing; malfunction in dialysis machine	Dyspnea, cyanosis, hypotension, respiratory distress	Oxygen, rapid transport; position patient on left side with head down

(Objective 7)

14. a. Epinephrine (1 mg IV), $NaHCO_3$ (1 mEq/kg IV), and atropine (1 mg IV)
(Objective 7)

b. Epinephrine can increase peripheral vascular resistance and is a sympathomimetic. Sodium bicarbonate should be given because the patient likely has hyperkalemia and severe acidosis related to his chronic renal failure and missed dialysis sessions. Atropine is a parasympatholytic and theoretically may help to initiate sinus activity.
(Objective 7)

c. Bicarbonate may inactivate epinephrine, therefore tubing should be flushed between drugs.
(Objective 7)

STUDENT SELF-ASSESSMENT

15. c. Because a twisted testicle causes blockage of the blood supply to the testis, intervention within 4 to 6 hours is essential.
(Objective 2)

16. c. Kidney infection is a renal cause, and prostatic enlargement and ureteral strictures are postrenal causes.
(Objective 6)

17. a. Do not assess blood pressure or start an IV on the side where the fistula or shunt is placed. Vascular access should not routinely be obtained through the shunt. In rare cases, because of an arrest situation, medical direction may authorize vascular access through the shunt.
(Objective 5)

18. c. Infection at the site of catheter insertion is common and may lead to peritonitis.
(Objective 7)

19. a. Peaked, tented T waves are associated with hyperkalemia, a common electrolyte imbalance.
(Objective 7)

20. b. Sodium bicarbonate may temporarily cause movement of potassium out of the vascular space and may relieve the cardiac effects until definitive care (dialysis) can be given.
(Objective 7)

21. a. Anemia secondary to lack of a substance needed for red blood cell production reduces the oxygen-carrying capacity of the blood.
(Objective 6)

WRAP IT UP

1. Hypertension, diabetes
(Objective 5)

2. c, e, f, j, k, m
(Objective 6)

3. d. If the fistula is damaged during the attempt to access it, the patient's emergency dialysis will be delayed. After venous access has been established, drugs can be given by this route. Patency can be verified by palpation of a bruit over the fistula. Blood pressure assessment and vascular access should not be performed in the arm with the fistula to avoid damaging the fistula.
(Objective 7)

4. a. During dialysis, hypotension can be caused by a rapid reduction in vascular volume, fast changes in electrolytes, or vascular instability.
b. Hypotension and mild hypoxia, in addition to the patient's high risk factors, can result in chest pain during dialysis.
c. Cardiac arrest could be a result of myocardial irritability related to occlusion of blood vessels or of acidosis and electrolyte imbalance related to the patient's week without dialysis.
(Objective 7)

5. a. Nitroglycerin was given to dilate his coronary blood vessels, improving blood flow to the heart, and to decrease preload and afterload, thereby reducing the work the heart must do.
b. Atropine was given to block parasympathetic stimulation because the patient had a pulseless arrest with a rate of less than 60/min.
c. Sodium bicarbonate was given because of the possibility that acidosis or hyperkalemia (or both) related to the renal failure caused the cardiac arrest.
(Objective 7)

CHAPTER

36

Toxicology

READING ASSIGNMENT

Chapter 36, pages 920-969, in *Mosby's Paramedic Textbook,* ed. 3

OBJECTIVES

Upon completion of this chapter, the paramedic student will be able to do the following:
1. Define poisoning.
2. Describe general principles for assessment and management of the patient who has ingested poison.
3. Describe the causative agents and pathophysiology of selected ingested poisons and management of patients who have taken them.
4. Describe how physical and chemical properties influence the effects of inhaled toxins.
5. Distinguish among the three categories of inhaled toxins: simple asphyxiants, chemical asphyxiants and systemic poisons, and irritants or corrosives.
6. Describe general principles of managing the patient who has inhaled poison.
7. Describe the signs, symptoms, and management of patients who have inhaled cyanide, ammonia, or hydrocarbon.
8. Describe the signs, symptoms, and management of patients injected with poison by insects, reptiles, and hazardous aquatic creatures.
9. Describe the signs, symptoms, and management of patients with organophosphate or carbamate poisoning.
10. Outline the general principles of managing patients with drug overdose.
11. Describe the effects, signs and symptoms, and specific management for selected drug overdose.
12. Describe the short- and long-term physiological effects of ethanol ingestion.
13. Describe signs, symptoms, and management of alcohol-related emergencies.
14. Identify general management principles for the most common toxic syndromes based on a knowledge of the characteristic physical findings associated with each syndrome.

SUMMARY

- A poison is any substance that produces harmful physiological or psychological effects.
- The toxic effects of ingested poisons may be immediate or delayed. This depends on the substance that is ingested. The main goal is to identify effects on the three vital organ systems most likely to produce immediate morbidity and mortality. These are the respiratory system, the cardiovascular system, and the central nervous system. The goal of managing serious poisonings by ingestion is to prevent the toxic substance from reaching the small intestine. This limits its absorption.
- Strong acids and alkalis may cause burns to the mouth, pharynx, esophagus, and sometimes the upper respiratory and GI tracts. Prehospital care is usually limited to airway and ventilatory support, IV fluid replacement, and rapid transport to the appropriate medical facility.

- The most important physical characteristic in the potential toxicity of ingested hydrocarbons is its viscosity. The lower the viscosity, the higher the risk of aspiration and associated complications. Hydrocarbon ingestion may involve the patient's respiratory, gastrointestinal, and neurological systems. The clinical features may be immediate or delayed in onset.
- Methanol is a poisonous alcohol. It is found in a number of products. Methanol itself is no more toxic than ethanol. Yet its metabolites (formaldehyde and formic acid) are very toxic. Ingestion can affect the central nervous system, the gastrointestinal tract, and the eyes. It also can cause the development of metabolic acidosis.
- Ethylene glycol toxicity is caused by the buildup of toxic metabolites, especially glycolic and oxalic acids after metabolism. This occurs mainly in the liver and kidneys. This toxicity may affect the central nervous system and cardiopulmonary and renal systems. It may result in hypocalcemia as well.
- The majority of isopropanol (isopropyl alcohol) is metabolized to acetone after ingestion. Isopropanol poisoning affects several body systems, including the central nervous, gastrointestinal, and renal systems.
- Infants and children are high-risk groups for accidental iron, lead, and mercury poisoning. This is due to their immature immune systems or increased absorption as a function of age. Ingested iron is corrosive to gastrointestinal tract mucosa. It may produce lethal GI hemorrhage, bloody vomitus, painless bloody diarrhea, and dark stools.
- Food poisoning is a term used for any illness of sudden onset (usually associated with stomach pain, vomiting, and diarrhea) suspected of being caused by food eaten within the previous 48 hours. Food poisoning can be classified as infectious. This results from a bacterium or virus. It also can be classified as noninfectious. This results from toxins and pollutants.
- The toxic effects of major poisonous plant ingestions are predictable. They are categorized by the chemical and physical properties of the plant. Most responses are consistent with the type of major toxic chemical component in the plant.
- The concentration of a chemical in the air helps to predict the severity of an inhalation injury. The duration of exposure helps to determine this as well. Solubility also influences the extent of an inhalation injury. Highly reactive chemicals cause more severe and rapid injury than less-reactive chemicals. Properties that determine chemical reactivity are chemical pH; direct-acting potential of chemicals; indirect-acting potential of chemicals; and allergic potential of chemicals.
- Cyanide refers to any of a number of highly toxic substances that contain the cyanogen chemical group. Regardless of the route of entry, cyanide is a rapidly acting poison. It combines and reacts with ferric ions of the respiratory enzyme cytochrome oxidase. This inhibits cellular oxygenation. This can produce a rapid progression from dyspnea to paralysis, unconsciousness, and death.
- Ammonia is a toxic irritant. It causes local pulmonary complications after inhalation. In severe cases, bronchospasm and pulmonary edema may develop.
- Hydrocarbon inhalation may cause aspiration pneumonitis. It also has the potential for systemic effects such as CNS depression and liver, kidney, or bone marrow toxicity.
- Simple asphyxiants cause toxicity by lowering ambient oxygen concentration. Chemical asphyxiants possess intrinsic systemic toxicity. This toxicity occurs after absorption into the circulation. Irritants or corrosives cause cellular destruction and inflammation as they come into contact with moisture in the respiratory tract.
- The general principles of managing inhaled poisons are the same as for any other hazardous materials incident.
- Hymenoptera and arachnida cause the highest incidence of need for emergency care. Arthropod venoms are complex and diverse in their chemistry and pharmacology. They may produce major toxic reactions in sensitized persons. Such reactions include anaphylaxis and upper airway obstruction.
- The two main families of venomous snakes indigenous to the United States are pit vipers and coral snakes. Pit viper venom can produce various toxic effects on blood and other tissues. These effects include hemolysis, intravascular coagulation, convulsions, and acute renal failure. The venom of the coral snake is mainly neurotoxic. Signs and symptoms range from slurred speech, dilated pupils, and dysphagia to flaccid paralysis and death.
- The marine animals most likely to be involved in human poisonings in U.S. coastal waters are coelenterates, echinoderms, and stingrays. Coelenterate envenomation ranges in severity from irritant dermatitis to excruciating pain, respiratory depression, and life-threatening cardiovascular collapse. Echinoderm toxins may cause immediate intense pain, swelling, redness, aching in the affected extremity, and nausea. Delayed effects may include respiratory distress, paresthesia of the lips and face, and in severe cases, respiratory paralysis and complete atonia. Locally, stingray venom produces a painful traumatic injury. It may cause bleeding and necrosis. Systemic manifestations range from weakness and nausea to seizures, paralysis, hypotension, and death.

- Organophosphates and carbamates inhibit the effects of acetylcholinesterase. A mnemonic aid that may help the paramedic to recognize this type of poisoning is *SLUDGE*. (This stands for *s*alivation, *l*acrimation, *u*rination, *defe*cation, *g*astrointestinal upset, and *e*mesis.) The most specific findings, however, are miosis, rapidly changing pupils, and muscle fasciculation.
- General principles for managing drug abuse and overdose include scene safety; ensuring adequate airway, breathing, and circulation; history; substance identification; focused physical exam; initiation of an IV; administration of an antidote if needed; prevention of further absorption; and rapid transport.
- Narcotics are CNS depressants. They can cause life-threatening respiratory depression. In severe intoxication, hypotension, profound shock, and pulmonary edema may be present. Naloxone is a pure narcotic antagonist effective for virtually all narcotic and narcotic-like substances.
- Sedative-hypnotic agents include benzodiazepines and barbiturates. Signs and symptoms of sedative-hypnotic overdose are chiefly related to the central nervous and cardiovascular symptoms. Flumazenil (Romazicon) is a benzodiazepine antagonist. It is useful in reversing the effects of these agents if they were given in a clinical setting.
- Commonly used stimulant drugs are those of the amphetamine family. Adverse effects include tachycardia, increased blood pressure, tachypnea, agitation, dilated pupils, tremors, and disorganized behavior. With sudden withdrawal, the patient becomes depressed, suicidal, incoherent, or near coma.
- Phencyclidine (PCP) is a dissociative analgesic with sympathomimetic and CNS stimulant and depressant effects. In low doses, PCP intoxication produces an unpredictable state that can resemble drunkenness (and rage). High-dose intoxication may cause coma. This may last from several hours to days. Respiratory depression, hypertension, and tachycardia may be present. PCP psychosis is a psychiatric emergency. It may mimic schizophrenia.
- Hallucinogens are substances that cause distortions of perceptions. Depending on the agent, overdose may range from visual hallucinations and anticholinergic syndromes, to more serious complications, including psychosis, flashbacks, and respiratory and CNS depression.
- Tricyclic antidepressant toxicity is thought to result from central and peripheral, atropine-like anticholinergic effects and direct depressant effects on myocardial function. A prolonged QRS complex, a GCS score less than 8, or both, should alert the paramedic to a major TCA toxicity.
- Lithium is a mood-stabilizing drug. Toxic ingestion can include CNS effects that can range from blurred vision and confusion to seizure and coma.
- Cardiac drugs are a common cause of poisoning deaths in children and adults. The drugs responsible for the majority of these fatalities are digitalis, beta blockers, and calcium channel blockers.
- MAO inhibitors block or diminish the activity of the monoamines (norepinephrine, dopamine, serotonin). Toxic effects include CNS depression and various neuromuscular and cardiovascular system manifestations.
- Nonsteroidal antiinflammatory drugs (NSAIDs) work by blocking the production of prostaglandins. The effects of overdose of ibuprofen are usually reversible, are seldom life-threatening, and include mild GI and CNS effects. Salicylate poisoning may cause CNS stimulation, GI irritation, glucose metabolism, fluid and electrolyte imbalance, and coagulation defects.
- Acetaminophen overdose may cause life-threatening liver damage. This results from formation of a hepatotoxic intermediate metabolite if it is not managed within 16 to 24 hours of ingestion.
- Some drugs are abused for sexual purposes or for sexual gratification. These are commonly classified by users as "uppers," "downers," and those that have more than one primary effect ("all-arounders"). Problems associated with their use vary widely.
- Alcohol dependence is a disorder characterized by chronic, excessive consumption of alcohol that results in injury to health or in inadequate social function and the development of withdrawal symptoms when the patient stops drinking suddenly. Alcohol causes multiple systemic effects. These include neurological disorders, nutritional deficiencies, fluid and electrolyte imbalances, gastrointestinal disorders, cardiac and skeletal muscle myopathy, and immune suppression. Several conditions caused by consumption or abstinence from alcohol that may require emergency care are acute alcohol intoxication, alcohol withdrawal syndromes, and disulfiram-ethanol reaction.
- The most common toxic syndromes are cholinergic, anticholinergic, hallucinogenic, opiate, and sympathomimetic. Using these classifications allows the paramedic to group similar toxic agents together. It allows him or her to more easily remember how to assess and treat the poisoned patient.

REVIEW QUESTIONS

Match the illnesses in Column II with the toxic syndromes in Column I. You may use the signs and symptoms more than once.

Column I

1. _____ Anticholinergic syndrome
2. _____ Cholinergic syndrome
3. _____ Opiate/sedative/ethanol syndrome
4. _____ Sympathomimetic syndrome

Column II

a. Bradycardia
b. Cardiac dysrhythmias
c. Dry mouth
d. Hypertension
e. Respiratory depression
f. Salivation
g. Tachycardia
h. Urination

Match the poisons in Column II with their descriptions in Column I. Use each poison only once.

Column I

5. _____ Metabolizes to formic acid and causes toxic visual effects
6. _____ Ingestion of odorless, sweet liquid in antifreeze causes central nervous system depression
7. _____ Inhalation, ingestion, and absorption prevents oxygen from reaching cells
8. _____ Inhalation produces lacrimation, dyspnea, and inflammation of the airway
9. _____ Vomiting should not be induced for phenol and others in this group
10. _____ These chemicals include lye and cause immediate damage to the mucosa
11. _____ The long duration of action requires treatment with atropine and pralidoxime

Column II

a. Acid
b. Alkali
c. Ammonia
d. Carbamate
e. Cyanide
f. Ethylene glycol
g. Hydrocarbon
h. Isopropanol
i. Methanol
j. Organophosphate

12. You are called to the home of a young child whose family states that he ingested some liquid from a bottle in the garage. He is arousable only to painful stimulation. After a rapid assessment of the patient, you contact the regional poison control center.

   a. What information should you be prepared to give the center?

   _____

   b. What general care measures should you take when caring for this patient if the source of the poisoning is unknown?

   _____

   _____

13. You insert a 36 to 40 French orogastric tube into a patient.

   a. What position should the patient be in?

   _____

   b. What precaution should be taken for the unconscious patient?

   _____

c. How should irrigation be performed?

_____

_____

14. Complete the information missing in the following table.

Ingested Poison	Charcoal (Yes/No)	Other Interventions
a. Bleach		
b. Ammonia		
c. Gasoline		
d. Methanol		
e. Ethylene glycol		
f. Isopropanol		
g. Cyanide		

15. A 65-year-old woman complains of food poisoning after eating at a local seafood restaurant 2 hours earlier.

a. What is the typical time onset for signs of food poisoning?

_____

b. What treatment should be provided for the patient with food poisoning?

_____

_____

Questions 16 to 18 refer to the following case study:

A 21-year-old man calls 911 after becoming extremely ill from eating some wild mushrooms. The patient is awake and complaining of nausea, vomiting, and diarrhea. He has pinpoint pupils and the following vital signs: BP 90/50 mm Hg, P 48, and R 24. His electrocardiogram rhythm shows a sinus bradycardia with occasional ventricular escape beats.

16. What type of toxic syndrome does this patient appear to be exhibiting?

_____

17. How can you find out more about the specific poison involved in this case?

_____

18. What treatment measures may be indicated for this patient in consultation with medical direction?

_____

19. Complete the information missing in the following table.

Toxic Chemical	Class of Toxin	Signs and Symptoms	Treatment
Copper welding fumes			
Hydrogen sulfide			
Methane gas			
Chlorine gas			

20. A worker in a chemical plant is exposed to ammonia gas and is dyspneic, choking, and wheezing. What treatment should be provided for this patient?

_____

_____

Questions 21 to 24 refer to the following case study:

A farmer calls you to his ranch after spraying pesticide on a windy day. On your arrival, he is coming out of the bathroom complaining of severe diarrhea and says he cannot stop urinating. Tears are running down his face, and he is coughing up large amounts of phlegm. His electrocardiogram is shown in Fig. 36-1.

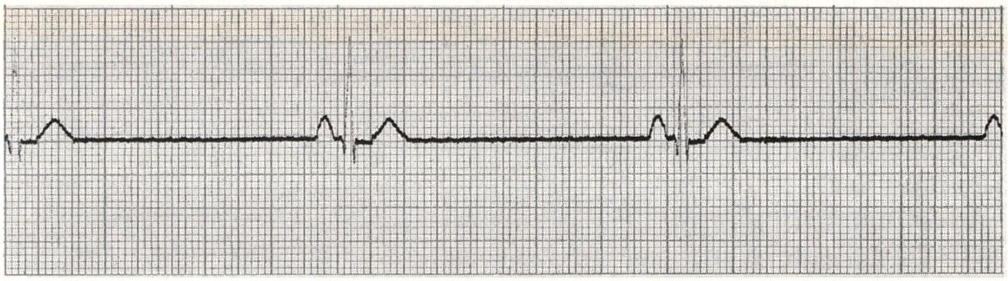

Figure 36-1

21. What poisoning do you suspect?

_____

22. What other signs or symptoms might be present?

_____

23. What is your interpretation of the electrocardiogram?

_____

24. List specific interventions to be used in his care.

_____

_____

_____

25. Interpret the following historical information presented to you at the scene of a potential drug overdose.

a. "He mainlined some China white."

_____

b. "She was space-basing angel dust and candy."

_____

c. "They were freebasing a rock."

_____

d. "He was skin-popping some M."

_____

e. "She snorted some PCP before she went crazy."

_____

Match the drugs in Column II with the appropriate overdose description in Column I. Use each drug only once.

Column I	Column II
26. _____ Central nervous system stimulant and depressant properties can produce violent, unpredictable behavior.	**a.** Acetaminophen
27. _____ It causes visual disturbances, dry mouth, seizures, and tachycardia with a wide QRS complex.	**b.** Cocaine
28. _____ It causes tachypnea, central nervous system depression, gastrointestinal irritation, and tinnitus.	**c.** Heroin
29. _____ Mild, influenza-like symptoms are followed by latent liver failure.	**d.** Iron
30. _____ This stimulant can cause dysrhythmias, myocardial infarction, and hyperthermia.	**e.** Phencyclidine
	f. Salicylate
	g. Tricyclic antidepressant

Questions 31 and 32 refer to the following case study:

A 32-year-old woman has overdosed on sleeping pills. She is awake but drowsy.

31. What information regarding the poisoning is critical to the care of this patient?

_____

_____

32. What dose of activated charcoal should be given?

_____

33. Complete the information missing in the following table.

Ingested Poison	Charcoal (Yes/No)	Other Interventions
a. Aspirin		
b. Acetaminophen		
c. Iron		

34. Give two examples of drugs commonly abused in each of the following categories.

a. Narcotics: _____

b. Central nervous system depressants: _____

c. Central nervous system stimulants: _____

d. Hallucinogens: _____

Questions 35 to 37 refer to the following case study:

Your patient injected heroin intravenously and arouses only to pain. He has pinpoint pupils and slow, snoring respirations.

35. What is the primary life threat that must be managed immediately in this patient?

_____

36. How will you manage this life threat until you can administer drugs?

_____

37. List the appropriate drug and dose used to improve this patient's condition.

_____

38. If this man is a chronic heroin abuser and the drug listed previously is administered, what signs and symptoms of narcotic withdrawal will you anticipate?

_____

Questions 39 to 41 refer to the following case study:

A 17-year-old has taken about 50 tablets of chlordiazepoxide and is comatose, with slow, irregular respirations.

39. What is the pupil response likely to be in this patient?

_____

40. Why would administration of flumazenil (Romazicon) to antagonize the effects of this ingestion be risky for this patient?

_____

41. Local college students call you to a party, where participants have been freebasing cocaine. One of the participants has lost consciousness. What life-threatening effects of this drug may have caused loss of consciousness in this patient?

_____

Questions 42 to 44 refer to the following case study:

A popular group is playing at a local club. Security calls you to the parking lot to care for a patient who has reportedly taken PCP (phencyclidine).

42. What should be your primary concern when caring for this patient?

_____

43. Describe the appropriate initial approach to this patient, who is alert and quiet.

_____

44. List signs and symptoms that may be displayed by this patient.

_____

Questions 45 to 48 refer to the following case study:

An 18-year-old woman took about 20 tablets of amitriptyline about 1 hour before your arrival at her home. She is drowsy and confused, has a dry mouth, and complains of blurred vision. Her electrocardiogram is shown in Fig. 36-2.

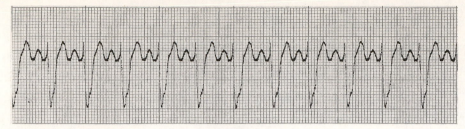

Figure 36-2

45. Should you perform gastric lavage on this patient? Why or why not?

_____

_____

46. What is your interpretation of the electrocardiogram?

_____

47. What drug and appropriate dose may be given to prevent deterioration of this patient's cardiac status?

_____

48. What additional signs and symptoms do you anticipate as this patient's condition deteriorates?

_____

Questions 49 and 50 refer to the following case study:

Your unit is on the scene of a two-car accident. You are caring for a 47-year-old man who appears to be intoxicated. His friend says that he is an alcoholic. The patient states that he drank three beers in the past 5 hours.

49. Should you accept this history of the number of drinks as reliable?

_____

50. If the patient is an alcoholic, what *chronic* physiological changes in the following areas will make it more difficult to assess his condition and more likely for severe injury to occur?

  a. Neurological changes:

_____

  b. Nutritional problems:

_____

  c. Fluid and electrolyte imbalances:

_____

  d. Coagulation disorders:

_____

51. Describe the management of a comatose patient suspected to be severely intoxicated by alcohol.

_____

_____

_____

52. Describe the management of a patient experiencing alcohol withdrawal accompanied by severe seizures.

_____

_____

_____

53. List signs and symptoms of delirium tremens.

_____

_____

54. You are at the first aid station for a church picnic. A 16-year-old boy comes to the station complaining of a bee sting. No signs of anaphylaxis are present.

    a. List general care measures for this person.

_____

    b. Describe the method for removing the stinger.

_____

55. List two diseases produced by ticks and possible signs and symptoms for each.

    a.

    b.

56. Describe the proper technique for removing a tick.

_____

57. A hysterical 20-year-old man states that he has just been bitten by a copperhead snake while camping.

    a. List signs and symptoms that would be present if a moderate envenomation had occurred.

_____

    b. Describe the appropriate prehospital management of this patient.

_____

_____

58. For each of the following marine animal classifications, list one example and outline general management principles for envenomation:

a. Coelenterates:

_____

b. Echinoderms:

_____

c. Stingrays:

_____

STUDENT SELF-ASSESSMENT

59. Any substance that produces harmful physiological or psychological effects is known as a(n):
    a. Overdose
    b. Poison
    c. Toxin
    d. Venom

60. Which toxic syndrome would present for the patient who has ingested cocaine?
    a. Anticholinergic syndrome
    b. Cholinergic syndrome
    c. Opiate/sedative/ethanol syndrome
    d. Sympathomimetic syndrome

61. What is the primary goal when assessing a poisoned patient?
    a. Begin decontamination of the poison as quickly as possible with activated charcoal.
    b. Determine the exact nature of the poison so that appropriate treatment can be given.
    c. Obtain a history to determine the exact time that the poisoning occurred.
    d. Identify the effects on the respiratory, cardiovascular, and central nervous systems.

62. Charcoal is effective in treating specific overdoses because it does which of the following?
    a. Reverses the effects of the ingested drug
    b. Binds the drug and prevents absorption
    c. Causes severe nausea and vomiting
    d. Makes the drug speed through the intestine

63. Which is true regarding syrup of ipecac?
    a. It is indicated for use in petroleum distillate ingestion.
    b. It is not associated with life-threatening complications.
    c. It may interfere with other methods of decontamination.
    d. It should be given within the first 2 hours after ingestion.

64. What should be your primary concern when caring for a patient who has ingested hydrocarbon?
    a. Aspiration
    b. Central nervous system effects
    c. Dysrhythmias
    d. Hypotension

65. Medical direction may advise administration of sodium bicarbonate in all of the following *except* which poisoning and overdose situation?
    a. Ethylene glycol
    b. Methanol
    c. Isopropanol
    d. Tricyclic antidepressant

66. Which of the following is true regarding poison plant ingestions?
    a. Dialysis is an effective treatment for most plant poisons.
    b. Ingestion of poisonous plants is common in the United States.
    c. Most signs and symptoms are delayed several days.
    d. Specific treatment should not begin until the plant is identified.

67. Symptoms commonly associated with poisonous mushroom ingestion are likely to include which of the following?
    a. Bradycardia
    b. Dry mouth
    c. Hypertension
    d. Hyperthermiaj

68. Which of the following hydrocarbon properties is associated with the greatest risk?
    a. Low adhesion of molecules along a surface
    b. Low surface tension
    c. High viscosity
    d. High volatility
69. Toxic hydrocarbon inhalation most often is associated with which of the following?
    a. Childhood ingestions
    b. Industrial exposures
    c. Mixing chemicals
    d. Recreational huffing
70. Which of the following overdose or poisoning typically will lead to bradycardia?
    a. Carbamates
    b. Cocaine
    c. Isopropanol
    d. Methanol
71. What should your first priority be when evaluating a patient contaminated with organophosphates?
    a. Administer atropine.
    b. Establish intravenous therapy.
    c. Put on protective gear.
    d. Suction excess secretions.
72. Atropine is supplied in a 10-mL syringe that contains 1 mg of the drug. You wish to administer 2 mg to a patient who has organophosphate poisoning. How many milliliters will you give?
    a. 1 mL
    b. 2 mL
    c. 10 mL
    d. 20 mL
73. Naloxone will antagonize the effects of all of the following except which drug?
    a. Diazepam
    b. Meperidine
    c. Morphine
    d. Propoxyphene
74. What should your highest priority be when caring for a patient at a methamphetamine lab?
    a. Administration of diazepam to control tremors
    b. Decontamination of the patient
    c. Maintaining scene safety
    d. Talking down the paranoid patient
75. The patient who has taken an overdose of oil of wintergreen most likely will have which of the following?
    a. Bradycardia, hyperglycemia, and nystagmus
    b. Seizures, hyperglycemia, and ventricular tachycardia
    c. Hypoglycemia, tachypnea, and tinnitus
    d. Hematemesis, metabolic alkalosis, and coma
76. What are the typical findings in patients within the first 24 hours of an overdose of acetaminophen?
    a. Dysrhythmias
    b. Hypoglycemia
    c. No symptoms
    d. Right upper quadrant abdominal pain
77. When ingestion of multivitamins is suspected in a child, it is critical to determine whether the preparation contains
    a. Ascorbic acid.
    b. Folic acid.
    c. Iron.
    d. Thiamine.
78. Which of the following drugs most likely will produce tachycardia if a patient overdoses?
    a. Digoxin (Lanoxin)
    b. Propranolol (Inderal)
    c. Sertraline (Zoloft)
    d. Verapamil (Calan)
79. An alert 4-year-old child ingested about 10 of his grandmother's blood pressure tablets 20 minutes ago. He is awake and alert. What drug should be administered in this situation?
    a. Activated charcoal
    b. Atropine
    c. Calcium chloride
    d. Dopamine
80. Intravenous therapy in the alcoholic with depleted thiamine stores may lead to which of the following?
    a. Disulfiram-ethanol reaction
    b. Guillain-Barré syndrome
    c. Mallory-Weiss tears
    d. Wernicke-Korsakoff syndrome
81. Which of the following is true regarding delirium tremens?
    a. It affects almost all alcoholics going through alcohol withdrawal.
    b. It is associated with a high mortality rate if untreated.
    c. It is characterized by bradycardia, hypotension, and hypothermia.
    d. It usually occurs 12 to 24 hours following cessation of alcohol ingestion.
82. Alcohol withdrawal seizures should be treated with which of the following?
    a. Dextrose 50%
    b. Diazepam
    c. Magnesium sulfate
    d. Thiamine

83. An 18-year-old man who attempts to extract honey from a beehive on a dare sustains 20 to 30 stings. He has a headache, fever, and involuntary muscle spasms and reports a syncopal episode. What type of reaction do you suspect?

a. Anaphylactic
b. Delayed
c. Local
d. Toxic

84. A 52-year-old man states that he was bitten by a spider at a woodpile. He now is complaining of back, chest, and abdominal pain and has a severe headache. What type of spider envenomation would produce these symptoms?

a. Black widow
b. Brown recluse
c. Tarantula
d. Wolf

85. A hiker states that he was bitten by a red and yellow snake and is now complaining of slurred speech and dysphagia. His pupils are dilated. You suspect envenomation by what kind of snake?

a. Copperhead
b. Cottonmouth moccasin
c. Coral
d. Massasauga

86. Which treatment may be harmful for the patient who has sustained a venomous coral snake bite to the ankle?

a. Applying ice to wound on affected extremity
b. Initiating an intravenous line in an affected extremity
c. Elevating the extremity above the heart
d. Wrapping the affected extremity with an elastic bandage

87. For which overdose would isoproterenol be indicated to treat symptomatic bradycardia?

a. Digoxin
b. Nortriptyline
c. Propranolol
d. Verapamil

Questions 88 and 89 relate to the following scenario.

Your patient is a 42-year-old found "asleep" in the park. Rangers were unable to wake him. He is unresponsive to pain and has snoring respirations at about 2 per minute. His pupils are pinpoint. He has track marks on his arms.

88. What type of overdose would be a likely cause of his decreased level of consciousness?

a. Cocaine
b. Heroin
c. Methamphetamine
d. Phencyclidine

89. Which intervention will be your first priority in his care?

a. Assist ventilations with bag-mask device.
b. Check his blood glucose level.
c. Deliver a fluid bolus of 200 mL normal saline.
d. Give naloxone (Narcan) 0.4 to 2.0 mg intravenously.

WRAP IT UP

You are dispatched to a home for a "possible overdose." On arrival, you find your 22-year-old male patient in the bathtub. He moans and flexes slightly in response to painful stimulus. Emesis is sprayed around the toilet, and a pile of pill bottles is in the sink. The pill bottles are prescribed to several persons and you find Tylenol, aspirin, Vicodin, Glucophage, vitamins with iron, Elavil, Ativan, Ritalin, metoprolol, and empty bottles of rubbing alcohol and vodka. You assess him and find his vital signs are BP 100/70 mm Hg, P 104, R 6, SaO$_2$ 65%. You assist his respirations with a bag-valve-mask, and he gags when you try to place an oral airway, so you insert a nasopharyngeal airway. You find his skin to be pale and dry, and his pupils are 2 mm. An IV is started, and his blood glucose reading is 25 mg/dL. You administer naloxone (Narcan) followed by D50W. An electrocardiogram tracing shows sinus tachycardia with occasional PVCs. His level of consciousness improves slightly, and he is somewhat combative on arrival to the ED.

1. Which of the substance(s) that he ingested can cause the following:

a. Hypoglycemia
b. Acidosis
c. Tachycardia
d. Respiratory depression
e. Decreased level of consciousness
f. Pupil constriction
g. Bradycardia
h. Cardiac dysrhythmias
i. Seizures

2. Place a check mark beside the drugs, or classifications of drugs, that this patient may have taken.
   a. _____ Acetaminophen
   b. _____ Benzodiazepine
   c. _____ Beta-blocker
   d. _____ Ethanol alcohol
   e. _____ Hypoglycemic
   f. _____ Salicylate
   g. _____ Isopropanol
   h. _____ Mineral
   i. _____ Opioid/narcotic
   j. _____ Organophosphate
   k. _____ Stimulant
   l. _____ Tricyclic antidepressant

3. For each of the following drugs this patient has taken, describe the action that is most likely to cause death.

   a. Acetaminophen:_____
   _____

   b. Metoprolol:_____
   _____

   c. Vodka:_____
   _____

   d. Metformin (Glucophage):_____
   _____

   e. Aspirin:_____
   _____

   f. Iron:_____
   _____

   g. Hydrocodone/acetaminophen (Vicodin):_____
   _____

   h. Tricyclic antidepressant:_____
   _____

4. Explain your rationale for the interventions that you performed.

   a. Bag-valve-mask:_____
   _____

   b. Naloxone:_____
   _____

   c. D50W:_____

5. Would other antidotes or therapeutic interventions be indicated for this patient if these drugs were taken individually?

   _____

6. Which of the following is true regarding the care of the overdosed patient?
   a. The most important goal for prehospital treatment is gastric emptying.
   b. Gathering of information from the scene is critical in toxicology emergencies.
   c. Administration of antidotes, when indicated, takes priority over all interventions.
   d. Syrup of ipecac should be given to all overdose patients if not contraindicated.

7. Which of the drugs he ingested, when taken individually, could cause the following toxidromes:
   a. Cholinergic
   b. Anticholinergic
   c. Hallucinogen
   d. Opioid
   e. Sympathomimetic

CHAPTER 36 ANSWERS

REVIEW QUESTIONS

1. c, g
2. a, b, f, h
3. b, e, g
4. b, d, g
   (Questions 1 to 4, Objective 2)

5. i
   (Objective 4)

6. f
   (Objective 4)

7. e
   (Objectives 4 and 6)

8. c
   (Objective 8)

9. g
   (Objective 4)

10. b
    (Objective 4)

11. j
    (Objective 9)

12. a. You should be prepared to tell the poison control center the specific agent ingested, amount of agent ingested, time ingested, age, patient weight, medical condition, and treatment rendered before arrival of emergency medical services personnel.
    (Objective 3)

    b. Ensure adequate airway, ventilation, and circulation. Obtain a history (especially specific to substance ingested), and perform a physical exam. Assess for hypoglycemia. Consult with medical direction for further treatment guidelines. Monitor vital signs and electrocardiogram. Transport rapidly for definitive treatment.
    (Objective 3)

13. a. Position the patient in the left lateral Trendelenberg's (swimmer's) position
    b. Peform rapid sequence endotracheal intubation before orogastric tube intubation if patient has a decreased level of consciousness with an absent gag reflex
    c. After assessment for proper tube placement, normal saline (preferably warmed) should be infused into the orogastric tube in 200- to 300-mL boluses, and the tube should be allowed to drain after each bolus. Continue this process until the gastric drainage returns clear.
    (Objective 3)

14. Indicated in alert patient if ingestion ≤ 1 hour prior

Ingested Poison	Charcoal (Yes/No)	Other Interventions
a. Bleach	No	Dilution with milk or water (200 to 300 mL for an adult or 15 mL/kg for a child)
b. Ammonia	No	Dilution with milk or water
c. Gasoline	No	Initiation of intravenous line, monitoring of airway, and electrocardiogram
d. Methanol	Controversial	Lavage, indicated in alert patient if ingestion ≤ 1 hour prior sodium bicarbonate intravenously (30 to 60 mL), and 80-proof ethanol by mouth
e. Ethylene glycol	Yes	Lavage, indicated in alert patient if ingestion ≤ 1 hour prior sodium bicarbonate intravenously (30 to 60 mL), 80-proof ethanol by mouth, and (rarely) furosemide, thiamine, and calcium gluconate
f. Isopropanol	Yes	Lavage indicated in alert patient if ingestion ≤ 1 hour prior
g. Cyanide	No	Amyl nitrite pearls, 3% sodium nitrite, and 25% sodium thiosulfate

(Objective 4)

15. a. Time varies: chemical, 1 to 2 hours; bacterial toxins, 1 to 12 hours; viral or bacterial, 12 to 48 hours.

    b. Take universal precautions, maintain airway and breathing, and initiate intravenous therapy with crystalloid solution to treat dehydration and fluid and electrolyte imbalance.
    (Objective 4)

16. Cholinergic syndrome
(Objective 2)

17. Ask the patient if he still has a sample of the mushroom and what time he took it. If he does not have a sample, have him describe the mushroom. Contact poison control and medical direction (per protocol) for help with identification and treatment information. Prehospital treatment likely will be guided by signs and symptoms rather than specific identification information.
(Objective 2)

18. Maintain airway and prepare to suction secretions if needed; administer high-concentration oxygen; monitor electrocardiogram and vital signs frequently; initiate an intravenous line and infuse fluids as ordered by medical direction; and prepare to administer atropine sulfate as ordered by medical direction.
(Objective 4)

19. Rescuers should wear appropriate personal protective equipment.

Toxic Chemical	Class of Toxin	Sign and Symptoms	Treatment
Copper welding fumes	Metal fumes	Chills, fever, myalgias; headache, cough, leukocytosis	Remove patient from source, treat symptoms.
Hydrogen sulfide	Chemical asphyxiant	Sudden collapse, rotten egg smell, rapid fatigue	Remove patient from source, oxygenate.
Chlorine gas	Irritant	Lacrimation, sore throat, stridor, tracheobronchitis, pulmonary edema	Remove patient from source, give humidified oxygen and bronchodilators, manage airway.

(Objective 6)

20. Ensure personal protection; open airway; administer high-flow oxygen; initiate an intravenous line to keep the vein open; and if pulmonary edema develops, consider administration of diuretics and bronchodilators. (Objective 8)

21. Carbamate or organophosphate (Objective 9)

22. Pupil constriction, muscle fasciculation, headache, weakness, dizziness, hypotension, bronchoconstriction, anxiety, seizures, and convulsions (Objective 9)

23. Sinus bradycardia (Objective 9)

24. Wear protective gear; decontaminate as appropriate; suction oral secretions as necessary; prepare to intubate if patient's condition deteriorates; initiate intravenous therapy with crystalloid to keep the vein open; administer atropine 2 to 4 mg intravenously every 5 to 15 minutes as necessary to induce relative tachycardia, flushing, and decreased secretions; monitor for dysrhythmias; administer pralidoxime; administer diazepam as necessary for seizures. (Objective 9)

25. a. He took fentanyl or heroin intravenously.
    b. She was smoking PCP and crack (cocaine).
    c. They were smoking purified crack cocaine.
    d. He injected morphine subcutaneously.
    e. She ingested PCP nasally.
    (Objective 10)

26. e
27. g
28. f
29. a
30. b
(Questions 26 to 30, Objective 11)

31. What was taken? Where is the container? How much was in it and how much is left (may need to estimate based on date prescription issued, amount prescribed daily, and amount left in bottle)? When was the drug taken? Has the patient vomited or taken anything to induce vomiting since the drug was taken? Has any antidote been given to the patient? Ask the patient the following: Why did you do this? Were you trying to hurt or kill yourself? (Objective 10)

32. 30 to 100 g activated charcoal (Objective 10)

33.

Ingested Poison	Charcoal (Yes/No)	Other Interventions
a. Aspirin	Yes	D50W if patient is hypoglycemic
b. Acetaminophen	Usually not (varies by medical direction)	Acetylcysteine (Mucomyst; varies by medical direction)
c. Iron	No	Monitor airway, initiate IV line

34. a. Heroin, morphine, oxycontin, vicodin, and methadone; b. barbiturates (secobarbital, phenobarbital) and benzodiazepines (diazepam, chlordiazepoxide); c. amphetamines and cocaine; d. lysergic acid diethylamide (LSD) and phencyclidine (PCP).
(Objective 10)

35. Respiratory depression (partial airway obstruction and decreased minute volume)
(Objective 11)

36. Assist ventilation with a bag-mask
(Objective 11)

37. Naloxone (Narcan) 0.4–2.0 mg intravenously or 0.4–0.8 mg IM or SC. Use smaller doses if known addiction. (Administer enough to ensure adequate airway reflexes and ventilation.)
(Objective 11)

38. Gooseflesh (piloerection), tachycardia, diaphoresis, irritability, insomnia, abdominal cramps, tremors, nausea, vomiting, cold sweats and chills, fever, and diarrhea
(Objective 11)

39. Bilaterally dilated and slow to react to light
(Objective 11)

40. Flumazenil (Romazicon) has serious side effects if patient is benzodiazepine dependent or if the patient has taken certain other medicines (e.g., TCA)
(Objective 11)

41. Cardiac dysrhythmias, seizures, or cerebrovascular accident (following intracranial hemorrhage)
(Objective 11)

42. Personal safety
(Objective 11)

43. Quiet, calm approach. Interview the patient while minimizing external sensory stimuli (for example, bright lights, noise).
(Objective 11)

44. Euphoria, disorientation, seizures, hypertensive crisis, dysrhythmias, catatonia, unresponsiveness, and bizarre and violent behavior. These patients are extremely difficult to manage and dangerous if found in or provoked into violent behavior.
(Objective 11)

45. She is drowsy and her level of consciousness could deteriorate further. Intubate using rapid-sequence intubation (if authorized) before gastric lavage to prevent aspiration
(Objective 11)

46. Sinus tachycardia with delayed ventricular conduction (wide QRS complex)
(Objective 11)

47. Sodium bicarbonate 1 to 2 mEq/kg intravenously and normal saline bolus of 500–1000 mL. Medical direction may also order magnesium sulfate.
(Objective 11)

48. Delirium, depressed respirations, hypertension or hypotension, hyperthermia or hypothermia, seizures, coma, and dysrhythmias
(Objective 11)

49. No. Alcoholics frequently underestimate the number of drinks they have had.
(Objective 13)

50. a. Short-term memory deficit, problems with coordination, and difficulty with concentration can mimic signs and symptoms of head injury
b. Nutritional deficiencies can cause muscle cramps, paresthesias, seizures, tremor or ataxia, and poor wound healing.
c. Chronic dehydration may be difficult to distinguish from a new onset of fluid loss. Patient will decompensate faster if acute fluid loss occurs resulting from trauma.
d. Clotting factors are suppressed by chronic alcohol abuse, resulting in increased risk of bleeding, especially subdural hematoma, with minor trauma.
(Objective 12)

51. Protect airway (high risk of aspiration); ventilate as necessary; initiate intravenous therapy; draw blood samples per protocol; determine blood glucose levels and if low, administer thiamine 100 mg intravenously and D50W 25 g intravenously; if opiate overdose is suspected or unknown, administer naloxone 2 mg intravenously; monitor airway, breathing, vital signs, and electrocardiogram.
(Objective 13)

52. Manage as in answer 51 and protect from injury; administer diazepam 2.5 to 5.0 mg or lorazepam 1 to 2 mg intravenously if additional seizures occur; examine for signs or symptoms of traumatic injury.
(Objective 13)

53. Hyperactive motor, speech, and autonomic activity; confusion; disorientation; delusion; hallucinations; tremor; agitation; insomnia; tachycardia; fever; hypertension; dilated pupils; profuse diaphoresis; and in severe cases, cardiovascular collapse
(Objective 13)

54. a. Assess for anaphylaxis, apply ice packs, and immobilize and elevate affected extremity.
b. Scrape or brush off. Do not squeeze because doing so will inject additional venom.
(Objective 14)

55. a. Lyme disease. Early signs are fever, lethargy, muscle pain, and general malaise; late signs are cardiac abnormalities, cranial nerve palsies, and arthritis
b. Tick paralysis. Signs include restlessness and paresthesia in hands and feet progressing to ascending symmetrical flaccid paralysis, which may include respiratory muscles.
(Objective 14)

56. Apply gloves and grasp tick as close to skin surface as possible (may use tweezers or forceps if available), pull out with steady pressure (avoid squeezing tick), and cleanse wound and observe for any remnants of tick.
(Objective 14)

57. a. Fang marks, pain and edema, weakness, diaphoresis, nausea, vomiting, and paresthesias
b. Ensure personal safety from another bite; monitor airway, breathing, and circulation; initiate intravenous therapy in unaffected extremity; immobilize affected extremity in dependent position; and keep patient at rest. (Objective 14)

58. a. Jellyfish, fire corals, and sea anemones. Rinse wound with seawater; apply vinegar, baking soda, isopropanol, ammonia, meat tenderizer (for 5 to 10 minutes only); remove visible tentacles with forceps; apply shaving cream, gently shave affected area or use knife or spatula to gently scrape remaining tentacles; and rinse again
b. Sea urchins, starfish, and sea cucumbers. Remove embedded spines with forceps and immerse affected extremity (and unaffected extremity to prevent thermal injury) in hot water during transport
c. Stingrays. Irrigate wound with saltwater or freshwater; remove venom apparatus if it is visible; and immerse the affected part in hot water. (Objective 14)

59. b
(Objective 1)

60. d
(Objective 2)

61. d. Life threats that will need immediate management usually are identified by assessing these areas. (Objective 3)

62. b. Charcoal binds the drug by adsorption. It often is given with a cathartic that speeds the bound drug through the gastrointestinal tract. (Objective 3)

63. c. Gastric lavage and charcoal generally are considered superior. Ipecac is contraindicated in petroleum distillate ingestions. Ipecac is associated with aspiration, Mallory-Weiss tear of the esophagus, pneumomediastinum, and fatal diaphragmatic or gastric rupture. If indicated, it should be given within 20 minutes after ingestion. (Objective 2)

64. a. Inducing emesis usually is contraindicated for these patients, unless the toxicity of the specific hydrocarbon is so great that the risks of absorption in the gastrointestinal tract outweigh the risks of aspiration. (Objective 4)

65. c. Methanol and ethylene glycol produce metabolic acidosis, so $NaHCO_3$ is indicated. In a tricyclic antidepressant overdose, $NaHCO_3$ will decrease the toxic cardiac side effects. No metabolic acidosis usually is associated with isopropanol ingestion. (Objective 4)

66. b. The second most common reported category of poisonings is from plants. Dialysis is not effective for most plant poisonings. Most signs and symptoms occur within several hours after ingestion. Treatment should be based on symptoms and not be delayed until the identity of the plant can be determined. (Objective 4)

67. a. Salivation and hypotension are likely to accompany the bradycardia. Symptoms vary according to the specific variety of mushroom ingested. (Objective 4)

68. d. The lower the viscosity, the higher the risk of aspiration. (Objective 5)

69. d. Huffing or sniffing substances such as carbon tetrachloride, methylene chloride, or aromatic hydrocarbons such as benzene and toluene is the most common method.
(Objective 8)

70. a. All of the other chemicals are more likely to cause tachycardia.
(Objective 9)

71. c. All other interventions are critical; however, rescuer safety should precede treatment because these poisons are absorbed readily through the skin, by ingestion, or by inhalation.
(Objective 9)

72. d
(Objective 9)

73. a. All of the others are narcotics.
(Objective 11)

74. c. Methamphetamine labs may produce hazards because of booby traps, explosive chemicals, a violent patient, or hazardous material contamination. Scene safety should be the highest priority.
(Objective 11)

75. c. Oil of wintergreen contains a large amount of salicylate and has produced many fatal ingestions.
(Objective 11)

76. c. Unless patients volunteer information regarding an overdose of acetaminophen, they may be asymptomatic or complain of only mild influenza-like symptoms for the first 24 hours after ingestion.
(Objective 11)

77. c. Ingestion of an overdose of iron is often lethal
(Objective 11)

78. c. All of the other drugs are more likely to produce bradycardia, although digoxin can produce bradycardia or tachycardia.
(Objective 11)

79. a. The immediate goal is to adsorb the drug and prevent its passage into the small intestine where it can be absorbed into the blood. Later, if signs and symptoms develop, they will be treated.
(Objective 11)

80. d. Wernicke-Korsakoff syndrome can lead to irreversible neurological problems and may be avoided by giving thiamine before administration of D50W.
(Objective 12)

81. b. The mortality rate has been reported as high as 15% for delirium tremens. It affects about 5% of hospitalized alcoholics undergoing withdrawal and usually occurs 72 to 96 hours after withdrawal of alcohol. Symptoms are associated with autonomic hyperactivity.
(Objective 13)

82. b. Diazepam in doses of 5 mg every 5 minutes up to a total of 30 mg may be needed. Lorazepam 1 to 2 mg intravenously is an alternative.
(Objective 13)

83. d. Anaphylaxis likely would include respiratory distress and urticaria. His reaction was immediate and generalized and involved a large exposure to venom.
(Objective 14)

84. a. The brown recluse spider produces a local reaction leading to delayed skin necrosis. Envenomation from most other spiders typically causes local versus systemic reactions.
(Objective 14)

85. c. This description matches a coral snake, which is the only neurotoxic snake listed.
(Objective 14)

86. d. Ice or cold packs may increase tissue damage. Establish IV in unaffected extremity.
(Objective 14)

87. c. Isoproterenol may induce or aggravate hypotension and ventricular dysrhythmias and should not be given for drug-induced bradycardia unless massive beta-blocker poisoning has occurred.
(Objective 11)

88. b. The other three are stimulants and the patient has pinpoint pupils, so an opiate overdose is more likely.
(Objective 11)

89. a. Assist ventilation and then give naloxone.
(Objective 10)

WRAP IT UP

1. a. Hypoglycemia: aspirin, Glucophage, acetaminophen (72 to 96 hours), ethanol (Vodka)
   b. Acidosis: aspirin
   c. Tachycardia: Ritalin, Elavil
   d. Respiratory depression: Vicodin, Ativan, Elavil, aspirin (late), ethanol alcohol
   e. Decreased level of conciousness: Glucophage (from hypoglycemia), Vicodin, Elavil, Ativan, rubbing alcohol, ethanol (Vodka)
   f. Pupil constriction: Vicodin, Ritalin
   g. Bradycardia: metoprolol
   h. Cardiac dysrhythmias: Elavil, metoprolol, Tylenol (4 to 14 days)
   (Objectives 2 and 11)
   i. Seizures: aspirin, Glucophage (hypoglycemia), Elavil, metoprolol

2. a, b, c, d, e, f, g, h, i, k, l
   (Objective 3)

3. a. Acetaminophen: respiratory depression or cardiac dysrhythmias
   b. Metoprolol: bradycardia, ventricular dysrhythmias
   c. Vodka (ethanol): airway obstruction
   d. Glucophage: hypoglycemic coma
   e. Aspirin: acidosis, convulsions, respiratory arrest, brain death
   f. Iron: gastrointestinal bleeding
   g. Vicodin: respiratory depression
   h. Tricyclic antidepressant: cardiac dysrhythmias, CNS depression
   (Objective 2, 10, and 11)

4. a. Support depressed, slow respirations.
   b. Naloxone is an antidote for narcotic (Vicodin) overdose and its accompanying respiratory depression.
   c. Blood glucose tests revealed hypoglycemia, which occurred as a result of his ingestions.
   (Objectives 10 and 11)

5. Flumazenil (Romazicon) is used to treat benzodiazepine overdose. However, it is only recommended after procedural sedation. It is not used in multiple-drug overdoses because life-threatening side effects can occur in patients who have taken certain other drugs, including tricyclic antidepressants.

Sodium bicarbonate is indicated in cases of tricyclic antidepressant overdose, and medical control may or may not have ordered it in this polydrug situation.

Glucagon can be administered in beta-blocker overdose.

Activated charcoal sometimes is indicated to adsorb drugs that are ingested; however, with the airway not yet secured, this could increase the risk of aspiration.
(Objective 11)

6. b. Gathering information related to the toxic ingestion is a key element in the prehospital care of the poisoned patient. Ipecac should not be used to treat ingestions. Antidotes are available for few poisonings.
(Objective 10)

7. a. None
b. Elavil
c. None
d. Vicodin
e. Ritalin
(Objective 14)

37

Hematology

READING ASSIGNMENT

Chapter 37, pages 970-982, in *Mosby's Paramedic Textbook,* ed. 3

OBJECTIVES

Upon completion of this chapter, the paramedic student will be able to:
1. Describe the physiology of blood and its components.
2. Discuss pathophysiology and signs and symptoms of specific hematological disorders.
3. Outline general assessment and management of patients with hematological disorders.

SUMMARY

- Blood is composed of cells and formed elements surrounded by plasma. About 95% of the volume of formed elements consists of RBCs (erythrocytes). The remaining 5% consists of WBCs (leukocytes) and cell fragments (platelets).

- Anemia is a condition in which the amount of hemoglobin or erythrocytes in the blood is below normal. Two common forms of anemia are iron deficiency anemia and hemolytic anemia. All forms of anemia share signs and symptoms. These signs and symptoms include fatigue and headaches, sometimes a sore mouth or tongue, brittle nails, and in severe cases, breathlessness and chest pain. Diagnosis is made by history and from blood tests and bone marrow biopsy.

- *Leukemia* refers to any of several types of cancer in which an abnormal proliferation of WBCs usually occurs in the bone marrow. The proliferation of leukemic cells crowds and impairs the normal production of RBCs, WBCs, and platelets. Leukemia is classified as acute or chronic. The proliferation of leukemic cells makes the patient highly susceptible to serious infections, anemia, and bleeding episodes. The diagnosis is confirmed by bone marrow biopsy.

- *Lymphoma* refers to a group of diseases that range from slowly growing chronic disorders to rapidly evolving acute conditions. Hodgkin's disease is one type; all others are called *non-Hodgkin's lymphomas*.

- Polycythemia is characterized by an unusually large number of RBCs in the blood as a result of their increased production by the bone marrow. Polycythemia may be a natural response to hypoxia. (This is known as secondary polycythemia.) Polycythemia also may occur for unknown reasons. (This is known as primary polycythemia.)

- Disseminated intravascular coagulopathy is a complication of severe injury, trauma, or disease. It disrupts the balance among procoagulants, thrombin formation, inhibitors, and lysis. Signs and symptoms of disseminated intravascular coagulation include dyspnea, bleeding, and those associated with hypotension and hypoperfusion. The treatment is aimed at reversing the underlying illness or injury that triggered the event.

- Hemophilia A is caused by a deficiency of a blood protein called *factor VIII*. Hemophilia B is caused by a deficiency of factor IX. Bleeding from hemophilia can occur spontaneously, after even minor injury, or during some medical procedures.

- Sickle cell disease is a debilitating and unpredictable recessive genetic illness. It affects persons of African descent. Less often, it affects persons of Mediterranean origin. Sickle cell anemia produces an abnormal type of hemoglobin. This is called *hemoglobin S*. This abnormal type has an inferior oxygen-carrying capacity. Complications of sickle cell disease include episodes of severe pain, fatigue, pallor, jaundice, stroke, delayed growth, hematuria, priapism, and splenomegaly.
- Multiple myeloma is a malignant neoplasm of the bone marrow. The tumor destroys bone tissue (especially flat bones). This causes pain, fractures, hypercalcemia, and skeletal deformities.
- In many cases of hematological disorders, the prehospital treatment is supportive. Treatment includes ensuring adequate airway, ventilatory, and circulatory support.

REVIEW QUESTIONS

Match the hematology terms in Column II with the description in Column I. Use each term only once.

Column I	Column II
1. _____ Include eosinophils, basophils, and neutrophils	a. Basophils
2. _____ Destroy red blood cells	b. Bilirubin
3. _____ Destroy invading organisms and include monophils	c. Erythrocytes
	d. Macrophages
4. _____ Waste product after destruction of hemoglobin	e. Phagocytes
5. _____ Activate chemicals that trigger inflammation	f. Plasma of hemoglobin
6. _____ Contains albumin, globulins, and fibrinogen	g. Platelets
7. _____ Composed of water and hemoglobin	h. White blood cell inflammation

8. Complete the information in the following table.

Condition	Cause	Signs and Symptoms
Anemia		
Leukemia		
Lymphomas		
Polycythemia		
Disseminated intravascular coagulation		
Hemophilia		
Sickle cell disease		
Multiple myeloma		

9. You respond to a private residence and find a 21-year-old black woman who is complaining of pain in her abdomen, hands, and feet. She said she had the flu and vomited 3 times yesterday. She tells you that she suffers from sickle cell disease.

  a. What type of sickle cell crisis may present in this manner?

b. What event may have triggered a crisis in this patient?

_____

c. What specific organ should you try to palpate on your physical examination of this patient?

_____

d. Outline the prehospital care of this patient.

_____

STUDENT SELF-ASSESSMENT

10. Which is true regarding red bone marrow?
    a. Only white blood cells are formed here.
    b. It is formed in the liver.
    c. It is composed mainly of connective tissue and fat.
    d. It is found in the vertebrae, pelvis, sternum, and ribs.
11. Which of the following is a normal value for hemoglobin?
    a. 10 g/100 mL   c. 35%
    b. 15 g/100 mL   d. 50%
12. Which type of anemia may be cured by splenectomy?
    a. Aplastic   c. Iron deficiency
    b. Hemolytic   d. Sickle cell
13. Which is true of acute myeloblastic leukemia?
    a. It affects mostly young children.
    b. Reed-Sternberg cells are present.
    c. Generalized itching may be present.
    d. It is difficult to cure.
14. Which hematological disorder is diagnosed using bone marrow biopsy?
    a. Disseminated intravascular coagulation
    b. Leukemia
    c. Hodgkin's disease
    d. Sickle cell anemia
15. Which of the following is a target organ in Hodgkin's lymphoma?
    a. Kidney   c. Spleen
    b. Liver   d. Testes
16. What can trigger secondary polycythemia?
    a. Blood loss   c. Hypoxia
    b. Hypothermia   d. Infection
17. Which of the following occurs when disseminated intravascular coagulation is present?
    a. Coagulation inhibition levels are increased.
    b. Fibrin is deposited in small vessels in multiple organs.
    c. Platelets and fibrinogen V, VIII, and XIII increase.
    d. Thrombin is destroyed.
18. What is needed to stop the bleeding that occurs during hemophilia?
    a. Factor VIII   c. Oxygen administration
    b. Intravenous fluids   d. Topical thrombin
19. Although all sickle cell disease emergencies can cause death, which one represents an immediate life-threatening situation?
    a. Aplastic crisis   c. Splenic sequestration
    b. Hemolytic crisis   d. Vasoocclusive crisis
20. In which hematological disorder of the bone marrow does the tumor destroy bone tissue?
    a. Hodgkin's disease   c. Lymphoma
    b. Leukemia   d. Multiple myeloma

21. Prehospital care for a conscious patient with a hematological problem should always include which of the following?

    a. Analgesics   **c.** Blood transfusion

    b. Antidysrhythmics   **d.** Emotional support

WRAP IT UP

You are dispatched to respond to a call for a person with difficulty breathing. Your patient is a 45-year-old white male who is the soccer coach at a local high school. He experienced shortness of breath and sweating during a practice drill with his team, and a player called 911. On arrival you note a pale man in moderate distress. He is alert and oriented and says he was fine until he started running. His initial SaO_2 is 89%, and his breath sounds are clear and equal bilaterally. You mention to him that he appears to have an unusual number of bruises on various areas of his body—ranging from old yellow or gray ones to purplish red newer ones. He appears nervous when you ask about his medical history and denies any significant illness, injury, or medications. His vital signs are BP 108/66 mm Hg, P 124, and R 24. You administer oxygen by non-rebreather mask and move him by stretcher into the ambulance. In the privacy of the ambulance, he confides to you that he has been ill and just this week saw his doctor because he has never had any medical problems but has been feeling tired all the time; has generalized bone pain, night sweats, and swollen "glands" in his neck; and has lost 25 lb in the last 8 weeks. This afternoon, his doctor called and said that his blood tests were grossly abnormal and he wanted to hospitalize him to run more tests to rule out leukemia. The coach confesses that he could not believe it and decided to go ahead with practice because he did not know what to tell the kids. His oxygen saturation is now 98%, and you initiate an IV and transport him, completing your physical exam en route. He subsequently is diagnosed with acute myeloblastic leukemia, and 6 months later you read of his death in the obituaries.

1. Which of the following blood cells increase or decrease in leukemia?

    a. Red blood cells   Increase/decrease

    b. White blood cells   Increase/decrease

    c. Platelets   Increase/decrease

2. What explains the following signs/symptoms that this patient experienced?

    a. Fatigue

    b. Swollen lymph nodes

    c. Difficulty breathing

    d. Bruising

3. What additional findings might you encounter when you assess the abdomen?

4. Place a check mark beside other hematological conditions you might have suspected, based on his history and presenting condition, if the patient had not confessed his presumed diagnosis.

    a. _____ Anemia   **e.** _____ Multiple myeloma

    b. _____ Hemophilia   **f.** _____ Polycythemia

    c. _____ Hodgkin's disease   **g.** _____ Sickle cell disease

    d. _____ Lymphoma

CHAPTER 37 ANSWERS

REVIEW QUESTIONS
1. h
2. d
3. e
4. b
5. a
6. f
7. c
(Questions 1 to 7, Objective 1)

8.

Condition	Cause	Signs and Symptoms
Anemia	Iron deficiency; decreased production and survival of red blood cells	Fatigue headaches, sore mouth or tongue, brittle nails, breathlessness, or chest pain
Leukemia	Abnormal chromosomes; disorganized proliferation of white blood cells in bone marrow	Bleeding, bone pain, frequent bruising, sternal tenderness, fatigue, headache, weight loss, height sweats; enlarged lymph nodes, liver, spleen; anemia, infections
Lymphomata	Proliferation of cells in lymph tissues (may be genetic link)	Swollen lymph nodes in neck, armpits, groin; fatigue, chills, and night sweats; severe itching, cough, weight loss, dyspnea, chest discomfort
Polycythemia	Unusually large number of red blood cells	Headache, dizziness, blurred vision, generalized itching; hypertension, splenomegaly, platelet disorders, red hands and feet, purple complexion, stroke and development of leukemias
Disseminated intra-vascular coagulation	Complication of severe injury, trauma, disease; imbalance of clotting mechanisms	Dyspnea, bleeding, hypotension, hypoperfusion
Hemophilia	Inherited bleeding disorder; deficiency of factor VIII or less often factor IX	Spontaneous bleeding (joints, deep muscles, urinary tract, and intracranial sites most common) after injury or during medical procedures
Sickle cell disease	Genetic illness; red blood cells are distorted into sickle shape that is easily destroyed and can clog blood vessels	Episodes of severe pain, fatigue, pallor, jaundice, stroke; delayed growth, development, and sexual maturation; hematuria, priapism, splenomegaly
Multiple myeloma	Malignant neoplasm of bone marrow	Pain, fractures, hypercalcemia, skeletal deformities, kidney failure, anemia, weight loss, rib fractures, recurrent infections

(Objective 2)

9. a. Possibly a vasoocclusive sickle cell crisis
    b. Dehydration or stress from her illness the day before may have triggered her crisis.
    c. The spleen may enlarge during a sickle cell crisis, so it should be evaluated.
    d. You should administer oxygen by non-rebreather mask at 12 to 15 L/min. You should initiate an intravenous line and administer a fluid bolus under medical direction. Although analgesia will be a high priority for this patient, medical direction may not order it until the abdomen can be examined to ensure that an urgent surgical condition does not exist.
    (Objective 2)

10. d. All types of blood cells are formed here. Yellow marrow is composed of connective tissue and fat.
    (Objective 1)

11. b. Normal hemoglobin ranges from 13.5 to 18 g/100 mL. Normal hematocrit ranges from 38% to 54%.
    (Objective 1)

12. b. Treatment for aplastic anemia may include blood transfusion, folic acid, and bone marrow transplantation. Iron deficiency anemia is treated with supplemental iron and folic acid.
    (Objective 2)

13. d. Acute myeloblastic anemia affects middle-aged adults. Reed-Sternberg cells are characteristic of Hodgkin's lymphoma. Itching is not a classic symptom.
    (Objective 2)

14. b. Disseminated intravascular coagulation is diagnosed based on clinical history and laboratory values that include clotting studies, platelet count, and fibrin degradation products. Sickle cell anemia is confirmed by laboratory testing.
    (Objective 2)

15. c. Hodgkin's lymphoma primarily affects lymphoid tissues.
    (Objective 2)

16. c. The body produces more red cells in an attempt to improve oxygenation in conditions such as high altitude and chronic lung disease.
    (Objective 2)

17. b. Coagulation inhibition levels are decreased. Platelets and coagulation factors are consumed, and thrombin is formed.
    (Objective 2)

18. a. Factor VIII is needed to reestablish a normal clotting cascade and stop bleeding.
    (Objective 2)

19. c. Splenic sequestration occurs in childhood and is caused by blood trapped in the spleen. Aplastic crisis occurs when the bone marrow temporarily stops making red blood cells. In hemolytic crisis, red blood cell breakdown exceeds production. Vasoocclusive sickle cell crisis occurs when the sickle-shaped cells block blood flow to organs and tissues.
    (Objective 2)

20. d. Hodgkin's disease is a type of lymphoma and affects the lymph tissue. Leukemia is similar to multiple myeloma, but in multiple myeloma, the primary target is bone.
    (Objective 2)

21. d. Acute or chronic hematological disorders produce tremendous emotional stress on patients and families. You should be empathetic and provide calm support during care and transport. Analgesics and antidysrhythmics occasionally may be indicated. Prehospital blood transfusion usually is done only during interfacility transfers.
(Objective 2)

WRAP IT UP

1. a. Decrease; b. increase; c. decrease
(Objective 2)

2. a. A decrease in red blood cells causes a decrease in oxygen delivery to the cells that could affect adenosine triphosphate (energy) production.
b. Lymph nodes help to rid the body of excess or damaged white blood cells, which are characteristic of leukemia.
c. The patient's decrease in red blood cells did not permit his body to transport enough oxygen to meet the increased demand during exertion at practice.
d. Platelets are essential to control bleeding in the body and are greatly decreased in leukemia.
(Objectives 1 and 2)

3. The liver and spleen likely will be greatly enlarged.
(Objective 3)

4. a. Because of his pallor and dyspnea
c and d. Although he is somewhat young, other signs and symptoms would not exclude Hodgkin's and other lymphomata.
e. His age and bone pain are consistent with multiple myeloma.
His history does not include hemophilia, which is present at birth; polycythemia is a problem of excess red cells and typically would produce red-purple skin, not pallor as in this patient (and this patient does not seem to have risk factors for polycythemia); this patient is white, so sickle cell anemia would be unlikely, and he has no known history of sickle cell disease that would be diagnosed early in life.
(Objective 2)

Environmental Conditions

READING ASSIGNMENT

Chapter 38, pages 984-1003, in *Mosby's Paramedic Textbook*, ed. 3

OBJECTIVES

Upon completion of this chapter, the paramedic student will be able to:
1. Describe the physiology of thermoregulation.
2. Discuss the risk factors, pathophysiology, assessment findings, and management of specific hyperthermic conditions.
3. Discuss the risk factors, pathophysiology, assessment findings, and management of specific hypothermic conditions and frostbite.
4. Discuss the risk factors, pathophysiology, assessment findings, and management of submersion and drowning.
5. Identify the mechanical effects on the body based on a knowledge of the basic properties of gases.
6. Discuss the risk factors, pathophysiology, assessment findings, and management of diving emergencies and high-altitude illness.

SUMMARY

- Body temperature is regulated by a thermoregulatory center in the posterior hypothalamus. The body temperature can be increased or decreased in two ways. One of these ways is through the regulation of heat production. (This is known as thermogenesis.) The other way is through the regulation of heat loss. (This is known as thermolysis.).

- Heat illness results from one of two basic causes. First, the normal temperature-regulating functions can be overwhelmed by conditions in the environment. These conditions can include heat stress. More often, though, they involve excessive exercise in moderate to extreme environmental conditions. The other cause is the failure of the body's thermoregulatory mechanism. This may occur in older adults or ill or debilitated individuals. Heat cramps are brief, intermittent, and often severe. They are muscular cramps that occur in muscles fatigued by heavy work or exercise. Heat exhaustion is characterized by minor aberrations in mental status, dizziness, nausea, headache, and a mild to moderate rise in the core body temperature (CBT) (up to less than 103° F [39° C]). Heat stroke occurs when the temperature-regulating functions break down entirely. This failure results in body temperature rises to 105.8° F (41° C) or higher. Temperatures this high damage all tissues and lead to collapse.

- Hypothermia (a CBT lower than 95° F [35° C]) can result from a decrease in heat production, an increase in heat loss, or a combination of these two factors. The progression of clinical signs and symptoms of hypothermia is divided into three classes based on the CBT: mild (CBT between 93.2° and 96.8° F [34° and to 36° C]), moderate

(CBT between 86° and 93° F [30° and 34° C]), and severe (CBT below 86° F [30° C]). Severely hypothermic patients have no vital signs, including respiratory effort, pulse, and blood pressure.

- Frostbite is a localized injury. It results from environmentally induced freezing of body tissues. This freezing leads to the damage to blood vessels. Ischemia often produces the most damaging effects of frostbite. In deep frostbite this can include mummification and sloughing of nonviable skin and deep structures.
- Drowning is a process that results in primary respiratory impairment from submersion/immersion in a liquid medium that presents the person from breathing air. Regardless of the type of water aspirated, the pathophysiology of drowning is characterized by hypoxia, hypercapnia, and acidosis, which result in cardiac arrest.
- The three laws pertaining to the basic properties of gases that are involved in all pressure-related diving emergencies are Boyle's law, Dalton's law, and Henry's law. Increased pressure dissolves gases into blood; oxygen metabolizes, and nitrogen dissolves.
- Barotrauma is tissue damage. It results from compression or expansion of gas spaces when the gas pressure in the body differs from the ambient pressure. The type of barotrauma depends on whether the diver is in descent or ascent. Air embolism is the most serious complication of pulmonary barotrauma. It is a major cause of death and disability among sport divers.
- High-altitude illness results from exposure to reduced atmospheric pressure, which results in hypoxia. Forms of high-altitude illness include acute mountain sickness, high-altitude pulmonary edema, and high-altitude cerebral edema.

REVIEW QUESTIONS

Match the terms related to environmental conditions in Column II with the appropriate description in Column I. Use each term only once.

Column I

1. _____ Goose bumps
2. _____ Dissipation of heat in the body by various mechanisms
3. _____ Sudden return of cold blood and wastes to the core
4. _____ Temperature difference between body and environment
5. _____ Gas volume inversely related to its pressure

6. _____ Decompression sickness
7. _____ Heat immersion causing hypotension from vasodilation
8. _____ Total pressure of gases equaling the sum of partial pressure of component gases
9. _____ Regulation of heat production in the body
10. _____ Amount of gas dissolved in fluid volume is proportional to pressure of gas with which it is in equilibrium

Column II

a. Afterdrop phenomenon
b. Boyle's law
c. Cold diuresis
d. Dalton's law
e. Dysbarism
f. Henry's law
g. Piloerection
h. Rewarming shock
i. Thermal gradient
j. Thermogenesis
k. Thermolysis

11. Briefly describe how each of the following contributes to heat production in the body.

   a. Chemical control:

   _____

   b. Musculoskeletal system:

   _____

c. Endocrine system:

_____

12. For each of the following situations, select the mechanisms of heat loss that apply (conduction, convection, evaporation, and radiation). You may use each answer more than once.

   a. On a windy autumn evening, you remove the clothing of a trauma patient to assess his injuries more accurately. On arrival to the emergency department, his temperature is 94° F (34.4° C). _____.

   b. During a multiple patient situation, you extricate a partially clothed patient onto a cold metal backboard. On arrival to the emergency department, her temperature is 96° F (35.6° C). _____.

   c. On a dry, cool spring evening you transport a wet patient who injured her neck after diving into a swimming pool. On arrival to the emergency department, her temperature is 94.6° F (34.8° C). _____.

   d. A patient with a 40% body surface area burn is cooled continuously with normal saline en route to the hospital. On arrival to the emergency department, his temperature is 93.5° F (34.2° C). _____.

13. You are on the scene of a multiple-car collision on a hot July day. List four ways your body will compensate to prevent your temperature from rising.

   a.

   b.

   c.

   d.

14. You are assisting with a search-and-rescue effort after a hurricane. It is cold, wet, and windy. List four ways your body will attempt to maintain a normal temperature.

   a.

   b.

   c.

   d.

15. For each of the following examples, identify the type of heat illness and briefly describe the appropriate prehospital patient care.

   a. You are working at an amusement park on a 95° F (35° C) humid day. A hot, sweaty 45-year-old woman comes to your aid station complaining of severe cramping in her calves. Her vital signs are BP 116/72 mm Hg, P 116, and temperature 98.6° F (37° C).

   Illness:

_____

   Management:

_____

b. A 55-year-old man is complaining of dizziness, nausea, and vomiting while participating in a long-distance walk fund-raiser. His vital signs while lying down are BP 104/70 mm Hg and P 108. His vital signs while standing are BP 86/50 mm Hg and P 128, and his temperature is 101° F (38.3° C).
Illness:

_____

Management:

_____

c. On a 100° F (37.8° C) day, an 80-year-old woman becomes confused and agitated and has a seizure in her apartment, which does not have air-conditioning. She is responsive to pain, has jugular venous distention, and is sweating profusely. Her vital signs are BP 92/70 mm Hg, P 120, R 24, and temperature 106° F (41.1° C).
Illness:

_____

Management:

_____

16. Why is the increased metabolic rate that is produced in mild hypothermia undesirable for a patient who already has an injury or medical illness?

_____

_____

Questions 17 to 19 refer to the following case study:

> You are caring for a snowmobiler whose rig broke through the ice 30 minutes ago. He pulled himself out of the water and collapsed before rescuers reached him 20 minutes later. He has been moved to a safe area.

17. Describe general measures of care to begin immediately on this patient.

_____

_____

18. You determine that he is apneic and pulseless. His electrocardiogram displays the rhythm shown in Fig. 38-1. What actions should be taken if the following occur?

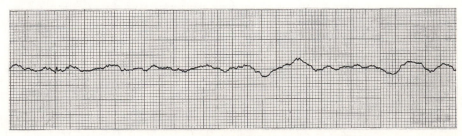

Figure 38-1

a. His core temperature is less than 86° F (30° C).

_____

_____

b. His core temperature is greater than 86° F (30° C).

_____

_____

19. When should resuscitation efforts be terminated?

_____

20. You are transporting a hiker who became lost on a trail. He is shivering and hungry and has a temperature of 97° F (36.1° C). How would you treat this patient?

_____

_____

21. A firefighter dives into an ice-covered pond to rescue a child who has fallen through the ice on a windy, cold January evening. On the 10-minute walk back to the firetruck, the firefighter develops slurred speech and ataxia and complains that his heart is pounding. At the ambulance, his temperature is 89.5° F (31.9° C). His electrocardiogram is shown in Fig. 38-2.

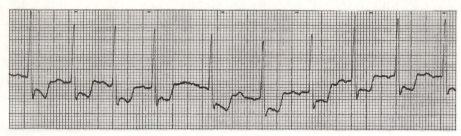

Figure 38-2

a. What is your interpretation of the electrocardiogram tracing?

_____

b. Describe your management of this patient.

_____

_____

_____

Questions 22 to 24 refer to the following case study:

During a cross-country ski meet, a participant complains of coldness, numbness, and extreme pain in the fingers of his right hand.

22. Differentiate between the findings you would anticipate for superficial frostbite and deep frostbite.

_____

_____

23. List four factors that increase susceptibility to frostbite that you should look for in this patient.

   a.

   b.

   c.

   d.

24. How would you treat frostbite in this patient?

_____

_____

Questions 25 to 27 refer to the following case study:

   A 2-year-old child pulled from a backyard pool is apneic and pulseless.

25. Identify four factors that will influence this patient's clinical outcome.

   a.

   b.

   c.

   d.

26. What complications do you anticipate if the patient is resuscitated?

_____

_____

_____

27. Describe prehospital management of this child.

_____

_____

28. List five body areas on the patient where pain may occur resulting from SQUEEZE.

   a.   **d.**

   b.   **e.**

   c.

29. A diver experiences acute distress immediately after rapidly surfacing from a deep dive.

   a. List five signs or symptoms of air embolism.

      a.   **d.**

      b.   **e.**

      c.

   b. Describe special considerations necessary for care of this patient while you are providing advanced life support and transport.

_____

_____

30. A tourist at a local resort complains of severe joint pain, fatigue, vertigo, and paraesthesia 12 hours after returning from his first dive.

    a. What diving injury do you suspect?

_____

    b. Describe prehospital management of this patient.

_____

_____

31. You respond to a mountain resort where a participant in a cycling event has become ill.

    a. List the three types of high-altitude illness.

        a.

        b.

        c.

    b. What single intervention is most critical to long-term improvement of the patient suffering from high-altitude illness after the ABCs have been managed?

_____

STUDENT SELF-ASSESSMENT

32. What is the most important organ that regulates body temperature?
    a. Heart   **c.** Pituitary gland
    b. Lungs   **d.** Skin

33. You are assessing firefighters in the rehab area of a major fire on a summer day. Your patient is dizzy and nauseated and has orthostatic hypotension. What should you do?
    a. Administer medication for his nausea.
    b. Ask him to rest for 15 minutes before returning to the fire.
    c. Have him drink a fluid-replacement beverage.
    d. Initiate an intravenous line and administer a fluid bolus.

34. What causes shock to develop in the patient with heat stroke?
    a. Fluid loss   **c.** Peripheral vasodilation
    b. Myocardial depression   **d.** All of the above

35. What is the most critical intervention for heat stroke?
    a. Fluid resuscitation   **c.** Rapid cooling in transit
    b. Medication administration   **d.** Rapid transport to a hospital

36. When does shivering stop in a hypothermic patient?
    a. The body temperature drops to 90° F (32.2° C).
    b. Glucose or glycogen is depleted.
    c. Excessive amounts of insulin are excreted.
    d. P_{CO_2} increases to more than 50 mm Hg.

37. Prehospital care of a frostbitten extremity should include which of the following?
    a. Application of a tourniquet
    b. Elevation of the affected extremity
    c. Rapid rewarming in hot water
    d. Refreezing of the injured extremity

38. All drownings are characterized by which of the following?
   a. Hypovolemia, hypoxia, and acidosis
   b. Hypoxia, acidosis, and hypothermia
   c. Hypoxia, acidosis, and hypercapnia
   d. Hypovolemia, acidosis, and hypercapnia
39. Which of the following best describes the term *drowning*?
   a. Death from submersion up to 24 hours after arrival in the emergency department
   b. Death related to submersion that occurs at any time after the incident
   c. Impaired breathing from submersion/immersion in a liquid
   d. Swimming-related distress sufficient to require support in the prehospital setting
40. What is the single most important factor in determining survival after submersion injury?
   a. Age of the patient
   b. Contaminants in the water
   c. Duration of submersion
   d. Water temperature
41. Which law of physics states that the volume of gas is related inversely to its pressure at a constant temperature?
   a. Boyle's law
   b. Dalton's law
   c. Henry's law
   d. Newton's law
42. A diver is in respiratory distress after ascent. You palpate subcutaneous emphysema. He is probably suffering from which of the following?
   a. Barotrauma of descent
   b. Decompression sickness
   c. Pulmonary air embolus
   d. Pulmonary overpressurization syndrome
43. What is the primary danger of nitrogen narcosis?
   a. Hypoxemia
   b. Impaired judgment
   c. Respiratory acidosis
   d. Shock resulting from hypovolemia
44. What is the critical sign or symptom that indicates deterioration in a patient with acute mountain sickness?
   a. Ataxia
   b. Headache
   c. Irritability
   d. Vomiting

WRAP IT UP

You are standing by with searchers who are trying to find a 50-year-old hunter who is evidently lost in a marshy area and has not been heard from in 18 hours. The weather is cold and windy, with temperatures the night before dropping to 40° F (4° C) and winds of up to 20 mph. An excited transmission on the radio lets you know that he has been found alive. Crews are going to bring him out to your staging area. He arrives in the bed of a pickup truck, conscious but confused. Rescuers tell you they found him staggering in the swamp. His overalls are soaked and his boots are full of water. You move him in the warm ambulance and quickly but gently remove his clothes and cover him with warm, dry blankets. Your partner puts a warm pack on his antecubital space to try to expose a vein to start an IV. Warmed, humidified oxygen is administered by mask, and his vital signs are taken. Because of the large number of exposure incidents in your area, you have a hypothermia thermometer and obtain a core temperature of 87° F (30.5° C), BP 100/60 mm Hg, P 56, R 16, SaO$_2$ unobtainable; and his skin is cool and pale. You initiate an IV of warmed normal saline and obtain a blood glucose, which is 78 mg/dL; electrocardiogram rhythm is sinus bradycardia. As you go en route to the hospital, medical direction asks you to infuse a fluid challenge of 250 mL and reassess the patient. You are sweating because of the heat in the patient compartment and check the heat packs you have placed in his armpits and groin to ensure they are still warm. While you perform your comprehensive exam, you note that his feet have a waxy, white appearance and that he appears to have severe pain when you palpate them. On arrival to the ED his vital signs are BP 110/64 mm Hg, P 58, R 20, and temperature 90° F (32° C).

1. What was the equivalent chill factor at the coldest part of the night?
2. Which of the following mechanisms of heat loss played a role in this situation?
   a. Conduction
   b. Convection
   c. Evaporation
   d. Radiation

3. Place a check mark sign beside symptoms that demonstrate moderate hypothermia that are found in this patient.

   a. ____ Atrial fibrillation   e. ____ Confusion
   b. ____ Ataxia   f. ____ Fixed, dilated pupils
   c. ____ Bradycardia   g. ____ Loss of deep tendon reflexes
   d. ____ Cardiac instability   h. ____ Shivering

4. Explain why the following interventions could be harmful in this patient.
   a. Vigorous movement

   b. Lactated Ringer's solution intravenously

   c. Placing the patient in a high Fowler's position

5. Which is true regarding the assessment findings of his feet?
   a. They are likely just cold and will rewarm last because of the distal circulation.

   b. This is evidence of extensive frostbite, and he will probably need amputations.

   c. Rewarming should not be attempted because of possible tissue damage.

   d. Trench foot is possible, and blisters may begin to form as he rewarms.

REVIEW QUESTIONS

1. g
   (Objective 1)

2. k
   (Objective 1)

3. a
   (Objective 3)

4. i
   (Objective 1)

5. b
   (Objective 5)

6. e
   (Objective 6)

7. h
   (Objective 3)

8. d
   (Objective 5)

9. j
   (Objective 1)

10. f
    (Objective 5)

11. a. Oxidation of energy sources; b. shivering can increase heat production by 400%; c. increased basal metabolic rate and vasoconstriction
    (Objective 1)

12. a. Conduction, convection, and radiation; b. conduction and radiation; c. conduction, radiation, convection, and evaporation; d. conduction, radiation, convection, and evaporation
    (Objective 1)

13. Skin vasodilation (becomes warm and flushed), sweating, decreased hormone secretion, and decreased muscle tone
    (Objective 1)

14. Peripheral vasoconstriction (cool, pale skin), goose bumps, shivering, increased voluntary activity, increased hormone secretion, and increased appetite
    (Objective 1)

15. a. Heat cramps. Remove patient from hot environment, replace sodium and water, and intravenously infuse saline solution if condition is severe.
    b. Heat exhaustion. Remove patient from hot environment and intravenously infuse saline solution.

c. Heat stroke. Secure airway, assess breathing, ventilate if indicated, administer high-flow oxygen, move patient to a cool environment, remove all clothing, wet the skin with cool fluid, fan the patient, initiate intravenous fluid therapy with normal saline, consult with medical direction regarding a fluid challenge, and monitor for signs of fluid overload. If seizures recur, administer diazepam, assess for hypoglycemia, and administer D50W if indicated. (Objective 2)

16. Increasing the metabolic rate increases the heart rate and contractility and increases the body's use of oxygen and other nutrients. The patient with preexisting trauma or illness will not tolerate these extra demands, which may compromise organ response to illness or injury. (Objective 3)

17. Assess and secure the airway, assess breathing, and assist with 100% oxygen (warmed and humidified if available); if indicated, assess circulation and begin cardiopulmonary resuscitation only after verifying that no pulse is present. Move the patient to a warm environment and remove all clothing. Assess the body temperature. Begin warming. (Objective 3)

18. a. Cardiopulmonary resuscitation; defibrillation at 360 J; monophasic; biphasic per manufacturer, usually 120-200 J intubation; ventilation with warm, humid oxygen; intravenous infusion of warm normal saline; withhold drugs until T >30°C (86°F); provide active internal rewarming and transport to the hospital
    b. Cardiopulmonary resuscitation, defibrillation at 360 J; monophasic; biphasic per manufacturer usually 120-200 J intubation; ventilation with warm, humid oxygen; intravenous infusion of warm normal saline; intravenous administration of medications as indicated for ventricular fibrillation with a delay between doses; and another defibrillation as core temperature rises. Provide active external rewarming. (Objective 3)

19. Resuscitation may be withheld if there are obvious lethal injuries or if the body is frozen, preventing chest compression or airway management. Resuscitation could stop when the patient's core temperature has reached 94° to 95° F (34° to 35° C) and all resuscitation efforts are still unsuccessful. (Objective 3)

20. Move patient to warm area, remove any wet clothing, and wrap patient in warm blanket. If he is awake and alert, administer warm, sugar-sweetened drinks (no alcohol, coffee, or tea). If necessary, apply hot packs wrapped in towels to the neck, armpits, and groin. (Objective 3)

21. a. Atrial fibrillation
    b. Put the patient at rest and move to a warm environment after ensuring adequate airway, breathing, and circulation. Carefully remove all wet clothing and wrap patient in a blanket. Administer 100% oxygen (heated and humidified if possible) by non-rebreather mask. Initiate intravenous therapy of normal saline (initial fluid challenge of 250 to 500 mL may be ordered by medical direction, and use warmed fluids if available). Transport gently, apply warm packs covered in towels to groin and axilla, and monitor the patient carefully en route. (Objective 3)

22. In deep frostbite the underlying tissue is hard and not compressible, whereas in superficial frostbite the underlying tissue springs back when palpated. (Objective 3)

23. No protective clothing; preexisting illness or injury (diabetes or vascular insufficiency); fatigue; tobacco; tight, constrictive clothing; alcohol ingestion; and vasodilatory medications (some antihypertensives) (Objective 3)

24. Elevate and protect the affected extremity, provide rapid transport to a medical facility, and assess for hypothermia. (Objective 3)

25. Temperature of water, length of submersion, cleanliness of water, and age of patient
(Objective 4)

26. Acute respiratory failure, dysrhythmias, decreased cardiac output, cerebral edema leading to central nervous system dysfunction, and renal dysfunction (rare)
(Objective 4)

27. Ensure scene safety, initiate cardiopulmonary resuscitation, secure the airway with an endotracheal tube and ventilate with 100% oxygen, assess cardiac rhythm and follow advanced life support protocols to manage appropriately, assess for hypothermia, and transport to appropriate medical facility.
(Objective 4)

28. Ears, sinuses, lungs and airways, gastrointestinal tract, thorax, and teeth
(Objective 6)

29. a. Focal paralysis or sensory changes, aphasia, confusion, blindness or another visual disturbance, convulsion, loss of consciousness, dizziness, vertigo, abdominal pain, and cardiac arrest
b. If the patient's trachea is intubated, fill the balloon with normal saline instead of air; evaluate for pulmonary over pressurization syndrome (POPS); and transport in the left lateral recumbent position with a 15-degree elevation of the thorax.
(Objective 6)

30. a. Decompression sickness
b. Administer high-flow oxygen, initiate intravenous therapy, and rapidly transport for recompression (follow local protocol so that patient can reach hyperbaric chamber as quickly as possible).
(Objective 6)

31. a. Acute mountain sickness, high-altitude pulmonary edema, and high altitude cerebral edema; b. descent to a lower altitude
(Objective 6)

32. d. Vasoconstriction and vasodilation of the blood vessels in the skin are the major ways the body releases or conserves heat.
(Objective 1)

33. d. Based on his symptoms, you suspect heat exhaustion. Because he is nauseated and has orthostatic hypotension, he needs intravenous rather than oral rehydration. He should be moved to a cool environment and not returned to the fire.
(Objective 2)

34. d
(Objective 2)

35. c. Damage to the body continues as long as the temperature remains elevated.
(Objective 2)

36. b. Shivering should continue until the core temperature reaches 86° F (30° C). A tremendous amount of energy is needed for shivering, so glucose and glycogen must be available to fuel this increased muscle activity.
(Objective 3)

37. b. Rapid rewarming in warm water is indicated only when sanctioned by medical direction if no chance of refreezing exists. Refreezing is damaging to the tissues.
(Objective 3)

38. c. The lack of ventilation causes a buildup of carbon dioxide, which coupled with the lack of oxygen intake (hypoxia) leads to acidosis.
(Objective 4)

39. c. The Utstein definition of drowning is now recommended.
(Objective 4)

40. c. Although each factor listed influences patient outcome after submersion, duration of submersion and degree of hypoxia are the critical elements that determine odds of survival.
(Objective 4)

41. a. Dalton's law states that the total pressure of a mixture of gases is equal to the sum of the partial pressures of the component gases. Henry's law states that the amount of gas dissolved in a given volume of fluid is proportional to the pressure of the gas with which it is in equilibrium. Newton's law states that a body at rest will remain at rest until acted on by an outside force, and a body in motion will remain in motion until acted on by an outside force.
(Objective 5)

42. d. As trapped air in the lungs expands on rapid ascent, it ruptures alveoli and allows gas to leak into the subcutaneous tissues.
(Objective 6)

43. b. The neurodepressant effects of nitrogen narcosis may lead to diving accidents resulting from impaired judgment.
(Objective 6)

44. a. Ataxia signals progression of the illness, and coma may result within 24 hours of its onset.
(Objective 6)

WRAP IT UP

1. 18° F (−8° C)
(Objective 1)

2. a, b, d. Conduction causes heat loss from warm skin to cold air or water; convection causes heat loss from the 20 mph wind blowing over; radiation is the heat radiating off his skin.
(Objective 1)

3. b, c, e. Loss of deep tendon reflexes and dilated pupils are signs of severe hypothermia. Shivering typically has stopped by when the patient has moderate hypothermia.
(Objective 3)

4. a. The heart become irritable in hypothermia, and vigorous movement can trigger ventricular fibrillation.
b. The cold liver is unable to metabolize the lactate.
c. Orthostatic hypotension may result if the patient is moved to a sitting position.
(Objective 3)

5. d. Prolonged exposure to very cold water can cause trench foot. He will likely develop signs and symptoms similar to frostbite as he rewarms.
(Objective 3)

Infectious and Communicable Diseases

READING ASSIGNMENT
Chapter 39, pages 1004-1041, in *Mosby's Paramedic Textbook,* ed. 3

OBJECTIVES
Upon completion of this chapter, the paramedic student will be able to:
1. Identify general public health principles related to infectious diseases.
2. Describe the chain of elements necessary for an infectious disease to occur.
3. Explain how internal and external barriers affect susceptibility to infection.
4. Differentiate the four stages of infectious disease: the latent period, the incubation period, the communicability period, and the disease period.
5. Describe the mode of transmission, pathophysiology, prehospital considerations, and personal protective measures to be taken for the human immunodeficiency virus (HIV), hepatitis, tuberculosis, meningococcal meningitis, and pneumonia.
6. Describe the mode of transmission, pathophysiology, signs and symptoms, and prehospital considerations for patients who have rabies or tetanus.
7. List the signs, symptoms, and possible secondary complications of selected childhood viral diseases.
8. List the signs, symptoms, and possible secondary complications of influenza, severe acute respiratory syndrome (SARS), and mononucleosis.
9. Describe the mode of transmission, pathophysiology, prehospital considerations, and personal protective measures for sexually transmitted diseases.
10. Identify the signs and symptoms and prehospital considerations for lice and scabies.
11. Outline the reporting process for exposure to infectious or communicable diseases.
12. Discuss the paramedic's role in preventing disease transmission.

SUMMARY
- National concerns regarding communicable disease and infection control have resulted in public law, standards, guidelines, and recommendations to protect health care providers and emergency responders against infectious diseases. The paramedic must be familiar with these guidelines. He or she also must take personal protective measures against exposure to these pathogens.

- The chain of elements needed to transmit an infectious disease includes the pathogenic agent, a reservoir, a portal of exit from the reservoir, an environment conducive to transmission of the pathogenic agent, a portal of entry into the new host, and susceptibility of the new host to the infectious disease.
- The human body is protected from infectious disease by external and internal barriers. These serve as lines of defense against infection. External barriers include the skin, GI system, upper respiratory tract, and genitourinary tract. Internal barriers include the inflammatory response and the immune response.
- The progression of infectious disease from exposure to the onset of symptoms follows four stages. These are the latent period, the incubation period, the communicability period, and the disease period.
- The human immunodeficiency virus is directly transmitted person to person. This occurs through anal or vaginal intercourse, across the placenta, by contact with infected blood or body fluids on mucous membranes or open wounds, through blood transfusion or tissue transplant, or by the use of contaminated needles or syringes. The virus affects the CD4 T cells. Secondary complications are usually related to opportunistic infections that arise as the immune system deteriorates. The disease progression can be categorized into category A (acute retroviral infection, seroconversion, and asymptomatic infection); category B (early symptomatic HIV); and category C (late symptomatic HIV and advanced HIV). Paramedics should observe strict compliance with universal precautions for protection against HIV. Patient care should include helping these patients feel that they can obtain acceptance and compassion from health care workers.
- Hepatitis is a viral disease. It produces pathologic changes in the liver. The three main classes of hepatitis virus are hepatitis A, hepatitis B, and hepatitis C.
- Tuberculosis is a chronic pulmonary disease. It is acquired by inhaling a tubercle bacilli. The infection is passed mainly by infected persons coughing or sneezing the bacteria into the air or from contact with sputum that contains virulent TB bacilli. The infection is characterized by stages of early infection (frequently asymptomatic), latency, and a potential for recurrent postprimary disease.
- Meningococcal meningitis refers to inflammation of the membranes that surround the spinal cord and brain. It can be caused by bacteria, viruses, and other microorganisms.
- Bacterial endocarditis is an inflammation of the endocardium and one or more heart valves. The disease can be fatal if untreated.
- Pneumonia is an acute inflammatory process of the respiratory bronchioles and alveoli. Agents responsible for this disease may be bacterial, viral, or fungal.
- Tetanus is a serious, sometimes fatal, disease of the CNS. It is caused by infection of a wound with spores of the bacterium *Clostridium tetani*. The most common symptom is trismus. This symptom makes it difficult to open the mouth.
- Rabies is an acute viral infection of the CNS. Humans are highly susceptible to the rabies virus after being exposed to saliva from a bite or scratch of an infected animal.
- Hantaviruses are carried by rodents. They are transmitted by inhaling material contaminated with rodent urine and feces. Many forms of this disease occur in specific geographical areas.
- Rubella is a mild, febrile, and highly communicable viral disease. It is characterized by a diffuse punctate macular rash. The CDC recommends that all health care providers receive immunization if they are not immune from previous rubella infection.
- Rubeola is an acute, highly communicable viral disease. (It is caused by the measles virus.) It is characterized by fever, conjunctivitis, cough, bronchitis, and a blotchy red rash.
- Mumps is an acute, communicable systemic viral disease. It is characterized by localized unilateral or bilateral edema of one or more of the salivary glands. There is occasional involvement of other glands.
- Chickenpox is highly communicable. It is characterized by a sudden onset of low-grade fever, mild malaise, and a maculopapular skin eruption for a few hours and vesicular for 3 to 4 days, leaving a granular scab. The virus may reactivate during periods of stress or immunosuppression. At that time, it may produce an illness known as *shingles*.
- Pertussis is an infectious disease that leads to inflammation of the entire respiratory tract. It causes an insidious cough. The cough becomes paroxysmal in 1 to 2 weeks and lasts for 1 to 2 months.
- Influenza is mainly a respiratory infection. It is spread by influenza viruses A, B, and C.
- Severe acute respiratory syndrome (SARS) is a viral illness. It is spread by exposure to infected droplets. It was first detected in 2003. The illness begins with a fever and mild respiratory symptoms. It can progress to respiratory failure and death.
- Mononucleosis is caused either by the Epstein-Barr virus or cytomegalovirus. Both of these are members of the herpesvirus family.

- Syphilis is a systemic disease. It is characterized by a primary lesion; a secondary eruption involving skin and mucous membranes; long latency periods; and eventual seriously disabling lesions of the skin, bone, viscera, CNS, and cardiovascular system.
- Gonorrhea is caused by the sexually transmitted bacterium *Neisseria gonorrhoeae*. Gonorrhea is treatable with antibiotics. However, some strains brought into the United States from other countries do not respond to the usual antibiotic therapy.
- Chlamydia is a major cause of sexually transmitted nonspecific urethritis or genital infection. Signs and symptoms are similar to gonorrhea.
- Herpes simplex virus is transmitted by skin-to-skin contact with an infected area of the body. The primary infection produces a vesicular lesion (blister). This lesion heals spontaneously. After the primary infection, the virus travels to a sensory nerve ganglion. It remains there in a latent stage until reactivated.
- Lice are small, wingless insects that are ectoparasites of birds and mammals. During biting and feeding, secretions from the louse cause a small, red macule and pruritus.
- The human scabies mite is a parasite. It completes its life cycle in and on the epidermis of its host. Scabies bites are usually concentrated around the hands and feet, especially between the webs of the fingers and toes.
- Reporting a possible communicable disease exposure permits immediate medical follow-up. It also enables the designated officer to make changes that might prevent exposures in the future. Moreover, it helps employees to get the proper evaluation and testing.
- Part of the paramedic's professional duty related to infectious disease transmission is to know when not to go to work. Paramedics also have a duty to use the proper BSI (universal precautions) at all times.

REVIEW QUESTIONS

Match the infectious diseases listed in Column II with their descriptions in Column I. Use each disease only once.

Column I	Column II
1. _____ Infection that produces influenza-like symptoms, dark-colored urine, and light-colored stools	a. Chlamydia
	b. Gonorrhea
	c. Hepatitis
2. _____ Macular rash that can cause severe birth defects if a susceptible mother is exposed in pregnancy	d. Herpes simplex
	e. Human immunodeficiency virus
3. _____ Bacterial pulmonary infection spread by airborne droplets	f. Meningitis
	g. Rubella
4. _____ Viral infection that impairs the ability of the body to fight other infectious disease	h. Syphilis
	i. Tuberculosis
5. _____ Sexually transmitted disease characterized in the early stage by a painless chancre	j. Varicella
6. _____ Inflammation of lining of the central nervous system that may produce headache, stiff neck, seizures, and coma	
7. _____ Bacterial infection that produces mucopurulent discharge but rarely causes septicemia	
8. _____ Generalized illness accompanied by vesicular lesions, fever, and malaise	

9. List the six components of the chain of elements that must be present for an infectious disease to occur.

a.   d.

b.   e.

c.   f.

10. Describe two situations that interfere with the external bodily barriers to infection, thereby increasing the risk of infection.

    a.

    b.

11. Name two factors that can affect the ability of the internal barriers of the body to fight infectious disease.

    a.

    b.

12. For each of the following patient care scenarios, describe the personal protective measures that you should take.

    a. A 23-year-old woman is about to deliver her fourth child. The baby's head is crowning, and you are preparing for delivery.

_____

    b. A 50-year-old man is complaining of severe substernal chest pain. You are preparing to initiate an intravenous line to administer medications.

_____

    c. You are preparing to administer epinephrine subcutaneously to a 25-year-old patient with dyspnea because of anaphylaxis.

_____

    d. A 17-year-old girl ingested a large amount of alcohol and barbiturates, vomited, and rapidly lost consciousness. You elect to intubate her trachea.

_____

    e. A 55-year-old man attempted suicide by holding a shotgun under his chin and firing. He is combative and thrashes about as you try to control the large amount of bleeding and secure his airway.

_____

    f. A butcher sustained a laceration to her hand at work. The wound is oozing a small amount of blood.

_____

Questions 13 to 16 refer to the following case study:

    While caring for a 40-year-old man who has nausea, vomiting, right upper quadrant abdominal pain, and jaundice, you puncture your finger with a needle contaminated with the patient's blood. The hospital notifies you the next day that he tested positive for hepatitis.

13. What type or types of hepatitis can produce the symptoms experienced by this patient?

_____

14. What are the most effective measures you can take to prevent yourself from becoming infected with hepatitis at work?

_____

15. Describe the modes of transmission for hepatitis B.

_____

16. Can you do anything now that you are exposed so that you will not get hepatitis?

_____

17. What signs and symptoms may be evident on the prehospital examination of a patient in each of the following stages of infection from the human immunodeficiency virus?

   a. Acute retroviral infection:

_____

   b. Asymptomatic infection:

_____

   c. Early symptomatic infection:

_____

   d. Late symptomatic infection:

_____

18. You are transporting a patient with human immunodeficiency virus to the hospital after he sustained a sprained ankle at a volleyball game. No other injuries are evident.

   a. What personal protective measures should you take while caring for this patient?

_____

   b. How should the ambulance be cleaned before transport of the next patient?

_____

19. What is the best way for emergency care workers to monitor whether they have been exposed to a patient with tuberculosis?

_____

20. A 23-year-old man has a severe headache and a temperature of 102° F (38.9° C) and complained earlier of a stiff neck. Now he is limp and arouses only to a loud voice. You suspect meningitis.

   a. What personal protective measures should you use on this call? (You plan to initiate an intravenous line and apply oxygen by mask.)

_____

   b. If the emergency department contacts you later to inform you that the patient has bacterial meningitis, should you report an exposure?

_____

   c. What is the likelihood that you will be given prophylaxis if you have used appropriate body substance isolation from the beginning of this call?

_____

21. List three chronic signs or symptoms that may develop if syphilis is untreated for a number of years.

   a.

   b.

   c.

22. What personal protective measures should be taken when examining the mouth of a child with an outbreak of herpes simplex on the lips?

23. For each of the following ailments, list the signs and symptoms and site of infestation:

   a. Pubic lice:

   _____

   b. Head lice:

   _____

   c. Scabies:

   _____

Questions 24 to 26 refer to the following case study:

   You transport a child who has a temperature of 101° F (38.3° C) and a generalized skin rash that began the previous day. Some lesions are flat and red, some are raised blisters, and others have scabbed. On arrival to the emergency department, the pediatrician confirms that the child has chickenpox.

24. Is this disease communicable at this stage?

   _____

25. If you have never had chickenpox, how long would you expect to wait before symptoms appear?

   _____

26. Are you contagious during this entire time?

   _____

Questions 27 to 35 refer to the following case study:

   During your care of a patient at the scene of a motor-vehicle crash, you had blood splash into your eyes while your partner was intubating the patient and you were holding in-line immobilization of the cervical spine. You had gloves on at the time.

27. Has a significant exposure to blood or body fluids occurred?

   _____

28. When should you report this exposure?

   _____

29. Besides evaluation for postexposure prophylaxis, what other emergency care will you need in this situation?

   _____

   The patient refuses to give permission to test for human immunodeficiency virus.

30. Can the emergency department ignore the patient's refusal and run a test for human immunodeficiency virus in this situation? Why?

_____

31. What other questions should you ask the patient?

_____

32. What are your options for postexposure prophylaxis if the patient refuses testing?

_____

_____

33. After counseling and examination by the emergency department staff, you are offered a course of medicine for postexposure prophylaxis. How will you decide whether to take the medicine?

_____

34. Why do you think some paramedics might need psychological counseling after this incident?

_____

35. How could this exposure have been prevented?

_____

STUDENT SELF-ASSESSMENT

36. Which agency is responsible for establishing the guidelines for body substance isolation and universal (standard) precautions?
    a. Centers for Disease Control
    b. Department of Health
    c. Department of Transportation
    d. Occupational Safety and Health Administration
37. Which of the following could be used to interrupt the portal of entry in the chain of elements of an infectious disease?
    a. Administering antibiotics to kill a bacterium
    b. Cleaning a blood spill with an appropriate agent
    c. Receiving immunizations at appropriate intervals
    d. Using gloves as defined in the body substance isolation guidelines
38. Which of the following is an internal barrier to infection?
    a. Flora
    b. Leukocytes
    c. Nasal hairs
    d. Prostatic fluid
39. The internal defense that provides antibodies to destroy invading organisms is produced by which of the following?
    a. Cell-mediated immunity
    b. Complement
    c. Humoral immunity
    d. Killer cells
40. The infectious disease phase that begins when the agent invades the body and ends when the disease process begins is which period?
    a. Communicability
    b. Disease
    c. Incubation
    d. Latent
41. Death caused by hepatitis is most likely to occur from which strain of the virus?
    a. Hepatitis A
    b. Hepatitis B
    c. Hepatitis C
    d. Non-A, non-B hepatitis

42. What type of organism causes hepatitis?
    a. Bacteria
    b. Fungus
    c. Parasite
    d. Virus
43. Which sign or symptom can help to distinguish pneumonia from other respiratory illness?
    a. Fatigue and loss of appetite
    b. Headache and muscle aches
    c. Shaking chills and chest pain
    d. Yellow mucus from productive cough
44. Which of the following is a classic sign or symptom of tetanus?
    a. Flaccid paralysis
    b. Seizures
    c. Trismus
    d. Urticaria
45. What is the reaction causing muscle spasms that prevents a patient with rabies from drinking called?
    a. Hydropenia
    b. Hydrophobia
    c. Polydipsia
    d. Polyuria
46. What is the primary mode of transmission for rubella, mumps, and varicella?
    a. Blood-to-blood contact
    b. Fecal contamination
    c. Lesion contact
    d. Respiratory droplets
47. Complications of varicella may include all of the following *except* which disease?
    a. Bacterial infection
    b. Croup
    c. Meningitis
    d. Reye's syndrome
48. Which treatment measure usually is given to patients with chickenpox, influenza, or herpes simplex?
    a. Antibiotic therapy
    b. Aspirin for pain and fever
    c. Comfort measures
    d. Intravenous therapy
49. Which childhood disease is characterized by a violent cough that can persist for 1 to 2 months?
    a. Influenza
    b. Mumps
    c. Pertussis
    d. Pneumonia
50. What secondary complication of influenza often is associated with severe illness or death?
    a. Aspiration
    b. Dehydration
    c. Meningitis
    d. Pneumonia
51. Which sign or symptom associated with mononucleosis could produce a life-threatening condition if the patient is not maintained at rest?
    a. Fever
    b. Lymphadenopathy
    c. Oral rash
    d. Splenomegaly
52. A patient has a headache, malaise, fever, lymphadenopathy, and a symmetrical rash that involves the palms and soles. He states that an ulcerated sore on his penis healed spontaneously 3 weeks earlier. Which infectious disease do you suspect?
    a. Chlamydia
    b. Gonorrhea
    c. Herpes
    d. Syphilis
53. Which body system harbors the dormant herpesvirus?
    a. Cardiovascular system
    b. Gastrointestinal system
    c. Integumentary system
    d. Nervous system
54. Which of the following is the most effective measure that you can take to prevent the spread of severe acute respiratory syndrome?
    a. Antibiotic treatment if exposure is suspected
    b. Hand washing and respiratory protection
    c. Immunization with a pneumonia vaccine
    d. Treatment with bronchodilator drugs

WRAP IT UP

You are dispatched to a store for "difficulty breathing." The patient is a thin 40-year-old who bystanders say lives in the adjacent park. The man is coughing vigorously, and you note a strong smell of whiskey as you approach him. His vital signs are BP 142/88 mm Hg, P 104, R28, SaO_2 92%, so you apply a nasal cannula. He is cooperative but has slurred speech and tells you that he just cannot seem to catch his breath, so you listen and hear diffuse, coarse crackles in his lungs. You note some purple skin lesions around his bare feet, which he says are numb, and his mouth is coated with white plaque. His arms and feet are scarred with old track marks. Although initially reluctant to tell you much about his history, when you move him to the ambulance, he discloses that he has AIDS. He says he has not been compliant with his medications and has not been to see a doctor for about 6 months. When you ask about this cough and dyspnea, the patient says that it has been going on for about 3 months and that he has lost weight, has night sweats, and now is coughing up blood. You and your partner don N-95 HEPA masks, replace the patient's nasal cannula with an oxygen face mask, and open the window in the back of the ambulance. As you move the patient to the ER stretcher, he has a coughing spasm and expectorates a large amount of bloody sputum, which sprays into your face and eyes. You immediately wash with soap and water and have the ED staff irrigate your eyes. After contacting your supervisor, the appropriate exposure reporting papers are completed, and after the patient's HIV and tuberculosis risk factors and health status is determined, the ED physician sits down to explain your options. You are told the benefits and risks of tuberculosis and HIV transmission by this exposure, and the side effects associated with the prophylactic drugs. You decide to take the prophylactic drugs, and subsequently miss the next 2 days of work sick from them. Your pregnant wife is upset and fearful that she may become HIV positive. In 6 months and finally a year, the HIV screening tests come back negative, and at last you stop waking in the night, fearful that you will contract this life-threatening illness.

1. What additional personal protective measure(s) could have decreased your risk for this exposure?

_____

2. Identify (a) each of the elements in the chain of transmission of infectious disease that are present on this call and (b) actions that were taken to reduce the risk of transmission at some links in the chain.

Link	How is it present on this call?	Actions taken to reduce the risk of transmission?
Pathogenic agent(s)		
Reservoir		
Portal of exit		
Transmission		
Host susceptibility		

3. Place a check mark beside the complications of human immunodeficiency virus or acquired immunodeficiency syndrome that are seen in this patient.
   a. _____ *Candida*
   b. _____ Dementia
   c. _____ Kaposi sarcoma
   d. _____ Pulmonary tuberculosis
   e. _____ *Pneumocystis carinii* pneumonia
   f. _____ Sensory neuropathy
   g. _____ Wasting syndrome

4. What risk factors does this patient have for tuberculosis?

_____

_____

5. Which is true regarding follow-up after infectious disease exposure?
   a. If proper immunizations have been obtained, medical follow-up is not needed.
   b. Prophylaxis should not be taken without information regarding risks and benefits.
   c. Reporting should be deferred until the end of the paramedic's shift.
   d. The final decision regarding prophylaxis is the choice of the treating physician.

CHAPTER 39 ANSWERS

REVIEW QUESTIONS

1. c
   (Objective 5)

2. g
   (Objective 7)

3. i
   (Objective 5)

4. e
   (Objective 5)

5. h
   (Objective 9)

6. f
   (Objective 5)

7. b
   (Objective 9)

8. j
   (Objective 9)

9. A pathological agent, a reservoir, a portal of exit from the reservoir, an environment conducive to transmission of the pathogenic agent, portal of entry, and susceptibility of the new host to the infectious disease
   (Objective 2)

10. Burns, lacerations, abrasions, intravenous therapy, and urinary catheter
    (Objective 3)

11. Human immunodeficiency virus, chemotherapy, and prolonged steroid therapy
    (Objective 3)

12. a. Gloves, gown, mask, and eyewear
    b. Gloves
    c. Nothing is necessary according to the Centers for Disease Control and Prevention; however, if bleeding is likely and because the prehospital setting is high risk, gloves are indicated.
    d. Gloves, mask, and eyewear
    e. Gloves, gown, mask, and eyewear
    f. Gloves
    (Objective 1)

13. Hepatitis A, B, or C
    (Objective 5)

14. Take hepatitis B virus vaccination, and use strict universal (body substance isolation) precautions as warranted by each situation.
    (Objectives 1 and 5)

15. Direct introduction of infected blood by needle or transfusion, introduction of serum or plasma through skin cuts, absorption of infected serum or plasma through mucosal surfaces, absorption of saliva or semen through mucosal surfaces, and transfer of infective serum or plasma via inanimate surfaces
(Objective 5)

16. Yes. If the patient is found to have hepatitis A, you may be given an immune globulin injection. If he has hepatitis B and if you are not immune to the hepatitis B virus, a hepatitis B virus vaccine will be given to protect against future exposures, and hepatitis B immune globulin will be given to provide temporary passive immunity to the hepatitis B virus. No immunization or immune globulin exists that is effective to prevent hepatitis C.
(Objective 5)

17. a. Fever, swollen lymph nodes, and sore throat; b. enlarged lymph nodes; c. bacterial pneumonia, oral lesions, shingles, and pulmonary tuberculosis; d. diarrhea, tumors, dementia, neurological symptoms, and opportunistic infections
(Objective 5)

18. a. You should take the same precautions you would take with any patient with this type of injury. If no open wounds are present, no body substance isolation is indicated.
b. Clean the ambulance as you would after any patient.
(Objectives 1 and 5)

19. Periodic skin test with purified protein derivative (of tuberculin) and chest x-ray study if purified protein derivative (of tuberculin) test is positive or other history exists indicating the need
(Objective 5)

20. a. Gloves and mask (respiratory spread); wear eye shield if risk of splash or spray exists (for example, if the patient vomits or needs to be intubated)
b. An exposure should be reported if you did not have appropriate personal protective equipment on or if you had contact with blood or body fluids.
c. The need for prophylaxis will be determined by your occupational health provider but is not likely indicated if all body substance isolation precautions were used for the entire call.
(Objective 5)

21. Paresis, wide gait, ataxia, psychosis, and signs of myocardial insufficiency
(Objective 9)

22. Gloves (mask and protective eyewear if any risk of splash or spray of body fluids exists)
(Objective 1)

23. a. Pubic lice look like crabs or gray-blue spots, and nits appear on abdomen, thighs, eyelashes, eyebrows, and axillary hair.
b. Head lice have an elongated body with narrow head and three pair of legs, and nits look like dandruff that cannot be brushed off.
c. Scabies produces bites concentrated around webs of hands and feet, a child's face and scalp, a female's nipples, and a male's penis, and vesicles and papules that become easily infected because of scratching.
(Objective 10)

24. Yes. Chickenpox is contagious for 1 to 2 days before the onset of the rash until all of the lesions are crusted and dry.
(Objective 7)

25. 13 to 17 days
(Objective 7)

26. Varicella can be transmitted 1 to 2 days before eruption of the rash until the lesions have all scabbed over.
(Objective 5)

27. Yes. Blood that came in contact with your mucous membranes is a significant exposure.
(Objective 5)

28. Immediately report the exposure as soon as you arrive at the hospital with the patient. If you did not transport the patient to the hospital, you should go there immediately (or follow your local protocol).
(Objective 5)

29. You should irrigate your eyes immediately after the eye splash exposure.
(Objective 5)

30. No. The emergency department cannot ignore the patient's request. The patient has the legal right to refuse a test for human immunodeficiency virus.
(Objective 5)

31. Ask if the patient has human immunodeficiency virus and assess for risk factors that would indicate the potential for such infection (intravenous drug use, unsafe sex practices).
(Objective 5)

32. The emergency department or occupational medicine staff still may offer you prophylactic drug treatment based on the nature of the exposure and the patient's risk factors (antiviral and possibly protease inhibitor drugs).
(Objective 5)

33. The benefits to you (risk of human immunodeficiency virus infection) versus complications of the prophylaxis therapy based on your personal health status will need to be weighed before you decide whether to take the medicine.
(Objective 5)

34. For a year, you will undergo periodic evaluation to determine whether you have converted to HIV-positive status. Until that time, you should alter your sexual practices and discontinue breast-feeding if you are lactating. This can be a difficult time for paramedics and their significant others, wondering if the next test will be positive. Counseling may provide an opportunity to verbalize those feelings in a healthful manner.
(Objective 5)

35. Use of eye shield and face mask likely would have prevented this exposure.
(Objectives 5 and 12)

36. a. The Centers for Disease Control and Prevention establishes guidelines that often are adopted by the Occupational Safety and Health Administration and are incorporated by agencies such as the Department of Health and Department of Transportation into other documents (for example, National Standard Paramedic Curriculum).
(Objective 1)

37. d. All of the answers reflect something that could break a link in the chain of transmission. Antibiotics can kill the pathogenic agent; cleaning agents with appropriate disinfectants destroy the environment conducive to transmission; immunizations decrease host susceptibility.
(Objective 2)

38. b. All other answers are external barriers to infection.
(Objective 3)

39. c. Antibodies can fix complement. Killer cells are part of cell-mediated immunity.
(Objective 3)

40. c. The communicability period begins when the latent period ends and continues as long as the agent is present and can spread to others. The latent period begins with invasion of the body and ends when the agent can be shed or communicated. The disease period follows the incubation period and has variable lengths.
(Objective 4)

41. b. Short- and long-term mortality is higher from hepatitis B.
(Objective 2)

42. d
(Objective 2)

43. c. The patient with pneumonia also may have all of the other signs and symptoms.
(Objective 5)

44. c. Trismus (lockjaw) often occurs and makes opening the mouth difficult. The patient often has muscle tetany and spasms but not urticaria or seizures.
(Objective 6)

45. b. Hydropenia is a lack of water in tissues; polydipsia is increased thirst; and polyuria is increased urination.
(Objective 6)

46. d
(Objective 7)

47. b
(Objective 7)

48. c. Antibiotic therapy would be indicated only if a secondary bacterial infection develops. Aspirin is contraindicated for children and patients with chickenpox. Intravenous therapy would be needed only if an acute complication of these viral illnesses develops.
(Objectives 7, 8, and 9)

49. c. Influenza and pneumonia can produce cough; however, they do not persist as long as pertussis.
(Objective 7)

50. d. Pneumonia is an especially dangerous secondary complication for patients who are elderly or have preexisting lung or heart disease.
(Objective 8)

51. d. The enlarged spleen increases the chance of injury if the patient sustains a blow to the abdomen.
(Objective 8)

52. d. Syphilis is associated with systemic and chronic signs and symptoms.
(Objective 9)

53. d. The virus migrates along the sensory nerve pathways and remains in a latent stage on the ganglion.
(Objective 9)

54. b. There is no vaccine to prevent severe acute respiratory syndrome, nor is the disease treatable with antibiotics. Bronchodilators may be used to manage signs and symptoms of severe acute respiratory syndrome but do not prevent its spread.
(Objective 8)

WRAP IT UP

1. Protective eyewear could have prevented this exposure.
   (Objective 5)

2.

Link	How is it present on this call?	Actions taken to reduce the risk of transmission?
Pathogenic agent(s)	Human immunodeficiency virus, tuberculosis (bacteria)	Face washed with soap and water; eyes irrigated
Reservoir	Patient in poor heath	Mask on patient
Portal of exit	Cough with bloody sputum	Mask on patient
Transmission	Cough with bloody sputum	Mask on patient, N-95 mask, gloves, on paramedics, window open in ambulance
Host susceptibility		Human immunodeficiency virus, tuberculosis prophylaxis drugs

   (Objective 2)

3. a (white, coated tongue), b (slurred speech, confusion), c (skin discoloration on feet), d (cough, hemoptysis, night sweats), f (numbness in feet), g (thin, wasted appearance)
   (Objective 5)

4. Alcohol use, intravenous drug user (or former user), positive for human immunodeficiency virus, homeless
   (Objective 5)

5. b. Follow-up should be initiated as soon as possible after the exposure for maximum effectiveness. The paramedic should make the decision after being given adequate information about risks/benefits of treatment.
   (Objective 11)

Behavioral and Psychiatric Disorders

READING ASSIGNMENT

Chapter 40, pages 1042-1061, in *Mosby's Paramedic Textbook,* ed. 3

OBJECTIVES

Upon completion of this chapter, the paramedic student will be able to:

1. Define what constitutes a behavioral emergency.
2. Identify potential causes for behavioral and psychiatric illnesses.
3. List three critical principles that should be considered in the prehospital care of any patient with a behavioral emergency.
4. Outline key elements in the prehospital patient examination during a behavioral emergency.
5. Describe effective techniques for interviewing a patient during a behavioral emergency.
6. Distinguish between key symptoms and management techniques for selected behavioral and psychiatric disorders.
7. Identify factors that must be considered when assessing suicide risk.
8. Formulate appropriate interview questions to determine suicidal intent.
9. Explain prehospital management techniques for the patient who has attempted suicide.
10. Describe assessment of the potentially violent patient.
11. Outline measures that may be used in an attempt to safely diffuse a potentially violent patient situation.
12. List situations when patient restraints can be used.
13. Discuss key principles in patient restraint.
14. Describe safety measures taken when patient violence is anticipated.
15. Explain variations in approach to behavioral emergencies in children.

SUMMARY

- A behavioral emergency is a change in mood or behavior. This change cannot be tolerated by the involved person or others. It calls for immediate attention.
- Physical or biochemical disturbances can result in significant changes in behavior. Psychosocial mental illness is often the result of childhood trauma, parental deprivation, or a dysfunctional family structure.
- Changes in behavior caused by interpersonal or situational stress are often linked to specific incidents, such as environmental violence, death of a loved one, economic or employment problems, or prejudice and discrimination.

- When dealing with behavioral emergencies, the paramedic should contain the crisis. He or she should provide the proper emergency care as well. Also, the paramedic should transport the patient to an appropriate health care facility.
- During the patient assessment, an attempt should be made to determine the patient's mental state, name and age, significant past medical history, medications (and compliance), and past psychiatric problems, as well as the precipitating situation or problem.
- Effective interviewing techniques include active listening, being supportive and empathetic, limiting interruptions, and respecting the patient's personal space.
- All cognitive disorders result in a disturbance in thinking that may manifest as delirium or dementia.
- Schizophrenia is characterized by recurrent episodes of psychotic behavior. This behavior may include abnormalities of thought process, thought content, perception, and judgment.
- Anxiety disorders may cause a panic attack. Anxiety disorders include phobias, obsessive-compulsive disorders, and posttraumatic syndrome.
- Depression is an impairment of normal functioning. A person with depression may have feelings of hopelessness, loss of appetite, decreased libido, and feelings of worthlessness and guilt.
- Bipolar disorder is a manic-depressive illness. In this illness, depressive and manic episodes alternate with one another.
- Somatoform disorders are conditions in which there are physical symptoms for which no physical cause can be found. The cause is thought to be psychological. These include somatization disorder and conversion disorder.
- Factitious disorders are disorders in which symptoms mimic a true illness. However, the symptoms have been invented. They are under the control of the patient.
- Dissociative disorders are a group of psychological illnesses. In these disorders, a particular mental function is separated from the mind as a whole.
- The most common eating disorders considered to be forms of psychiatric illness are anorexia nervosa and bulimia nervosa.
- Impulse control disorders are characterized by the inability to resist an impulse or temptation to do some act that is unlawful, socially unacceptable, or self-harmful.
- Personality disorders are conditions characterized by failing to learn from experience or adapt appropriately to changes. This results in personal distress and impairment of social functioning.
- A threat of suicide is an indication that a patient has a serious crisis. This crisis requires immediate intervention.
- Questions that determine the patient's ideation, plan, intent, and means to commit suicide should be asked.
- After ensuring scene safety, the first priority in patient management after a suicide attempt is medical care. If the patient is conscious, developing rapport as soon as possible is crucial.
- Assessment of a potentially violent patient should include past history of violence, posture, vocal activity, and physical activity.
- When trying to defuse a situation involving a potentially violent patient, the paramedic should ensure a safe environment, gather the patient's history, try to gain the patient's cooperation, avoid threats, and explain the paramedic's role in providing care.
- Severely disturbed patients who pose a threat to themselves or others may need to be restrained.
- Reasonable force to restrain a patient should be used as humanely as possible. An adequate number of personnel is needed. This will ensure patient and rescuer safety during restraint. The risk of personal injury and legal liability is always present.
- Personal safety measures while responding to a behavioral emergency should include not allowing the patient to block the exit, keeping large furniture between you and the patient, working as a team, avoiding threatening statements, and using soft objects to absorb the impact of thrown objects.
- When caring for children with behavioral emergencies, the paramedic should attempt to gain their trust, tell them they won't be hurt, keep questions brief, be honest, involve parents (if appropriate), and take threats of violence seriously.

REVIEW QUESTIONS

Match the psychiatric conditions in Column II with their descriptions in Column I. Use each condition only once.

	Column I		Column II
1. ____	Feelings of worthlessness and guilt	**a.**	Conversion hysteria
2. ____	Unfounded fear of situation or object	**b.**	Depression
3. ____	Loss of touch with reality in this major mental disorder	**c.**	Mania
4. ____	Loss of sensory or motor function without organic cause	**d.**	Neurosis
5. ____	Excessive elation, irritability, talkativeness, and delusions	**e.**	Panic attack
6. ____	Logical, highly developed delusions	**f.**	Paranoia
		g.	Phobia
		h.	Psychosis

7. You arrive at the home of a 60-year-old man whose behavior is erratic. He alternates between hysterical bursts of laughter, irritability, sitting quietly, and crying. You find metformin HCL (Glucophage), hydralazine, and thyroxine in the medicine chest and note an ecchymotic area on his left temple. His skin is hot and moist. Based on this patient's history, what are some likely organic causes of his behavior that must be ruled out before assuming that this is a behavioral emergency?

_____

_____

_____

8. a. List three psychosocial causes of mental illness.

_____

b. List three sociocultural causes of mental illness.

_____

Questions 9 to 11 refer to the following patient case study:

You are called to a private residence to care for a behavioral emergency. Police report that the patient is "OBS." On arrival, you find a 34-year-old woman sitting quietly in a living room chair. She is complaining of depression.

9. What four general management principles should you consider on this and all behavioral calls?

a.

b.

c.

d.

10. What should your scene survey include?

_____

_____

11. What minimum patient data should be obtained if possible?

_____

_____

12. Should a detailed secondary survey be performed on a patient with a behavioral emergency?

_____

13. Complete the missing information in the following table.

Illness	Classification	Clinical Presentation	Treatment (Medical or EMS)
Dementia			
Schizophrenia			
Posttraumatic syndrome			
Bipolar disorder			
Somatization disorder			
Bulimia nervosa			

14. A patient with a phobia of heights must be rescued by ladder from a high bridge. What measures can you take to prevent a panic attack?

_____

15. A manic patient is being transported to the hospital for psychiatric evaluation. Describe effective patient management techniques in this situation.

_____

16. Family members call you to the home of a 25-year-old man who has become increasingly out of touch with reality. He feels that aliens are trying to kidnap him so that they can remove his brain. He tells you that they are trying to control his thoughts. He states, "They're here. Can't you hear them laughing?"

a. What behavioral illness does this presentation suggest?

_____

b. What approach will enable therapeutic communication with this patient?

_____

17. You are on the scene with a 25-year-old woman who cut her wrist with a razor blade. She is crying, "Let me go. Why didn't you let me do it?" She has a small laceration with controlled bleeding, minimal blood loss, and stable vital signs.

a. How can you best assess the patient's suicidal risk?

_____

b. What are your goals in caring for this patient during transport?

_____

Questions 18 to 22 refer to the following case study:

A distraught family calls you to take their son to the hospital for a court-ordered, involuntary psychiatric evaluation. They state that he has been breaking furniture for the past few hours and refuses to take his antipsychotic drugs.

18. What four factors should you assess rapidly to determine the potential for violence in this patient?

a.

b.

c.

d.

Your patient is pacing, is verbally abusive, and is threatening injury to those who approach. He is not armed.

19. You elect to restrain him. What help should you request?

_____

20. When approaching the patient to prepare for restraint, what should you note about the physical environment?

_____

21. Assuming that the patient meets the standard for involuntary detention in your state, how should he be restrained (including position and ways to secure extremities and torso)?

_____

_____

22. After restraints are applied, what should you monitor en route to the hospital?

_____

STUDENT SELF-ASSESSMENT

23. What is a change in mood or behavior that cannot be tolerated by the involved person or others and needs immediate attention called?
    a. Behavioral emergency
    b. Delusion
    c. Neurosis
    d. Psychosis

24. What is the characteristic of abnormal (maladaptive) behavior?
    a. Deviates from the person's normal behavior
    b. Does not conform to your idea of normal behavior
    c. Interferes with a person's ability to function
    d. Violates a societal law

25. Which of the following questions would be most appropriate to begin a conversation with a mentally ill patient?
    a. Did you start feeling this way today?
    b. Are you feeling bad now?
    c. How did this all begin?
    d. Are you okay?

26. Which response by the paramedic is most likely to lead to an effective interview in the prehospital setting?
    a. Everything will be fine.
    b. I know exactly how you feel.
    c. Yes, I see those scary bugs too.
    d. You look very sad.

27. Which condition is a state of acute mental confusion commonly brought on by a physical illness?
    a. Delirium
    b. Delusions
    c. Dementia
    d. Depression

28. A middle-aged woman suddenly loses the ability to speak after catching her husband in an extramarital affair. What behavioral illness may have caused her problem?
    a. Conversion hysteria
    b. Depression
    c. Panic attack
    d. Phobia

29. Which of the following feelings commonly characterizes depression?
    a. Hopelessness
    b. Hunger
    c. Increased libido
    d. Restlessness
30. You are transporting a man who believes he is Elvis Presley. His wife states that he quit his job, keeps calling her Priscilla, and is preparing to move to Graceland. You suspect that he is suffering from which of the following?
    a. Delusions
    b. Neurosis
    c. Paranoia
    d. Phobia
31. A panic attack typically occurs with any of the following *except* which symptom?
    a. Chest pain and vertigo
    b. Hyperventilation
    c. Suicidal intent
    d. Trembling and sweating
32. What is the highest priority on a suicide call?
    a. Ensuring safety of crew members
    b. Managing life threats
    c. Talking the person out of it
    d. Listening empathetically
33. Which of the following statements regarding suicide is true?
    a. Those who talk about killing themselves rarely do it.
    b. Men commit suicide more often than women.
    c. Suicide is an inherited tendency.
    d. When depression lifts, suicide risk disappears.
34. When should a violent patient be released from physical restraints?
    a. Immediately after administration of haloperidol intramuscularly
    b. As soon as the patient assures cooperation
    c. When the police have adequate personnel to control the patient
    d. When a physician at the hospital determines the patient is no longer dangerous
35. You are caring for a violent psychiatric patient. Which of the following drugs would *not* be appropriate for chemical restraint?
    a. Diazepam
    b. Diphenhydramine
    c. Haloperidol
    d. Lorazepam
36. Which strategy should be used to maintain emergency medical services crew safety when on a behavioral emergency call?
    a. Be firm and tell the patient to behave or you will have to use restraints.
    b. Interview the patient privately while your partner waits outside of the room.
    c. Kneel and put your arm on the patient's shoulder to show you care.
    d. Stay closer to the exit than the patient, with furniture between you and the patient.
37. Which strategy will be helpful when caring for a child who is experiencing a behavioral emergency?
    a. Avoid having the parents present during care.
    b. Do not be concerned about the possibility of violence.
    c. Keep the interview questions brief.
    d. Lie if you need to gain cooperation.

WRAP IT UP

You immediately recognize your patient when you arrive at the call. "Herb" is a 30-year-old homeless man with a history of schizophrenia. He is in and out of treatment facilities, and he is difficult to predict. When he is taking his medications, he is usually reasonable, but when he runs out of his medications or chooses not to take them, he can be dangerous. The police are with him and have called because he was threatening to kill himself. You introduce yourself, call him by name, and ask how he is feeling. He says, "The voices are telling me to end it all." "What do you mean by end it all?" you ask. "Kill myself you silly, x#@$er, he replies, "What did you think I meant?" His voice tone gets louder as he speaks, and he begins to lean forward menacingly toward you. "I'm here to help you, Herb," you tell him. "Have you thought about how you would do it?" you ask. "Hanging, it's what the voices say I should do," he replies, "that's why I'm headed to the park, lots of good trees for it over there." "Herb, we'd like to take you to the hospital to get you some medicine so you don't hurt yourself, you explain. With that, he suddenly lunges toward you, screaming, "You'll never get me to go back to that place." With police assistance, you subdue him and restrain him supine on your cot, where he continues to struggle forcefully. Then, with the approval of online medical direction, you administer haloperidol intramuscularly. You manage to get a pulse oximeter reading every few minutes and monitor his respirations carefully. Just as you arrive at the hospital, 30 minutes later, you note marked relaxation, and his voice calms. You give report to the ED staff and assist them to secure him to their stretcher after the physician briefly examines him. As you return to the station, you express your frustration about this patient to your partner: it just doesn't seem right that they can't find a treatment to make him well for more than a month or so at a time.

1. What clues led you to believe that the patient's behavior might become violent?

_____

2. Which of the following is true regarding schizophrenia?
   a. It is more common in men than women.

_____

   b. It typically resolves when the patient is in his or her 40s.

_____

   c. Delusions and auditory hallucinations are common.

_____

   d. Suicide rarely is associated with this disease.

_____

3. Explain why asking a patient directly about suicidal intent would or would not be a helpful strategy.

_____

4. Explain your rationale for administering haloperidol.

_____

CHAPTER 40 ANSWERS

REVIEW QUESTIONS

1. b
2. g
3. h
4. a
5. c
6. f

(Questions 1 to 6, Objective 5)

7. Metformin (Glucophage) indicates that he is diabetic; assess for hypoglycemia or hyperglycemia. Thyroxine is prescribed for thyroid disorders, which can cause behavioral alterations. Treatment with hydralazine suggests he has a history of hypertension or heart disease, so he may have had a transient ischemic attack, stroke, or cardiac dysrhythmia. The ecchymotic area on his head could indicate cerebral injury from trauma, causing his behavior. His warm, moist skin could indicate many problems. If he has a fever, an infectious process will have to be ruled out as a cause for his mental status change.
(Objective 2)

8. a. Childhood trauma, parental deprivation, or a dysfunctional family structure
   b. War, riots, rape, assault, death of a loved one, economic and employment problems, or prejudice and discrimination
   (Objective 2)

9. a. Ensure scene safety.
   b. Contain the crisis.
   c. Render appropriate emergency care.
   d. Transport to the appropriate medical facility.
   (Objective 3)

10. Look for evidence of violence, substance abuse, a suicide attempt, and any weapons that may be accessible to the patient.
    (Objective 4)

11. The patient's mental status, name, age, significant medical history, medications, allergies, and the precipitating event for this crisis should be ascertained from the patient, family, or other bystanders.
    (Objective 4)

12. The need to perform a physical assessment should be guided by your initial patient interview. If no possibility to exacerbate a violent situation arises and no life threat exists, the survey can be deferred until you arrive at the hospital. Bulky clothing and bags should be examined for the presence of weapons by law enforcement before transport.
    (Objective 4)

13.

Illness	Classification	Clinical Presentation	Treatment (Medical or EMS)
Dementia	Cognitive disorder	General decline in mental functioning; inability for self-care	Medical interventions
Schizophrenia	Schizophrenia	Recurrent psychotic behavior; abnormal thought processes, delusions, hallucinations, poor judgment	Drug therapy; paramedic should be friendly but neutral; do not respond to anger or speak to family in hushed tones; be firm, maintain personal safety.

Illness	Classification	Clinical Presentation	Treatment (Medical or EMS)
Posttraumatic syndrome	Anxiety disorder	Reaction to severe psychosocial event producing depression, sleep disturbances, nightmares, survivor guilt	Psychotherapy; medication
Bipolar disorder	Mood disorder	Alternating depressive and manic behaviors	Medications; paramedic should be calm and provide firm emotional support; minimize stimulation (no lights or sirens)
Somatization disorder	Somatoform disorder	Chronic physical complaints without any physical problems identified; associated with anxiety, depression	Psychotherapy
Bulimia nervosa	Eating disorder	Binge eating followed by purging (vomiting or laxatives), depression, self-deprivation	Medication, psychotherapy, hospitalization

(Objective 5)

14. Talk through the steps (rehearse) of the rescue slowly and calmly with the patient.
(Objective 5)

15. Provide calm, firm, emotional support, and minimize sensory stimuli.
(Objective 6)

16. a. Schizophrenia or paranoia is suggested by this presentation.
b. Be friendly but neutral; modulate your voice so that it does not get louder if the patient does. Do not talk to the family in whispers. Use firmness and tact to guide the patient to the ambulance. Consider asking for police assistance if you suspect a risk of violence.
(Objective 5)

17. a. Ask, "Why did you do that? Were you trying to kill yourself?" Determine whether she had a plan (did she leave a note or call significant others to say good-bye?).
b. Ensure safety (protect the patient from escape or injury), listen in a nonjudgmental way, observe the dressing to ensure bleeding is controlled.
(Objectives 7 to 9)

18. a. Does the patient have a history of violent, aggressive, or hostile behavior?
b. What is the patient's posture? Is he sitting or standing? Does he appear tense or rigid?
c. What does his voice sound like? Is his speech loud, obscene, or erratic?
d. Is he pacing or agitated or displaying aggressive behaviors?

19. Ask for police assistance.
(Objective 14)

20. Look for any objects that the patient could use as a weapon.
(Objective 14)

21. A minimum of two rescuers should move swiftly toward the patient and position themselves close to and slightly behind the patient. Each rescuer then should position an inside leg in front of the patient's leg to force the patient into a prone position if needed. The least restrictive restraints needed for a given situation should be used.
(Objective 13)

22. Monitor the patient's level of consciousness, airway, breathing, circulation, vital signs, oxygen saturation (if available), and peripheral pulses while the patient remains in restraints.
(Objective 13)

23. a. Delusional behavior, neurosis, or psychosis may be present during a behavioral emergency.
(Objective 1)

24. c. Many persons break laws without demonstrating abnormal behavior. One person (the paramedic) does not establish norms for society. A person may deviate from usual, normal behavior and not meet the standard for abnormal behavior.
(Objective 1)

25. c. All of the other questions elicit a yes or no answer and yield limited information.
(Objective 5)

26. d. You may acknowledge and label a patient's feelings, but do not patronize or give false reassurances. Correct cognitive misconceptions or distortions in a nonconfrontational manner.
(Objective 4)

27. a. Common signs and symptoms include inattention, memory impairment, disorientation, clouding of consciousness, and vivid visual hallucinations.
(Objective 5)

28. a. In conversion hysteria, painful emotions are converted unconsciously into physical symptoms.
(Objective 5)

29. a. The depressed patient has low self-worth, a loss of appetite, and decreased libido and is tense and irritable.
(Objective 5)

30. a. Neurosis is a faulty or inefficient way of coping. Paranoia is an abnormal way of thinking, characterized by delusions of persecution or grandeur usually centered on a theme. A phobia occurs when a person transfers feelings of anxiety onto a situation or object in the form of an irrational, intense fear.
(Objective 5)

31. c
(Objective 5)

32. a. A small percentage of suicidal patients also will be homicidal. All of the other options are important, but crew safety is your primary responsibility.
(Objective 9)

33. b. Women attempt suicide more often, but men succeed at a higher rate. All talk or threats of suicide should be taken seriously. When depression lifts, the person finally may have the energy to follow through on a suicide plan.
(Objective 7)

34. d. Releasing a patient from restraints en route can place the crew in great danger.
(Objective 13)

35. b. Diphenhydramine is an antihistamine and would not be effective in this situation.
(Objective 13)

36. d. Be sure you can exit quickly if the situation deteriorates. Do not threaten the patient. Do not allow the patient to be alone or to be alone with an emergency medical services crew member on the scene. Remain a safe distance from the patient until your assessment reveals no danger.
(Objective 14)

37. c. Usually the parents can be helpful in the interview and help to relieve anxiety in children (if the situation worsens when they are present, immediately remove them). Children can become violent and injure themselves or others. Do not lie to children.
(Objective 15)

WRAP IT UP

1. His voice was getting louder, his posture became more threatening, and he started to use profane language.
(Objective 10)

2. c. The disease occurs as often in woman as in men. Schizophrenia is a chronic, lifelong disease that is associated with about a 10% risk of suicide.
(Objective 6)

3. It is important to determine suicide risk by asking patients direct questions about their intent, method, and timing of when they intend to commit suicide. This often is not associated with an escalation of the patient's violent behavior.
(Objectives 5, 7, and 8)

4. Haloperidol is an antipsychotic drug that can help control violent, aggressive behavior.
(Objective 11)

Gynecology

READING ASSIGNMENT
Chapter 41, pages 1062-1071, in *Mosby's Paramedic Textbook*, ed. 3

OBJECTIVES
Upon completion of this chapter, the paramedic student will be able to:
1. Describe the physiological processes of menstruation and ovulation.
2. Describe the pathophysiology of the following nontraumatic causes of abdominal pain in females: pelvic inflammatory disease, ruptured ovarian cyst, cystitis, dysmenorrhea, mittelschmerz, endometriosis, ectopic pregnancy, vaginal bleeding.
3. Describe the pathophysiology of traumatic causes of abdominal pain in females, including vaginal bleeding and sexual assault.
4. Outline the prehospital assessment and management of the female with abdominal pain.
5. Outline specific assessment and management for the patient who has been sexually assaulted.
6. Describe specific prehospital measures to preserve evidence in sexual assault cases.

SUMMARY
- Menstruation is the normal, periodic discharge of blood, mucus, and cellular debris from the uterine mucosa. Ovulation is the release of a secondary oocyte from the ovary.
- Pelvic inflammatory disease (PID) results from infection of the cervix, uterus, fallopian tubes, and ovaries and their supporting structures.
- Ruptured ovarian cyst occurs when a thin-walled, fluid-filled sac located on the ovary ruptures. This can cause internal hemorrhage.
- Cystitis is inflammation of the inner lining of the bladder. It usually is caused by a bacterial infection.
- Dysmenorrhea is characterized by painful menses. It may be associated with headache, faintness, dizziness, nausea, diarrhea, backache, and leg pain.
- Mittelschmerz is German for "middle pain." This pain may occur from the rupture of the graafian follicle and bleeding from the ovary during the menstrual cycle.
- Endometritis is inflammation of the uterine lining. Endometriosis is characterized by endometrial tissue growing outside of the uterus.
- An ectopic pregnancy is one that develops outside the uterus.
- Vaginal bleeding is the loss of blood from the uterus, cervix, or vagina.
- Traumatic causes of vaginal bleeding include straddle injuries, blows to the perineum, blunt forces to the lower abdomen, foreign bodies in the vagina, injury during intercourse, abortion attempts, and soft tissue injuries from sexual assault.
- The goal of prehospital care of lower abdominal pain in the female is to obtain a history (including a gynecological history); provide airway, ventilatory, and circulatory support as needed; and provide transport for physician evaluation.

- Sexual assault is a crime of violence. It can have serious physical and psychological effects.
- Paramedics should be aware of the need to preserve evidence from a sexual assault crime scene.

REVIEW QUESTIONS

Match the gynecological problems in Column II with their description in Column I. Use each term only once.

Column I	Column II
1. _____ Abdominal pain at ovulation	**a.** Dysmenorrhea
2. _____ Beginning of menses	**b.** Endometriosis
3. _____ Intraabdominal growth of the uterine lining	**c.** Endometritis
4. _____ Infection of the female pelvic organs	**d.** Menarche
5. _____ Menstrual cramps	**e.** Mittelschmerz
6. _____ Fluid sac that ruptures	**f.** Pelvic inflammatory disease
	g. Ruptured ovarian cyst

7. The normal menstrual cycle is about **(a)** _____ days. The average menstrual flow is

(b) _____ to _____ mL and usually lasts from **(c)** _____

to _____ days. During the menstrual cycle, some of the primary follicles become

(d) _____. These enlarge and form a lump on the surface of the ovary and when mature are

known as the **(e)** _____ or _____ The release of the oocyte from the follicle

is called **(f)** _____ After ovulation, the follicle turns into a glandular structure called the

(g) _____ the cells of which secrete large amounts of **(h)** _____ and some

(i) _____ If pregnancy occurs, the fertilized oocyte **(j)** (_____) begins

releasing a hormonelike substance called **(k)** _____ that keeps the corpus from degenerating.

8. Other than pain, list three signs or symptoms that a woman may experience during menses.

   a.

   b.

   c.

Questions 9 to 12 refer to the following case study:

> You are called to a private residence to evaluate a 19-year-old woman who is complaining of severe pelvic pain. Her pain began yesterday, and she says it is unbearable now. She has no allergies, takes no medicines, and has no significant medical history.

9. What specific questions related to her obstetrical history should you ask her?

   a. _____

   b. _____

   c. _____

   d. _____

563

e. _____

f. _____

g. _____

h. _____

i. _____

j. _____

She tells you that she has never been pregnant, that she presently has her menstrual period, and that it is of normal color and amount. She denies vaginal discharge or the possibility of pregnancy because she uses birth control pills. She states that she has not had intercourse in 4 months. She denies other symptoms of pregnancy and any history of gynecological problems.

10. What should you specifically assess on the physical examination?

_____

_____

Her lower abdomen is diffusely tender. Vital signs are within normal limits, and her skin is warm and dry.

11. What are some potential causes of her pain?

_____

_____

12. What prehospital interventions will you provide for this patient?

_____

_____

13. What measures can be taken in the prehospital environment to minimize the fear and stress experienced by a victim of sexual abuse?

_____

14. Describe five guidelines for evidence preservation on a sexual abuse call.

a.

b.

c.

d.

e.

STUDENT SELF-ASSESSMENT

15. How often does a typical woman have menstrual flow?
 a. Every 14 days   **c.** Every 28 days
 b. Every 21 days   **d.** Every 35 days

16. Which hormone initiates the ovarian cycle leading to ovulation?
    a. Estrogen
    c. Luteinizing hormone
    b. Follicle-stimulating hormone
    d. Progesterone
17. What is the most common cause of pelvic inflammatory disease?
    a. Gonorrhea
    b. Herpes virus
    c. Human immunodeficiency virus
    d. Syphilis
18. Which of the following factors increases the incidence of dysmenorrhea?
    a. Increased age
    c. Childbirth
    b. Frequent exercise
    d. Infection
19. A ruptured ovarian cyst may mimic all of the following *except* which disorder?
    a. Appendicitis
    c. Ectopic pregnancy
    b. Cholecystitis
    d. Salpingitis
20. Which of the following is a normal sign or symptom of cystitis?
    a. Blood in the urine
    c. Inability to urinate
    b. Flank pain
    d. Painless urination
21. Which of the following is true regarding endometriosis?
    a. It is an inflammation of the uterine lining.
    b. It is common in young women.
    c. It has no effect on fertility.
    d. Its pain may increase during menstruation.
22. Which of the following gynecological problems may cause severe internal hemorrhage?
    a. Dysmenorrhea
    c. Salpingitis
    b. Mittelschmerz
    d. Ruptured ovarian cyst
23. Which of the following is a traumatic cause of vaginal bleeding?
    a. Abortion attempts
    c. Onset of labor
    b. Disorders of the placenta
    d. Pelvic inflammatory disease
24. What is your most important role in caring for a victim of sexual abuse?
    a. Allow only a paramedic of the same gender to care for the patient.
    b. Provide a safe and secure environment for the patient.
    c. Preserve evidence exactly as outlined by protocol.
    d. Perform a complete history and thorough examination.
25. Which of the following should you do to preserve evidence on a sexual abuse call?
    a. Ask the patient to shower.
    c. Place the clothing in a paper bag.
    b. Thoroughly clean wounds.
    d. Search the scene for evidence.

WRAP IT UP

"Unit twelve, respond to one-two-five-six Weston, cross-street Thames, abdominal pain." You and your partner look hungrily at the dinner you have just set on the table, and you quickly move to the ambulance. Your patient is a 26-year-old female whose abdominal pain began 2 hours ago. She is pale and her skin is cool. She is anxious and appears to be in significant pain, especially guarding her left lower quadrant when you palpate her abdomen. Her vital signs are BP 90/50 mm Hg, P 128, R 20, and SaO₂ 95%. She has been pregnant 4 times but has miscarried each within the first 8 weeks. Her last normal menstrual period was 8 weeks ago, so she is concerned that her pain may be related to the pregnancy. She started spotting yesterday but has not soaked a pad yet. You quickly apply oxygen by mask, elevate her legs, and tell your partner to start en route. During transport, you start one IV of normal saline with blood tubing and another with macrodrip tubing using lactated Ringer's. When you reassess her vital signs, her blood pressure is 74/50 mm Hg, P 134, R 28, so you open the IVs to administer a fluid challenge. You call the receiving hospital so that they can prepare to resuscitate this patient. On arrival, uncrossmatched blood is given to her, and within 20 minutes, they are rushing her to surgery to treat her ectopic pregnancy.

1. Place a check mark beside the gynecological condition that you might suspect if this patient's pregnancy status were not known.
   a. _____ Cystitis
   b. _____ Dysmenorrhea
   c. _____ Endometriosis
   d. _____ Mittelschmerz
   e. _____ Pelvic inflammatory disease
   f. _____ Ruptured ovarian cyst

2. Which is true of ectopic pregnancy?
   a. It usually occurs in the fallopian tube.
   b. It is a fluid-filled sac on the ovaries.
   c. Uterine inflammation occurs because of placental tissue retention.
   d. There is ectopic growth and functioning of uterine tissue.

3. Why was it critical to evaluate the possibility of pregnancy in this patient?

   _____

   _____

4. Explain your rationale for the following interventions.
   a. Elevation of her legs

   _____

   _____

   b. Intravenous fluid bolus

   _____

   _____

   c. Oxygen therapy

CHAPTER 41 ANSWERS

GYNECOLOGY

1. e
2. d
3. b
4. f
5. a
6. g
(Questions 1 to 6, Objective 2)

7. a. 28; b. 25, 60; c. 4, 6; d. secondary follicles; e. vesicular, graafian follicles; f. ovulation; g. corpus luteum; h. progesterone; i. estrogen; j. zygote; k. chorionic gonadotropin.
(Objective 1)

8. Headache, faintness, dizziness, nausea, diarrhea, backache, leg pain, chills, nausea, and vomiting
(Objective 2)

9. a. Have you ever been pregnant? If yes, how many pregnancies and how many have you carried to term?
b. Have you ever had a cesarean delivery?
c. When was your last menstrual period? How long did it last? Was it normal? Do you have a regular menstrual cycle? Have you had any bleeding between your periods?
d. Could you be pregnant now? Is your period late or did you miss one? Do you have any breast tenderness, increased need to urinate, or morning sickness? Have you had any unprotected sexual activity?
e. Do you have a history of any gynecological (female) problems such as bleeding, infections, pain during intercourse, miscarriage, abortion, or ectopic pregnancy?
f. Are you having any bleeding now? If you are, what color is it, how many pads have you soaked, and how long have you been bleeding?
g. Do you have any vaginal discharge? What color and how much is there? Does it smell bad?
h. What kind of birth control do you use? Have you ever forgotten to use it?
i. Have you had any injury to your genital area?
j. How are you feeling now?
(Objective 4)

10. Evaluate vital signs and check for signs of blood loss (skin signs, orthostatic vital signs). Palpate the abdomen to assess for masses, tenderness, guarding, distention, and rebound tenderness.
(Objective 4)

11. Pelvic inflammatory disease, ruptured ovarian cyst, dysmenorrhea, endometritis, endometriosis, or appendicitis are potential causes. Ectopic pregnancy and miscarriage should not be discounted completely because sometimes patients do not give a completely accurate sexual history.
(Objective 4)

12. Consider oxygen administration; however, because no signs of shock exist, this may not be necessary. Consider initiating intravenous therapy. Transport in a position of comfort.
(Objective 4)

13. Move to a private, safe location; allow paramedic who is the same sex as the patient to provide care if possible; minimize questions and physical examination as appropriate; and listen and provide comfort.
(Objective 5)

14. Handle clothes as little as possible, do not clean wounds, use paper bags for clothing and bag each item separately, ask the victim not to change clothing, and try not to disturb the crime scene.
(Objective 6)

15. c. Menstrual flow varies according to each individual.
(Objective 1)

16. c. Follicle-stimulating hormone stimulates development of the follicle. Estrogen causes a surge in the production of luteinizing hormone, which initiates the ovarian cycle.
(Objective 1)

17. a. *Chlamydia* organisms and *Chlamydia trachomatis* also often are associated with pelvic inflammatory disease.
(Objective 2)

18. d. All of the other factors often decrease the severity of this condition.
(Objective 2)

19. b. The pain of cholecystitis is usually in the right upper quadrant of the abdomen. All other conditions cause lower abdominal pain.
(Objective 2)

20. a. Urination is usually painful and frequent in cystitis. Flank pain may indicate that the infection has moved to the kidneys.
(Objective 2)

21. d. Endometriosis is an ectopic placement of uterine lining and causes inflammation of the endometrium. It is common in women in their late 30s and is associated with infertility.
(Objective 2)

22. d
(Objective 2)

23. a. All other answers are nontraumatic causes of vaginal bleeding.
(Objective 3)

24. b. Having a paramedic of the same sex as the patient perform care is desirable but may not always be possible. You should attempt to preserve evidence, but this is not always possible if a life-threatening condition exists that requires rapid intervention. Perform only the necessary history and physical examination.
(Objective 5)

25. c. Bag items separately if possible. The patient should not shower, wash, or have wounds cleansed until evidence can be gathered.
(Objective 6)

WRAP IT UP

1. f. She gave no urinary signs or symptoms, so cystitis would not be a consideration. Pelvic inflammatory disease is possible, but there is no report of vaginal discharge. The pain of dysmenorrhea and mittelschmerz is not usually so severe and are not associated with shock.

2. a. It can occur less often in the ovary, abdominal cavity, or cervix.
(Objective 2)

3. If the pregnancy status is known, the differential diagnosis can be narrowed.
(Objective 2)

4. a. Elevating her legs may improve her shock temporarily.
b. An intravenous fluid bolus will increase the preload and temporarily increase the blood pressure.
c. Because this patient is in shock, oxygenation is critical, especially because she has internal bleeding.
(Objective 2)

42

Obstetrics

READING ASSIGNMENT

Chapter 42, pages 1072-1097, in *Mosby's Paramedic Textbook,* ed. 3

OBJECTIVES

Upon completion of this chapter, the paramedic student will be able to do the following:

1. Describe the organization and function of the specialized structures of pregnancy.
2. Outline fetal development from ovulation through adaptations at birth.
3. Explain normal maternal physiological changes that occur during pregnancy and how they influence prehospital patient care and transportation.
4. Describe appropriate information to be elicited during the obstetrical patient's history.
5. Describe specific techniques for assessment of the pregnant patient.
6. Describe general prehospital care of the pregnant patient.
7. Discuss the implications of prehospital care after trauma to the fetus and mother.
8. Describe the assessment and management of patients with preeclampsia and eclampsia.
9. Explain the pathophysiology, signs and symptoms, and management of the processes that cause vaginal bleeding in pregnancy.
10. Outline the physiological changes that occur during the stages of labor.
11. Describe the role of the paramedic during normal labor and delivery.
12. Compute an Apgar score.
13. Describe assessment and management of postpartum hemorrhage.
14. Discuss the identification, implications, and prehospital management of complicated deliveries.

SUMMARY

- The placenta is a disklike organ. It is composed of interlocking fetal and maternal tissues. It is the organ of exchange between the mother and fetus. Blood flows from the fetus to the placenta through two umbilical arteries. These arteries carry deoxygenated blood. Oxygenated blood returns to the fetus through the umbilical vein. The amniotic sac is a fluid-filled bag. It completely surrounds and protects the embryo.
- The developing ovum is known as an embryo during the first 8 weeks of pregnancy. After that time and until birth it is called a fetus. Gestation (fetal development) usually averages 40 weeks from the time of fertilization to the delivery of the newborn.
- The pregnant woman undergoes many physiological changes that affect the genital tract, breasts, gastrointestinal system, cardiovascular system, respiratory system, and metabolism.
- The patient history should include obstetrical history; presence of pain; presence, quantity, and character of vaginal bleeding; presence of abnormal vaginal discharge; presence of "bloody show"; current general health and prenatal care; allergies and medicines taken; and maternal urge to bear down.

- The goal in examining an obstetrical patient is to rapidly identify acute life-threatening conditions. A part of this involves identifying imminent delivery. Then the paramedic must take the proper management steps. In addition to the routine physical examination, the paramedic should assess the abdomen, uterine size, and fetal heart sounds.
- If birth is not imminent, the paramedic should limit prehospital care for the healthy patient. It should be limited to basic treatment modalities. It should include transport for physician evaluation as well.
- Causes of fetal death from maternal trauma include death of the mother, separation of the placenta, maternal shock, uterine rupture, and fetal head injury.
- Preeclampsia occurs after 20 weeks' gestation. The criteria for diagnosis include hypertension, proteinuria, and excessive weight gain with edema. Eclampsia is characterized by the same signs and symptoms with the addition of seizures or coma.
- Vaginal bleeding during pregnancy can result from abortion (miscarriage), ectopic pregnancy, abruptio placentae, placenta previa, uterine rupture, or postpartum hemorrhage. Abortion is the termination of pregnancy from any cause before 20 weeks' gestation. Ectopic pregnancy occurs when a fertilized ovum implants anywhere other than the uterus. Abruptio placentae is partial or complete detachment of the placenta at more than 20 weeks' gestation. Placenta previa is placental implantation in the lower uterine segment partially or completely covering the cervical opening. Uterine rupture is a spontaneous or traumatic rupture of the uterine wall.
- The first stage of labor begins with the onset of regular contractions. It ends with complete dilation of the cervix. The second stage of labor is measured from full dilation of the cervix to delivery of the infant. The third stage of labor begins with delivery of the infant and ends when the placenta is expelled and the uterus has contracted.
- One of the primary responsibilities of the EMS crew is to prevent an uncontrolled delivery. The other is to protect the infant from cold and stress after birth.
- Criteria for computing the Apgar score include appearance (color), pulse (heart rate), grimace (reflex irritability), activity (muscle tone), and respiratory effort.
- More than 500 mL of blood loss after the delivery of the newborn is called a postpartum hemorrhage. It often results from ineffective or incomplete contraction of the uterus.
- Paramedics should be alert to factors that point to a possible abnormal delivery.
- Cephalopelvic disproportion produces a difficult labor because of the presence of a small pelvis, an oversized uterus, or fetal abnormalities. Most infants are born head first (cephalic or vertex presentation). However, sometimes a presentation is abnormal. In breech presentation, the largest part of the fetus (the head) is delivered last. Shoulder dystocia occurs when the fetal shoulders impact against the maternal symphysis pubis. This blocks shoulder delivery. Shoulder presentation (transverse presentation) results when the long axis of the fetus lies perpendicular to that of the mother. The fetal arm or hand may be the presenting part. Cord presentation occurs when the cord slips down into the vagina or presents externally.
- A premature infant is born before 37 weeks' gestation.
- A multiple gestation is a pregnancy with more than one fetus. It is accompanied by an increased complication rate.
- A precipitous delivery is a rapid spontaneous delivery with less than 3 hours from onset of labor to birth. The main danger to the fetus is from cerebral trauma or tearing of the umbilical cord.
- Uterine inversion is a rare complication of childbirth. It is a serious complication. With this condition, the uterus turns "inside out."
- The development of pulmonary embolism during pregnancy, labor, or the postpartum period is one of the most common causes of maternal death.
- Premature rupture of the membranes is a rupture of the amniotic sac before the onset of labor, regardless of gestational age.
- An amniotic fluid embolism may occur when amniotic fluid enters the maternal circulation during labor or delivery or immediately after delivery.

REVIEW QUESTIONS

Match the types of abortion in Column II with their description in Column I. Use each term only once.

Column I

1. _____ Abortion before 12 weeks not externally induced
2. _____ Legal termination of pregnancy to preserve the mother's health
3. _____ All the products of conception passed before 12 weeks
4. _____ Symptoms of impending abortion with a closed cervix
5. _____ Failure to pass a fetus after 4 weeks of fetal death
6. _____ Intentional termination of pregnancy

Column II

a. Complete abortion
b. Incomplete abortion
c. Induced abortion
d. Missed abortion
e. Spontaneous abortion
f. Therapeutic abortion
g. Threatened abortion

Match the problems of pregnancy in Column II with their description in Column I. Use each problem only once.

Column I

7. _____ Painless bleeding in third trimester of pregnancy
8. _____ Hypertension, proteinuria, and visual disturbance in the third trimester
9. _____ Severe abdominal pain, shock, and easily palpable fetal parts
10. _____ Painful third-trimester bleeding
11. _____ Third-trimester seizure after a new onset of hypertension
12. _____ Abdominal pain, scant vaginal bleeding, and shock in the first trimester

Column II

a. Abortion
b. Abruptio placentae
c. Eclampsia
d. Ectopic pregnancy
e. Placenta previa
f. Preeclampsia
g. Uterine rupture

13. In what lunar month do the following fetal development characteristics typically occur?

a. Fetal movement felt by the mother:

_____

b. Fetal heart beat:

_____

c. Distinct fingers and toes:

_____

d. Eyebrows and fingernails:

_____

e. Possible viability if born:

_____

14. What causes the arteriovenous shunts to close at birth?

_____

_____

15. What do the following pregnancy terms mean?

a. A patient is gravida 6 para 5 (G6 P5).

_____

b. She is a multipara.

_____

c. The patient has postpartum bleeding.

_____

d. You are called to care for a nullipara who is term.

_____

16. A woman in her fortieth week of pregnancy complains of heartburn, dizziness, and frequency of urination. Her heart rate is 100; respirations are 20 and deep; and blood pressure is 90/60 mm Hg. (She says her normal is 100/70 mm Hg.) She has slight edema of the ankles and tortuous varicose veins. Explain how the physiological alterations of pregnancy cause each of the signs or symptoms she is experiencing.

a. Heartburn:

_____

_____

b. Dizziness:

_____

_____

c. Frequency of urination:

_____

_____

d. Hypotension:

_____

_____

e. Pedal edema and varicose veins:

_____

_____

17. Briefly explain why each of the following historical findings would cause concern if delivery is imminent in the field:

a. No prenatal care:

_____

_____

b. Diabetic mother:

_____

_____

c. Vaginal bleeding:

_____

_____

d. Current heroin intoxication:

_____

_____

Questions 18 to 20 refer to the following case study:

A 28-year-old woman who is in her third trimester complains of abdominal pain after an automobile accident in which she was the unrestrained driver. She is pale, and her vital signs are blood pressure, 90/60 mm Hg; pulse, 134; and respirations, 28. Her abdomen is tender to palpation, and you note some vaginal bleeding.

18. What other subjective information do you need from the mother?

_____

_____

19. How can you determine whether the infant is in distress?

_____

_____

20. Describe prehospital care and transport of this patient.

_____

_____

_____

Questions 21 to 24 refer to the following case study:

A 30-year-old woman says she is 9 weeks' pregnant and complains of severe cramping pain in the lower abdomen and vaginal bleeding. She states that she has saturated six sanitary napkins and passed some "white, stringy stuff" that her husband shows you in the toilet.

21. What condition of pregnancy do you suspect?

_____

22. What actions should you take so that the physician can determine whether she has had a complete abortion?

_____

23. Estimate her blood loss if you feel the history was accurate.

_____

24. Why might this patient be exhibiting a grief reaction?

_____

_____

25. An obstetrician calls you to his office to transport a 28-year-old woman who has an ectopic pregnancy (determined by ultrasound). She complains of severe abdominal pain and has frank signs of shock.

    a. What other signs or symptoms might she experience?

_____

    b. Describe interventions you will use on your 20-minute trip to the emergency department.

_____

_____

26. What general patient care measures should be taken for any patient who has third-trimester bleeding without shock?

_____

_____

_____

Questions 27 to 31 refer to the following case study:

    A 40-year-old primipara in the third trimester complains of headache, dizziness, and nausea. Vital signs are blood pressure, 160/100 mm Hg; pulse, 110; and respirations, 20. Her hands and feet are considerably swollen, and you note intermittent facial twitching. She says her doctor was worried about protein in her urine.

27. What complication do you suspect?

_____

28. In what position should you transport this patient?

_____

29. List two drugs with appropriate doses that may be ordered by medical direction to stop seizure activity in these types of patients.

_____

30. Besides medication, what emergency medical services actions can minimize the risk of seizures?

_____

31. What risks to the fetus exist with this condition?

_____

_____

Questions 32 to 36 refer to the following case study:

    You are called to a private residence 30 minutes from the nearest hospital to care for a woman in labor.

32. What information in the patient's medical history is important to help gauge how quickly labor will progress?

_____

_____

33. What specific signs or symptoms during labor would lead you to believe that delivery is imminent?

_____

_____

34. As the baby's head delivers, what assessment and interventions should you perform?

_____

_____

35. Describe the procedure to clamp the umbilical cord.

_____

_____

36. When should the Apgar score be calculated?

_____

37. If necessary, when should oxytocin be administered, and what is the proper dose and route?

_____

38. Labor fails to progress after a baby in breech position is delivered to the level of the chest. Describe the steps you should take in this situation.

_____

_____

39. After the head of a baby with shoulder dystocia is delivered, what can you do to deliver the shoulders while minimizing fetal injury?

_____

_____

40. A 35-year-old woman who is G6 P5 states that she is ready to deliver her baby at home. Her membranes have ruptured, her contractions are frequent, and she wants to push. When you examine her perineum, you see the umbilical cord protruding from the vagina.

a. What actions should you take immediately to prevent fetal hypoxia?

_____

_____

b. Should you attempt to deliver this baby on the scene?

_____

STUDENT SELF-ASSESSMENT

41. Functions of the placenta include all except which of the following?
    a. Excretion of wastes
    b. Hormone production
    c. Metabolism of drugs
    d. Transfer of gases

42. The primary role of amniotic fluid is which of the following?
    a. Excretion
    b. Hydration
    c. Nutrition
    d. Protection

43. The fetal structure that allows blood to bypass the liver and go directly into the inferior vena cava is which of the following?
    a. Ductus arteriosus
    b. Ductus venosus
    c. Foramen ovale
    d. Umbilical vein

44. The umbilical cord carries which of the following?
    a. Deoxygenated blood by one umbilical artery and oxygenated blood by one umbilical vein
    b. Deoxygenated blood by two umbilical arteries and oxygenated blood by one umbilical vein
    c. Oxygenated blood by one umbilical artery and deoxygenated blood by one umbilical vein
    d. Oxygenated blood by two umbilical arteries and deoxygenated blood by one umbilical vein

45. Where should the uterus be palpable at week 20 of gestation?
    a. At the lower border of the umbilicus
    b. Between the symphysis pubis and umbilicus
    c. Halfway between the umbilicus and the xiphoid
    d. Just above the symphysis pubis

46. Which of the following is the normal fetal heart rate?
    a. 80 to 120 beats/min
    b. 120 to 160 beats/min
    c. 160 to 200 beats/mine
    d. 200 to 240 beats/min

47. In which of the following positions should the hypotensive pregnant patient who is more than 4 months gestation be transported?
    a. High Fowler's
    b. Left lateral recumbent
    c. Prone
    d. Supine

48. Immediately after the delivery of a healthy baby, your patient's eyes roll back and she becomes pulseless. She has no previous medical history. Which of the following may have caused her cardiac arrest?
    a. Abruptio placentae
    b. Amniotic fluid embolism
    c. Aortic dissection
    d. Congestive cardiomyopathy

49. When attempting to resuscitate a patient in cardiac arrest who is 8 months pregnant, what special care measures should you use to be most effective?
    a. Decrease ventilation volumes to minimize gastric distention.
    b. Increase the dose of epinephrine to maximize vasoconstriction.
    c. Perform chest compressions lower on the sternum.
    d. Tilt her torso laterally to prevent compression of the vena cava.

50. By which of the following signs is eclampsia distinguished from preeclampsia?
    a. Edema
    b. Glucosuria
    c. Hypertension
    d. Seizures

51. The primary complication from administration of magnesium sulfate is which of the following?
    a. Increased hypertension
    b. Precipitous delivery
    c. Respiratory depression
    d. Ventricular dysrhythmias

52. Excessive traction on the umbilical cord during placental delivery may cause which of the following?
    a. Fetal distress
    b. Placenta previa
    c. Uterine inversion
    d. Uterine rupture

53. Which of the following occurs in the second stage of labor?
    a. Cervical dilation
    b. Delivery of the infant
    c. Expulsion of the placenta
    d. Fetal descent into the birth canal

54. When delivering a baby's head, you note that the umbilical cord is wrapped around the baby's neck. Which of the following is the first action you should take?
    a. Cut the cord in two places, clamp, and proceed with delivery.
    b. Elevate the mother's hips and have her pant until you reach the hospital.
    c. Gently unloop the cord around and over the baby's head.
    d. No special action is needed; the cord will free itself as the shoulders deliver.

55. A minute after delivery, a baby has a weak cry, a pink body with blue extremities, and a pulse of 128; he actively moves about and sneezes when a catheter is introduced into his nose. The Apgar score is which of the following?

 a. 6
 b. 7
 c. 8
 d. 9

56. Hemorrhage control in the postpartum period may include all of the following *except* which?

 a. Elevation of the mother's hips
 b. Delivery of oxytocin intravenously
 c. Breast-feeding of the baby
 d. Vigorous uterine massage

57. For which of the following is the premature infant at risk?

 a. Gestational diabetes
 b. Hypothermia
 c. Placenta previa
 d. Prolapsed umbilical cord

58. Which of the following is a frequent complication of multiple gestation?

 a. Eclampsia
 b. Placenta previa
 c. Premature delivery
 d. Uterine rupture

59. Which of the following complications of pregnancy is most likely to require delivery by cesarean section?

 a. Breech presentation
 b. Cephalopelvic disproportion
 c. Shoulder dystocia
 d. Vaginal bleeding

60. A 30-year-old woman develops dyspnea and severe chest pain 24 hours after delivery of her third child. She is hypotensive and in acute distress. Based on her history, you suspect which of the following?

 a. Eclampsia
 b. Myocardial infarction
 c. Pneumonia
 d. Pulmonary embolism

61. Which of the following is the primary danger to an infant delivered during a precipitous delivery?

 a. Abruptio placentae
 b. Cerebral trauma
 c. Nuchal cord
 d. Placenta previa

62. Which of the following describes chorioamnionitis?

 a. Amniotic fluid embolism
 b. Excessive amniotic fluid
 c. Infection of fetal membranes
 d. Premature rupture of the membranes

WRAP IT UP

At 1630 your crew is sitting around the kitchen table, reviewing some QI data with your supervisor, when you are dispatched for a "maternity case." When you arrive, your 30-year-old patient is on the sofa, saying, "I've got to push!" As you prepare to check her perineum, you obtain a quick history: She is due in 8 weeks, her bag of waters ruptured with clear fluid, there is one fetus, and she denies using narcotic drugs. Her perineum is bulging, and there is evidence of mucousy bloody show, so you call for additional personnel. Your partner listens for fetal heart tones, which he finds inferior to the umbilicus at 150 beats/min. The patient has another contraction, moaning loudly, "the baby's coming." The baby's head is now visible at the perineum so you prepare for imminent delivery and open the OB kit. You continue to obtain her history and note that she has two children at home, and no miscarriages or other health problems. Your partner moves to the ambulance to open the pediatric resuscitation bag and set up for neonatal resuscitation. You don a face shield, gown, and a clean pair of gloves, and then the patient's next contraction begins—you estimate they are 2 to 3 minutes apart. You encourage her to push, and see the baby's forehead appear and then retract slightly when the contraction ends. Coaching her breathing, you arrange towels under her buttocks, elevating them slightly, and prepare some clean towels and blankets for the baby. With the next contraction, the baby's head delivers face down. While supporting the baby's head with one hand, you insert a finger in the vagina and sweep around the neck to feel for the presence of the cord; there is none. Then, taking the bulb syringe from your kit, you suction the fluids from the baby's mouth and then nose, clearing the thick clear mucus. As the next contraction begins, the baby rotates laterally, and you guide it downward to deliver the first shoulder and up to free the other; then the baby slips quickly from the birth canal. It's a girl, and she is very slippery and hard to hold on to. You hold her level with her mother's perineum, as you again suction her nose and mouth and then begin to warm and dry her, vigorously rubbing her back to stimulate the floppy baby to breathe. The cord is clamped and cut, and at 1 minute, you note the baby is still pale and blue, her heart rate is 100 beats/min, she grimaces when you put the bulb syringe in her nose, she has some flexion, but her muscle tone is generally floppy, and she has slow, irregular respirations. You apply oxygen, position her on her back with her shoulders slightly elevated, and flick her feet to stimulate her. She is becoming pinker and has brisk capillary refill, and at 5 minutes her heart rate is 140 beats/min, but even though she is breathing, there is no brisk cry or cough, she grimaces to suction, and her body is now completely pink, in fact it looks very red. You remove the wet towel and cover her (including her head) with warm blankets, apply an oxygen saturation monitor and continue the blowby oxygen, continually monitoring her respiratory effort. She is very small, around 5 lb you guess. In the meantime, your partner has been caring for the mother, who by now has delivered the placenta. She has brisk bleeding from the vagina and cramping. He has started an IV and administered oxytocin intramuscularly. Her vital signs are stable, and she is asking about her baby. Your partner massages the mother's fundus, which she finds uncomfortable. You arrive at the hospital in 8 minutes, where the neonatal resuscitation team is awaiting your arrival. They immediately take the baby, evaluate her in the ED, where her saturation and heart rate are good, allow the mother to hold her for a moment, then take her to the neonatal ICU, where they tell the mother they will intubate her because of her premature status. A week later, baby is discharged to home in good health.

1. What stage of labor is the mother in when you arrive?

    _____

2. Why is this baby at risk for complications during or after delivery?

    _____

3. What was the baby's Apgar score?
    a. At 1 minute:

    _____

    b. At 5 minutes:

    _____

4. What additional resuscitation measures would you have performed immediately if the baby's color and heart rate did not improve after oxygen administration?
    a. Begin ventilation using a bag-mask device and oxygen.
    b. Give epinephrine 0.01 mg/kg.
    c. Initiate vascular access by cannulation of the umbilicus.
    d. Intubate the trachea and ventilate at a rate of 20 per minute.
5. a. What head presentation did you note at delivery?
    b. Is this normal or abnormal?

    _____

6. What action would you have taken if you palpated the cord around his neck?

    _____

7. Why did you hold the baby at the level of the mother's perineum until the cord was cut?

    _____

8. What should be done with the placenta?

    _____

9. Where should the cord be cut?

    _____

10. Explain your rationale for the following interventions:
   a. Stimulation of the baby

   _____

   b. Suctioning of fluids from the mouth and nose

   _____

   c. Elevation of the baby's shoulders

   _____

   d. Massage of the mother's abdomen

   _____

   e. Administration of oxytocin

CHAPTER 42 ANSWERS

REVIEW QUESTIONS

1. e
(Objective 9)

2. f
(Objective 9)

3. a
(Objective 9)

4. g
(Objective 9)

5. d
(Objective 9)

6. c
(Objective 9)

7. e
(Objective 9)

8. f
(Objective 8)

9. g
(Objective 9)

10. b
(Objective 9)

11. c
(Objective 8)

12. d
(Objective 9)

13. a. Fifth
b. Fourth
c. Third
d. Sixth
e. Eighth
(Objective 2)

14. The rapid increase in systemic vascular resistance, aortic pressure, and left ventricular and left atrial pressures after placental flow stops and the decrease in pulmonary vascular resistance resulting from expansion of the lungs cause atrioventricular shunts to close within a few hours after birth.
(Objective 2)

15. a. She has had six pregnancies and delivered five children.

b. She has had two or more deliveries.

c. The patient had bleeding after delivery of her baby.

d. You are called to care for a woman who has never delivered and whose pregnancy has reached 40 weeks of gestation.

(Objective 4)

16. a. Decreased tone and motility of the gastrointestinal tract, which leads to slow gastric emptying and relaxation of the pyloric sphincter

b. Decreased PCO_2 caused by increased respiratory rate and tidal volume late in pregnancy

c. Pressure that the gravid uterus places directly on the bladder when the fetal head moves down in the pelvis near term

d. Blood pressure decreases 10 to 15 mm Hg during the second semester and gradually increases to prepregnant levels near term. (The patient should be questioned about her normal blood pressure.)

e. Impaired venous return resulting from the pressure the uterus exerts

(Objective 3)

17. a. Problems such as maternal nutrition, growth of fetus, maternal diabetes, and preeclampsia would not have been managed; an increased risk of fetal and maternal problems at birth exists.

b. Increased birth weight of the baby may make field delivery difficult or impossible if cephalopelvic disproportion is present.

c. Vaginal bleeding may indicate abruptio placentae, placenta previa, or uterine rupture. All of these conditions cause an increase in fetal mortality rate and pose a risk of maternal shock and death.

d. Recent maternal narcotic intoxication causes neonatal respiratory depression and increases the risk of complications in the field.

(Objective 4)

18. When did she last feel fetal movement? What other medical problems does she have? What other medications does she take? Is she having any contractions?

(Objective 7)

19. Assess fetal heart tones. (A persistent fetal heart rate of greater than 160 or less than 120 is an early sign of fetal distress and fetal or maternal hypoxia.) Ask the mother to report fetal movement to you.

(Objective 7)

20. Administer 100% oxygen by non-rebreather mask (monitoring oxygen saturation with pulse oximeter, if available). Immobilize the patient on a backboard and roll the backboard to the left side. Consider applying pneumatic antishock garments in case the patient's condition deteriorates (controversial). Initiate intravenous lactated Ringer's solution or normal saline (two large-bore lines) en route to the nearest appropriate trauma center and frequently reassess vital signs, fetal heart tones, and the amount of vaginal bleeding en route.

(Objective 7)

21. Spontaneous abortion

(Objective 9)

22. Retrieve the tissue from the toilet and give it to the emergency department staff so that a pathologist can examine it for completeness.

(Objective 9)

23. 6 sanitary napkins × 20 to 30 mL/pad = 120 to 180 mL of blood lost.

(Objective 9)

24. Pregnant women are often attached to the fetus and grieve when they know that their baby has died. This fact is especially true if a similar event has happened to the patient in the past.

(Objective 9)

25. a. Vaginal bleeding, shoulder pain, nausea, vomiting, and syncope

b. Administer 100% oxygen by non-rebreather mask. Consider use of pneumatic antishock garments (controversial). While en route, initiate two large-bore intravenous lines and infuse boluses of normal saline or lactated Ringer's solution. Place the patient in modified Trendelenburg's position if signs and symptoms of shock do not improve, and report her condition and diagnosis to the receiving hospital so that operative preparations can be made.
(Objective 9)

26. Administer 100% oxygen by a non-rebreather mask. Place the patient in left lateral recumbent position. Initiate precautionary intravenous lactated Ringer's solution or normal saline en route to the hospital. Rapidly transport the patient to the closest appropriate medical center and monitor maternal vital signs and fetal heart tones.
(Objective 6)

27. Preeclampsia
(Objective 8)

28. Left lateral recumbent
(Objective 8)

29. Magnesium sulfate 10% (1 to 4 g slow intravenous infusion) and diazepam (5 mg slow intravenous) over 2 minutes
(Objective 8)

30. Minimized stimulation and gentle patient handling
(Objective 8)

31. Abruptio placentae is a complication, and maternal apnea during a seizure may cause fetal hypoxia.
(Objective 8)

32. How many previous deliveries has she had, and how quickly did they progress? How long has she been in labor, and how close are the contractions?
(Objective 11)

33. Contractions lasting 45 to 60 seconds at 1- to 2-minute intervals; measurement from beginning of one contraction to the beginning of the next; patient who wants to bear down or have a bowel movement; large amount of bloody show; crowning; and mother's feeling that delivery is imminent
(Objective 11)

34. Examine for the presence of a nuchal cord. If this cord is present, gently slip it over the infant's head or, if this is not possible, clamp it in two places and cut between the clamps to release the cord. If the cord is cut, ensure that the rest of the delivery proceeds rapidly because the baby has no source of oxygen. Suction the fluids from the baby's mouth and nose with a bulb syringe. Deliver the shoulders.
(Objective 11)

35. Clamp 6 to 9 inches from the infant in two places. Cut between the clamps with sterile scissors or a scalpel. Examine the cord to ensure that no bleeding exists.
(Objective 11)

36. At 1 minute and 5 minutes of age
(Objective 12)

37. After delivery of the baby, 10 units of oxytocin in 1000 mL of lactated Ringer's solution infused at 20 to 30 gtt/min on microdrip tubing
(Objectives 11 and 13)

38. If the head does not deliver immediately, place a gloved hand in the vagina with the palm toward the baby's face. Form a V, with the index and middle fingers on either side of the baby's nose, and push the vaginal wall from the face until delivery. If the head does not deliver within 3 minutes, maintain the airway as described and transport the patient to the receiving hospital.
(Objective 14)

39. Position the mother on her left side in the knee-chest position. Guide the baby's head downward to allow the anterior shoulder to slip under the symphysis pubis; avoid excess force. Rotate the fetal shoulder girdle into the wider oblique pelvic diameter and deliver the posterior and then the anterior shoulders.
(Objective 14)

40. a. Elevate the mother's hips, administer oxygen, and ask the mother to pant with contractions to avoid bearing down. With gloved hand, gently push the baby's presenting part back into the vagina and elevate it to relieve pressure on the cord. Maintain this position while rapidly transporting the patient to the receiving hospital.
b. No, this baby will have to be delivered by cesarean section.
(Objective 14)

41. c
(Objective 1)

42. d. Although amniotic fluid originates from fetal urine and secretions from the respiratory tract, skin, and amniotic membranes, its primary function is protection.
(Objective 1)

43. b. The ductus arteriosus connects the aorta and pulmonary artery, and the foramen ovale provides a passageway for blood directly from the right to the left atrium. The umbilical cord connects the placenta to the embryo and is its lifeline.
(Objective 2)

44. b
(Objective 1)

45. a. At week 12, the uterus is just above the symphysis pubis; at week 16, between the symphysis pubis and the umbilicus; and at week 28, halfway between the umbilicus and the xiphoid.
(Objective 5)

46. b. A persistent rate greater than 160 or below 120 is a sign of fetal distress and fetal or maternal hypoxia.
(Objective 5)

47. b. This position prevents pressure from being exerted on the inferior vena cava.
(Objective 6)

48. b. Maternal mortality from pregnancy-related causes is rare. If the patient had abruptio placentae, a healthy delivery would be unlikely. Aortic dissection and congestive cardiomyopathy may cause maternal death, but amniotic fluid embolism is more likely at the time of delivery.
(Objective 6)

49. d. Drug doses and ventilations do not need to be modified. Chest compressions should be performed higher on the sternum.
(Objective 6)

50. d. Edema and hypertension are found in both.
(Objective 8)

51. c. Magnesium also can cause clinically significant hypotension.
(Objective 8)

52. c. Uterine inversion also may happen, although less frequently, after a contraction, cough, or sneeze.
(Objective 14)

53. b. During the prodromal period, the fetus descends into the birth canal. In the first stage the cervix dilates completely, and in the third stage the placenta is delivered.
(Objective 10)

54. c. Usually the cord can be freed in this manner. If this action fails and the decision is made to cut the cord after your medical direction protocols, delivery must be expedited or the baby will suffer severe hypoxia and risk of death.
(Objectives 11 and 14)

55. c. Weak cry (1); plus pink body and blue extremities (1); plus pulse at 128 (2), plus active movement (2); plus sneeze (2) = 8
(Objective 12)

56. a. Having the baby suckle stimulates the production of oxytocin.
(Objective 13)

57. b. The premature infant has a large surface area-to-mass ratio and is susceptible to hypothermia. In addition, a potential for cardiorespiratory dysfunction exists because of immaturity.
(Objective 14)

58. c. Other complications include abruptio placentae, postpartum hemorrhage, and abnormal presentation.
(Objective 14)

59. b. In this condition the pelvic ring is too small to allow passage of the baby's head.
(Objective 14)

60. d. Pulmonary embolism or, more rarely, amniotic fluid embolism can cause these signs and symptoms.
(Objective 14)

61. b. Tearing of the umbilical cord is also a risk.
(Objective 14)

62. c. This condition often occurs after prolonged premature rupture of the membranes.
(Objective 14)

WRAP IT UP

1. Stage II (expulsion stage)
(Objective 10)

2. Baby is premature based on mother's history
(Objective 14)

3. a. 1-minute Apgar: 4
b. 5-minute Apgar: 7
(Objective 12)

4. a. Assisted ventilation may be all that is necessary to open the small airway and stimulate normal breathing in the infant.
(Objectives 7 and 14)

5. a. Vertex (cephalic); this is normal
(Objective 10)

6. Gently try to slip the cord over the head.
(Objective 14)

7. Elevation of the baby below the perineum could result in undertransfusion of blood from the cord; lowering the baby below the perineum could result in overtransfusion of cord blood.
(Objective 11)

8. The placenta surface should be inspected to see whether it is intact (retained fragments can cause postpartum hemorrhage); and then it should be placed in a plastic bag and transported with the mother to the hospital.
(Objective 11)

9. Clamp the cord in two places 4 to 6 inches from the baby and then cut between the clamps.
(Objective 11)

10. a. Stimulation of the baby is designed to promote effective respiratory effort.
b. Suctioning of fluids from the mouth and nose clears the upper airway of mucus and other secretions to promote normal unobstructed breathing
c. Elevation of the baby's shoulders positions the airway in the most effective manner to promote effective ventilation.
d. Massage of the mother's abdomen stimulates uterine contractions that help to slow vaginal bleeding.
e. Administration of oxytocin causes uterine contraction and slows vaginal bleeding.
(Objective 11)

PART NINE

IN THIS PART

Neonatology

READING ASSIGNMENT

Chapter 43, pages 1100-1115, in *Mosby's Paramedic Textbook,* ed. 3

OBJECTIVES

Upon completion of this chapter, the paramedic student will be able to:
1. Identify risk factors associated with the need for neonatal resuscitation.
2. Describe physiological adaptations at birth.
3. Outline the prehospital assessment and management of the neonate.
4. Describe resuscitation of the distressed neonate.
5. Discuss postresuscitative management and transport.
6. Describe signs and symptoms and prehospital management of specific neonatal resuscitation situations.
7. Identify injuries associated with birth.
8. Describe appropriate interventions to manage the emotional needs of the neonate's family.

SUMMARY

- When oxygenation and continued ventilations do not improve the infant's condition or they begin to deteriorate further, ET intubation and administration of drugs may be required. The drugs most often used during neonatal resuscitation are epinephrine, volume expanders, and naloxone.
- Some of the more common congenital anomalies include choanal atresia, cleft lip, diaphragmatic hernia, and Pierre Robin syndrome.
- At birth, newborns make three major physiological adaptations necessary for survival: (1) emptying fluids from their lungs and beginning ventilation, (2) changing their circulatory pattern, and (3) maintaining body temperature.
- The initial steps of neonatal resuscitation (except for those born through meconium) are to prevent heat loss, clear the airway by positioning and suctioning, provide tactile stimulation and initiate breathing if necessary, and further evaluate the infant.
- The three most common complications during the postresuscitation period are endotracheal position change (including dislodgment), tube occlusion by mucus or meconium, and pneumothorax. During transport of the neonate, it is important to maintain body temperature, oxygen administration, and ventilatory support.
- Specific situations that may require advanced life support for the neonate include meconium staining, apnea, diaphragmatic hernia, bradycardia, premature infants, respiratory distress and cyanosis, hypovolemia, seizures, fever, hypothermia, hypoglycemia, and vomiting and diarrhea.
- Premature infants have an increased risk of respiratory suppression, hypothermia, and head and brain injury. In addition to low birth weight, various antepartum and intrapartum risk factors may affect the need for resuscitation.
- About 2% to 7% of every 1000 live births result in avoidable and unavoidable mechanical and anoxic trauma during labor and delivery.

- The paramedic should be aware of the normal feelings and reactions of parents, siblings, other family members, and caregivers while providing emergency care to an ill or injured child.

REVIEW QUESTIONS

Match the structures described in Column I with the correct term in Column II.

	Column I		Column II
1.	_____ A vertical split in the lip	**a.**	Choanal atresia
2.	_____ Abnormalities that include a small mandible and defects of the eyes and ears	**b.**	Cleft lip
		c.	Diaphragmatic hernia
3.	_____ Occlusion that blocks the passage between the nose and pharynx	**d.**	Gastroesophageal reflux
		e.	Pierre Robin syndrome
4.	_____ Protrusion of stomach through the diaphragm		

5. List two risk factors that may indicate the need for neonatal resuscitation in each of the following categories:

    a. Antepartum risk factors

_____

    b. Intrapartum risk factors

_____

6. What three major adaptations are necessary for the survival of the neonate at birth?

    a.

    b.

    c.

7. List three actions that help maintain body warmth of the neonate.

    a.

    b.

    c.

8. Arrange the following steps in neonatal resuscitation (assuming you have a blue infant with slightly decreased respirations and a heart rate of 70 that does not improve at each step) in the correct order in the following table.

Incorrect Order	**Correct Order**
Administer epinephrine.	
Obtain vascular access.	
Administer oxygen at 5 L/min.	
Ventilate with bag-mask device.	
Perform chest compressions.	
Warm, dry, suction, and stimulate.	

Questions 9 to 14 pertain to the following case study:

    A 3-kg baby is delivered, his airway has been suctioned, and he has been positioned properly. Tactile stimulation has been provided; however, he is still not breathing.

9. At what rate should you ventilate the neonate?

_____

After ventilations are initiated, you detect a pulse of 70 per minute.

10. Where should you palpate the pulse on a neonate?

_____

11. What steps should you take now?

_____

After you initiate chest compressions, there is no improvement. Your partner has intubated the baby.

12. What size of endotracheal tube would be appropriate for this infant?

_____

13. What are your options to obtain vascular access?

_____

14. What drug/dose should you administer when vascular access has been established?

_____

15. List an intervention for each of the following neonatal postresuscitation complications:

   a. Endotracheal tube dislodgment

_____

   b. Endotracheal tube occlusion by mucus

_____

   c. Pneumothorax

_____

STUDENT SELF-ASSESSMENT

16. In which of the following situations will you anticipate the need for neonatal resuscitation?
   a. Contractions have been occurring for 6 hours.
   b. Physician states the baby weighs 3600 g (7½ lb).
   c. Rupture of the membranes occurred 12 hours ago.
   d. The baby is at 36 weeks' gestation.
17. What initiates respiration in the newborn?
   a. Chemical and temperature changes
   b. Chest compression
   c. Closure of the patent ductus
   d. Cutting the umbilical cord
18. What is a proper position to maximize the airway of a neonate?
   a. Prone with neck slightly extended
   b. Supine with neck slightly flexed
   c. Supine with towel under the shoulders
   d. Supine with towel under the head
19. Which neonatal suctioning technique is appropriate after delivery if no meconium has been observed?
   a. Cut the umbilical cord before suctioning.
   b. Suction secretions from the mouth first and then the nose.
   c. Suction secretions from the nose first and then the mouth.
   d. Suctioning is unnecessary if meconium is not observed.

20. Priorities of care for neonatal resuscitation are as follows:
    a. Prevent heat loss, administer intravenous fluids, and allow the infant to feed at the breast.
    b. Position the neonate, suction to clear the airway, minimize external stimulation, and initiate intravenous fluids.
    c. Prevent heat loss, position the neonate, suction to clear the airway, and provide stimulation.
    d. Position the infant, suction to clear the airway, administer intravenous fluids, and provide stimulation.
21. Deep suctioning of the posterior pharynx of the neonate may cause which of the following?
    a. Bradycardia
    b. Central nervous system depression
    c. Hypocarbia
    d. Tachypnea
22. After delivery the infant is warmed, dried, and stimulated. Respirations are 30 per minute and heart rate is 110, but the baby's lips and ears are still blue. What should you do?
    a. Administer oxygen at 5 L/min by holding the tubing ½ inch from the nose.
    b. Begin bag-mask ventilation with 100% oxygen until the color improves.
    c. Initiate bag-mask ventilation and chest compressions.
    d. No intervention is needed; this is a normal finding in the newborn.
23. Which of the following is an acceptable method of neonatal stimulation?
    a. Shouting loudly close to the baby's ear
    b. Holding the baby by the ankles and slapping the buttocks
    c. Slapping or flicking the soles of the feet or rubbing the back
    d. Vigorously shaking the baby by firmly grasping the shoulders
24. When should the paramedic consider intubation of the neonate?
    a. If the heart rate increases after bag-mask ventilation is performed
    b. If prolonged ventilation is likely to be needed
    c. Immediately after absent respirations are noted
    d. When the gestational age is less than 39 weeks
25. What is the normal heart rate of an infant?
    a. 60 beats/min
    b. 80 beats/min
    c. 120 beats/min
    d. 160 beats/min
26. Which finding may indicate a postresuscitation complication related to intubation in the neonate?
    a. Decreased resistance to ventilation
    b. Diminished breath sounds
    c. Increase in chest expansion
    d. Return of tachycardia
27. Apnea in infants may be related to which of the following?
    a. Central nervous system disorders
    b. Excessive stimulation
    c. Meconium aspiration
    d. Use of stimulants
28. The most common factor for respiratory distress and cyanosis in a neonate is prematurity. Which of the following factors also can be responsible for this condition?
    a. Cleft lip congenital anomaly
    b. Mucus obstruction of the nasal passages
    c. Premature rupture of membranes
    d. Postterm delivery
29. What is the correct first drug and dose used for the treatment of neonatal bradycardia in the presence of adequate ventilation and oxygenation?
    a. Atropine 0.01 mg/kg IV
    b. Atropine 0.02 mg/kg IV
    c. Epinephrine 0.01 mg/kg (1:1000) IV
    d. Epinephrine 0.01 mg/kg (1:10,000) IV
30. Which of the following is a risk factor associated with cardiac arrest in the newborn?
    a. Amniotic fluid aspiration
    b. Gestational diabetes
    c. Intrauterine asphyxia
    d. Premature cutting of the cord after birth

31. Which is true regarding vomiting in the neonate?
    a. An intravenous line should be established if this is observed.
    b. It is unusual and is associated with serious illness.
    c. It is a frequent occurrence and should be of no concern.
    d. Persistent bile-stained vomit may indicate a bowel obstruction.
32. What sign or symptom can be found following phototherapy for hyperbilirubinemia?
    a. Bradycardia   c. Seizures
    b. Diarrhea   d. Vomiting
33. You are called to evaluate a 4-day-old breast-fed infant whose mother states the child has diarrhea. When asked, she says the child is having five or six "loose" yellow stools per day. What is your assessment of this situation?
    a. This number of stools is normal for a breast-fed baby.
    b. This indicates a serious situation that requires immediate intravenous therapy.
    c. This indicates bowel obstruction from a congenital defect.
    d. The yellow stools could indicate hepatitis, and the mother should be assessed for risk.
34. A mother states that she has observed repetitive eye deviation and blinking and sucking and swimming movements of the 2-day-old infant's arms. This may indicate which of the following?
    a. Focal clonic seizures   c. Subtle seizures
    b. Multifocal seizures   d. Tonic seizures
35. What should be assessed in the prehospital setting when evaluating an infant with apparent seizures?
    a. Blood glucose level   c. Child's ability to feed normally
    b. Blood pressure   d. Glasgow Coma Scale
36. Which is true of a temperature of 100.4° F (38.0° C) in a neonate?
    a. It is a normal result of immature temperature control and does not require treatment.
    b. It may indicate a life-threatening infection and requires immediate transport.
    c. It often results in the development of febrile seizures that are difficult to control.
    d. Prehospital care should involve ice packs in the groin area to lower temperature.
37. A 3-kg infant delivered at home yesterday is limp and has irregular respirations. You assess the child, maintain warmth, assist ventilations, and initiate vascular access. The blood glucose drawn when the intravenous line was started is 40 mg/dL. What should you administer?
    a. 3 g of a $D_{10}W$ solution   c. 6 g of a $D_{10}W$ solution
    b. 3 g of a D50W solution   d. 6 g of a D50W solution
38. Which of the following injuries may occur during childbirth?
    a. Clavicle or extremity fracture   c. Spine or spinal cord injury
    b. Liver or spleen injury   d. All of the above
39. Which of the following statements by the paramedic would be helpful when speaking to the parents of an infant who is being resuscitated in the prehospital setting:
    a. Everything's going to be okay.
    b. Everything possible is being done for your baby.
    c. I can't tell you anything at all about your baby.
    d. I think your baby's going to make it; this is a great crew.

WRAP IT UP

You hear the dispatcher say, "Respond to a call for maternity ... ," and you figure this will just be another person who thinks she is in labor. However, when you arrive, the father meets you at the door yelling, "The baby, the baby." You find an 18-year-old woman squatting by the bed, pants around her ankles, screaming, and can see thick, chunky, green liquid running down her legs and a baby's head crowning at her perineum. You quickly pull out the OB kit, while your partner calls for a pumper assist and hurries to get the pediatric resuscitation bag from your ambulance. As the head delivers, you suction secretions from the mouth and then nose with the bulb syringe, pulling out thick meconium with each aspiration. The chest delivers, and there is no immediate spontaneous respiration, so you insert an endotracheal tube, quickly applying suction to the end. As you pull it out some residual green meconium is aspirated, and you repeat it twice until there is no aspirate. Your partner holds an oxygen mask close to the baby's face and checks his heart rate after you position him on his side, dry him, and stimulate him; it is 50 per minute, and he is floppy and does not grimace to suction, so your partner begins ventilation with a bag mask. After 30 seconds, there is no improvement in heart rate, so you have a firefighter perform chest compressions while you intubate the baby's trachea and verify placement. You explain quickly to the mother that the baby has not responded to initial treatment, so you are helping his blood circulate with chest compressions and are going to give him some medicines to help stimulate his heart. There is still no improvement, so you initiate a scalp vein IV and administer epinephrine. Reassessment shows a heart rate of 150 beats/min, which quickly slows when you stop ventilation for a moment. You continue ventilation with frequent reevaluation of tube placement and cover him to keep him warm until you arrive at the ED 10 minutes later. After a month in NICU, he is released home and his mother brings him to visit 2 months later.

1. What scene finding made you prepare for neonatal resuscitation?
   a. Age of the mother
   b. Baby crowning on arrival
   c. Presence of meconium on the mother's legs
   d. Resuscitation is needed on most field deliveries
2. What four newborn characteristics, assessed immediately after birth, would suggest that no resuscitation is needed?
   a.
   b.
   c.
   d.
3. What physiological change at birth explains the
   a. Presence of secretions in the baby's nose and mouth that need suctioning.

   _____

   b. Need to dry and warm the infant. _____

   c. Circulatory changes after the cord is cut. _____
4. Place a check mark beside the steps in the neonatal resuscitation pyramid that you performed on this baby.
   a. _____ Position, suction, stimulate   d. _____ Chest compression
   b. _____ Oxygen   e. _____ Intubation
   c. _____ Bag-mask ventilation   f. _____ Medication
5. Why was the baby intubated and secretions suctioned before any other resuscitation measures?
   a. All babies with meconium in the amniotic fluid need intubation.
   b. If the paramedic is skilled at intubation, it should be done first.
   c. It takes longer to insert an umbilical catheter, so it is left until later.
   d. The baby was depressed, and the meconium was thick.
6. Why is it important to give the family some preliminary information about the baby's condition?

_____

CHAPTER 43 ANSWERS

Review Questions

1. b
   (Objective 1)

2. e
   (Objective 1)

3. a
   (Objective 1)

4. c
   (Objective 1)

5. a. Multiple gestation, inadequate prenatal care, mother's age, history of perinatal morbidity or mortality, postterm gestation, drugs/medication, toxemia, hypertension, and diabetes
   b. Premature labor, meconium-stained amniotic fluid, rupture of membranes more than 24 hours before delivery, use of narcotics within 4 hours of delivery, abnormal presentation, prolonged labor or precipitous delivery, prolapsed cord, bleeding
   (Objective 1)

6. a. Emptying fluid from the lungs and beginning ventilation
   b. Changing the circulatory pattern
   c. Maintaining body temperature
   (Objective 2)

7. a. Dry the infant's head and body thoroughly; remove any wet coverings; cover the head and body of the baby with warm blankets; turn the heat up high in the ambulance; use chemical warm packs (with blankets between the pack and the infant). Wrap low-birth-weight infants in plastic food wrap.
   (Objective 3)

8.

Incorrect Order	Correct Order
Administer epinephrine.	Warm, dry, clear airway, and stimulate.
Obtain vascular access.	Administer oxygen at 5 L/min.
Administer oxygen at 5 L/min.	Ventilate with bag-mask device.
Ventilate with bag-mask device.	Perform chest compressions.
Perform chest compressions.	Obtain vascular access.
Warm, dry, clear airway, and stimulate.	Administer epinephrine.
(Objective 4)	

9. Initiate positive pressure breathing with 100% oxygen by bag mask at 40 to 60 breaths/min.
   (Objectives 3 and 4)

10. At the brachial artery, at the umbilical cord, or by auscultation
    (Objective 3)

11. Continue positive pressure ventilations for 30 seconds; if heart rate does not begin to improve, start chest compressions ½ to ¾ inch at 120 per minute.
    (Objective 4)

12. 2.5 or 3.0
(Objective 4)

13. Initiate a peripheral intravenous line, an intraosseous line, or an umbilical vein cannulation (if specially trained and authorized).
(Objective 4)

14. Epinephrine 0.01-0.03 mg/kg (1:10,000)
(Objective 4)

15. a. If breath sounds are audible only on the right, pull back slightly and reevaluate; if tube is in the correct location, secure. If breath sounds are absent, remove the tube and reintubate.
(Objective 5)

b. Suction the tube with a suction catheter and reevaluate.
(Objective 5)

c. Assess for presence of tension pneumothorax, and treat if present. If at hospital, prepare to assist with chest tube placement.
(Objective 5)

16. d. A premature infant refers to a baby born before 37 weeks' gestation (weight usually 0.6 to 2.2 kg [1½ to 5 lb]). The incidence of complications increases as gestational age (and weight) decreases. A normal birth weight is 7½ lb; 6 hours is not a lengthy labor. Rupture of membranes more than 24 hours before birth would be a concern.
(Objective 1)

17. a. As the chest recoils during delivery, chemical and temperature changes initiate the first breath. Cutting the umbilical cord initiates changes in fetal circulation.
(Objective 2)

18. c. The torso should be elevated ¾ to 1 inch so that the neck is slighted extended.
(Objective 3)

19. b. The mouth should be suctioned before the nose, and then the cord can be cut.
(Objective 3)

20. c. Intravenous fluids are rarely necessary in the normal infant if appropriate resuscitation is done.
(Objective 3)

21. a
(Objective 3)

22. a. Continue the oxygen administration until the color improves (keep the baby warm).
(Objective 3)

23. c. The goal is to stimulate the neonate without risk of injury.
(Objective 3)

24. b. Often the infant will initiate adequate spontaneous respirations after a brief period of bagging and will not require intubation. Increasing heart rate is a positive indicator.
(Objective 4)

25. c. A heart rate greater than 100 beats/min is desirable. Chest compressions should be initiated for a persistent heart rate less than 80 beats/min that does not respond to ventilation.
(Objective 3)

26. b. Decreased chest wall movement, return of bradycardia, unilateral decrease in chest expansion, altered intensity to pitch or breath sounds, and increased resistance to hand ventilation are signs that may point to tube migration, occlusion, or pneumothorax.
(Objective 5)

27. a. Other causes include narcotic/central nervous system depressant use, airway or respiratory muscle weakness, oxyhemoglobin dissociation curve shift, septicemia, and metabolic disorders.
(Objective 6)

28. b. Infants are obligate nose breathers; suctioning of mucus from the nasal passages will correct this problem.

29. d. Inadequate ventilations and oxygenation are the most common causes of bradycardia and should be reassessed continually.
(Objective 6)

30. c. Other causes are drugs taken by the mother, congenital diseases or malformations, and intrapartum hypoxemia.
(Objective 6)

31. d. Some vomiting is normal; however, if it is persistent or bile-stained or contains dark blood, a serious underlying illness may exist. Vascular access would not be indicated unless needed to treat dehydration or bradycardia because of the vagal stimulation this can produce.
(Objective 6)

32. b. Other causes of diarrhea in the neonate are gastroenteritis, lactose intolerance, neonatal abstinence syndrome, thyrotoxicosis, and cystic fibrosis
(Objective 6)

33. a. The baby should be assessed for clinical signs of dehydration or other signs of illness (e.g., fever, lethargy, and feeding habits), but typically this stool pattern is normal in this situation.
(Objective 5)

34. c. All types of seizures in this age group are considered pathological.

35. a. Hypoglycemia may produce seizure activity. Determining the presence of this condition and correcting it are urgent matters.
(Objective 6)

36. b. Even small temperature elevations in this age group can signal impending sepsis. Febrile seizures are unusual in this age group and would not be expected (especially at this temperature). Ice packs should never be applied to a neonate.
(Objective 6)

37. a
(Objective 6)

38. d. Brain and hypoxic injuries may occur as well.
(Objective 7)

39. b. Honest, frequent updates about the baby's condition should be given during the resuscitation so that family members can prepare themselves for the outcome.
(Objective 7)

WRAP IT UP

1. c. Meconium points to a high-risk delivery, especially if it is thick and dark. Other indicators of birth complications are early delivery, maternal use of drugs, and multiple births.
   (Objective 1)

2. a. Full-term baby
   b. No meconium or signs of infected amniotic fluid
   c. Baby is breathing or crying
   d. Baby has good muscle tone

3. a. Fluid is squeezed from the chest into the nose and mouth during delivery and should be suctioned.
   b. Infants have a large body surface area, immature temperature regulation mechanisms, and are born into a cool, wet environment. Maintaining warmth is a critical aspect of neonatal resuscitation.
   c. Cutting the cord shuts down placental circulation, closing some of the circulatory pathways established in utero.
   (Objective 2)

4. a, b, c, d, e, f. On most deliveries, progression past (a) or (b) is never needed.
   (Objectives 3 and 4)

5. d. This is the only situation when intubation would be near the first step.
   (Objectives 4 and 6)

6. Family should be given brief, accurate information often to give them a realistic idea of the condition of their baby.
   (Objective 8)

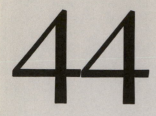

CHAPTER 44

Pediatrics

READING ASSIGNMENT

Chapter 44, pages 1116-1159, in *Mosby's Paramedic Textbook,* ed. 3

OBJECTIVES

Upon completion of this chapter, the paramedic student will be able to:
1. Identify the role of the Emergency Medical Services for Children program.
2. Identify modifications in patient assessment techniques that assist in the examination of patients at different developmental levels.
3. Identify age-related illnesses and injuries in pediatric patients.
4. Outline the general principles of assessment and management of the pediatric patient.
5. Describe the pathophysiology, signs and symptoms, and management of selected pediatric respiratory emergencies.
6. Describe the pathophysiology, signs and symptoms, and management of shock in the pediatric patient.
7. Describe the pathophysiology, signs and symptoms, and management of selected pediatric dysrhythmias.
8. Describe the pathophysiology, signs and symptoms, and management of pediatric seizures.
9. Describe the pathophysiology, signs and symptoms, and management of hypoglycemia and hyperglycemia in the pediatric patient.
10. Describe the pathophysiology, signs and symptoms, and management of infectious pediatric emergencies.
11. Identify common causes of poisoning and toxic exposure in the pediatric patient.
12. Describe special considerations for assessment and management of specific injuries in children.
13. Outline the pathophysiology and management of sudden infant death syndrome.
14. Describe the risk factors, key signs and symptoms, and management of injuries or illness resulting from child abuse and neglect.
15. Identify prehospital considerations for the care of infants and children with special needs.

SUMMARY

- The Emergency Medical Services for Children program was designed to enhance and expand emergency medical services for acutely ill and injured children. The program has defined 12 basic components of an effective Emergency Medical Services for Children system.
- Children have unique anatomical, physiological, and psychological characteristics, which change during their development.
- Some childhood diseases and disabilities can be predicted by age group.
- Many elements of the initial evaluation can be done by observing the child. The child's parent or guardian also should be involved in the initial evaluation. The three components of the pediatric assessment triangle are appearance, work of breathing, and circulation.

- Obstruction of the upper or lower airway by a foreign body usually occurs in toddlers or preschoolers. Obstruction may be partial or complete.
- Croup is a common inflammatory respiratory illness. It usually is seen in children between the ages of 6 months and 4 years. Symptoms are caused by inflammation in the subglottic region.
- Bacterial tracheitis is an infection of the upper airway and subglottic trachea usually seen in infants and toddlers; it often occurs with or after croup.
- Epiglottitis is a rapidly progressive, life-threatening bacterial infection. It causes edema and swelling of the epiglottis and supraglottic structures. It often affects children between 3 and 7 years of age.
- Asthma is common in children over 2 years of age. Asthma is characterized by bronchoconstriction that results from autonomic dysfunction or sensitizing agents.
- Bronchiolitis is a viral disease frequently caused by respiratory syncytial virus infection of the lower airway; it usually affects children age 6 to 18 months of age.
- Pneumonia is an acute infection of the lower airways and lungs involving the alveolar walls and the alveoli.
- Several special differences must be remembered when caring for a child in shock. These include circulating blood volume, body surface area and hypothermia, cardiac reserve, and vital signs and assessment. A child in shock may appear normal and stable until all compensatory mechanisms fail. At that point, pediatric shock progresses rapidly, with serious deterioration.
- When dysrhythmias occur in children, they usually result from hypoxia or structural heart disease.
- The most common causes of seizure in adult and pediatric patients are noncompliance with a drug regimen for the treatment of epilepsy, in addition to head trauma, intracranial infection, metabolic disturbance, or poisoning. The most common cause of new onset of seizure in children is fever.
- Hypoglycemia and hyperglycemia should be suspected whenever a child has an altered level of consciousness with no explainable cause.
- Children with infection may have a variety of signs and symptoms. These depend on the source and extent of infection and the length of time since the patient was exposed.
- Most poisoning events in the United States involve children. Signs and symptoms of accidental poisoning vary, depending on the toxic substance and the length of time since the child was exposed.
- Blunt and penetrating trauma is a chief cause of injury and death in children. Head injury is the most common cause of death in pediatric trauma patients. Early recognition and aggressive management can reduce morbidity and mortality caused by traumatic brain injury in children.
- Because of the pliability of the chest wall, severe intrathoracic injury can be present without signs of external injury. The liver, kidneys, and spleen are the most frequently injured abdominal organs. Extremity injuries are more common in children than adults.
- Sudden infant death syndrome is the leading cause of death in American infants under 1 year of age. The syndrome is defined as the sudden death of a seemingly healthy infant. The death cannot be explained by history and an autopsy.
- Child abuse and neglect is the maltreatment of children by their parents, guardians, or other caregivers. Forms of maltreatment include infliction of physical injury, sexual exploitation, and infliction of emotional pain and neglect.
- Some infants and children are born with or develop conditions that pose special needs. These children may require special medical equipment to sustain life. Often these children are cared for at home. Many are dependent on specialized medical equipment such as tracheostomy tubes, home artificial ventilators, central venous lines, gastrostomy tubes, and shunts.

REVIEW QUESTIONS

Match the drugs in column II with their appropriate initial *pediatric* dose in column I. Use each drug only once.

Column I	Column II
1. _____ 0.1 mL/kg	a. Adenosine
2. _____ 2 to 20 µg/kg/min	b. Amiodarone
3. _____ 1 mEq/kg per dose	c. Atropine sulfate
4. _____ 0.1 mg/kg	d. Diazepam
5. _____ 1 mg/kg	e. Dopamine hydrochloride
6. _____ 0.02 mg/kg	f. Epinephrine (1:10,000)
7. _____ 5 mg/kg	g. Lidocaine
	h. Sodium bicarbonate

8. In what pediatric age group(s) are you most likely to see the following illness or injuries?

   a. Sepsis:

_____

   b. Febrile seizures:

_____

   c. Jaundice:

_____

   d. Ingestions:

_____

   e. Falls:

_____

   f. Child abuse:

_____

   g. Drowning or near drowning:

_____

   h. Suicidal gestures:

_____

Questions 9 to 12 pertain to the following case study:

A 7-year-old boy is in acute respiratory distress after visiting a friend's home. He gives a history of asthma and allergy to dogs (his friend has three). His home medicines include an Atrovent inhaler, montelukast sodium (Singulair) tabs, which he takes daily, and pirbuterol (Maxair) by nebulizer as necessary, which he has not used for a week. He has circumoral cyanosis, is working very hard to breathe, and has faint inspiratory and expiratory wheezes.

9. What interventions are appropriate for this child? Include two possible beta-agonist drugs you could administer (with appropriate doses and routes).

_____

10. What side effects do you anticipate from the administration of these drugs?

_____

11. In 15 minutes, you see no clinical improvement and your estimated arrival time is still 20 minutes. What do you do?

_____

12. What aspects of the physical examination will change when the patient improves?

_____

_____

13. List three characteristic signs or symptoms of epiglottitis.

a.

b.

c.

14. A 20-month-old with croup is in mild respiratory distress on a cool October evening.

a. What intervention should you try before entering the ambulance that may cause rapid improvement in the patient's signs and symptoms?

_____

b. When in the ambulance, how will you care for this child?

_____

_____

Questions 15 to 19 pertain to the following case study:

A limp, 11-month-old boy is carried into the ambulance base by his mother. She states that he has had a fever with vomiting and diarrhea for 3 days. His eyes are sunken, his tongue is furrowed, and his lips are cracked. Physical examination reveals rapid respirations; cold, mottled extremities; and the electrocardiogram shown in Fig. 44-1.

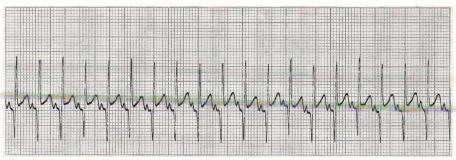

Figure 44-1

15. What condition does this child have?

_____

16. Interpret the electrocardiogram.

_____

17. Describe management of this child, assuming a 45-minute transport time.

_____

_____

18. What are the appropriate vital signs for this child?

_____

19. What clinical signs of improvement will you watch for in addition to improvement in vital signs?

_____

Questions 20 to 23 refer to the following case study:

A 3-year-old, 33 pound (15 kg)-child is found unconscious after suffocation with a plastic bag. On arrival, you find a dusky, pale child who is unresponsive and apneic. Occasionally you can palpate a faint pulse at the carotid artery, but you obtain no blood pressure reading. The electrocardiogram is shown in Fig. 44-2.

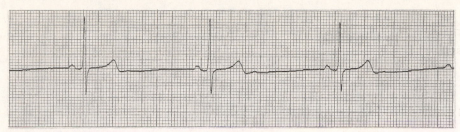

Figure 44-2

20. Interpret the electrocardiogram tracing.

_____

21. What actions will you take immediately, up to and including the first drug (with appropriate dose and route).

_____

_____

22. If an intravenous line cannot be immediately established, what two actions can be taken?

   a.

   b.

23. After your initial interventions result in no patient improvement, what is the next drug (and dose and route) indicated?

_____

24. A 3-week-old, 5 kg infant with a history of congenital heart defects suddenly loses consciousness and stops breathing. On arrival, you find him pulseless and apneic. Cardiopulmonary resuscitation is initiated by the police emergency medical responders. The electrocardiogram tracing in Fig. 44-3 is noted.

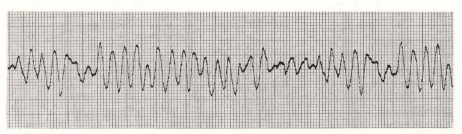

Figure 44-3

a. Outline your continued care of this patient, up to and including the first two drugs (including doses and routes).

_____

_____

_____

b. If a repeat dose of epinephrine is necessary, what is the correct dose and concentration?

_____

Questions 25 to 27 refer to the following case study:

A frightened mother tells you that when she put her 4-year-old, 14-kg child to bed, he complained of a slight earache and had a low-grade temperature. She heard a noise several hours later and found her child having a grand mal seizure, which stopped after approximately 1 minute. The child's temperature is 105.5° F (40.8° C). He appears to be postictal at this time.

25. After you have ensured that the child is stable, what history should you obtain from the mother?

_____

_____

26. What care should be provided en route to the hospital?

_____

_____

27. If the child has a seizure during transport, list two anticonvulsant drugs that may be given, including the appropriate doses and routes.

a.

b.

28. You are called to an elementary school to care for a 6-year-old who is "acting funny." She is responsive only to pain. The nurse says the child has a history of diabetes. You check a finger-stick glucose level and determine that this child's blood sugar is 35 mg/dL.

a. What drug should you administer (including dose and route)?

_____

b. What other signs or symptoms may this child have had before becoming this ill?

_____

_____

29. Your 3-year-old patient weighs 17 kg. He was involved in a head-on motor vehicle collision and was restrained only by a lap belt. He says his "tummy hurts." The physical examination reveals an anxious, pale child with a rigid, tender abdomen. Discuss the significance of the following physiological differences in children and specific ways they will influence your care of this child.

a. Children have a greater percentage of circulating blood volume than adults.

_____

_____

b. Children have a large body surface area in proportion to body weight.

_____

_____

c. Children's hearts function at near-maximal performance in a normal, healthy state.

_____

_____

d. Volume replacement in children is weight related.

_____

_____

_____

_____

e. Intravenous access is difficult to establish in children.

_____

_____

30. How do you determine whether an intraosseous needle has been properly placed?

_____

Questions 31 to 33 pertain to the following case study:

At 1 AM on a cool February morning, you are dispatched for a "baby choking." On arrival you find a well-nourished 4-month-old baby boy apneic and pulseless in his crib. There is frothy sputum in the nose and mouth, and his diaper is wet and full of stool. The child is cold, and dependent lividity is present. The hysterical mother states that he and his older sister have both had a slight cold but that otherwise he was healthy.

31. What characteristics of sudden infant death syndrome are consistent with this call?

_____

32. What other findings should you document in this situation?

_____

You spend some time at the scene comforting the family and making the appropriate notifications and then ride back quietly to the firehouse with your normally talkative partner. You ask if he is OK, and he says, "Of course, I'm fine." Then he immediately rushes to the phone, where you hear him awaken his wife and ask her to check on their 6-month-old daughter.

33. Should you ignore your partner's unusual behavior, since he told you he is OK? If not, what action(s) can you take?

_____

_____

Questions 34 to 36 pertain to the following case study:

A mother tells you that her 8-month-old son fell off his tricycle early in the day but seemed to be feeling fine. Later, she could not wake him from his nap. On physical examination you find a dirty child who has agonal respirations, a slow pulse, and extension posturing. No visible signs of trauma are present on the head, although small bruises are noted on the shoulders.

34. What should your immediate interventions be for this child?

_____

_____

35. What findings might lead you to suspect child abuse?

_____

_____

36. After you deliver the child to the appropriate medical center, what are your responsibilities?

_____

_____

37. What history and physical examination should be performed on a child who is a victim of sexual abuse?

_____

_____

STUDENT SELF-ASSESSMENT

38. Which of the following is a component of an effective EMSC system?
   a. Access to care   **c.** Legislative committees
   b. Immunization programs   **d.** Medical direction

39. Which examination strategy can help reduce anxiety in school-age children?
   a. Allow them to take part in decisions about their care.
   b. Reassure them that they are not being punished.
   c. Let them play with equipment.
   d. Use deep breathing and relaxation techniques.

40. Which age group fears bodily injury and mutilation and interprets words literally?
   a. Adolescents   **c.** School-age children
   b. Preschoolers   **d.** Toddlers

41. You are called to care for a 6-month-old child who has respiratory distress. Which of the following would be the most likely cause of this complaint in this age group?
   a. Asthma
   b. Bronchiolitis
   c. Epiglottitis
   d. Foreign body airway obstruction

42. A great deal of the child's physical examination can be done by which step?
 a. Assessing the skin temperature and moisture.
 b. Auscultating the breath sounds.
 c. Observing the child's behavior.
 d. Palpating the central and distal pulses.
43. Which of the following is a sign of respiratory distress in a child?
 a. Crying
 b. Elevated temperature
 c. Flushed skin
 d. Head bobbing
44. Which of the following is a bacterial infection of the upper airway and subglottic trachea that occurs during or after croup?
 a. Bronchiolitis
 b. Epiglottitis
 c. Pneumonia
 d. Tracheitis
45. Which of the following may be indicated for the management of severe respiratory distress associated with bronchiolitis?
 a. Albuterol, 0.15 mg/kg by inhalation
 b. Atropine, 0.01 mg/kg by inhalation
 c. Epinephrine, 0.1 mg/kg subcutaneously
 d. Terbutaline, 0.2 mg/kg subcutaneously
46 Which of the following is an appropriate intervention for a child in whom epiglottitis is suspected?
 a. Lay the child supine on the mother's lap.
 b. See if the epiglottis is swollen.
 c. Infuse intravenous normal saline fluids at 20 mL/kg.
 d. Give humidified oxygen by mask.
47. Which drug may be administered to relieve respiratory distress in a child with bronchiolitis?
 a. Albuterol
 b. Alupent
 c. Epinephrine
 d. Diphenhydramine
48. Which of the following findings would be your first indication that an infant is developing dehydration and needs a fluid bolus?
 a. Decreasing blood pressure and poor skin turgor
 b. Flat fontanelle and warm skin
 c. Loss of appetite and nausea
 d. Very dry mucous membranes and tachycardia
49. A 20-kg child is lethargic and tachycardic and has dry mucous membranes after a 3-day history of "flu." Medical direction asks for a fluid bolus of normal saline. How much will you administer initially?
 a. 20 mL
 b. 100 mL
 c. 200 mL
 d. 400 mL
50. You are caring for a child who has fatigue, difficulty breathing, and peripheral edema. Crackles are audible in the bases of both lungs. Which illness do you suspect?
 a. Anaphylaxis
 b. Asthma
 c. Cardiomyopathy
 d. Pneumonia
51. A 5-year-old, 44-lb child is in ventricular fibrillation. Which is the correct *initial* energy level for defibrillation?
 a. 20 joules
 b. 40 joules
 c. 80 joules
 d. 88 joules
52. What is the maximum single dose of atropine that should be given to a 6-year-old child?
 a. 0.05 mg
 b. 0.01 mg
 c. 0.1 mg
 d. 0.5 mg
53. What is the correct sequence of interventions for a bradycardic, hypotensive child after the airway has been secured, an intravenous line has been established, and cardiopulmonary resuscitation has been initiated?
 a. Atropine and epinephrine
 b. Epinephrine and atropine
 c. Atropine only
 d. Epinephrine only
54. An infant who "wasn't acting right" has a heart rate of 230/min. He is awake but lethargic, and his skin is pale with delayed capillary refill. He has SVT, and vagal maneuvers do not convert the rhythm. Your partner has established vascular access. What is the initial treatment of choice for this child?
 a. Adenosine
 b. Digoxin
 c. Synchronized cardioversion
 d. Verapamil

55. Which of the following is *not* likely to cause seizures?
   a. CNS infection
   b. Metabolic abnormalities
   c. Prolonged dehydration
   d. Serious head trauma

56. After intravenous administration of diazepam, you should monitor closely for which of the following?
   a. Decreased pulse
   b. Increased blood pressure
   c. Respiratory depression
   d. Vomiting or nausea

57. Your 7-year-old patient is lethargic and has a blood pressure of 70/50 mm Hg and a pulse of 138/min. Respirations are 40/min and smell fruity. His mother says he has been losing weight and has had increased urination and thirst for several weeks. What condition should you consider?
   a. Head injury
   b. Hydrocarbon ingestion
   c. Hyperglycemia
   d. Hyperthermia

58. What life-threatening condition may be found in a child after ingestion of alcohol?
   a. Hypoglycemia
   b. Hypothermia
   c. Hypokalemia
   d. Hypocalcemia

59. What clinical finding may be present in a child who has ingested a large amount of aspirin?
   a. Bradycardia
   b. Hiccoughs
   c. Hypothermia
   d. Tachypnea

60. You are caring for a teenager who was "huffing" toluene. What effects could this produce?
   a. Pulmonary edema
   b. Renal failure
   c. Uncontrolled bleeding
   d. Visual disturbances

61. A 14-year-old is experiencing anxiety, tremors, and chest pain after smoking crack cocaine. His vital signs are BP, 180/100 mm Hg; P, 130/min; and R, 20/min. Which of the following drugs would *not* be indicated in the initial care of this child?
   a. Aspirin
   b. Epinephrine
   c. Lorazepam
   d. Nitroglycerin

62. A 4-year-old has taken 10 tricyclic antidepressant tablets. Her BP is 60 mm Hg by palpation; P is 130/min; and she is drowsy. Which intervention would be indicated to improve her cardiac output?
   a. Lidocaine (1 mg/kg)
   b. Dopamine (5mcg/kg/min)
   c. Oxygen (2 L/min)
   d. Sodium bicarbonate (1 mEq/kg)

63. Glucagon may be helpful as an antidote to an overdose of
   a. Beta blockers
   b. Calcium channel blockers
   c. Cocaine
   d. Tricyclic antidepressants

64. Which mechanism of injury accounts for the largest number of trauma deaths in children?
   a. Drowning
   b. Falls
   c. Fire
   d. Motor vehicle crashes

65. Which is a sign of increasing intracranial pressure unique to an infant?
   a. Bulging fontanelle
   b. Cheyne-Stokes respirations
   c. Hypotension
   d. Tachycardia

66. Why is the child more vulnerable to liver and splenic injuries?
   a. Those organs are larger in children under the age of 8 years.
   b. Mechanisms of injury in children are more likely to affect these areas.
   c. The abdominal musculature is minimal and does not protect these organs.
   d. These organs are more fragile in a child and injure more easily.

67. Which is a risk factor associated with a higher incidence of SIDS?
   a. High maternal or paternal age
   b. Rank of first in the birth order
   c. Premature birth and low birth weight
   d. Higher socioeconomic groups

68. Which of the following injuries should be considered the result of possible abuse?
   a. Any fractures in a child less than 5 years of age.
   b. Injuries localized to one area of the body.
   c. Bruises or burns in unusual patterns.
   d. Lacerations on the forehead of a toddler.

69. You are called to care for a 10-month-old child who "didn't wake up from his nap." He is unconscious and has vomited. What other physical findings may indicate abuse?
   a. Dirty diaper
   b. Increased respiratory rate
   c. Other children in the room
   d. Retinal hemorrhage

70. Respiratory distress is reported in a child who has a tracheostomy. The tube appears to be partly obstructed. Which of the following should be your first intervention?
   a. Intubate the child orally.
   b. Insert a tracheal dilator to enlarge the hole.
   c. Remove and replace the tracheostomy.
   d. Suction the tracheostomy.

71. A child is experiencing signs and symptoms of hypoxia while on a home ventilator. On arrival you should immediately perform which of the following?
   a. Begin ventilation with a bag-valve device.
   b. Check the connections on the machine and oxygen.
   c. Contact medical direction to help trouble-shoot.
   d. Request that the home health agency repair the ventilator.

72. A frantic mother calls you to check her son's central venous catheter because it is leaking. On arrival you note that the catheter is cracked and leaking. The child's condition is stable. What action should you take?
   a. Clamp the line
   b. Flush the line
   c. Remove the line
   d. Tape around the crack

73. A child with a gastric feeding tube develops respiratory distress. For what complication should you assess?
   a. Allergic reaction
   b. Aspiration
   c. Hypoglycemia
   d. Pulmonary embolism

WRAP IT UP

You are dispatched to a home for an "unresponsive child." As you pull up to the house, a woman runs toward your ambulance with a limp, 3-week-old infant in her arms. "He's had a runny nose and been listless today," she explains, "then he started shaking all over, and now I can't wake him." "Febrile seizure," you hear your partner mutter under his breath. In the ambulance, oxygen is administered as you begin to assess the baby. He is floppy and limp, but he grimaces, whines weakly, and opens his eyes when you rub his sternum, and his arms flex. You note rapid breathing, with retractions of the ribs. The skin is pale and cool and shows sluggish capillary refill (about 3 seconds). Vital signs are BP, 70/50 mm Hg; P, 168/min; and R, 40/min. Oxygen saturation is intermittently showing about 95%, and the infant's lungs are clear. A temperature shows 99° F (37° C) axilla, and the diaper is wet when you remove it. Pupils are 3 mm and react to light; skin turgor seems normal; ECG shows a rapid, narrow complex tachycardia; and blood glucose is 98 mg/dL. No other significant findings are noted on the detailed exam. The baby's mother says he was term with no birth complications and no illnesses or injuries that she is aware of. You are able to start a 22 g IV in the AC space TKO and continue to monitor the baby's condition, which is unchanged en route. In the ED a determination of sepsis is made, and the infant is admitted to the ICU.

1. Put a ✓ beside some possible causes of this baby's condition, based on your initial impression.
   a. _____ Abuse
   b. _____ Croup
   c. _____ Dehydration
   d. _____ Febrile seizure
   e. _____ Jaundice
   f. _____ Meningitis
   g. _____ Sepsis

2. Which aspects of the physical examination indicated that the baby was in distress?

_____

_____

3. What treatment should have been given to treat the heart rate/rhythm?
   a. Adenosine
   b. Diltiazem
   c. Vagal maneuvers
   d. None of the above

4. What was the baby's score on the Glasgow Coma Scale?

_____

5. What should you monitor most closely as you continue transport?

_____

_____

6. a. List at least three possible causes of seizure in a baby this age.

_____

_____

    b. What interventions would you consider if the child has another seizure?

_____

_____

7. Why should you assess the blood glucose level in this child even though you know that the onset of type 1 diabetes does not usually occur until later in childhood?

_____

_____

CHAPTER 44 ANSWERS

REVIEW QUESTIONS

1. f
2. e
3. h
4. a
5. g
6. c
7. b

(Questions 1-7: Objective 7)

8. a. Neonate
   b. Infant, toddler, and preschooler
   c. Neonate
   d. Infant and toddler
   e. Infant, toddler, and school-age child
   f. Young infant, infant, toddler, school-age child, and adolescent (sexual abuse)
   g. Preschooler and school-age child
   h. Adolescent

   (Objective 3)

9. Humidified oxygen by nonrebreather mask, position of comfort (to maximize respiratory efficiency), albuterol 0.01 to 0.03 mL (0.05 to 0.15 mg)/kg/dose to maximum of 0.5 mL/dose diluted in 2 mL of 0.9% NS, or epinephrine 0.01 mL/kg subcutaneous (1:1000), maximum 0.3 mL

   (Objective 5)

10. Tachycardia and anxiousness

    (Objective 5)

11. Repeat drugs, initiate IV, and continue to reassess.

    (Objective 5)

12. Patient will state improvement, respiratory rate will decrease, oxygen saturation will improve, use of accessory muscles will decrease, wheezing will diminish (inspiratory wheeze and then expiratory wheeze should dissipate), and heart rate may decrease (although possibly not because of the effects of beta agonists).

    (Objective 5)

13. Drooling, stridor, sudden onset of high fever, and dysphagia

    (Objective 5)

14. a. Take the patient into the cool night air or into a steam-filled bathroom. b. Allow the child to assume a position of comfort and administer high-flow oxygen (humidified) by whatever means is least threatening to the child.

    (Objective 5)

15. Moderate to severe dehydration

    (Objective 6)

16. Sinus tachycardia

    (Objective 6)

17. Open airway, ventilate with 100% oxygen; initiate lactated Ringer solution or normal saline intravenously (intraosseously if intravenous line cannot be established), and infuse initial fluid bolus of 20 mL/kg; reassess and repeat until perfusion improves.
(Objective 6)

18. BP, 82/44 mm Hg; P, 80 to 140/min; R, 30 to 40/min
(Objective 4)

19. Improved level of consciousness, skin color, and temperature
(Objective 6)

20. Sinus bradycardia, rate 30/min
(Objective 7)

21. Assess ABCs, secure airway, administer 100% oxygen using bag-mask device, perform chest compressions, start an intravenous or intraosseous line, assess vital signs, and if bradycardia continues, administer epinephrine 0.1 mL/kg (1:10,000) intravenously or intraosseously.
(Objective 7)

22. Infuse the medication intraosseously or administer epinephrine 0.1 mL/kg (1:1000) endotracheally diluted to 3 to 5 mL. NOTE: Endotracheal dose is 10 times greater than the intravenous dose.
(Objective 7)

23. Atropine 0.02 mg/kg intravenously to a maximum single dose of 0.5 mg (child) and 1 mg (adolescent); minimum dose: 0.1 mg
(Objective 7)

24. a. Defibrillate at 2 J/kg; give 5 cycles of CPR; defibrillate 4 J/kg; CPR; start IV; give epinephrine 0.01 mg/kg (1:10,000)$^{IV/IO}$ every 3-5 min; secure airway when possible; confirm placement; defibrillate 4 J/kg, CPR; consider amiodarone or magnesium sulfate
b. 0.01 mg/kg (0.1 mL/kg 1:10,000)
(Objective 7)

25. Description of seizure activity, vomiting during seizure, history of epilepsy or another major medical illness, other current medicines, potential for toxic ingestion, recent head injury, and complaints of headache or stiff neck
(Objective 8)

26. Maintain airway and breathing; monitor vital signs; cool child with tepid water and fanning; monitor electrocardiogram and oxygen saturation (if available); depending on patient's vital signs and level of consciousness, initiate lactated Ringer solution intravenously to keep vein open and obtain blood sample; assess blood sugar and treat if it is below 60 mg/dL.
(Objective 8)

27. a. Diazepam 1 mg every 2 to 5 minutes by slow IV; if intravenous or intraosseous infusion is not possible, administer medication rectally at higher dose (0.5 mg/kg).
b. Lorazepam 0.05 to 0.15 mg/kg/dose intramuscularly, intravenously, or intraosseously to maximum dose 4 mg (rectal dose: 0.1 to 0.2 mg/kg)
(Objective 8)

28. a. 50% dextrose 1 to 2 mL/kg/dose or 25% dextrose 2 to 4 mL/kg/dose intravenously
(Objective 9)

b. Presenting symptoms of mild hypoglycemia may be hunger, weakness, tachypnea, and tachycardia. Presenting symptoms of moderate hypoglycemia may be sweating, tremors, irritability, vomiting, mood swings, blurred vision, stomachache, headache, and dizziness.
(Objective 9)

29. a. Because a relatively small loss of blood can be devastating, fluid resuscitation should be anticipated for blood volume losses that would seem small in an adult.
b. This makes children susceptible to hypothermia. Measures should be used on the scene to maintain body warmth.
c. This leaves them little reserve for a stressed situation such as shock. Energy and oxygen requirements should be reduced to a minimum by assisting ventilations and using measures to decrease anxiety and promote body warmth.
d. Volume replacement with lactated Ringer solution or normal saline should be initiated at 20 mL/kg given rapidly and repeated if no response is seen. If good response is obtained, the fluids should be continued at a weight-related maintenance rate obtained from medical direction.
e. Intravenous access should first be attempted in a peripheral vein in the arms, hands, or feet. If access cannot be easily established and the patient's condition deteriorates, intraosseous infusion should be used.
(Objectives 6, 12)

30. Aspiration of marrow may rarely be obtained. The intravenous fluid will run freely with no evidence of infiltration.
(Objectives 4, 6)

31. Occurrence between midnight and 6 AM, male child under 6 months, occurrence between October and March, frothy sputum, wet diaper with stool, second child, and recent mild viral illness.
(Objective 13)

32. Document death as required by protocol and observe carefully for any obvious external signs of trauma.
(Objective 13)

33. Encourage your partner to verbalize, perhaps stating, "It's frightening to go on a call like this when you have a baby at home." Listen if he wants to talk; if he does not, check on him again in the morning. Initiate the CISD team, following local protocol (if available).
(Objective 13)

34. Protect the cervical spine while opening the airway; hyperventilate with 100% oxygen and consider intubation; verify perfusion with slow pulse; if it is inadequate, initiate cardiopulmonary resuscitation; en route to the hospital initiate an intravenous or intraosseous line and administer medicines if indicated.
(Objective 12)

35. The story does not match the physical findings or the child's developmental stage. An 8-month-old child is too young to ride a tricycle. A fall from a tricycle is unlikely to produce intracerebral bleeding. The child had no external signs of head trauma but had bruises at the shoulders that may suggest shaking. The child was dirty (this could be normal).
(Objective 14)

36. Report the suspected abuse to the receiving facility and to other authorities as indicated by local protocol. Carefully document all physical findings and statements made by the mother, using exact quotes if possible. This document is likely to be questioned in court if abuse is suspected.
(Objective 14)

37. Only enough data to address the immediate threats to the health of the sexually abused child should be elicited. The child should be made to feel safe and secure, and the detailed history and physical examination should be performed by child sexual abuse specialists if they are available in your area.
(Objective 14)

STUDENT SELF-ASSESSMENT

38. a. The other 11 components are system approach, education, data collection, quality improvement, injury prevention, prehospital care, emergency care, definitive care, rehabilitation, finance, and ongoing health care from birth to young adulthood.
(Objective 1)

39. b. Have them repeat things back to you in their words to be sure they understand. Give them choices when possible. Anticipate questions about the long-term effect of care, injuries, and so on.
(Objective 2)

40. b. Toddlers fear separation and loss of direction; school-age children fear bodily injury and mutilation but are less likely to interpret words literally.
(Objective 2)

41. b. Asthma is usually not diagnosed until a child is 3 to 5 years of age. Epiglottitis is more common in children 3 to 5 years of age. Foreign body airway obstruction would be unlikely in this age group because children usually do not eat solid food at this age.
(Objective 3)

42. c. Each component is important, but information about level of consciousness, color, respiratory effort, and muscle tone often can be assessed by observing children before touching them.
(Objective 4)

43. d. Other signs are use of accessory muscles, nasal flaring, tachypnea, bradypnea, irregular breathing pattern, grunting, and absent or abnormal breath sounds.
(Objective 4)

44. d. It may produce stridor and complete airway obstruction.
(Objective 5)

45. a. The correct dose of epinephrine is 0.01 mL/kg subcutaneously (1:1000), and the correct dose of terbutaline is 0.01 mg/kg of a 1 mg/mL solution subcutaneously.
(Objective 5)

46. d. The child should be permitted to assume a position of comfort, which typically is sitting up with the chin jutted forward to maximize airflow. Examination of the airway can produce obstruction and is contraindicated. Initiation of an intravenous infusion will not improve the child's condition and may cause the child to become agitated and cry, increasing the respiratory distress.
(Objective 5)

47. a. Albuterol can provide temporary symptomatic relief with limited side effects.
(Objective 5)

48. d. Fluid resuscitation should not be delayed until the blood pressure drops, or resuscitating the child may be difficult. The fontanelle likely would be flat and the skin cool.
(Objective 6)

49. d. The recommended fluid bolus is 20 mL/kg.
20 mL/kg × 20 kg = 400 mL
(Objective 6)

50. c. Crackles and edema are characteristics of congestive heart failure associated with cardiomyopathy.
(Objective 6)

51. b. 44 lb = 20 kg; initial defibrillation is 2 joules/kg; 2 joules × 20 kg = 40 joules
(Objective 7)

52. d. Atropine 0.02 mg/kg to a maximum dose of 0.5 mg in a child
(Objective 7)

53. b. Epinephrine is the drug of choice in patients with bradycardia with hemodynamic compromise, followed by atropine if no improvement results.
(Objective 7)

54. a. If his condition deteriorates, synchronized cardioversion may be considered.
(Objective 7)

55. c. Unless the dehydration produces severe electrolyte imbalance, it is much more likely to produce shock and death than seizures.
(Objective 8)

56. c. Ventilatory equipment should be available, and the respiratory rate and depth should be closely monitored. Pulse oximetry should be used if available.
(Objective 8)

57. c. Undiagnosed type 1 diabetes can manifest in this manner with severe hyperglycemia and ketoacidosis. This child is critical and needs urgent transport with airway management, oxygenation, and fluid resuscitation.
(Objective 9)

58. a. Hypoglycemia can lead to death if left uncorrected.
(Objective 11)

59. d. Tachypnea, GI irritation, hypoglycemia, cardiac dysrhythmias (ventricular), seizure, coma, coagulation defects, and death can occur from salicylate poisoning.
(Objective 11)

60. d. Changes in color perception, hallucinations, and blindness can occur, as well as other CNS and GI effects.
(Objective 11)

61. b. Epinephrine would be indicated only if cardiac arrest ensues. Aspirin may be given to counteract the platelet aggregation property of cocaine; lorazepam is administered to treat anxiety and/or seizures; and nitroglycerin is used as a vasodilator to treat chest pain.
(Objective 11)

62. d. Sodium bicarbonate may be given to improve myocardial contractility and cardiac output. Lidocaine would be given to treat ventricular dysrhythmias (if present). Normal saline 10 mL/kg bolus may be given to improve cardiac output. Oxygen should be given at high flow based on the patient's physical findings.
(Objective 11)

63. a. Other prehospital interventions may include oxygen administration, ventilatory support (if indicated), ECG monitoring, treatment for shock, epinephrine infusion, sodium bicarbonate, and calcium chloride (controversial).
(Objective 11)

64. d. Motor vehicle crashes are the leading cause of death and serious injury in children.
(Objective 12)

65. a. Other findings include hypertension, bradycardia, and Cheyne-Stokes respirations.
(Objective 12)

66. c
(Objective 12)

67. c. Low maternal/paternal age, low socioeconomic group, and rank of second or third in the birth order are associated with an increased incidence.
(Objective 13)

68. c. Fractures in a child less than 2 years of age should be cause for suspicion.
(Objective 14)

69. d. Retinal hemorrhage is a sign of a shaken baby.
(Objective 14)

70. d. If suctioning does not improve the situation, removing and replacing the tracheostomy may be necessary. If this is not possible or proves unsuccessful, oral intubation or intubation through the stoma may be necessary.
(Objective 15)

71. a. Correcting the hypoxia is the priority. The machine can be checked and fixed after the hypoxia has been corrected.
(Objective 15)

72. a. If the child develops signs of air embolism, position him on the left side with his head lowered and administer high-flow oxygen.
(Objective 15)

73. b. If the tube becomes dislodged, the feeding could be delivered to the lung, causing aspiration.
(Objective 15)

WRAP IT UP

1. a, c, f, g. The baby is too young for croup and for febrile seizures (and the temperature is not high). No evidence of yellow skin or eyes was noted, which would be apparent in jaundice. Dehydration is less likely because skin turgor is normal and the diaper is wet.
(Objective 3)

2. Decreased muscle tone and level of consciousness; labored, rapid breathing; rapid heart rate; skin color.
(Objective 4)

3. d. Based on the information available, this baby's rapid heart rate probably is sinus tachycardia. If the rhythm were SVT, the heart rate could be expected to be about 220/min. Treatment should focus on the underlying cause of the tachycardia.
(Objective 7)

4. Opens eyes to pain (2) + flexion to pain (4) + whines (3) = 9
(Objective 4)

5. Respiratory status should be monitored closely by observing rate, effort, Sao_2, skin color, heart rate, and, if available, end-tidal CO_2.
(Objective 4)

6. a. Head trauma, intracranial infection, metabolic disturbance, poisoning, epilepsy
b. Secure the airway, manage breathing, and consider administration of lorazepam or diazepam.
(Objective 8)

7. Blood glucose can be altered by other illnesses and should be assessed in any child with altered level of consciousness.
(Objective 4)

Geriatrics

READING ASSIGNMENT

Chapter 45, pages 1160-1183, in *Mosby's Paramedic Textbook,* ed. 3

OBJECTIVES

Upon completion of this chapter, the paramedic student will be able to:

1. Explain the physiology of the aging process as it relates to major body systems and homeostasis.
2. Describe general principles of assessment specific to older adults.
3. Describe the pathophysiology, assessment, and management of specific illnesses that affect selected body systems in the geriatric patient.
4. Identify specific problems with sensations experienced by some geriatric patients.
5. Discuss effects of drug toxicity and alcoholism in the older adult.
6. Identify factors that contribute to environmental emergencies in the geriatric patient.
7. Discuss prehospital assessment and management of depression and suicide in the older adult.
8. Describe epidemiology, assessment, and management of trauma in the geriatric patient.
9. Identify characteristics of elder abuse.

SUMMARY

- The aging process proceeds at different rates in different persons. Respiratory function in the older adult generally is compromised. This is a result of changes in pulmonary physiology that go along with the aging process. Cardiac function also declines with age. This is a result of normal physiological changes and the high incidence of coronary artery disease. Renal blood flow falls an average of 50% between 30 and 80 years of age. A gradual decrease in neurons, decreased cerebral blood flow, and changes in the location and amounts of specific neurotransmitters probably contribute to changes in the CNS. As the body ages, muscles shrink, muscles and ligaments calcify, and the intervertebral disks become thin. Other physiological changes that occur with aging include changes in body mass and total body water, a decreased ability to maintain internal homeostasis, a decrease in the function of immunological mechanisms, nutritional disorders, and decreases in hearing and visual acuity.
- Normal changes with aging and existing illnesses may make evaluation of an ill or injured geriatric patient a challenge.
- Pneumonia is a leading cause of death in the geriatric age group. It often is fatal in frail adults. Chronic obstructive pulmonary disease (COPD) is a common finding in the geriatric patient who has a history of smoking. The disease usually is associated with various other diseases that result in reduced expiratory airflow. Pulmonary embolism is a life-threatening cause of dyspnea. Pulmonary embolism is associated with venous stasis, heart failure, COPD, malignancy, and immobilization. All of these are common in older adults.
- A lack of the typical chest pain can cause MI to go unrecognized in the geriatric patient. Heart failure is more frequent in geriatric patients and has a larger incidence of noncardiac causes. The most common cause of

dysrhythmias in the geriatric patient is hypertensive heart disease. Abdominal aortic aneurysm affects 2% to 4% of the U.S. population over 50 years of age. This aneurysm is most prevalent between 60 and 70 years of age. The incidence of hypertension in the geriatric patient increases when atherosclerosis is present.

- Risk factors for cerebral vascular disease in the older adult include smoking, hypertension, diabetes, atherosclerosis, hyperlipidemia, polycythemia, and heart disease.
- Delirium is an abrupt disorientation of time and place. Delirium is commonly a result of physical illness.
- Dementia is a slow, progressive loss of awareness of time and place. It usually involves an inability to learn new things or remember recent events. This condition often is a result of brain disease. Alzheimer's disease is the most common cause of dementia. Alzheimer's disease is a condition in which nerve cells in the cerebral cortex die and the brain substance shrinks.
- Parkinson's disease is a brain disorder. It causes muscle tremor, stiffness, and weakness.
- About 20% of older adults have diabetes. Almost 40% have some impaired glucose tolerance. Hyperglycemic hyperosmolar nonketotic coma is a serious complication of elderly type 2 diabetic patients. It has a mortality rate of 20% to 50%. Thyroid disease is more common in geriatric patients. It may not present in the classic manner.
- Gastrointestinal bleeding most often affects patients between 60 and 90 years of age. It has a mortality rate of about 10%. Bowel obstruction generally occurs in patients with prior abdominal surgeries or hernias. It also occurs in those with colonic cancer. Some geriatric patients may have problems with continence or with elimination as well.
- Aging results in a gradual decrease in epidermal cellular turnover. It also results in loss of deep and dermal vessels. Capillary circulation leads to changes in thermal regulation and skin-related complications.
- Osteoarthritis is a common form of arthritis in geriatric patients. It results from cartilage loss and wear and tear on the joints. The loss in bone density from osteoporosis causes bones to become brittle. These bones may fracture easily.
- As persons age, they may experience problems with vision, hearing, and speech.
- Geriatric patients are at an increased risk for adverse drug reactions. This is due to age-related changes in body makeup and drug distribution. It also is the result of metabolism and excretion. Moreover, the risk for adverse drug reactions often stems from multiple prescribed drugs. Alcohol abuse is a common problem in geriatric patients.
- The geriatric patient may develop hypothermia while indoors. This may be the result of cold surroundings and/or an illness that alters heat production or conservation. Hyperthermia most likely results from exposure to high temperatures that continue for several days.
- Depression is common in geriatric patients. It can result from physiological and psychological causes. The rate of completed suicides for geriatric patients is higher than that of the general population.
- One third of traumatic deaths in persons 65 to 74 years of age result from vehicular trauma. Twenty-five percent result from falls. In those older than 80 years of age, falls account for 50% of injury-related deaths. The risk of fatality from multiple trauma is estimated to be 3 times greater at 70 years of age than at 20 years of age.
- Elder abuse is classified as physical abuse, psychological abuse, financial or material abuse, and neglect.

REVIEW QUESTIONS

1. An 85-year-old woman falls down an escalator at a department store. Explain how age-related changes in each of the following areas increase her risk of suffering a traumatic injury or influence her body's response to a major injury.

   a. Respiratory system:

   _____

   _____

   b. Cardiovascular system:

   _____

   _____

c. Renal system:

_____

_____

d. Musculoskeletal system:

_____

_____

e. Thermoregulation:

_____

_____

2. A woman calls you to the home of her 70-year-old father, who has fallen. He says he is just fine. On your arrival, she states that he has a history of diabetes, a heart attack, heart failure, and lung disease. His home medications include Lanoxin, insulin, furosemide, Slow-K, Theo-Dur, and a number of vitamins and laxatives. He is on oxygen at 2 L/min by nasal cannula.

   a. What factors will make it difficult to assess and determine the nature of his acute problem?

_____

_____

_____

_____

   b. List eight possible causes of his fall.
   a.   e.
   b.   f.
   c.   g.
   d.   h.

Questions 3 to 5 pertain to the following case study:

   A 70-year-old man calls you to his home complaining of dyspnea and weakness. He has no underlying pulmonary problems. His ECG is shown in Fig. 45-1.

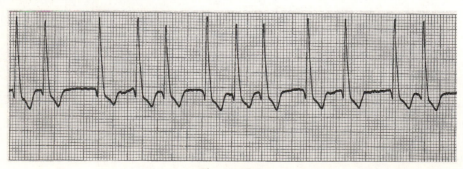

Figure 45-1

3. Why should you assess the appropriate history and physical examination for myocardial infarction and pulmonary embolism on this patient?

_____

4. What is your interpretation of the ECG rhythm?

_____

5. List two complications associated with this dysrhythmia.

   a.

   b.

6. A 76-year-old woman complains of diffuse abdominal pain. Identify four conditions that can cause this symptom.

   a.

   b.

   c.

   d.

7. Briefly describe the following characteristics of delirium:

   a. Onset:

_____

   b. Duration:

_____

   c. Metabolic causes:

_____

8. List four reversible causes of dementia.

   a.   **c.**

   b.   **d.**

Questions 9 to 11 pertain to the following case study:

   An 80-year-old man experiences a syncopal episode in church. He is conscious but pale and diaphoretic. His blood pressure is 80/50 mm Hg. His ECG is shown in Fig. 45-2.

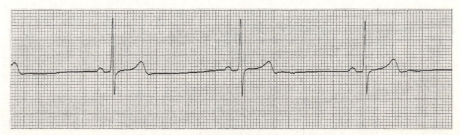

Figure 45-2

9. What is your interpretation of the rhythm?

_____

10. a. State the dose and route of administration of the drug used to treat this rhythm.

_____

b. What other intervention should be considered if drug therapy is unsuccessful?

_____

11. List two possible causes of the signs and symptoms this patient is experiencing.
a.
b.

Questions 12 to 15 pertain to the following case study:

On arrival at a call for "difficulty breathing," you find a 69-year-old woman complaining of dyspnea and chills. She states that she has been ill with a mild cough and weakness for approximately 1 week. Her skin is cold and clammy. Vital signs are BP, 108/70 mm Hg; P, 135/min; and R, 30/min. Breath sounds in the right base are diminished with scattered crackles. Her ECG is shown in Fig. 45-3.

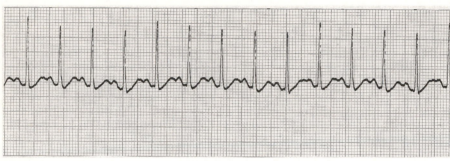

Figure 45-3

12. Identify the rhythm.

_____

13. What illness do you suspect?

_____

14. Should you use synchronized cardioversion or adenosine to treat the rhythm?

_____

15. What other interventions would be indicated for this patient?

_____

_____

16. An older man with a history of chronic lung disease is being transferred to another hospital. He has applied a Venturi mask that supplies oxygen at 24%. His vital signs are within normal limits. His ECG tracing is shown in Fig. 45-4.

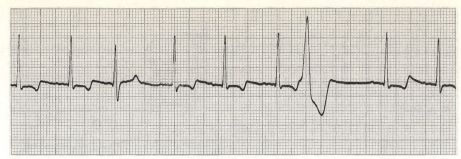

Figure 45-4

a. Identify the rhythm strip.

_____

b. What interventions are indicated with this rhythm?

_____

c. For what signs and symptoms of acute decompensation of COPD will you observe?

_____

17. An older patient who had a syncopal episode is now awake and has the following vital signs: BP, 108/70 mm Hg; P, 50/min; and R, 18/min and unlabored. The lungs are clear. The ECG is shown in Fig. 45-5.

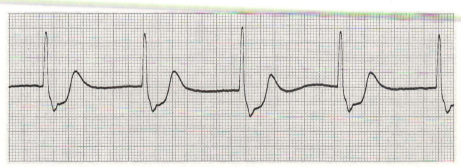

Figure 45-5

a. Identify the rhythm strip.

_____

b. After oxygen has been administered and intravenous therapy started, what interventions should be performed en route to the medical center?

_____

c. What age-related changes predispose this patient to developing this rhythm?

_____

Questions 18 to 21 refer to the following case study:

The family of a 72-year-old man states that he suddenly became confused and disoriented to time and place over the past few hours. His vital signs are BP, 168/110 mm Hg; P, 100/min; and R, 20/min. His ECG is shown in Fig. 45-6.

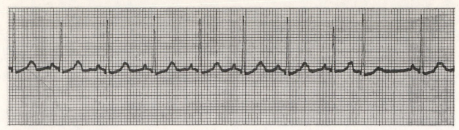

Figure 45-6

18. Is he likely experiencing dementia or delirium?

_____

19. Identify the rhythm strip.

_____

20. Are his symptoms related to his ECG tracing?

_____

21. List two factors that could cause this change in behavior.
    a.

    b.

Questions 22 and 23 refer to the following case study:

An 80-year-old woman complains of dizziness and shortness of breath. Her vital signs are BP, 82/50 mm Hg; P, 50/min; and R, 24/min. Her ECG tracing is shown in Fig. 45-7.

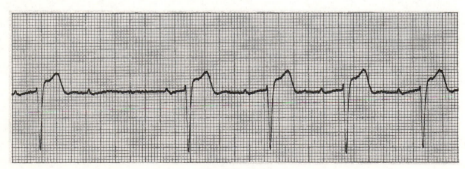

Figure 45-7

22. Identify the rhythm strip.

_____

23. **a.** What illness may be causing her signs and symptoms?

_____

b. List prehospital interventions that you will consider for this patient.

_____

24. A 94-year-old woman who was found in her apartment is confused and difficult to arouse. You note that it feels very cold inside, and her temperature is 95° F (35° C). List at least nine reasons (physiological, social, or medical) that she is at risk for hypothermia.

_____

_____

_____

25. Adverse drug reactions are common in older adults. For each of the following drugs or drug groups, list two signs or symptoms associated with overdose or adverse effects.

   a. Anticoagulants:

_____

_____

   b. Diuretics:

_____

_____

   c. Digitalis:

_____

_____

   d. Tricyclic antidepressants:

_____

_____

   e. Sedative-hypnotic drugs:

_____

_____

   f. Propranolol:

_____

_____

   g. Theophylline:

_____

_____

h. Quinidine:

_____

_____

Questions 26 to 29 refer to the following case study:

You are on the scene of a single-car accident in which a compact car struck a bridge abutment at high speed. The driver, an anxious 75-year-old man, complains of mild abdominal discomfort. Vital signs are BP, 90/70 mm Hg; P, 70/min; and R, 24/min and somewhat labored. His skin is pale and clammy, and his nail beds are dusky.

26. What vital sign assessment does *not* fit with this man's clinical picture?

_____

27. What aspect of his history may explain this discrepancy?

_____

28. Because he has just mild abdominal pain, should you be concerned?

_____

29. What prehospital treatment should be given after the cervical spine has been appropriately immobilized?

_____

_____

30. You are at the home of an older patient who appears dehydrated and very dirty. You note large ecchymotic areas on the back and hips. The daughter, who lives with the patient, says these were caused by a fall.

a. If you suspect elder abuse, what should you do?

_____

_____

b. Does the caregiver have any characteristics of an elder abuser?

_____

STUDENT SELF-ASSESSMENT

31. Alterations in lung and chest wall compliance in the older adult result in a decrease in which of the following?
  a. Alveolar diameter
  b. Residual volume
  c. Total lung capacity
  d. Vital capacity

32. Humpback posture that develops as a result of osteoporosis is known by which of the following terms?
  a. Kyphosis
  b. Lordosis
  c. Osteoarthritis
  d. Scoliosis

33. An elderly patient awoke with a sudden onset of dyspnea. The patient has crackles and wheezes. He had an MI 3 years ago and has no other history. Vital signs are BP, 170/94 mm Hg; P, 124/min; R, 28/min; and SaO_2, 90% on room air. You administer oxygen. What drug is indicated next?
  a. Albuterol
  b. Aspirin
  c. Epinephrine
  d. Furosemide

34. An elderly patient, whose only past medical history is metastatic breast cancer, has been on bed rest. She suddenly develops dyspnea and tachycardia. Which of the following would be the *least* likely cause of her symptoms?
    a. Chronic obstructive pulmonary disease
    b. Myocardial infarction
    c. Pneumonia
    d. Pulmonary embolus

35. Which of the following are possible causes of dementia?
    a. Alzheimer disease   c. Hyperglycemia
    b. Epilepsy   d. Pneumonia

36. Which illness causes trembling, a rigid posture, slow movement, and a shuffling, unbalanced walk?
    a. Alzheimer disease   c. Dementia
    b. Delirium   d. Parkinson disease

37. Administration of which of the following would be a critical prehospital intervention for an unconscious diabetic patient suffering from hyperglycemic hyperosmolar nonketotic coma?
    a. Dextrose   c. IV fluids
    b. Glucagon   d. Sodium bicarbonate

38. Which of the following is a consequence of thyroid dysfunction that might lead to a call for EMS?
    a. Altered mental status   c. Diarrhea
    b. Bradycardia   d. Weight gain

39. Your elderly male patient complains that he is unable to urinate. What condition should you inquire about specifically when obtaining his history?
    a. Constipation   c. Kidney stones
    b. Epididymitis   d. Prostate enlargement

40. Pressure ulcers are caused by which of the following?
    a. Burns   c. Infection
    b. Tissue hypoxia   d. Tears of the tissue

41. Which eye condition causes damage to the optic nerve and can result in blindness if untreated?
    a. Cataracts   c. Corneal abrasion
    b. Conjunctivitis   d. Glaucoma

42. A patient is being treated for Parkinson disease. What sign, if present, might you attribute to drug toxicity?
    a. Altered vision   c. Paresthesias
    b. Hypokalemia   d. Tardive dyskinesia

43. Which of the following medications may increase the elderly patient's risk of hyperthermia?
    a. Amitriptyline (Elavil)   c. Cimetidine (Tagamet)
    b. Aspirin   d. Coumadin

44. Which of the following may be a physiological cause of depression in an elderly patient?
    a. Hyperglycemia   c. Hyponatremia
    b. Hypertension   d. Hypothermia

45. What is the most common psychiatric disorder in older adults?
    a. Bipolar disorder   c. Hysteria
    b. Depression   d. Schizophrenia

46. Why might the symptoms of increased intracranial pressure be delayed in an older patient?
    a. Altered blood-brain barrier   c. Decreased cerebral blood flow
    b. Cerebral atrophy   d. Fragile bridging veins

47. Which of the following is most often fractured in falls by older adults?
    a. Ankle   c. Hip
    b. Clavicle   d. Wrist

48. Which of the following home medications increases the older person's risk of falling?
    a. Alprazolam   c. Hydrochlorothiazide
    b. Digoxin   d. Dipyridamole

WRAP IT UP

Your partner groans as your dispatcher sends you to a familiar address for a "person down with possible forcible entry." The 80-year-old patient is well known because of her frequent 9-1-1 calls to "assist the invalid" when she misses her walker and slides to the floor. Since her stroke 3 months ago, she has been calling 9-1-1 several times a week despite attempts to identify appropriate social services. Her home is locked up tight, and you can see that she is sitting on the floor, but she oddly won't acknowledge the knocking on the window. The fire captain quickly breaks out a pane of glass on a rear door and unlocks it, permitting you to enter her steamy home. "Mabel, what's going on today?" you call out. As you approach her, you recognize that something is wrong; instead of her typical crooked smile, she is staring blankly ahead, showing no sign she recognizes you. Her skin color isn't right either; she looks pale and sweaty, and her usually neatly coifed hair is disheveled and dirty. As you grasp her wrist, you feel her rapid, irregular pulse and note that her breathing seems labored and fast. The oxygen saturation monitor is registering only 89%, much lower than her normal reading, and you can hear some basilar crackles when you listen to her lungs. A quick scan of her body reveals no obvious injuries. "Mabel, what's wrong? Are you in pain? Did you fall?" you ask. She looks blankly at you, and the usually polite and articulate woman mumbles some obscenities and pushes you away. You administer oxygen and assess her vital signs, which are BP, 102/60 mm Hg; P, 124/min; and R, 24/min. Her pupils are 3 mm, equal, and reactive to light. By then your partner has the cot at her side, and you guide her onto it and secure the straps. In the ambulance her ECG shows atrial fibrillation, and a blood sugar reading of 78 mg/dL is obtained as you start her IV. As you look through her sack of familiar medicines (furosemide, Persantine, aspirin, Glucophage, Lipitor, Lanoxin, Paxil), you realize that some of them are empty and, based on the date they were prescribed, they should not be. Her Sao_2 is improving on oxygen, and her vital signs are unchanged, but she is still muttering obscenities. You look more carefully head to toe to see if you've missed something on your initial exam, but you find nothing additional. As you sit writing your report at the hospital, you recall your last visit, 3 days ago, and try to think of anything unusual that may have occurred, but nothing seemed out of place.

1. Based on the information given, list five chronic problems this patient is likely to have.
    a.

    b.

    c.

    d.

    e.

2. Place a ✓ beside some possible causes for this patient's altered level of consciousness.

    a. _____ Delirium   f. _____ Hypoxia

    b. _____ Dementia   g. _____ Hypoglycemia

    c. _____ Head injury   h. _____ Overdose

    d. _____ Hyperthermia   i. _____ Sepsis

    e. _____ Depression   j. _____ Stroke

3. a. Would this patient be a candidate for fibrinolytic therapy if an acute stroke were diagnosed? Yes/No

    b. Explain your answer: _____

    _____

    _____

4. Which of the patient's social or medical conditions would *not* put her at high risk for complications related to her diabetes?
    a. Aspirin use
    b. Decreased ability to care for herself
    c. Living alone
    d. Other illnesses

5. If you think she has taken an overdose, what problems should you anticipate during transport based on your knowledge of her prescription drugs.

CHAPTER 45 ANSWERS

REVIEW QUESTIONS

1. a. Because the baseline Pao_2 is lower, the body is less able to compensate if chest trauma is sustained or if the patient is hypoxic because of trauma (e.g., inhalation injury). The chest wall is less elastic and more susceptible to injury.

    b. Myocardial contusion can cause pump failure stemming from poor cardiac reserve. Decreased ability to increase the heart rate can result in a decreased ability to compensate for shock, and dysrhythmias can cause syncope and precipitate a fall.

    c. Renal blood flow is decreased, therefore a sudden traumatic event that causes shock and hypoperfusion to the kidneys can precipitate the onset of renal failure; decreased renal function can make an older adult more susceptible to toxic drug effects, leading to CNS depression, disturbances in balance, hypotension, and dysrhythmias, all of which can increase the risk of falls.

    d. Kyphosis may alter balance and predispose a person to falls, and osteoporosis increases the incidence of fractures after falls.

    e. Advancing age can result in decreased peripheral vasoconstriction, a lowered metabolic rate, and poor peripheral circulation and can impair the body's ability to regulate temperature effectively, especially during stressful events such as traumatic injury. Hypothermia may occur rapidly.
    (Objective 1)

2. a. His multiple illnesses and drugs make it difficult to assess for new onset of signs or symptoms. Diabetes: Impairs pain perception and retards healing. Heart attack and heart failure: Cardiac output may be impaired from chronic conditions, and dysrhythmias may be chronic. Lung disease: Patient's baseline must be determined. Cyanosis, increased respiratory rate, and abnormal lung sounds may be chronic. Lanoxin: Therapeutic effects slow heart rate; patient may not become tachycardic in response to trauma, and toxic effects may cause dysrhythmias. Insulin: Excessive amounts may cause hypoglycemia and produce CNS impairment. Furosemide: Diuretics may cause an electrolyte imbalance that can affect muscle strength and may precipitate dysrhythmias that can cause syncope and falls. His baseline SaO_2 may be lower than normal.
    (Objective 2)

    b. Dysrhythmias, visual impairment, neurological disabilities, arthritis, changes in gait, postural hypotension, syncope, cerebrovascular accident or transient ischemic attack, medications, slippery surfaces, loose rugs, objects on floors, poor lighting, pets, low beds or toilet seats, defective walking equipment, and lack of handrails on stairs.
    (Objective 8)

3. In an older adult, dyspnea and weakness may be the only presenting history for myocardial infarction. Carefully obtain a patient history; perform a physical examination, including a 12-lead ECG; and treat with a high index of suspicion for myocardial infarction (these signs and symptoms also accompany pulmonary embolus).
    (Objective 3)

4. Atrial fibrillation
    (Objective 3)

5. Cerebrovascular accident and pulmonary embolism
    (Objective 3)

6. Cholecystitis, colonic diverticular disease, appendicitis, aortic abdominal aneurysm, mesenteric artery occlusion, and mesenteric vein thrombosis
    (Objective 2)

7. a. Rapid

b. Variable: It is usually self-limited and can be corrected quickly when the cause is identified.

c. Electrolyte imbalance, hypoglycemia, hyperglycemia, acid-base imbalance, hypoxia, vital organ failure, and Wernicke encephalopathy

(Objective 3)

8. Hypothyroidism, Cushing syndrome, vitamin deficiencies, and hydrocephalus

(Objective 3)

9. Sinus bradycardia, rate 30/min

(Objective 3)

10. a. Atropine 0.5 IV

(Objective 3)

b. Transcutaneous pacing

(Objective 3)

11. Acute myocardial infarction, drug toxicity, or vagal response

(Objective 3)

12. Sinus tachycardia

(Objective 3)

13. Bacterial pneumonia or pulmonary embolus

(Objective 3)

14. No to both; you must treat the patient and her underlying problem.

(Objective 3)

15. Administer high-flow oxygen via nonrebreather mask, initiate intravenous therapy, and monitor the patient's response and vital signs closely en route.

(Objective 3)

16. a. Normal sinus rhythm with a premature atrial contraction and a premature ventricular contraction

b. Continue to monitor the patient and the electrocardiographic rhythm.

c. Assess for limited airflow, increased work of breathing, dyspnea, hypoxemia, or hemodynamic compromise. Measure for excessive increases in $EtCO_2$ if available.

(Objective 3)

17. a. Junctional rhythm

b. Observe the patient for any signs of hemodynamic compromise related to the slow rhythm (monitor vital signs and electrocardiogram). Consider drug administration or pacing if unstable.

c. Functional cells are lost in the SA and AV nodes during aging, which contributes to dysrhythmias.

(Objectives 2, 3)

18. Delirium (sudden onset)

(Objective 3)

19. Normal sinus rhythm with a premature atrial contraction

(Objective 3)

20. There is no reason for this ECG to cause these symptoms.

(Objective 3)

21. Intoxication or poisoning, withdrawal from drugs, metabolic disturbances, infectious processes, CNS trauma, and stroke.
(Objective 3)

22. Second-degree heart block Mobitz type II
(Objective 3)

23. a. Myocardial infarction is the most likely cause.
(Objective 3)

b. Administer high-concentration oxygen. Continue assessment to include breath sounds and observe for signs of congestive heart failure; perform head to toe survey. Initiate IV therapy at a TKO rate. Consider atropine 0.5 mg IV. Prepare to apply transcutaneous pacing. Consult with medical direction regarding administration of sedation (with caution because of dyspnea and hypotension). Provide rapid transport for definitive cardiac care. Perform a 12-lead ECG if available.
(Objective 3)

24. Decreased ability to sense changes in ambient temperature, less total body water to store heat, reduced likelihood of becoming tachycardic to compensate for cold stress, decreased ability to shiver, inability to pay utilities for heat, insufficient insulation, malnutrition, arthritis, drug overdose, hepatic failure, hypoglycemia, infection, Parkinson disease, stroke, thyroid disease, and uremia.
(Objective 6)

25. a. Bleeding problems, increased hemorrhage from trauma, multiple contusions, and allergic reactions.
b. Electrolyte abnormalities (sodium and potassium) and dehydration.
c. Influenza-like symptoms, multiple dysrhythmias, and bradycardia.
d. Dry mouth, tachycardia, ventricular dysrhythmias, seizures, and impaired level of consciousness.
e. Impaired perception (increased risk of falls) and decreased level of consciousness with respiratory depression.
f. Decreased heart rate (excessive), bronchoconstriction, and mood alteration.
g. Tachycardia, dysrhythmias, and CNS stimulation.
h. Dysrhythmias and clotting abnormalities.
(Objective 5)

26. His heart rate is slow relative to the rest of his clinical picture (everything else indicates impending shock or hypoxia).
(Objective 8)

27. He may have a pacemaker or may be taking medications (e.g., digitalis or beta blockers) that prevent his heart rate from becoming tachycardic in response to a decrease in cardiac output.
(Objective 8)

28. Yes, abdominal injuries are frequently lethal in older adults. His perception of pain may be impaired, and this situation could deteriorate quickly, especially with signs of shock.
(Objective 8)

29. Ensure a patent airway; deliver high-flow oxygen by nonrebreather mask; apply pneumatic antishock garments (if indicated by local protocol); en route to a trauma center, start two large-bore intravenous lines and administer small fluid challenges in consultation with medical direction; frequently monitor vital signs and lung sounds (for increased rales [crackles]) to make sure the patient is not developing a volume overload.
(Objective 8)

30. a. Follow local protocols and report to appropriate authority (e.g., local law enforcement, abuse hotline, medical direction) as indicated; report findings to receiving hospital and document findings thoroughly on prehospital run report.
b. Yes, daughter lives with parent.
(Objective 9)

31. d. Total lung capacity remains unchanged because the loss of chest wall compliance balances the weakened respiratory muscles. The residual volume increases as a result of variable increases in alveolar diameter and the tendency for distal airways to collapse on expiration.
(Objective 1)

32. a. *Lordosis* is the normal S curve of the spine. *Osteolysis* is degeneration of bone. *Scoliosis* is lateral curvature of the spine, usually found in childhood.
(Objective 3)

33. d. The patient has no history of COPD. His history and clinical presentation point to left-sided heart failure. Furosemide would be the drug of choice.
(Objective 3)

34. a. The risk of myocardial infarction increases in postmenopausal women. Myocardial infarction may manifest without pain in elderly patients. Pneumonia is a complication seen in immunocompromised patients or those who have other chronic illnesses, and it may have an atypical presentation in older adults. Pulmonary embolus is a higher risk in patients with cancer and in bedridden patients.
(Objective 3)

35. a. The other conditions may cause delirium.
(Objective 3)

36. d. These signs can be reduced or eliminated with drug therapy.
(Objective 3)

37. c. This condition results from excessive glucose in the blood and causes serious dehydration; IV fluids are indicated in the prehospital setting to treat the severe dehydration. Sodium bicarbonate may be indicated after arterial blood gas analysis or if the patient experiences cardiac arrest.
(Objective 3)

38. a. Thyroid dysfunction may also cause tachydysrhythmias, constipation, weight loss, anemia, or muscu-loskeletal complaints.
(Objective 3)

39. d. Prostate enlargement is a cause of dysuria commonly found in this age group.
(Objective 3)

40. b. The ulcers often become infected because of the poor blood supply to the area.
(Objective 3)

41. d. *Cataracts* are a loss in transparency of the lens of the eye. *Conjunctivitis* is an inflammation of the conjunctiva of the eye. *Corneal abrasion* is a scraping-off of the outer layer of the cornea.
(Objective 4)

42. d. Some of the older drugs prescribed for patients with Parkinson disease may produce this reaction.
(Objective 5)

43. a. Cyclic antidepressants, antidysrhythmics, and beta blockers may increase the risk of hyperthermia.
(Objective 6)

44. c. This may result from diuretic or other drug therapy and can have a very slow onset.
(Objective 7)

45. b. It may be caused by physiological or psychological factors.
(Objective 7)

46. b. The venous blood of a subdural hematoma takes longer to fill the larger space between the skull and the brain.
(Objective 8)

47. c
(Objective 8)

48. a. Sedative-hypnotic drugs put older patients at greater risk for falls.
(Objective 8)

WRAP IT UP

1. Stroke (in history and Coumadin); congestive heart failure (Lanoxin, furosemide); atrial fibrillation (Lanoxin); type 2 diabetes (Glucophage); high cholesterol (Lipitor); depression or anxiety (Paxil).
(Objectives 2, 3)

2. a (sudden onset of confusion); c (altered level of consciousness); d (house is hot); e (age and Paxil); f (Sao$_2$ and crackles); h (missing pills); i (elders are at high risk; crackles in lungs); j (prior stroke, atrial fibrillation)
(Objective 3)

3. a. No
b. Unknown time of onset of symptoms (must be less than 3 hours)
(Objective 2)

4. a. All of the other factors listed increase her risk of having poorly controlled diabetes.
(Objective 3)

5. Possibility for bleeding (Coumadin, aspirin); acidosis (aspirin); hypoglycemia (Glucophage); bradycardia or dysrhythmias (Lanoxin); depressed respirations (Paxil).
(Objective 2)

CHAPTER
46

Abuse and Neglect

READING ASSIGNMENT
Chapter 46, pages 1184-1195, in *Mosby's Paramedic Textbook,* ed. 3

OBJECTIVES
Upon completion of this chapter, the paramedic student will be able to do the following:
1. Define battering.
2. Describe the characteristics of abusive relationships.
3. Outline findings that indicate a battered patient.
4. Describe prehospital considerations when responding to and caring for battered patients.
5. Identify types of elder abuse.
6. Discuss legal considerations related to elder abuse.
7. Describe characteristics of abused children and their abusers.
8. Outline the physical examination of the abused child.
9. Describe the characteristics of sexual assault.
10. Outline prehospital patient care considerations for the patient who has been sexually assaulted.

SUMMARY
- Battering is the establishment of control and fear in a relationship through violence and other forms of abuse.
- Domestic violence follows a cycle of three phases. Phase one involves arguing and verbal abuse. Phase two progresses to physical and sexual abuse. Phase three consists of denial and apologies. Certain personality traits may predispose a person to abusive relationships.
- The paramedic may have a hard time identifying the battered patient. Injuries from domestic violence often involve contusions and lacerations of the face, neck, head, breast, and abdomen.
- The paramedic must ensure scene and personal safety in domestic violence events. The paramedic should manage physical injuries according to standard protocols. The paramedic should direct special attention toward the emotional needs of the victim as well.
- Elder abuse is classified into four categories: physical abuse, psychological abuse, financial or material abuse, and neglect.
- All 50 states have elder abuse statutes. Reporting of suspected elder abuse also is mandatory under law in most states.
- Most child abusers are the child's parents (77%). Eleven percent are other relatives of the victim. Abused children often exhibit behavior that provides key clues about abuse and neglect. The paramedic should observe carefully the child under 6 years of age who is passive or the child over 6 years of age who is aggressive.
- If the child volunteers the history of the event without hesitation and matches the history that the parent provides (and the history is suitable for the injury), child abuse is unlikely.

- Injuries may include soft tissue injuries, fractures, head injuries, and abdominal injuries.
- *Sexual assault* generally refers to any genital, anal, oral, or manual penetration of the victim's body by way of force and without the victim's consent. The highest incidence of sexual assault occurs in women who live alone in isolated areas.
- After managing all threats to life, the paramedic should provide emotional support to the victim. The paramedic should deliver care in a way that preserves evidence.

REVIEW QUESTIONS

Questions 1 to 5 pertain to the following case study:

> You are called to a private residence by a woman who says her husband "beat her up." On arrival, you hear loud shouting coming from the house.

1. What measures should be taken before entering the home?

_____

_____

2. When you begin your examination, what measures should you take to enhance safety and allow for a better history and examination?

_____

_____

The patient's vital signs are stable. She has several bruises around her face, but she is alert and oriented and does not want further care. You contact medical direction, and despite both your and their recommendations, the patient refuses transport.

3. What reasons might someone have for staying with an abusive partner?

_____

_____

4. If you tell her to move out immediately, would that be the safest course of action without planning on her part? Why or why not?

_____

_____

5. What advice and resources can you offer her before you leave the scene?

_____

_____

Questions 6 to 8 refer to the following case study:

> You are dispatched to a residence in a middle-class neighborhood for an "accidental injury." On arrival, you find an 80-year-old widow with a tender, swollen, ecchymotic left upper arm. She is awake and alert but very withdrawn. You note multiple other bruises on both arms and her back that are yellow, brown, and green. Her 60-year-old daughter lives with her and says that her mother tripped and fell. When you ask the patient to confirm this, she nods slowly; when you ask about the old bruises, she just shrugs. She has a history of heart disease, emphysema, and Type 2 diabetes. Her vital signs are normal.

6. What characteristics typical of an "average" victim of elder abuse does this woman have?

_____

7. What physical findings suggest possible abuse?

_____

8. What action should you take if you suspect abuse on this call?

_____

_____

_____

Questions 9 to 12 refer to the following case study:

> You are dispatched to an address in your district that is well-known to you and your partner. Both the woman that lives at this address and her boyfriend are heavy drinkers, and you have responded to multiple calls at their home. When you arrive, you find a 2-year-old girl with bilateral circumferential second-degree burns to her feet, lower legs, and buttocks. The mother says that when she was filling the tub to bathe the child after she dirtied her pants, the child stepped into the tub and got burned. You take the child to the ambulance to provide care and notice that she does not cry for her mother to be with her. She shudders when you touch her to begin your assessment and jumps every time someone approaches or opens a door.

9. What characteristics of an abusive family situation are present in this situation?

_____

_____

10. What specific characteristics of the injuries increase your suspicion of possible abuse?

_____

_____

11. How does the child's behavior suggest the possibility of an abusive family situation?

_____

_____

12. What are your legal responsibilities with regard to this situation?

_____

_____

13. List five measures to help preserve evidence on a sexual assault call.
   a.

   b.

   c.

   d.

   e.

14. List at least four injuries that may accompany sexual assault.

a.

b.

c.

d.

STUDENT SELF-ASSESSMENT

15. The establishment of control and fear in a relationship through violence and other forms of abuse is known by which of the following terms?
  a. Assault
  b. Battering
  c. Intimidation
  d. Terrorism

16. What typically occurs in the third phase of the domestic violence cycle?
  a. An argument occurs, and the situation escalates.
  b. Threats of violence and harm are made to the victim.
  c. Physical or sexual abuse occurs.
  d. The abuser apologizes for what has happened.

17. What does the victim of domestic violence often fear most?
  a. That her children will be harmed or taken away.
  b. That she will be humiliated in front of their friends.
  c. That she will not be able to achieve financial independence.
  d. That the abuser will hurt himself if the victim leaves.

18. Which of the following characteristics may an abuser or victim of domestic violence have?
  a. Alcohol or drug dependence
  b. Dislike of discipline
  c. Fear of love and affection
  d. Rigid personal boundaries

19. Which of the following injury patterns is more suggestive of domestic abuse?
  a. Contusions of the breast
  b. Fracture of the ankle
  c. Laceration of the finger
  d. Scald burn of the hand

20. What is an effective way to treat a patient whom you suspect has been injured in a domestic violence situation?
  a. Ask the police to speak to her partner so that you can examine her privately.
  b. Don't pry if she doesn't volunteer any information about abuse.
  c. If she won't talk, ask her, "You've been abused, haven't you?"
  d. Force her to go to the hospital even if she doesn't want to.

21. Which is an example of psychological abuse of an elder?
  a. Sexual molestation
  b. Theft of property
  c. Verbal threats
  d. Withholding food

22. What action should the paramedic take if elder abuse is suspected?
  a. Confront the suspected abuser about the abusive behavior and threaten to report it.
  b. Report your suspicions to medical direction and the appropriate state agency.
  c. Discuss the patient's rights and ways to follow up with authorities.
  d. Wait to see whether it happens again before you take action so that you can be sure.

23. Which of the following descriptions is most characteristic of a child abuser?
  a. 20-year-old mother
  b. 45-year-old female neighbor
  c. 50-year-old father
  d. 70-year-old uncle

24. What is helpful in most cases in assessing whether a child's injury is accidental or inflicted by an adult?
  a. Assessing the family for the characteristics of abusers
  b. Checking with the police to see whether a record of abuse exists
  c. Matching the description of the event to the injury
  d. Performing a careful, detailed physical examination

25. Which of the following statements about sexual assault is true?
  a. All victims of sexual assault are women.
  b. Rape is motivated by sexual desire.
  c. Threats of harm or use of weapons during the attack are rare.
  d. Victims often know their attackers.

26. What statement by the paramedic may be most helpful to a child who has been sexually assaulted?

    a. "Don't worry about anything; you are OK."

    b. "They'll probably get the person who did this."

    c. "You didn't do anything wrong; this wasn't your fault."

    d. "You're really lucky; it could have been a lot worse."

WRAP IT UP

You are dispatched to a large, elegant home for a "maternity case." En route, the dispatcher notes that the caller requests no lights and sirens and that the crew use a rear entrance. The patient's husband meets you; you recognize him, from his frequent television commercials, as a prominent injury claims attorney. He tells you that his wife has gone into labor. The patient is crying and telling you, "It's too early." She has two other children, has miscarried several times, and is at 30 weeks' gestation. She tells you her contractions began about an hour ago, are very painful, and are coming every 3 minutes. You note her pale skin and assess her vital signs, which are BP, 80/50 mm Hg; P, 132/min; and R, 28/min. The Sao_2 does not register. When you drape the patient and examine her perineum during a contraction to determine if she is crowning, you are alarmed to see that her undergarments are soaked with dark red blood, much different from the mucousy bloody show you've seen in the past. Your partner looks alarmed when she is unable to dopple fetal heart tones. The patient grimaces in pain when the Doppler is pressed against her abdomen, where you note an ecchymotic area lateral to her umbilicus. When you ask the patient if she has any risk factors for abruption, toxemia, high blood pressure, or trauma, she glances nervously at her husband but denies all. He quickly interrupts and says, "Well, she did fall down a couple of steps this morning." As you administer oxygen, she whispers to you that her husband punched her in the abdomen during an argument earlier today. As you quickly secure the patient to your cot and raise her legs, you explain to her that her pain and blood pressure concern you, therefore you will be staring an IV and transporting her to the closest hospital with high-risk OB services. The husband is crying and telling her that he loves her as you wheel her out the door. The patient appears embarrassed and tells you, "I should have left him years ago, but I know he'll take the other kids. He's really a good person, but he just has a bad temper. It's all my fault." You start an IV line en route and deliver her to the labor and delivery unit, where a team is waiting with four units of blood to rush her for an emergency C-section based on your report. Subsequently you learn that the patient survived but her baby did not. Her husband plea bargained, so you are thankful you did not have to testify at trial.

  1. Which is true about battered women?

    a. City dwellers are at higher risk of abuse.

    b. Domestic abuse calls pose little threat to rescuers.

    c. Fifteen percent to 25% of pregnant women are battered.

    d. Wife batterers do not usually abuse their children.

  2. What clues to abuse did you note before the patient told you she had been assaulted?

_____

_____

  3. Which action or actions could have increased the potential for violence directed at the EMS crew?

_____

_____

_____

  4. Put a ✔ beside interventions related to this patient's abuse that would have been appropriate for you to provide during transport.

    a. _____ Listen with a nonjudgmental attitude

    b. _____ Encourage the patient to get control of her life

    c. _____ Provide access to community resources

    d. _____ Provide a written list of community resources for the patient

    e. _____ Confirm that she is not at fault

    f. _____ Treat her in a sensitive manner

CHAPTER 46 ANSWERS

REVIEW QUESTIONS

1. Request and await police to help assess and maintain scene safety. Domestic violence calls are very dangerous. (Objective 4)

2. Move the patient to the ambulance as soon as possible. Do not ask about the violence until you have the patient alone. Have police remain with the alleged abuser while you perform your examination. (Objective 4)

3. The patient may fear for her own safety or the safety of her children if she leaves. A victim often believes that the offender's behavior will change. She may not have money or emotional support to help her leave. She may believe that she is the cause of the behavior or that abuse is a normal part of marriage. (Objective 2)

4. Often the perpetrator is released from jail within several hours. A woman who leaves is 75% more likely to be killed by her partner. A woman who leaves should be directed to community support agencies that can maximize her safety. Sometimes it is more prudent for her to stay and carefully plan a safe departure than to leave suddenly. (Objective 4)

5. Accept her decision and support her by confirming that she is not at fault and doesn't deserve to be abused. Give her written information (preferably on something small enough to hide) about community agencies that can provide financial, emotional, safety-related, and legal resources to assist her. Help her prepare a quick way out. Identify safety precautions for her. (Objective 4)

6. The victim is a widow who is over 75 years of age. She has multiple chronic health problems and lives with a child. (Objective 7)

7. The patient seems hesitant to confirm the source of the injury and has aging bruises. (Objective 5)

8. If you suspect abuse, you should report your suspicions to medical direction and call the agency mandated by law to report suspected elder abuse. (Objective 6)

9. This child is with a parent, and alcohol abuse is evident, which greatly increases the risk of physical abuse. You also have received many calls to this home. (Objective 7)

10. The burns involve both extremities and the buttocks and are circumferential, indicating that the child was probably forcibly held in the hot water. (Objective 8)

11. The child does not mind separation from the parents, appears fearful, and does not like to be touched. (Objective 7)

12. This case should be reported to the appropriate state agency for child abuse on arrival at the hospital (refer to local reporting protocols). (Objective 7)

13. a. Take steps to preserve evidence.
    b. Do not allow the patient to urinate, defecate, douche, or bathe.
    c. Do not remove evidence from areas of sexual contact.
    d. Notify law enforcement immediately.
    e. Maintain a chain of evidence with clothing and other items.
    (Objective 10)

14. a. Abrasions or bruises on the upper limb, head, and neck
    b. Forcible signs of restraint
    c. Petechiae of the face and conjunctiva
    d. Broken teeth, swollen jaw or cheekbone, or eye injuries
    e. Muscle soreness or stiffness of the shoulder, neck, knee, hip, or back
    (Objective 9)

STUDENT SELF-ASSESSMENT

15. b. Battering may include physical abuse (assault) or psychological abuse such as intimidation, isolation, or threats to control another person.
    (Objective 1)

16. d. This is known as the *honeymoon phase*.
    (Objective 2)

17. a. Usually all these fears exist, but children most often are the most compelling reason for the victim to stay.
    (Objective 2)

18. a. Abusers may feel that abuse is a form of discipline. Abusers or victims often have an intense need for love and affection and are unable to set personal boundaries.
    (Objective 2)

19. a. Abusive injuries are more commonly found on the face, head, neck, breasts, and abdomen.
    (Objective 3)

20. a. The partner may be reluctant to leave the victim alone and may need to be distracted for you to be able to conduct an effective history. If the victim does not volunteer information, you could say something nonthreatening, such as, "I'm concerned for you because I've seen these types of injuries in people who have been hit by others." Do not intimidate or accuse the victim. You cannot insist on transport if the adult patient is competent.
    (Objective 4)

21. c. Sexual molestation is physical abuse, theft is financial or material abuse, and withholding food is neglect.
    (Objective 5)

22. b. Report it to the authorities so that they will have complete information if a pattern of abuse exists.
    (Objective 6)

23. a. Most perpetrators are a parent, female, and under 40.
    (Objective 7)

24. c. If the child volunteers the same story as the parents without prompting and the story is consistent with the injuries you see, abuse is not likely. You probably will not have time in the field to assess the family or check police records.
    (Objective 8)

25. d. About 49,000 men report sexual assault each year. Rape is a crime of violence, not a sexual act. Threats of harm or the use of weapons for intimidation are common.
(Objective 9)

26. c. Abused children should understand that the assault was not their fault and that they won't be punished. False reassurances serve no purpose.
(Objective 10)

WRAP IT UP

1. c. Abuse is also common in rural and suburban areas. Domestic violence calls pose a high risk of violence toward police and EMS. More than half of wife batterers also abuse their children.
(Objective 2)

2. The request to respond on the quiet; the obvious trauma to the abdomen (characteristic of abuse); a pregnant patient with possible abruption (trauma is a possible cause); the changing story (no mention of trauma initially); and the high incidence of abuse during pregnancy.
(Objective 3)

3. Confronting or questioning the husband about the abuse.
(Objective 4)

4. a, e, f. The patient is experiencing a life-threatening injury, and the other interventions would not be appropriate at this time. A detailed report to hospital staff members, who can refer her to the appropriate social services after her recovery, would also be indicated.
(Objective 4)

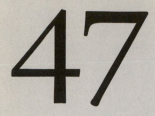

CHAPTER 47

Patients with Special Challenges

READING ASSIGNMENT
Chapter 47, pages 1196-1209, in *Mosby's Paramedic Textbook,* ed. 3

OBJECTIVES
Upon completion of this chapter, the paramedic student will be able to do the following:
1. Identify considerations in prehospital management related to physical challenges such as hearing, visual, and speech impairments; obesity; and patients with paraplegia or quadriplegia.
2. Identify considerations in prehospital management of patients who have mental illness, are developmentally disabled, or are emotionally or mentally impaired.
3. Describe special considerations for prehospital management of patients with selected pathological challenges.
4. Outline considerations in management of culturally diverse patients.
5. Describe special considerations in the prehospital management of terminally ill patients.
6. Identify special considerations in management of patients with communicable diseases.
7. Describe special considerations in the prehospital management of patients with financial challenges.

SUMMARY
- Certain accommodations may be needed for a hearing-impaired patient. These include helping with a patient's hearing aid, providing paper and pen to aid in communication, speaking softly into the patient's ear, and speaking in clear view of the patient.
- When caring for the visually impaired patient, the paramedic should help the patient use his or her glasses or other visual aids. The paramedic also should describe all procedures before performing them.
- Allow extra time for the history of a patient with a speech impairment. If appropriate, provide aids such as a pen and paper to assist in communication.
- When caring for an obese patient, use the proper sized diagnostic devices. Also, secure extra personnel if needed to move the patient for transport.
- When transporting patients with paraplegia or quadriplegia, extra personnel may be needed to move special equipment.
- Once rapport and trust have been established with a patient who has mental illness, the paramedic should proceed with care in the standard manner.
- When caring for a patient with developmental delays, the paramedic should allow enough time to obtain a history, perform an assessment, deliver care, and prepare for transport.
- The challenge in assessing patients with emotional impairments is distinguishing between symptoms produced by stress and those caused by serious medical illness.

- Pathological conditions may call for special assessment and management skills. The paramedic should ask about current medications and the patient's normal level of functioning.
- Diversity refers to differences of any kind. These include race, class, religion, gender, sexual preference, personal habitat, and physical ability. Good health care depends on sensitivity toward these differences.
- Often, calls involving the care of a terminally ill patient will be emotionally charged. They require a great deal of empathy and compassion for the patient and his or her loved ones.
- Some infectious diseases will take a toll on the emotional well-being of affected patients, their families, and loved ones. Paramedics should be sensitive to the psychological needs of the patient and his or her family.
- Financial challenges can deprive a patient of basic health care services. These patients may be reluctant to seek care for illness or injury.

REVIEW QUESTIONS

Match the pathological condition in column II with the appropriate description in column I. Use each condition just once.

Column I		Column II
1. _____ Nonprogressive disorders of movement and posture		a. Arthritis
2. _____ Inherited disorder that causes slow muscle deterioration		b. Cerebral palsy
3. _____ Congenital defect that exposes part of the spinal cord		c. Cystic fibrosis
4. _____ Autoimmune disorder that weakens the muscles of the		d. Multiple sclerosis
head and extremities		e. Muscular dystrophy
5. _____ Inflammation of the joints		f. Myasthenia gravis
6. _____ Inherited disease of the lungs and digestive tract		g. Poliomyelitis
7. _____ Autoimmune disease that affects the CNS		h. Spina bifida

For the patient situations in questions 8 to 20, identify which of the following prehospital considerations may be necessary to accommodate the patient's special needs. More than one answer may be required.

- **a.** Provide communication aids
- **b.** Allow additional time for history and management
- **c.** Obtain detailed information about the preexisting condition
- **d.** Determine baseline level of functioning
- **e.** Obtain additional resources and manpower to prepare for transport

8. _____ The patient had a stroke 6 months ago, has weakness on the right side, and speaks slowly and with a stutter. He called you today complaining of inability to urinate.

9. _____ Your patient complains of crushing chest pain. He weighs approximately 375 lb (170 kg).

10. _____ You are providing an interfacility transfer for a quadriplegic patient who is in halo traction.

11. _____ A man with a history of schizophrenia is having difficulty breathing because of his asthma.

12. _____ A 12-year-old girl with Down syndrome is having extreme weakness after chemotherapy for her leukemia.

13. _____ A moderately retarded man lacerated his finger at his job in the cafeteria.

14. _____ A severely arthritic patient was involved in a motor vehicle crash.

15. _____ A 14-year-old patient with quadriplegic spastic paralysis and mental retardation caused by cerebral palsy is febrile and congested.

16. _____ A child with cystic fibrosis has vomiting and diarrhea.

17. _____ A 43-year-old woman with multiple sclerosis complains of severe vertigo.

18. _____ An 8-year-old boy with Duchenne muscular dystrophy says he can't breathe.

19. _____ A 45-year-old patient who suffered a head injury 5 years ago is confused and pale.

20. _____ A 65-year-old man tells you he is being treated for tuberculosis.

STUDENT SELF-ASSESSMENT

21. Which of the following accommodations might be helpful to many patients with hearing impairment?
    a. No accommodation is necessary.
    b. Speaking very loudly into the patient's ear
    c. Speaking very slowly with very exaggerated lip movements
    d. Writing key questions or instructions on a piece of paper

22. Which of the following fits the definition of obesity?
    a. A person who is impaired as a result of excessive weight
    b. A person who weighs 20% or more than the maximum desirable weight relative to height
    c. A person who weighs 50 lb (23 kg) more than the average weight for someone of that age
    d. A person who weighs more than 250 lb (114 kg)

23. During the initial examination of a patient with a mental illness, what is your priority?
    a. To determine whether the patient is aware of the mental illness
    b. To determine whether the patient is dangerous
    c. To determine the patient's specific form of mental illness
    d. To determine the type of medications the patient is taking

24. What challenge is posed by caring for a patient who is emotionally impaired?
    a. Determining whether symptoms are produced by stress or medical illness
    b. Determining whether the patient is lying or telling the truth
    c. Obtaining an accurate medical history from caregivers
    d. Winning the patient's trust so that you can perform the examination

25. A patient with severe arthritis of the spine falls down some steps. What is likely to be the most significant challenge in caring for this patient?
    a. Communicating so that you can understand the patient
    b. Determining whether the patient has any serious injuries
    c. Obtaining a reliable patient history and medication list
    d. Securing the patient to a spine board to minimize pain

26. Which of the following terms describes the involuntary writhing movements found in some patients with cerebral palsy?
    a. Ataxia
    b. Athetosis
    c. Diplegia
    d. Mucoviscidosis

27. During transport of a patient with severe cystic fibrosis, you should anticipate the need for which of the following?
    a. Antidysrhythmic treatment
    b. Blood glucose monitoring
    c. Nitrous oxide inhalation
    d. Suctioning

28. Which of the following is true about cultural diversity in prehospital patient care?
    a. All generations in a culture share the same beliefs.
    b. Personal prejudices and belief systems should not interfere with patient care.
    c. People must accept your explanation of the cause of their illness.
    d. You should agree with every aspect of a patient's cultural beliefs.

29. What is a primary consideration during transport of a terminally ill patient?
    a. The family should be encouraged to deal with the imminent death.
    b. Talking to the family may interfere with their grieving process.
    c. Pain management is usually the priority of care.
    d. Rapid transport is essential for definitive care.

30. How can you show respect for the dignity of a patient with AIDS during transport?
    a. Don't discuss their disease process.
    b. To keep the patient from feeling ashamed, don't use BSI.
    c. Encourage the patient to express feelings related to the disease.
    d. Respecting the patient's dignity should not be a primary concern during prehospital care.

31. What statement may be helpful when transporting a patient who has serious financial concerns?
    a. "Don't worry; the ambulance bill won't come for a couple of months."
    b. "I don't see why you're worried. You're sick now—worry about the money later."
    c. "I'll ask the nurse to contact social services to see whether there is a program to help you."
    d. "We have people who never pay a dime for our service, and they abuse us all the time."

WRAP IT UP

You could have predicted it; a light, drizzly rain always causes multiple "fender benders" at this very busy corner. As you approach the scene, you can see that a van has struck the rear of a large dump truck. There is almost no visible damage to the truck, but the van has considerable front-end damage. The van's driver, a woman in her thirties, is crying and calling out to her rear-seat passenger, a 13-year-old boy who was thrown out of his wheelchair, which had been secured in the specialized van. He is crying, making a high-pitched, moaning sound. As you approach him, the driver, his mother, tells you that his name is Michael, he has cerebral palsy with diplegic spasticity, and he is blind and has mental retardation. She tries to calm him, but his persistent cries pierce the environment, making it difficult to concentrate and impossible to hear anything on your assessment. You find him recumbent with his arms and legs drawn toward his chest in a fetal-like position. "Michael," you say loudly as you grasp one wrist and place the other hand on his shoulder, "I'm here to help you." His pulse is rapid, breathing is normal, and his skin is warm and dry. He has a laceration on the left temporal area of his head but no other visible soft tissue injury or any evidence of deformity or crepitus distally. Vital signs are BP, 96 mm Hg by palpation; P, 120/min; R, 20/min; and Sao_2, 97%. His pupils are 3 mm, equal, round, and react to light. By now your partner has evaluated the mother; her vital signs are stable, she denies any injury, and she refuses any care. You ask her to help you to calm her son. She moves close to him and rubs his back while singing a familiar song into his ear, and the moaning begins to slow. After realizing that standard spinal immobilization would be impossible because of the rigid spasticity of the boy's limbs, you and your partner determine that applying a cervical collar and a half spine board device will provide stabilization of the spine. Medical direction concurs. In simple language you explain each step of the process, which his mother relays to him. Although his agitation increases, it is manageable. After the immobilization has been applied, you position him on the stretcher in a semisitting position with blankets and pillows supporting his legs. You allow his mother to sit seat belted in the CPR seat beside him, where she continually soothes him on the way in and tells you that she thinks his behavior is appropriate for the situation. He is treated in the ED and released several hours later.

1. What difficulties were posed by the assessment of this patient?

2. Why is it appropriate to have the parent remain with the child in this situation?

3. What does *diplegic spasticity* mean?
   a. It affects both arms and legs.
   b. It is intermittent.
   c. It affects both limbs on one side of the body.
   d. It causes involuntary writhing movements.

4. Explain why it would be appropriate to deviate from standard spinal immobilization protocol in this situation.

CHAPTER 47 ANSWERS

REVIEW QUESTIONS

1. b
2. e
3. h
4. f
5. a
6. c
7. d
   (Questions 1-7: Objective 3)

8. a, b, c, d
   (Objective 1)

9. c, e
   (Objective 1)

10. b, c, d, e
    (Objective 1)

11. c, d
    (Objective 2)

12. b, c, d
    (Objective 2)

13. b, d
    (Objective 2)

14. b, c, e (possibly)
    (Objective 3)

15. c, d, e
    (Objective 3)

16. c, d
    (Objective 3)

17. c, d
    (Objective 3)

18. c, d
    (Objective 3)

19. c, d
(Objective 3)

20. c
(Objective 6)

STUDENT SELF-ASSESSMENT

21. d. Speak in low tones into the patient's ear if residual hearing exists. Otherwise, if the patient reads lips, speak at a regular speed in view of the patient.
(Objective 1)

22. b
(Objective 1)

23. b. The safety of the patient, crew, and bystanders should always be prioritized.
(Objective 2)

24. a. Anxiety can produce a host of symptoms that mimic serious medical illness.
(Objective 2)

25. d. The arthritic pain and deformity can make spinal immobilization challenging.
(Objective 3)

26. b. Ataxia is a loss of coordination and balance. Diplegic cerebral palsy affects all four limbs, the legs more severely than the arms. Mucoviscidosis is cystic fibrosis.
(Objective 3)

27. d. These patients often have excessive secretions, and the paramedic should anticipate the need for suctioning.
(Objective 3)

28. b. Individual beliefs exist even within specific cultures. People may choose to have their own beliefs about the cause of their illness despite your explanations. You need not agree with all aspects of a patient's cultural beliefs, but do not let your opinion interfere with patient care or interaction.
(Objective 4)

29. c. Some families will not be fully prepared for the death regardless of the length of illness. The paramedic should support the patient and family with honest and empathetic care. Talking to the patient and family should be encouraged if the patient's condition permits.
(Objective 5)

30. c. There is no reason not to mention the disease to the patient, but the condition should remain confidential with regard to others. Use BSI as you would for any other patient care situation. The dignity of each patient is an important part of prehospital patient care delivery.
(Objective 6)

31. c. The patient may worry about receiving poor credit ratings, adding to a mounting debt, and being a deadbeat. Offer constructive suggestions related to their financial concerns rather than empty statements.
(Objective 7)

WRAP IT UP

1. He is unable to communicate effectively, he is blind and so is probably terrified because he has no idea what happened to him, and he is mentally retarded.
(Objective 2)

2. The mother knows how to communicate with her child, can calm him, and can tell medical providers what behaviors are normal or abnormal for her son.
(Objective 1)

3. a. All four limbs are affected, the legs more than the arms. *Athetosis* describes writhing movements.
(Objective 3)

4. Positioning this patient supine on a long spine board would be impossible. Adaptations in care should take into consideration the physical needs of the patient and the potential for injury. Consultation with medical direction can be helpful.
(Objective 3)

CHAPTER

48

Acute Interventions for the Home Health Care Patient

READING ASSIGNMENT

Chapter 48, pages 1210-1229, in *Mosby's Paramedic Textbook*, ed. 3

OBJECTIVES

Upon completion of this chapter, the paramedic student will be able to:

1. Discuss general issues related to the home health care patient.
2. Outline general principles of assessment and management of the home health care patient.
3. Describe medical equipment, assessment, and management of the home health care patient with inadequate respiratory support.
4. Identify assessment findings and acute interventions for problems related to vascular access devices in the home health care setting.
5. Describe medical equipment, assessment, and management of the patient with a gastrointestinal or genitourinary crisis in the home health care setting.
6. Identify key assessments and principles of wound care management in the home health care patient.
7. Outline maternal/child problems that may be encountered early in the postpartum period in the home health care setting.
8. Describe medical therapy associated with hospice and comfort care in the home health care setting.

SUMMARY

- About 25% of home health care patients have heart and circulatory diseases as their primary diagnosis. Other common diagnoses of home health care patients include cancer, diabetes, and hypertension. Typical EMS calls to a home health care setting may include respiratory failure, cardiac decompensation, septic complications, equipment malfunction, and other medical problems.
- After arrival at the scene of a home health care patient, the scene size-up should include standard precautions, elements of scene safety, and environmental setting. The initial assessment should focus on illness or injury that poses a threat to life. The paramedic should take appropriate measures as indicated.

- Patients with diseases of the respiratory system being cared for at home are at increased risk for airway infections. In addition, the progression of their illnesses may lead to difficulty breathing, making current support equipment inadequate.
- Assessment findings that may require acute interventions in patients with VADs include infection, hemorrhage, hemodynamic compromise from circulatory overload or embolus, obstruction of the vascular device, and catheter damage with leakage of medication.
- Patients with diseases of the digestive or genitourinary system may have medical devices such as urinary catheters or urostomies, indwelling nutritional support devices (e.g., percutaneous endoscopic gastrostomy tube or gastrostomy tube), colostomies, and nasogastric tubes. Acute interventions required for these patients can result from UTI, urosepsis, urinary retention, and problems with gastric emptying or feeding.
- Home health care patients with acute infections have an increased death rate from sepsis and severe peripheral infections. Many also have a decreased ability to perceive pain or perform self-care.
- Maternal/child conditions that one may encounter in the home health care setting during the postpartum period include postpartum hemorrhage, infection, pulmonary embolism, postpartum depression, septicemia in the newborn, infantile apnea, and failure to thrive.
- Hospice services include supportive social, emotional, and spiritual services for the terminally ill. They also provide support for a patient's family. Palliative care is directed mainly at providing relief to a terminally ill person. They do this through symptom and pain management.

REVIEW QUESTIONS

Questions 1 to 4 refer to the following case study:

> You are called to care for a patient who has difficulty breathing. When you arrive at his home, you find a man who has a tracheostomy and is on a ventilator. The low pressure alarm is sounding.

1. What signs and symptoms might the patient have if he were hypoxic?

_____

_____

2. What should your first action be?

_____

_____

3. What will you check on the ventilator to assess the problem?

_____

_____

4. How can you calm the patient before reconnecting him to the ventilator?

_____

_____

_____

Questions 5 to 7 refer to the following case study:

> An elderly patient has a home IV infusion. You are called to treat her for difficulty breathing. She has a history of multiple myeloma. Her husband thinks the pump hasn't been working correctly and too much has run in.

5. What specifically would you assess to check for fluid overload?

_____

The patient has crackles bilaterally in the bases of her lungs, and her neck veins are slightly distended. Her vital signs are 160/84 mm Hg; P, 100/min; and R, 24/min. Her Sao_2 is 93% on room air.

6. What interventions should you perform in cooperation with medical direction?

_____

_____

7. Should you transport the patient for evaluation by a physician?

_____

Questions 8 to 13 pertain to the following case study:

You are called to a home for an "assist invalid" call. An elderly woman greets you, and after you help her husband to bed (he couldn't get off the commode), she asks you to check his arm. She says that he burned it 4 days ago. When you remove the dressing, you note a green wound bed surrounded by black tissue. The drainage is green and foul smelling.

8. What does the appearance of this wound suggest?

_____

9. How would it look if it were healing normally?

_____

10. What should you look for in the surrounding skin?

_____

The skin around the wound is reddened and warm to the touch.

11. What does this assessment suggest?

_____

_____

12. What systemic assessment should you perform on this patient?

_____

The patient's vital signs are BP, 150/80 mm Hg; P, 110/min; and R, 16/min. His skin feels hot to the touch. The rest of the exam is normal.

13. What action should you take?

_____

_____

Questions 14 to 17 refer to the following case study:

You respond to a call for "baby not breathing." On arrival you find a woman sobbing while holding her 4-day-old infant in her arms. The baby is awake, lying quietly in her mother's arms. The parents state that they had just put her down for a nap, when they noticed that she wasn't breathing and her color looked bad. They state that the episode lasted about 15 to 20 seconds.

14. What assessments should you perform?

_____

_____

_____

The baby's examination looks normal. While you are on the phone with medical direction, your partner shouts at you. She states that the baby stopped breathing for approximately 15 seconds and was very pale, and the heart rate dropped to 80/min on the monitor. Now she is breathing normally.

15. What are some possible causes of infantile apnea?

_____

_____

16. What interventions should you perform?

_____

_____

17. What equipment should you prepare and keep easily accessible during transport?

_____

_____

STUDENT SELF-ASSESSMENT

18. What was the historical focus of home health care?
  a. To benefit the rich
  b. To care for rural patients
  c. To provide wider physician care
  d. To provide preventative care
19. Home health care services in the United States include which of the following?
  a. Diagnostic radiology
  b. Minor surgical procedures
  c. IV antibiotic therapy
  d. Physician visits for acute illness
20. The Haddon matrix states that any injury or disease can be broken down into three components. Which of the following shows the correct three?
  a. Agent, host, environment   **c.** Patient, host, environment
  b. Agent, host, mechanical force   **d.** Agent, disease, environment

21. What type of infection control standards should be practiced in the home health setting?
    a. No precautions are needed.
    b. Use precautions only for HIV patients.
    c. Wear reusable rubber gloves.
    d. Observe universal precautions.
22. Assessment of the milieu in home care includes evaluation to ensure which of the following?
    a. Infectious waste is disposed of properly.
    b. Dogs and other pets are contained.
    c. No hazards are present in the home.
    d. The home has heat, water, and electricity.
23. On arrival at a call in which home care is provided, your priority (after making sure the scene is safe) is to assess for which of the following?
    a. Abusive caregivers
    b. Equipment failure
    c. Life-threatening illness or injury
    d. Medical device malfunction
24. Which of the following systems will not work during a power failure?
    a. Demand valve
    b. Liquid oxygen
    c. Oxygen concentrators
    d. Oxygen cylinders
25. You are called because the high pressure alarm keeps sounding on a home care ventilator. What might this indicate?
    a. Cuff leak
    b. Disconnected tubing
    c. Insufficient oxygen
    d. Water in tubing
26. Which of the following is a peripheral vascular access device?
    a. Groshon
    b. Hickman
    c. Intracath
    d. Mediport
27. Which of the following complications of vascular access devices does not pose an immediate life threat?
    a. Circulatory overload
    b. Embolus
    c. Hemorrhage
    d. Site infection
28. Which of the following is a sign of air embolus that may occur if air enters a vascular access device?
    a. Distended neck veins
    b. Fever
    c. Hypotension
    d. Pulmonary congestion
29. How much heparin should be used when flushing a peripheral vascular device?
    a. 2.5 to 3 mL (10 U/mL)
    b. 2.5 to 3 mL (100 U/mL)
    c. 3 to 5 mL (10 U/mL)
    d. 3 to 5 mL (100 U/mL)
30. What complication can result from an untreated urinary tract infection in a patient with a urinary catheter?
    a. Kidney stones
    b. Prostatic hypertrophy
    c. Sepsis
    d. Urinary retention
31. Which complication of tube feedings can cause serious skin breakdown and fluid and electrolyte imbalances?
    a. Bowel obstruction
    b. Choking
    c. Diarrhea
    d. Irritable bowel syndrome
32. What is a critical step in the insertion of a urinary catheter?
    a. Do not retract the foreskin, if present.
    b. Inflate the balloon with 10 to 15 mL of sterile saline after insertion.
    c. Use aseptic technique until the catheter is inserted and the balloon inflated.
    d. Use significant force to overcome resistance during catheter insertion.
33. Which of the following enhances wound repair?
    a. Environmental contamination
    b. Eschar
    c. Moisture
    d. Necrotic tissue
34. Your patient delivered a baby 3 days ago. She is complaining of severe abdominal pain, weakness, and shaking chills. What postpartum complication should be anticipated?
    a. Appendicitis
    b. Endometritis
    c. Hemorrhage
    d. Pulmonary embolism
35. You are called to the home of a woman who appears to have signs and symptoms of postpartum depression. Your priority should be to assess for which of the following?
    a. Depressive psychosis
    b. Forgetfulness or memory loss
    c. Severe sleep disturbances
    d. The well-being of the baby

36. A mother calls you to evaluate her 11-day-old infant. She says she has been nursing him, but he doesn't "seem right." He is difficult to awaken and pale, and he has dry mucous membranes and a sunken fontanelle. She thinks he hasn't wet a diaper in about 18 hours. What do you suspect?
   a. Apnea
   b. Dehydration
   c. Jaundice
   d. Sepsis

37. Which of the following terms describes abnormal retardation of growth and development in an infant caused by maternal deprivation or malnutrition?
   a. Cerebral palsy
   b. Cystic fibrosis
   c. Failure to thrive
   d. Muscular dystrophy

38. What is the primary goal of palliative care?
   a. To make sure that optimal nutritional requirements are met
   b. To help families accept the reality of impending death
   c. To improve the quality of a person's life as death approaches
   d. To provide complete relief of any pain or discomfort

WRAP IT UP

When you walk into the neat, single-story home, you are surprised to see your patient, a 35-year-old man, sitting upright in a wheelchair using a ventilator. With great difficulty he tells you that he is a high-level quadriplegic, and he directs you to some papers that describe his medical history. He has a ventilator, a G tube, a urinary catheter, and several splints on his extremities. You note that he has an oral antibiotic that was prescribed today. He says he is "sick; just doesn't feel well," and his doctor would like him transported to the ED for evaluation. His skin is hot, and his pulse is rapid. His vital signs are T, 102.6° F (38.8 ° C) axilla; BP, 90/68 mm Hg; and P, 128/min. His ventilator is set at a rate of 12 with a tidal volume of 500 mL on room air; his Sao$_2$ is 90%. You can hear some wheezes in his lungs, so you connect some oxygen to the ventilator. You note that the urine in his catheter bag is a milky color. The rest of his exam is unremarkable. It takes a few moments for you and your partner to plan how to effectively move him to the cot without disturbing the ventilator. You make sure the G tube is clamped securely and move the urinary catheter so that you won't pull on it. The patient says he can breathe spontaneously for several minutes on his own, so you momentarily disconnect him as you perform the lift. In the ambulance, you administer bronchodilator updraft treatment while your partner starts an IV and delivers a 200 mL fluid bolus. Reassessment in a few minutes shows that his vital signs are now BP, 100/70 mm Hg; P, 120/min; and Sao$_2$, 97%.

1. Why is it important to review the medical papers of the home care patient if they are available?

_____

2. Put a ✔ beside the type(s) of home care services this patient is likely to need on an ongoing basis.
   a. _____ Cardiopulmonary care
   b. _____ Dermatological or wound care
   c. _____ Catheter management
   d. _____ Gastroenterological care
   e. _____ Hospice care
   f. _____ Orthopedic care
   g. _____ Pain management
   h. _____ Rehabilitative care

3. What complications requiring emergency care could occur based on this patient's use of a
   a. Ventilator
   b. G tube
   c. Foley catheter

4. If you could not transport the patient with his ventilator, what should you do?

_____

_____

CHAPTER 48 ANSWERS

REVIEW QUESTIONS

1. A hypoxic patient may be restless, confused, tachycardic, hypertensive, dyspneic, or cyanotic or may have a headache. When you monitor the patient, you may find a low Sao$_2$ or cardiac dysrhythmias. (Objective 3)

2. If he appears to be in distress, immediately begin ventilation with a bag-valve device and 100% O$_2$. Then you can evaluate the equipment problem. Determine the need for suctioning. (Objective 3)

3. Check the ventilator for disconnected tubing or power cords; check the settings; make sure the tracheostomy tube is in the proper place and the balloon is adequately inflated. (Objective 3)

4. Reassure the patient that the problem has been fixed, perhaps showing him how you fixed it. Tell him you will remain with him for several minutes after you reconnect him to the ventilator to make sure that everything continues to work properly. (Objective 3)

5. Assess the patient's level of consciousness and level of distress; respiratory rate and lung sounds; neck for signs of JVD; skin color, temperature, and moisture; and vital signs. (Objective 4)

6. Slow the infusion to a keep-open rate; provide high-concentration oxygen; elevate the patient's head; maintain body warmth; monitor vital signs; reassess. If her condition does not improve, consider the need for a diuretic. (Objective 4)

7. The need to transport depends on the patient's response to your interventions, other anticipated complications based on the contents of the infusion, and the patient's wishes with regard to transport. The decision should be made in consultation with medical direction. (Objective 4)

8. The wound has many signs of infection and necrosis. (Objective 6)

9. A properly healing wound has a pink or red wound bed, clear or serosanguineous drainage, and no odor. (Objective 6)

10. The surrounding skin should be assessed for color, warmth, and swelling. (Objective 6)

11. The redness and warmth of the surrounding skin suggest infection. (Objective 6)

12. A full assessment is necessary. Specifically, vital signs, including temperature and lung sounds, should be evaluated. (Objective 6)

13. His physical examination suggests systemic infection. You should administer high-concentration oxygen, start IV fluids, assess his temperature, and transport. (Objective 6)

14. A full assessment is indicated, including initial assessment, vital signs, blood glucose, and ECG and oxygen saturation monitoring.
(Objective 7)

15. Infantile apnea may be caused by hypoglycemia, hypocalcemia, hypothermia, sepsis, pneumonia, meningitis, CNS hemorrhage, hypoxic injury, seizures, respiratory distress, hyaline membrane disease, and obstruction.
(Objective 7)

16. Keep the baby warm; administer dextrose if the glucose level is low; administer high-concentration oxygen by mask or blow-by; start an IV line (in consultation with medical direction); continually monitor breathing, color, oxygen saturation, and ECG; transport.
(Objective 7)

17. Make sure that resuscitation equipment is within easy reach. Open the appropriate size bag-mask for the child and connect it so that it is easily accessible should another apneic episode occur.
(Objective 7)

STUDENT SELF-ASSESSMENT

18. d. The growing population of immigrants in large cities stimulated the growth of nurse-provided home care for the poor.
(Objective 1)

19. c. The home health field may continue to expand, perhaps offering these services in the future.
(Objective 1)

20. a. These factors occur in three phases: preinjury, injury, and postinjury.
(Objective 1)

21. d. The same precautions should be used as in the hospital setting.
(Objective 1)

22. d. Environmental assessments include infectious waste, pets, and hazards.
(Objective 2)

23. c. Life threats should be identified before further assessment is done.
(Objective 2)

24. c. The patient should keep an oxygen cylinder on hand in case this happens.
(Objective 3)

25. d. Cuff leakage and disconnected tubing trigger a low pressure alarm. The oxygen alarm sounds if the oxygen supply is inadequate.
(Objective 3)

26. c. The rest are central venous access devices.
(Objective 4)

27. d. Although a site infection is not an immediate life threat, it can cause sepsis and possibly death if it spreads and becomes systemic.
(Objective 4)

28. c. Fever is a sign of infection. Distended neck veins and pulmonary congestion are signs of fluid overload. Other signs and symptoms of embolus include cyanosis; weak, rapid pulse; and loss of consciousness. (Objective 4)

29. b (Objective 4)

30. c. Urosepsis is managed with antibiotic therapy. (Objective 5)

31. c. Excessive diarrhea can cause skin to break down rapidly, as well as dehydration and electrolyte imbalances. A change in the volume or type of tube feeding may remedy the problem. (Objective 5)

32. c. The foreskin should be retracted to visualize the urethra. The balloon should be inflated with 3 to 5 mL of sterile water. Excessive force should not be necessary and may injure the urethra. (Objective 5)

33. c. An adequate blood supply and sufficient oxygen and nutrition are also essential. (Objective 6)

34. c. Fever and abdominal pain are the most common signs and symptoms of postpartum hemorrhage. (Objective 7)

35. d. Some women who suffer from this condition fantasize about harming their babies. All the other symptoms should be assessed after the physical well-being of the mother and baby have been ensured. (Objective 7)

36. b. Further evaluation is necessary, but the patient's clinical presentation suggests severe dehydration, which requires immediate fluid resuscitation and rapid transport. (Objective 7)

37. c. This condition can also be caused by chromosomal abnormalities and major organ system defects. (Objective 7)

38. c. Palliative care customizes treatment for patients and their families, providing pain and symptom management if needed and mental and spiritual guidance with the goal of improving quality of life. (Objective 8)

WRAP IT UP

1. To determine his normal state of functioning, other medical conditions, home medications, any special instructions regarding care, legal papers, including advanced directives, normal vital signs, and private physician and hospital of choice. (Objective 2)

2. a, b, c, d, h (Objective 1)

3. a. The ventilator could fail as a result of power loss, kinks or water in the tubing, and excessive secretions. Patients can develop pneumothorax or experience anxiety attacks if they feel as if they are not being ventilated. Oxygen supply (if present) can fail.

b. G tube: Aspiration and severe diarrhea can occur.

c. A urinary catheter can become infected, resulting in sepsis. It can cause urethral trauma if pulled out forcefully with the balloon inflated, and the patient can develop serious signs and symptoms if the catheter is removed and urinary retention occurs.

(Objectives 3, 5)

4. Ventilate the patient with a bag-mask device or place on an automatic transport ventilator adjusted closely to the settings the patient was on at home.

(Objective 3)

PART TEN

IN THIS PART

Ambulance Operations

READING ASSIGNMENT
Chapter 49, pages 1230-1239, in *Mosby's Paramedic Textbook*, ed. 3

OBJECTIVES
Upon completion of this chapter, the paramedic student will be able to do the following:
1. List standards that govern ambulance performance and specifications.
2. Discuss the tracking of equipment, supplies, and maintenance on an ambulance.
3. Outline the considerations for appropriate stationing of ambulances.
4. Describe measures that can influence safe operation of an ambulance.
5. Identify aeromedical crew members and training.
6. Describe the appropriate use of aeromedical services in the prehospital setting.

SUMMARY
- The federal KKK A-1822 standards provide the foundation of uniformity for the design of ambulance vehicles.
- Completing an equipment and supply checklist at the start of every work shift is important. It is essential for safety, patient care, and risk management. It also helps to ensure proper handling and safekeeping of scheduled medications.
- The methods for estimating ambulance service needs and placement in a community have changed. Compliance in providing EMS services within time frames that meet national standards is the method that now is commonly used.
- Factors that influence safe ambulance operation include proper use of escorts, environmental conditions, proper use of warning devices, proceeding safely through intersections, parking at the emergency scene, and operating with due regard for the safety of all others.
- The staffing of air ambulances includes a pilot and various health care professionals. These individuals undergo specialized training in flight physiology and the use of special medical equipment and procedures.
- When paramedics request aeromedical service, the flight crew should be advised of the type of emergency response, the number of patients, and the location of the landing zone and any prominent landmarks and hazards. Paramedics should always follow strict safety measures during helicopter landings. This helps to prevent injury to air medical crews, ground crews, the patient, and bystanders.

REVIEW QUESTIONS

1. Cite the standard that defines ambulance design or performance.

   _____

2. List three types of prehospital care supplies that should be routinely checked on an ambulance.

   a. _____

   b. _____

   c. _____

3. What would be a consequence of the following supply/equipment problems?

   a. The batteries aren't charged on the portable suction unit, and your patient is trapped in a car with a mouth full of blood and vomit.

   _____

   b. The defibrillator doesn't work, and the patient is in ventricular fibrillation.

   _____

   c. You run out of strips to check blood glucose levels on a call with an elderly man who has an altered level of consciousness and no available history.

   _____

   d. Someone forgot to replace the OB (delivery) kit after the last delivery.

   _____

   e. You run out of oxygen while on a call for pulmonary edema.

   _____

4. EMS and community planners must consider a number of factors when determining ambulance placement to provide acceptable availability and response times. List four of these factors.

   a.

   b.

   c.

   d.

5. Explain how you can reduce the risk of vehicle accidents in each of the following situations:

   a. You are being followed by a police escort.

   _____

   b. It's 0500, and driving conditions include a light rain and heavy fog.

   _____

   c. The lights and sirens are on, and you are preparing to proceed through a red light at an intersection.

   _____

Questions 6 to 10 refer to the following case study:

You respond to a rollover MVC with a patient ejected at 0800. On arrival you find a 4-year-old girl who was thrown 20 feet from the vehicle. She is unconscious, has rapid, shallow respirations, and shows signs of shock. The nearest hospital is 40 minutes away; a pediatric trauma center is 45 minutes away by ground, 20 minutes by air. Air medical ETA to your location would be 10 minutes.

6. Give two reasons why this is an appropriate situation for use of air medical transport.

a.

b.

7. What information should you give the dispatcher when you call to activate the air medical transport?

_____

_____

_____

8. Describe landing zone selection and preparation for this air medical response.

_____

_____

The crash occurred across from a baseball diamond that is easily accessible, and the LZ is set up there.

9. What patient management procedures should be performed before the helicopter arrives?

_____

_____

10. List three safety measures that should be taken as you approach the helicopter to load the patient when it lands.

a.

b.

c.

STUDENT SELF-ASSESSMENT

11. Which of the following is true of the KKK A-1822 standards?
    a. They contradict the AMD 001-009 performance standards.
    b. They designate design standards for types I, II, and III ambulances.
    c. They define performance specifications for air ambulances.
    d. They outline ambulance driving standards and qualifications.

12. Why are routine ambulance equipment checks essential?
    a. So that accurate patient billing and reimbursement can occur in a timely manner
    b. So that disciplinary action will not be necessary if an equipment failure occurs
    c. So that essential equipment is available and in working order during patient care
    d. So that state laws and regulations can be met and licensure can be maintained

13. Emergency vehicle placement in a community should be determined by which of the following?
    a. Average response times that meet national standards
    b. The number of receiving hospitals in the region
    c. The projected revenue flow from reimbursement
    d. Where the citizens would like to have ambulances

14. Which of the following help promote safety when driving an ambulance?
    a. Drive no faster than 20 miles per hour over the speed limit on routine calls.
    b. Make sure that only the driver and the patient are always restrained.
    c. Use extreme caution at intersections, especially when using lights and sirens.
    d. Use lights and sirens often so that other drivers will yield the right of way.

15. How can the paramedic promote safety when responding to a vehicle crash on the highway?
    a. Park 100 feet past the crash.
    b. Park downhill from hazardous materials.
    c. Park on the opposite side of the road.
    d. Turn off emergency lights.

16. All air medical crew members should receive specialized training in which of the following areas?
    a. Airway management techniques
    b. Flight physiology
    c. Medication administration
    d. Vascular access techniques

17. Which of the following situations would justify the use of air medical transport by an advanced life support unit with an ETA of 40 minutes?
    a. Possible fractured tibia with good pulses
    b. Possible aneurysm with absent pedal pulses
    c. Home delivery with both patients stable
    d. Asthma patient with P, 100/min; R, 20/min

18. Which of the following safety measures should be used when approaching the helicopter to load patients?
    a. Approach the aircraft as soon as it lands.
    b. At least six people should help load the aircraft.
    c. Long objects should be carried vertically to maintain control.
    d. The aircraft should be approached from the front.

WRAP IT UP

"C-crew," your partner mutters as you begin your morning ambulance check. It's frustrating, because things just don't seem as neat and clean as you like them, and there's always some little thing missing or out of place. You complete the equipment checklist and then go to the office to fill out a maintenance request for the broken latch on the medication drawer. Because it's the first day of the month, the sealed pediatric bag is opened and checked to make sure that none of the drugs have expired. Just as break time begins, you are dispatched to a call for an electrocution. The pumper is responding with you, so you and your partner follow it at a distance, taking care to change the siren as you pass motorists that have pulled to the right. At each light you change your siren and sound the air horn, stop, and make sure all traffic has stopped before you proceed. En route, you ask dispatch to place the air medical team on standby because the burn center is an hour away. You are thankful that your new engine house is so close to the scene; it will probably save you a couple of minutes on this response.

When you arrive on the scene, you find that the patient touched some high-voltage wires with a tree trimmer and is critically burned, so you immediately ask that the aircraft be launched. Your captain sends two of his crew members to set up the landing zone in an adjacent parking lot while the rest of the team works to assess and treat the patient. When the flight crew lands, you give a report, explaining that intubation is impossible because the man's jaw is clenched. After assessing the patient, the air crew performs rapid sequence induction and intubates the patient, ensuring a secure airway in flight. You help them with loading, being careful to stay to the front of the aircraft, away from the tail rotor. Back at the station, you restock and document the call and then get your well-deserved cup of coffee.

1. Put a ✔ beside the consequences of failing to check the ambulance equipment or to maintain it properly.
   a. _____ Batteries dead in saturation monitor
   b. _____ Inability to defibrillate
   c. _____ Break down en route to hospital
   d. _____ Drugs expired
   e. _____ Traction splint unavailable
   f. _____ No oxygen available
   g. _____ Appropriate drug not on ambulance
   h. _____ Ambulance tire blowout

2. What advantage of constructing a new station is described here?

3. List two additional safe driving considerations that were not mentioned in this case study.

_____

_____

4. List two advantages of aeromedical transport that were described in this situation.

_____

_____

CHAPTER 49 ANSWERS

REVIEW QUESTIONS

1. KKK A-1822D
   (Objective 1)

2. a. Supplies (airway, vascular access, dressings)
   b. Medications (number and expiration dates, oxygen supply)
   c. Equipment (including routine maintenance, battery loads, supplementary supplies)
   (Objective 2)

3. a. The patient may aspirate and die.
   b. You will be unable to defibrillate until another unit arrives, and the patient may deteriorate into asystole and die.
   c. You will be unable to determine whether the altered consciousness is due to hypoglycemia. If you administer glucose and the patient's altered level of consciousness is related to a stroke, this action may worsen his condition.
   d. You will have to search for other appropriate supplies, wasting time to care for the patient and baby. What will you use to cut the cord and then clamp it?
   e. The patient's hypoxia may worsen, resulting in death.
   (Objective 2)

4. a. National response time standards
   b. Geographical area
   c. Population and patient demand
   d. Traffic conditions
   Others include time of day and appropriate placement of vehicles.
   (Objective 3)

5. a. Make sure that the police follow at a safe distance. Use a siren tone different from that used by the police.
   b. Slow the ambulance to a safe speed and use the low beam lights.
   c. Remember that not all drivers will hear your sirens or see your lights. Stop and look to make sure that all traffic is stopping (make eye contact if possible). Use the yelp mode of the siren and remain vigilant as you proceed.
   (Objective 4)

6. Your patient is critical and requires specialized resources, and you are far from a hospital.
   (Objective 6)

7. Advise the flight crew that you are at an MVC with a critically ill child. Let them know the location of the landing zone and any prominent landmarks or hazards.
   (Objective 6)

8. The landing zone should be 100 × 100 feet. It should have few vertical structures and should be relatively flat and free of high grass, crops, debris, or rough terrain (check local standards for specific variations).
   (Objective 6)

9. As many patient care procedures as possible should be done, depending on the ETA of the helicopter. The airway should be secured, and the patient ventilated appropriately. The patient should be secured to a long spine board with straps and cervical immobilization. Vascular access should be obtained, and other patient assessment and care continued (e.g., maintain warmth) until the helicopter arrives.
   (Objective 6)

10. Do not approach the aircraft unless directed to do so by the crew. Approach from the front of the aircraft and stay clear of the tail rotor. Allow a minimal number of people to help load. Secure loose objects. Walk in a crouched position. Carry objects at waist height. Depart from the front in view of the pilot. Wear eye protection.
    (Objective 6)

STUDENT SELF-ASSESSMENT

11. b. The AMD 001-009 performance standards have been incorporated into the latest KKK standards.
    (Objective 1)

12. c. Lack or failure of essential patient equipment could mean the difference between life and death.
    (Objective 2)

13. a. A number of factors will affect those times, and they can vary by time of day and other variables. This should be monitored on a continuing basis.
    (Objective 3)

14. c. Paramedics driving an ambulance should remain at or below the speed limit except in extreme circumstances. For maximal safety, the paramedic attendant should also be restrained except when patient care requires movement. Lights and sirens should be used only on emergency responses (as dictated by policy) and when a patient in critical condition is being transported.
    (Objective 4)

15. a. Ideally, the ambulance should be on the same side of the road as the crash. Emergency lights should be left on. Ambulances should be parked uphill and upwind from hazardous materials incidents.
    (Objective 4)

16. b. Some air medical services require training in specialized airway and vascular access techniques, as well as expanded medication administration knowledge. This varies by agency.
    (Objective 5)

17. b. Unless inclement weather or impassable roads prohibit transport, all the other patients could be appropriately transported by ground ALS service.
    (Objective 6)

18. d. No one should approach the aircraft until a crew member signals that it is OK. A minimal number of people should approach the aircraft. No objects should be held up.
    (Objective 6)

WRAP IT UP

1. a (are replacements available on the ambulance, are the batteries fully charged on the defibrillator, and are there defibrillator pads on truck); c (is preventive maintenance being done); d (what effect would giving an expired drug have); e (how will that affect the patient's pain and further damage/bleeding); f (what if your patient is critical; would you have to call another ambulance); g (how would you explain that in court); h (what might the consequence be; are you checking the tires each day and reporting wear)
   (Objective 2)

2. Reduction in response time
   (Objective 3)

3. Wearing seatbelts; driving the speed limit, except as allowed by law; parking safely at the scene.
   (Objective 4)

4. The crew is trained and authorized to perform advanced techniques; a specialized resource center can be reached more quickly.
   (Objectives 5, 6)

Medical Incident Command

READING ASSIGNMENT
Chapter 50, pages 1240-1256, in *Mosby's Paramedic Textbook*, ed. 3

OBJECTIVES
Upon completion of this chapter, the paramedic student will be able to:
1. Identify the components of an effective incident command system.
2. Outline the activities of the preplanning, scene management, and postdisaster follow-up phases of an incident.
3. Identify the five major functions of the incident command system.
4. List command responsibilities during a major incident response.
5. Describe the section responsibilities in the incident command system.
6. Identify situations that may be classified as major incidents.
7. Describe the steps necessary to establish and operate the incident command system.
8. Given a major incident, describe the groups and/or divisions that would need to be established and the responsibilities of each.
9. List common problems related to the incident command system and to mass casualty incidents.
10. Outline the principles and technology of triage.
11. Identify resources for the management of critical incident stress.

SUMMARY
- The ICS organizational structure should be adaptable to any agency or to any incident requiring emergency management. The ICS also must be expandable. It must be able to expand from dealing with a nonmajor incident to a major one in a logical way.
- All participating response agencies must agree to the preplan (phase 1 of the ICS). The preplan must address common goals and the specific duties of each group. Phase 2 requires the development of a strategy to manage the emergency scene. Phase 3 includes a postdisaster review of lessons learned from the incident and the determination of ways to improve.
- The five major functions of the ICS organization are command, planning, operations, logistics, and finance/administration.
- The responsibility of command should belong to one person. This should be a person who can effectively manage the emergency scene. In multiagency and/or multijurisdictional incidents, unified command may be used.
- The planning section should provide past, present, and future information about the incident and the status of resources. The operations section directs and coordinates all operations. It also ensures the safety of all personnel.

The logistics section is responsible for providing supplies and equipment (including personnel to operate the equipment), facilities, services, food, and communications support. The finance/administration section tracks incident and reimbursement costs.
- The need to expand the ICS at a medical incident is based on the number of casualties and the nature of the event.
- The first EMS unit to arrive at the scene should make a quick and rapid assessment of the situation. Command must immediately establish radio contact with the communications center or emergency operations center. Additional units should be requested as soon as the need has been identified.
- Common divisions or groups that may need to be established include extrication/rescue, treatment, and transportation. A staging area and support branch may also be needed. The rescue/extrication group is responsible for managing trapped patients at the scene. The treatment group provides advanced care and stabilization until the patients are transported to a medical facility. The transportation group communicates with the receiving hospital, ambulances, and aeromedical services for patient transport. The staging area is used in large incidents to prevent vehicle congestion and delays in response. The rehabilitation area allows rescue personnel to receive physical and psychological rest. The support branch coordinates the gathering and distribution of equipment and supplies for all divisions and groups.
- Problems of mass casualty incidents and incident command systems stem from numerous issues related to communication, resource allocation, and delegation.
- Triage is a method used to categorize patients for priorities of treatment. START triage uses a 60-second assessment. It focuses on the patient's ability to walk, respiratory effort, pulses/perfusion, and neurological status. The METTAG system is one of a number of tape, tag, and label systems used to categorize patients during triage.
- Critical incident stress debriefing is part of a critical incident stress management program. Such debriefing should be part of postdisaster standard operating procedures.

REVIEW QUESTIONS

Match the terms in column II with their definitions in column I. Use each term only once.

Column I	Column II
1. _____ Contracts agreeing to interagency exchange of resources when necessary	a. Apparatus
2. _____ Pumpers, ladder trucks, rescue trucks	b. Command
3. _____ Rendezvous location for all arriving EMS, fire, and rescue equipment	c. Command post
4. _____ Responsible for coordination of major incident situation	d. Communication center
	e. Mutual aid
	f. Sector
	g. Staging area

Questions 5 to 13 refer to the following case study:

Dispatch radios your crew to respond to a local sports stadium for a bleacher collapse at a college football game. During your initial size-up, you determine that 50 to 100 people are injured, with a substantial number of victims still trapped under the fallen concrete seats. It is rush hour, and traffic conditions will be heavy for at least 2 more hours.

5. List three actions that should be taken by the first unit arriving at the scene.

_____

_____

6. a. How will command be determined?

_____

_____

b. Will single or unified command be used?

_____

_____

7. List nine command responsibilities during this incident.

   a.

   b.

   c.

   d.

   e.

   f.

   g.

   h.

   i.

8. Fill in Fig. 50-1 with the appropriate positions needed in this incident command situation.

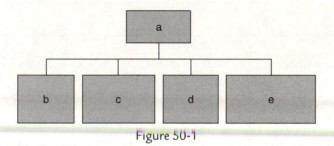

Figure 50-1

9. Briefly describe the responsibilities of each of the following sectors that command has established for this incident.

   a. Support branch:

_____

_____

   b. Staging area:

_____

_____

   c. Extrication group:

_____

_____

   d. Treatment group:

_____

_____

e. Transportation:

_____

_____

_____

10. Explain how communications can be initiated in an effective manner in this situation.

_____

_____

_____

11. a. What special resources will be needed during this incident?

_____

_____

    b. How will command know where to obtain those resources?

_____

_____

12. Triage each of the following patients injured at this scene using START triage and METTAG categories.

    a. A man walks over to you complaining of chest pain.

_____

    b. A woman has a respiratory rate of 20/min and no radial pulse, but a carotid pulse is present.

_____

    c. A man is lying under a bleacher. His respiratory rate is 24/min; a radial pulse is present; he can't touch his nose with his index finger; he knows his name but not the date or year.

_____

    d. A woman is leaning against a bleacher, unable to walk. Her respiratory rate is 16/min; a radial pulse is present; she can stick out her tongue and touch her nose with her index finger; she knows her name, the date, and the year.

_____

    e. A man has a respiratory rate of 8/min. He has no radial pulse, but a carotid pulse is present.

_____

    f. A woman is trapped under a post. She is not breathing and has no pulse.

_____

13. During triage, what care should be provided to the patients in question 12?

_____

STUDENT SELF-ASSESSMENT

14. An ideal incident command system would have which of the following characteristics?
    a. It would be able to expand to a larger incident in a logical manner.
    b. It would be used only for large or complex mass casualty situations.
    c. It would provide for just single jurisdiction involvement.
    d. It would respond to one specific incident or situation.

15. Which phase of major incident planning involves establishing an inventory of community resources needed for selected disasters?
    a. Logistics operations
    b. Postdisaster follow-up
    c. Scene management
    d. The preplan

16. What are the five major components of FEMA's ICS organization?
    a. Communications, logistics, operations, staging, support
    b. Communications, finance, staging, support, treatment
    c. Command, finance, logistics, operations, planning
    d. Command, operations, planning, transportation, treatment

17. Which of the following should have the highest priority when the incident commander is considering whether to expand the ICS organization during an incident?
    a. Cost
    b. Incident stability
    c. Life safety
    d. Property conservation

18. What is the primary responsibility of the section chiefs in an MCI situation?
    a. To assume overall accountability for the MCI situation
    b. To make sure that section members are working toward a common goal
    c. To operate rescue equipment and supervise staff in the area
    d. To provide patient care and stabilization within a defined area

19. Which section has overall responsibility for the areas that provide care to medical staff?
    a. Finance
    b. Logistics
    c. Operations
    d. Planning

20. Which of the following situations would be *least* likely to be declared a major incident?
    a. Rural EMS service, motor vehicle collision requiring four EMS units
    b. City EMS service, train derailment, possible hazardous materials leak
    c. Rural EMS service, two-patient incident with high-angle rescue
    d. City EMS service, two-person motor vehicle collision, no patient trapped

21. Except in unusual circumstances, patient care and stabilization should be provided by which group?
    a. Extrication
    b. Support
    c. Treatment
    d. Triage

22. What is an appropriate role for a physician brought to the scene from a local hospital?
    a. Incident commander
    b. Extrication group resource
    c. Staging area resource
    d. Transport group resource

23. The most appropriate *radio* communication during a mass casualty incident would be between which of the following crew members?
    a. Command and sector officers
    b. Individuals within each unit
    c. Treatment group and hospital
    d. Public information officer and press

24. Which of the following may create a problem at an MCI?
    a. Organizing patients rapidly at a treatment area
    b. Transporting patients prematurely
    c. Performing rapid "initial" stabilization of patients
    d. Wearing identification vests

25. Patient classification during mass casualty incidents should be based on which of the following?
    a. Physiological signs, mechanism of injury, and anatomical injury
    b. Mechanism of injury, anatomical injury, and patient age
    c. Chief complaint, physiological signs, and anatomical injury
    d. Physiological signs, anatomical injury, and concurrent disease

26. Your patient has a gunshot wound to the chest, is conscious, and has a respiratory rate of 36/min. Which of the following would be the appropriate triage category, using the triage systems discussed in the text?
    a. Urgent, yellow
    b. Critical, red
    c. Dead/dying, black
    d. Delayed, green
27. Mental status examination during START triage should include which of the following?
    a. Asking the patient to touch his nose
    b. AVPU
    c. Glasgow coma scale
    d. Observing for arm drift
28. What information should be included on the patient tracking log?
    a. Patient's age
    b. Patient's injuries
    c. Patient's next of kin
    d. Patient's priority
29. Which of the following is *not* typically provided in a critical incident stress management program?
    a. Advice to command during large-scale incidents
    b. Defusing services immediately after a large-scale incident
    c. Long-term psychiatric counseling
    d. On-scene support for distressed personnel

WRAP IT UP

At 0828 on this foggy morning, a large passenger aircraft runs off runway M2R, striking the perimeter fence around the airport. Your ambulance is the first to arrive on the scene. The local fire chief is the incident commander, and he immediately delegates your supervisor to assume EMS command. She, in turn, asks that you lead the rescue/extrication group. You send your partner to do a quick size-up of the patients who are out of the aircraft. The initial assessment reveals that the pilot was found not breathing and pulseless; three crew members and three passengers are noted to have inhalation injury and severe respiratory distress; the other 19 patients appear on initial exam to be walking, complaining of minor injuries. The next several hours are frantic and chaotic at times as the patients are sorted, treated, and finally transported.

During an incident debriefing 3 days later, you review the whole situation. The incident commander shows how he laid out the groups: rescue/extrication (triage, treatment, transport), staging, and transportation. A PIO officer was definitely an asset for dealing with the huge media presence, and a liaison officer helped to communicate with the unified command. Problems identified in the situation included difficulty with communication, a delay in getting ambulances to the scene, a traffic jam at the scene, difficulty identifying branch leaders, and failure to update the hospitals about incoming patients. Some suggestions are offered for remedying these problems, and another planning meeting is scheduled for 2 weeks later.

1. What additional support staff person should have been appointed by command, in addition to the public relations and liaison officers?

2. What are some possible causes of the difficulties identified in this situation, and which sectors or branches are responsible for identifying solutions?

Problem	Possible Causes	Sector or Branch Responsible for Solution
a. Difficulty with communication		
b. Delay in ambulance arrival		
c. Traffic jam on scene		
d. Difficulty identifying command		
e. Failure to update hospitals		

3. Based on the limited information you have, how many patients would you triage as
   a. Dead or dying
   b. Critical
   c. Urgent
   d. Delayed

CHAPTER 50 ANSWERS

REVIEW QUESTIONS

1. e
2. a
3. g
4. b
(Questions 1-4: Objective 1)

5. A rapid scene assessment should be performed. Communication should be established with the communications center or emergency operations center (as dictated by local policy). Additional units should be requested as soon as the need has been identified.
(Objective 7)

6. a. Command is determined by the preplanned system of arriving emergency units. The person assuming command must be familiar with ICS structure and the operating procedures of responding units.
(Objective 7)

b. It will likely be a unified command involving EMS, fire/rescue, and police. Some communities have public safety departments that incorporate all three functions. In that case, a single command will likely be used.
(Objective 4)

7. Assuming an effective command position that has a good vantage point and is away from any danger of the bleachers, some responsibilities would be: transmitting initial radio reports to the communications center; evaluating the scene rapidly (visually and with reports of other first responders); developing a strategy to safely extricate, triage, treat, transport, and provide security on scene; requesting additional equipment and personnel resources and assigning command roles; assigning sectors and identifying objectives in cooperation with section chiefs; evaluating information to determine the progress of the event; sending units no longer needed back into service; terminating command at an appropriate time; and evaluating the effectiveness of operations (may be done retrospectively).
(Objective 4)

8. Incident command organizational chart completed. a. Command b. Finance c. Logistic d. Operation e. Planning
(Objective 3)

9. a. Procuring and distributing supplies (medicine, food, water, protective gear) and resources (heavy equipment, special tools).
b. Designating and staffing a safe helicopter landing zone and designating and staffing a staging area where all arriving apparatus will report and be assigned to areas where needed.
c. Triaging victims and moving them to a designated treatment area; securing necessary experts to determine the safest extrication procedures for this structure; coordinating physical rescue operations (including direction of heavy equipment); and ensuring scene safety.
d. Selecting a site close to but at a safe distance from the collapse site; categorizing patients on arrival and sending them to the appropriate segment of the treatment area or immediate or delayed zones; providing patient care and stabilization until transport can be provided; and communicating frequently with the transportation sector so that appropriate patient transfers can be facilitated.
e. Coordinating patient transport with the staging area manager and treatment groups; communicating with receiving hospitals so that appropriate resources can be selected; and assigning patients to ambulances or helicopters and directing them to the appropriate facilities.
(Objective 8)

10. Effective communications can be enhanced by using a common frequency (command frequency) for interdisciplinary communication when necessary; using the radio frequencies designated in the plan; using different frequencies for fire, EMS, and other support agencies; making sure that common terminology is used; ensuring clear, concise radio traffic; preparing messages before transmitting; limiting use of radios; and identifying the speaker only by sector.
(Objective 7)

11. a. Air medical transport, because of heavy traffic and heavy equipment needed to extricate victims from under the bleachers.
(Objective 8)

b. The preplan should identify the availability and location of specialized resources that may be needed during an MCI situation.
(Objective 2)

12. a. Delayed, yellow (may be upgraded after retriage in treatment sector)
    b. Critical, red
    c. Critical, yellow
    d. Delayed, green
    e. Critical, red
    f. Dead/dying, black
(Objective 10)

13. The airway may be opened if necessary and hemorrhage controlled.
(Objective 10)

STUDENT SELF-ASSESSMENT

14. a. The ICS should be adaptable to small or large situations involving one or more jurisdictions as the need arises.
(Objective 1)

15. d. Preidentification of resources ensures rapid deployment by logistics during a disaster.
(Objective 2)

16. c. Command, finance, logistics, operations, and planning (C-FLOP) are the foundations on which the ICS is built.
(Objective 3)

17. c. The priority is always the safety of the emergency responders and the public.
(Objective 4)

18. b. The incident commander has overall responsibility. The section chiefs should be directing staff in their sectors, not performing physical tasks or providing patient care.
(Objective 3)

19. b. The rehab branch falls under the command of the logistics section.
(Objective 3)

20. d. In most city EMS systems, this type of patient situation should not overwhelm the system, requiring a mass casualty plan.
(Objective 6)

21. c. In triage, patients are sorted, airways are opened, and hemorrhage is controlled.
(Objective 8)

22. b. Physicians are probably not appropriately trained for command. Their services may be more useful in assisting with triage and providing emergency surgery to facilitate extrication (all extrication sector responsibilities). A physician may also be assigned to the treatment sector.
(Objective 3)

23. a. As much verbal communication as possible should take place during the mass casualty incident to permit essential communication on the airwaves.
(Objective 7)

24. b
(Objective 9)

25. d. Abnormal vital signs, obvious anatomical injury, and other obvious preexisting illnesses and injuries should be considered when triaging patients.
(Objective 10)

26. b. A respiratory rate over 30/min indicates critical status in the START triage method. This patient obviously has a serious anatomical injury and abnormal physiological signs, indicating that urgent care is necessary.
(Objective 10)

27. a. The patient should also be asked to state his name and the current date, including the year.
(Objective 10)

28. d. Patient identification, transporting unit, and hospital destination should also be noted.
(Objective 10)

29. c. The services provided depend on the local CISM team.
(Objective 11)

WRAP IT UP

1. There should always be a safety officer.
   (Objective 1)

2.

Problem	Possible Causes	Sector or Branch Responsible for Solution
a. Difficulty with communication	Failure to designate specific channels in preplan and/or early in incident Excessive talking on the radio; failure to use face-to-face communication	Incident command Sector officers
b. Delay in ambulance arrival	Possible failure to request resources early Possible failure to adequately control the perimeter and access roads	Incident command
c. Traffic jam on scene	Failure to designate staging area early; failure to designate areas spread apart (e.g., transportation, staging, command)	Law enforcement Incident command
d. Difficulty identifying command	Possible failure to declare who is in command on the radio Failure to wear identification vests or to mark the command area adequately	Incident command
e. Failure to update hospitals	Failure to give hospitals a brief report when wounded are leaving	Transportation group leader

   (Objective 9)

3. a. 1
   b. 3
   c. 0
   d. 19

   (Objective 10)

Rescue Awareness and Operations

READING ASSIGNMENT

Chapter 51, pages 1256-1275 in *Mosby's Paramedic Textbook,* ed. 3

OBJECTIVES

Upon completion of this chapter, the paramedic student will be able to do the following:

1. Describe factors that must be considered to ensure appropriate timing of medical and mechanical skills during a rescue.
2. Outline each phase of a rescue operation.
3. Identify the appropriate personal protective equipment (PPE) for rescue operations.
4. Describe important considerations for emergency medical services (EMS) crews in a surface water rescue.
5. Discuss important considerations for EMS crews in rescues associated with hazardous atmospheres, including confined spaces and trench or cave-in situations.
6. Describe hazards that may be present during an EMS rescue operation on a highway.
7. Describe important considerations for EMS crews in a rescue involving hazardous terrain.
8. Outline special considerations for prehospital assessment and management during a rescue operation.

SUMMARY

- Rescue is a patient-driven event. It calls for specialized medical and mechanical skills. The right amount of each must be applied at the right time. The main role of the paramedic in rescues is to have the proper training and the appropriate PPE. These allow safe access to the patient and the provision of treatment at the site and throughout the incident.
- The seven phases of a rescue operation are arrival and scene size-up, hazard control, gaining access to the patient, medical treatment, disentanglement, patient packaging, and transportation.
- The standards for protective clothing and personal protection equipment established by the National Fire Protection Association and OSHA have been adopted by many fire and EMS agencies. The appropriate PPE depends on the level of rescuer involvement and the nature of the incident.
- Water rescue should never be attempted by a single rescuer or by one who is untrained.
- Water hazards include obstructions to flow and foot or extremity pins that can trap victims and drag them under water. Some factors that contribute to flat water drowning are alcohol or other drug use. Also, cool water temperatures contribute to such drownings.

- Hazardous atmospheres are environments with low oxygen. These environments can occur in confined spaces. The six major hazards associated with confined spaces are oxygen-deficient atmospheres, chemical/toxic exposure and explosion, engulfment, machinery entrapment, electricity, and structural concerns.
- Traffic flow is the biggest hazard in EMS highway operations. Other scene hazards associated with highway operations include fuel or fire hazards, electrical power, unstable vehicles, airbags and supplemental restraint systems, and hazardous cargoes.
- Hazardous terrain can create major difficulties during rescue events. Three common classifications of hazardous terrain are low-angle, high-angle, and flat terrain with obstructions.

REVIEW QUESTIONS

Questions 1 and 2 refer to the following case study:

> A woman who is kayaking on a winter day is swept under the ice. You can see her about 3 feet (1 meter) from the edge of the ice where the water is rolling up over a large rock. Her team is frantically screaming at you to do something.

1. What hazards do you face if you enter the water to attempt a rescue?

_____

Additional equipment is requested, and a cut is made in the ice to retrieve the woman. However, she does not survive the 90-minute submersion.

2. What services of the local CISM team might your crew need after this incident?

_____

Questions 3 to 8 refer to the following case study:

> A party-goer falls into an open sewer standpipe. You estimate that he is approximately 30 feet down the 48-inch pipe. Bystanders report that he was talking to them when they arrived, but you hear him moaning only occasionally at this time.

3. What additional assistance will you request?

_____

4. What potential injuries should you worry about in this patient?

_____

5. Why must the rescue team test the air quality at several levels in the pipe?

_____

6. Why might the rescuer who enters the pipe wear an SABA instead of an SCBA during this rescue?

_____

7. What can cause problems when using an SABA?

_____

8. Aside from a confined-space rescue, what other hazardous rescue situation exists here?

_____

_____

Questions 9 to 18 refer to the following case study:

You are called to the scene of a motor vehicle collision at a busy urban shopping center. On arrival, you find that a large sedan has hit the side of a compact car, wedging it between the sedan and a storefront. A large crowd of spectators has gathered and is impeding your access to the patient. You note a trickle of gasoline coming from one of the vehicles. No other equipment or law enforcement personnel have been dispatched.

9. What should you be looking for as you do your scene size-up?

_____

10. What information/assistance did you receive on your response?

_____

_____

11. What steps should you take to gain control of the crowd?

_____

_____

_____

One patient was pulled from the sedan by bystanders before your arrival. He is pale and complains of abdominal pain. Your partner begins care. A second patient in the compact car is unconscious. He is trapped and inaccessible.

12. List the additional equipment and other resources you should request at this time.

_____

13. What hazards have you identified that should be reported to incoming crews?

_____

14. What actions can be taken to reduce the risks associated with the hazards you identified?

_____

_____

A rescue truck arrives, and the crew breaks a window in the compact car, providing limited access to the patient while rescue operations proceed.

15. What can you do for your patient at this time?

_____

16. How can you ensure patient safety during the rescue?

_____

_____

A brief primary survey reveals an unconscious patient with gurgling respirations and a strong radial pulse of 70/min. You observe a large ecchymotic area on the temporal region of the patient's head.

17. You have limited time and access to the patient. What are your priorities of care?

_____

_____

18. Describe the disentanglement, packaging, and removal segments of the rescue operation and your responsibilities to the patient during these phases.

_____

_____

_____

_____

_____

19. At the scene of an accident in which an energized wire is in contact with an involved automobile, what safety measures should be taken for

a. Rescuers:

_____

_____

b. People trapped in the involved automobile:

_____

_____

20. Give two examples of equipment that may be used to disentangle a person who is trapped inside a vehicle.

a.

b.

STUDENT SELF-ASSESSMENT

21. Aside from ensuring safety, the rescue operations should be guided by which of the following?
   a. Performance of techniques in the standardized manner
   b. The desire of the rescue team to complete the task
   c. The medical and physical needs of the patient
   d. The number of bystanders observing the scene

22. What is the responsibility of the paramedic in any rescue situation?
   a. To coordinate overall scene safety
   b. To direct scene and tactical operations
   c. To know when it is safe to attempt rescue
   d. To operate all rescue and extrication equipment
23. The safety of which of the following should be the *first* priority at the scene of any rescue?
   a. Bystanders **c.** Injured
   b. Crew **d.** Trapped
24. When does scene size-up begin on a call for rescue?
   a. On arrival to the scene **c.** When the call is received
   b. When specialized teams arrive **d.** When the patient is visible
25. Which is true regarding medical treatment during a rescue situation for a safely accessible patient?
   a. All standardized procedures should be followed.
   b. Medical treatment should be directed by the rescue commander.
   c. No treatment should be attempted until the patient has been freed.
   d. Rapid assessment and basic stabilization should be attempted.
26. What routine safety measures should be used to protect the patient during a vehicle rescue that does not involve fire or hazardous materials?
   a. Blanket **c.** Surgical mask
   b. Air bags **d.** An SCBA
27. According to NFPA and OSHA standards, EMS rescue personnel should have access to all the following personal protective equipment *except*
   a. Ear plugs **c.** Rubber boots
   b. Protective helmet **d.** Waterproof gloves
28. Which is true when responding to a rescue in swift water?
   a. A foot trapped in water should be freed the opposite way it went in.
   b. Do not walk through fast-moving water that is over knee deep.
   c. Flat water does not create any serious hazard.
   d. High dams create more dangerous situations than low dams.
29. What factors contribute to drowning?
   a. Cool water temperature **c.** PFDs worn properly
   b. Advanced patient age **d.** Swimming after eating
30. What factor would be an acceptable reason *not* to resuscitate a person who has drowned?
   a. More than 5 minutes of submersion was documented by witnesses.
   b. Evidence of activation of the mammalian diving reflex exists.
   c. Patient is cold, and temperature can't be detected on a regular thermometer.
   d. Rigor mortis or dependent lividity is present.
31. What is the first measure that should be used to attempt rescue for a person in the water?
   a. Go **c.** Row
   b. Reach **d.** Throw
32. Which of the following oxygen levels is considered hazardous?
   a. Over 19.5% **c.** Over 21%
   b. Over 22% **d.** Under 21%
33. Which is a clue to help identify an oxygen-limiting silo?
   a. An audible tone will sound.
   b. The color is usually blue.
   c. The placard states this information.
   d. The smell will be sweet.
34. You arrive at the scene of a trench collapse. When do you enter the trench to rescue the patient without specialized rescue equipment?
   a. The patient is unconscious.
   b. The patient is completely covered.
   c. The trench is less than waist deep.
   d. The trench is more than 3 feet wide.

35. Which of the following techniques may be used to increase safety at the scene of a vehicle accident with a gasoline leak at night?
    a. Put flares adjacent to the involved vehicles to alert motorists.
    b. Stage all apparatus on the highway and not on side roads.
    c. Use all warning lights and headlights to increase visibility.
    d. Wear high-visibility clothing, such as orange highway vests.
36. To reduce the risk of fire at the scene of a motor vehicle collision in which gasoline is leaking, a paramedic should *always* do which of the following?
    a. Disconnect the battery cable
    b. Douse the vehicle with foam
    c. Place a tarp over the spilled fuel
    d. Turn off the automobile ignition
37. Which type of extinguisher can be used to suppress a combustible metal fire?
    a. Class A   c. Class C
    b. Class B   d. Class D
38. What type of equipment is helpful for vehicle stabilization during rescue?
    a. Chain saws   c. Hurst tools
    b. Cribbing   d. Pry bars
39. You respond to a vehicle crash involving an undeployed air bag. What measure may create a hazard for rescuers?
    a. Using tools that generate sparks
    b. Cutting the steering column to disable the system
    c. Disconnecting or cutting both battery cables
    d. Cutting into the air bag module
40. What is the primary risk associated with hazardous terrain rescue?
    a. Avalanche of debris   c. Injury from falls
    b. Dropping the patient   d. Injury from projectiles
41. Which term describes rescue on steep terrain that can be walked on without use of the hands?
    a. Graded terrain rescue
    b. High-angle rescue
    c. Low-angle rescue
    d. Rescue on flat terrain with obstructions
42. Which of the following factors that can interfere with a paramedic's ability to adequately assess and treat a patient is unique to a rescue situation?
    a. Cumbersome personal protective equipment
    b. Lack of cooperation among your team members
    c. Hostile, uncommunicative patient
    d. Unstable vital signs and neurological status
43. Which is a complication of crush syndrome?
    a. Hypertension   c. Myoglobinemia
    b. Metabolic alkalosis   d. Sepsis
44. You are trying to free a driver involved in a head-on crash who is seriously injured. The car shows major front-end damage; also, the passenger air bag has deployed, but the driver-side air bag has not. How will this affect your approach to the rescue?
    a. When the ignition is off, the bag will not open unless there is a fire.
    b. It will not affect your approach to this patient.
    c. You will put a board between the patient and the unopened bag.
    d. You will keep at least 10 inches or more away from the path of the bag.

WRAP IT UP

You can sense the panic as you pull up to the scene of a mine explosion. Six men were down in the narrow shaft when a rumbling noise was heard, and then a plume of dark smoke slowly wound out of the mine. The incident commander and mine supervisor are reviewing the situation, trying to determine the best approach. An alternate shaft is available, but there is a fear of secondary danger. One garbled radio transmission from below indicates that there are survivors, but several are trapped under the rubble. It is determined that you and your partner will go in first because of your advanced, confined-space rescue training. The two of you don an SABA and rappelling harness and are lowered slowly down the secondary shaft. At the bottom, water is slowly creeping up the walls of the enclosure. Your lamps provide a glimpse of some movement through the haze, and you carefully move along the side of the wall, taking care not to catch your air hoses on the protruding rocks. When you reach the miners, two are dead, three are in good condition, and one is entangled in some twisted rebar. Over the next 4 hours, first the three men in good condition are lifted up the narrow shaft in a rescue harness; then the rebar is cut, the fourth miner is removed from the wreckage, his wounds are treated, and he is pulled to the top wrapped securely in a Stokes basket. Finally, the agonizing job of respectfully packaging and lifting the bodies is undertaken.

1. Put a ✓ beside potential hazards faced by the rescuers in this situation.
   a. _____ Collapse/engulfment
   b. _____ Electrical
   c. _____ Explosion
   d. _____ Hypothermia
   e. _____ Oxygen deficiency
   f. _____ Toxic gases

2. Identify steps that should be taken to minimize the risks you indicated for the trapped miners and for the rescuers.

_____

_____

_____

3. What personal protective equipment should the rescuers be using in this situation?

_____

4. Which phase of the rescue operation was it when the rescuers cut the rebar and freed the miner?
   a. Disentanglement
   b. Gaining access to the patient
   c. Hazard control
   d. Patient packaging

5. Which elements of low- or high-angle rescue did the rescuers need to consider during this situation?

_____

_____

6. Why should only specially trained rescuers be sent down the shaft on this type of call?

_____

_____

CHAPTER 51 ANSWERS

REVIEW QUESTIONS

1. Drowning, foot/extremity entrapment, hypothermia, recirculating current
   (Objective 4)

2. Defusing immediately after the incident if the emotional impact is high; critical incident stress debriefing 24 to 72 hours after the incident; follow-up to ensure that specific crew members are recovering; specialty debriefing for the people with the patient (if your team provides that service)

3. Rescue truck, possibly specialized hazardous materials team, high-angle rescue specialists
   (Objective 2)

4. Asphyxiation, toxic inhalation, trauma, drowning, and exposure (depending on time of year)
   (Objective 5)

5. Toxic gas may exist, or oxygen levels may be low, and these conditions may vary at different levels in the pipe.
   (Objective 5)

6. It may be difficult to maneuver in the pipe with a standard air tank, and the time required for the rescue may exceed the tank capacity.
   (Objective 5)

7. The line may kink or tangle, or the equipment may fail.
   (Objective 5)

8. High-angle rescue probably will be necessary to retrieve the patient.
   (Objective 7)

9. During arrival and scene size-up, you should look for environmental risks, the number of patients, and the need for medical care and/or rescue and then request additional resources.
   (Objectives 2, 6)

10. Information was limited to location and the fact that a crash had occurred. No additional equipment was dispatched (or has arrived).
    (Objective 2)

11. Immediately delegate several crowd members to move the crowd to a safe distance to allow for patient care and the arrival of additional equipment. Call for law enforcement officers to take charge of crowd control.
    (Objective 2)

12. Advanced life support ambulance, rescue truck, pumper, and law enforcement officers
    (Objective 2)

13. Hazards identified are a crowd and the gasoline spill.
    (Objective 2)

14. Make sure no one is smoking near the crash. Also, disconnect the vehicle battery cables.
    (Objective 2)

15. Begin initial patient assessment and airway management (if indicated).
    (Objective 8)

16. Protect the patient with blankets, shields, or flame-retardant coverings.
(Objective 8)

17. Securing an open airway, protecting the cervical spine, and assisting ventilations with high-concentration oxygen if possible.
(Objective 8)

18. Disentanglement involves removing the wreckage from the patient. Rescuers must protect the patient and maintain the airway, cervical spine immobilization, and breathing to the best of their ability. Packaging involves immobilization and removal of the patient from the scene to the emergency response vehicle. Rescuers must protect the patient's spine, splint or bandage injuries if appropriate (based on the acuteness of the patient's condition), and make sure that the patient is adequately secured before removal begins. The paramedic should oversee safe transport of the patient by the rescue team to the ambulance.
(Objective 2)

19. a. Contact utility workers to move downed wires or shut off power, keep bystanders away, and secure energized wires with a dry fire hose or other appropriate means.
b. Advise occupants to stay in the car.
(Objective 6)

20. Ropes, air bags, pry bars, jacks, wedges, cutters, spreaders, and winches
(Objective 6)

STUDENT SELF-ASSESSMENT

21. c. Other than safety, the patient is the primary focus of the rescue.
(Objective 1)

22. c. Unless responding as part of a specialized fire/rescue team, the paramedic is not responsible for coordinating the rescue, serving as the safety officer, or operating equipment. Although everyone on the scene should be alert for overall safety considerations, the paramedic's responsibilities are to recognize when a rescue is safe before arrival of specialized teams and to provide patient care and monitoring during a rescue situation.
(Objective 1)

23. b. Initial efforts should ensure that the crew is uninjured so that their EMS functions can be maintained.
(Objective 1)

24. c. The dispatch call can provide the first information paramedics need to size up a rescue situation and respond to it with the appropriate safety measures.
(Objective 2)

25. d. Moving all standardized equipment into the rescue area is not practical. Basic assessment and stabilization should be attempted until the patient is in the ambulance. In certain situations, when the surroundings are unsafe or the patient is inaccessible, delivery of care may not be possible.
(Objective 2)

26. a. Ear and eye protection may also be necessary. A face mask with supplemental air or oxygen would be needed only in situations in which the oxygen supply is inadequate or toxic fumes are present.
(Objective 2)

27. a. Although ear plugs are helpful during the response, they may impair communication on a rescue.
(Objective 3)

28. b. Walking in swift water could result in a foot becoming trapped, and the paramedic could be dragged under the surface.
(Objective 4)

29. a. Alcohol and drug use also contribute to drowning. Properly worn PFDs reduce the risk of drowning.
(Objective 4)

30. d. Survival after cold water drowning is difficult to predict; rigor mortis, dependent lividity, or putrefaction indicates death.
(Objective 4)

31. b. If the person is close enough, the rescuer should reach out with a long device. The next measure would be to throw a device to the person. Then, if this is unsuccessful, a boat should be taken to rescue the person. Finally, if no other option exists, a trained rescuer with appropriate PPE should enter the water in an attempt to rescue the individual.
(Objective 4)

32. b. High oxygen concentrations create a risk of rapid combustion to fuel fire or explosion. Concentrations below 19.5% are considered an atmospheric hazard.
(Objective 5)

33. b. Personnel on the scene may be helpful and may also provide that information.
(Objective 5)

34. c. Rescuer safety should be the primary concern.
(Objective 5)

35. d. Flares would be dangerous in the presence of a gasoline leak. Apparatus should be staged off the highway if possible. Placing one large apparatus in front of the scene so that safe loading can occur may be helpful. Use warning lights cautiously and make sure that headlights are not pointed at oncoming traffic.
(Objective 6)

36. d. In some cases the battery may be left connected. The other measures would be unnecessary in the absence of flames.
(Objective 6)

37. d. Class A is used to extinguish ordinary combustibles; class B, flammable liquids; and class C, energized electrical equipment.
(Objective 6)

38. b. The other tools are used for disentanglement.
(Objective 6)

39. c. The steering column should not be cut.
(Objective 6)

40. c. Both the rescuers and patient are at risk for falls during rescue from hazardous terrain.
(Objective 7)

41. c. *High angle* refers to cliffs or the sides of buildings or other structures; rope or aerial apparatus is needed for such rescues. Flat terrain with obstacles may include large rocks, loose soil, and waterbeds or creeks.
(Objective 7)

42. a. Ideally, team cooperation is a standard on all scenes. Hostile or unstable patients are not unique to rescue situations.
(Objective 8)

43. c. When the muscles are crushed, they release their pigment (myoglobin), which can cause renal failure. Hypotension and metabolic acidosis may also occur.
(Objective 8)

44. d. If possible, avoid that side of the car for your safety.
(Objective 8)

WRAP IT UP

1. a, b, c, d, e, f
(Objective 5)

2. Collapse: The incident commander should confer with the site engineer to determine the risk of further collapse.
Electrical: The incident commander and site engineer should make sure that power is disabled if the risk of electrical injury exists.
Explosion: The cause of the initial explosion should be identified, if possible, and the risk of secondary explosion determined. Measurements should be taken in the shaft to determine if explosive gas levels are present.
Hypothermia: The depth of the cold water and the potential for the water to rise to a dangerous level, posing the risk of hypothermia and/or drowning, should be determined.
Oxygen deficiency and toxic gases: Gas levels should be monitored.
(Objective 5)

3. Helmet, light, face shield or goggles, gloves, boots with steel toe shank, Nomex jumpsuit, PFD if risk of water rising exists
(Objective 3)

4. a. Gaining access to the patient was accomplished if the patient were accessible at first contact. Hazard control should have started before the rescuers entered the shaft and continued until conclusion of the rescue. Packaging covered the activities involved in securing the patient in the Stokes basket.
(Objective 2)

5. Low-angle rescue considerations would develop as the rescuers moved through the obstructions and hazards in the shaft. High-angle rescue principles would have been applied when the rescuers were lowered into the shaft and the miners were removed.
(Objective 7)

6. Confined space rescue is a very hazardous, specialized rescue. Attempting to enter the shaft without proper training would be very dangerous. It would likely violate OSHA rules.
(Objective 8)

CHAPTER

52

Crime Scene Awareness

READING ASSIGNMENT
Chapter 52, pages 1276-1285, in *Mosby's Paramedic Textbook*, ed. 3

OBJECTIVES
Upon completion of this chapter, the paramedic student will be able to:
1. Describe general techniques for determining whether a scene is violent and choosing the appropriate response to a violent scene.
2. Outline techniques for recognizing and responding to potentially dangerous residential calls.
3. Outline techniques for recognizing and responding to potentially dangerous calls on the highway.
4. Describe signs of danger and emergency medical services (EMS) response to violent street incidents.
5. Identify characteristics of and EMS response to situations involving gangs, clandestine drug labs, and domestic violence situations.
6. Outline general safety tactics that EMS personnel can use if they find themselves in a dangerous situation.
7. Describe special EMS considerations when providing tactical patient care.
8. Discuss EMS documentation and preservation of evidence at a crime scene.

SUMMARY
- A key point in ensuring scene safety is to identify and respond to dangers before they threaten. If the scene is known to be violent, the EMS crew should remain at a safe and out-of-sight distance from the area. They should remain at this distance until the scene has been secured.
- The paramedic should look for warning signs of violence during response to a residence. He or she should retreat from the scene if danger becomes evident.
- A response to a highway incident may present the dangers associated with traffic and extrication. However, it may present danger from violence as well. Occupants may be armed, wanted or fleeing felons, intoxicated or drugged, or violent/abusive from an altered mental state.
- The paramedic should monitor for warning signs of danger in violent street incidents. He or she should retreat from the scene if necessary.
- A gang is any group of people who take part in socially disruptive or criminal behavior. Some gangs are involved in violent criminal activities. EMS personnel often look like law enforcement officers. Thus, they should be very cautious about personal safety when working in gang areas.

- Clandestine lab activities can produce explosive and toxic gases. Other risks include booby traps that can maim or kill an intruder, and armed or violent occupants.
- EMS personnel who respond to a scene of domestic violence should be aware that acts of violence may be directed toward them by the perpetrator; they should take all safety precautions.
- Tactics for safety include avoidance, tactical retreat, cover and concealment, and distraction and evasive maneuvers.
- Tactical patient care refers to care activities that occur inside the scene perimeter. This is known as the "hot zone." Providing care in this area calls for special training and authorization, body armor and a tactical uniform, compact and functional equipment, and in some operations, personal defensive weapons.
- The paramedic's observations at a crime scene are important. They should be carefully documented. Evidence should be protected while caring for the patient. This can be done by not unnecessarily disturbing the scene or destroying evidence.

REVIEW QUESTIONS

Questions 1 and 2 apply to the following case study:

You are responding to a routine call in a residential neighborhood.

1. When should your scene size-up begin?

_____

2. List six warning signs of danger that you should look for on this call.

   a.

   b.

   c.

   d.

   e.

   f.

3. List strategies to increase safety as you approach each of the following:
   a. A darkened residence:

_____

_____

   b. A vehicle stopped on the side of the highway:

_____

_____

4. For each of the situations below, indicate which of the following tactics would best increase your safety and describe how you would use it.

   Avoidance   Cover and concealment
   Tactical retreat   Distraction and evasive maneuvers

   a. You respond to a school shooting. En route, you determine that several shots fired in a school classroom have been reported; however, there is no confirmation that the perpetrator has been apprehended.

_____

_____

b. You are providing care to an injured fan at a large soccer match when irate fans begin to hurl bottles at you and your partner.

_____

_____

c. You are on bike patrol at a community picnic. You respond to a call for a "person injured." You find a teenager dressed in known gang attire who was punched in the face. As you begin your care, you hear the sound of gunfire nearby.

_____

_____

d. During assessment of a patient with an altered level of consciousness in the living room of a small home, his behavior escalates suddenly and he starts yelling and threatening to hurt you as he lunges toward you.

_____

_____

5. List six types of physical evidence that may be found at a crime scene.

a.

b.

c.

d.

e.

f.

STUDENT SELF-ASSESSMENT

6. When should assessment of the potential for violence at the scene begin?
   a. If the patient threatens the crew
   b. On arrival at the scene
   c. When the patient is encountered
   d. En route to the call

7. Which of the following may indicate that the residence you are about to enter is potentially dangerous?
   a. Darkened residence   **c.** No car in the driveway
   b. History of multiple calls   **d.** Person waving you in

8. Which represents the safest approach to a single vehicle stopped on the highway?
   a. Approach from the passenger side of the vehicle
   b. Simultaneous approach by both crew members
   c. Ambulance lights turned off to eliminate glare
   d. Walking between the ambulance and the other vehicle

9. Which of the following is most likely to protect the paramedic from danger during a violent street scene?
   a. Allow police to control the scene and proceed as usual.
   b. Attempt to disperse the crowd while providing care.
   c. Retreat immediately from the scene with the patient.
   d. There is no danger; crowds will not attack paramedics.

10. How can you learn about gang-related activity in your EMS response area?
   a. Police   **c.** Social service agencies
   b. School officials   **d.** All of the above

11. Which of the following drugs are commonly produced or altered in drug labs?
    a. Codeine
    c. Methamphetamine
    b. Marijuana
    d. Morphine
12. Which of the following may signal a situation that includes domestic violence?
    a. Darkened rooms
    c. Inaccurate medical history
    b. Excessive nervous talking
    d. Inconsistent injuries
13. Which of the following is a common EMS safety strategy in a dangerous situation?
    a. Avoidance
    c. Negotiation
    b. Contact
    d. Use of weapons
14. Which is an appropriate location for cover during gunfire?
    a. Bushes
    c. Large tree
    b. Car door
    d. Wooden sign
15. Which of the following provides a clue that a patient may become violent?
    a. Crossed legs
    c. Quiet dialogue
    b. Hands on hips
    d. Verbal abuse
16. Body armor is least effective against which of the following weapons?
    a. Air guns
    c. Ice picks
    b. Handguns
    d. Knives
17. Which of the following does tactical paramedic training usually include?
    a. HAZMAT decontamination
    b. Minor surgical techniques
    c. Radiographic interpretation
    d. Suturing and advanced wound care
18. Which of the following is an appropriate way to approach a crime scene?
    a. Document any suspicions you may have.
    b. Follow the same path to and from the victim.
    c. Move visible evidence so that police can find it.
    d. Save patient items in a plastic bag.

WRAP IT UP

As you respond to a call for a suicidal patient, dispatch notifies you that this address is flagged because the occupant is heavily armed and has shown violent behavior in the past. The dispatcher notifies you that the police are en route. The 9-1-1 call was placed by the patient's girlfriend, who said that he was threatening to "blow his brains out." You stage a block away from the home, out of sight of the scene, until dispatch notifies you, "The scene is safe; you may proceed in." You enter the darkened house and find your patient, a very tall, muscular man in his sixties. He is a retired police officer and has many weapons, which are evident to you. You hear loud barking from behind a closed bedroom door. Police tell you that a German shepherd that had been trained as an attack dog was secured in that room. As you begin to question the patient, he somehow escapes the grip of the police and grabs a gun. You and your partner quickly flee the house and run behind the ambulance engine-block, where you seek cover. A prolonged standoff with the police ensues, until finally the tactical police squad throws a stun grenade into the home, subduing the patient, and the incident is over.

1. What is the rationale for staging a block away from this scene?

2. Aside from known information about previous violent episodes, what are some other situational clues that this may be a violent scene?

3. Put a ✓ beside the safety tactics that were used at this scene.
   a. _____ Avoidance
   c. _____ Distraction and evasive maneuvers
   b. _____ Cover and concealment
   d. _____ Tactical retreat

4. If you were to hide behind the ambulance box, which of the following would be true?
   a. It would provide cover.
   b. It would protect you from gunfire.
   c. It would provide protection from any potential danger.
   d. It would provide temporary concealment.

5. a. Is this a crime scene? Yes/No
   b. If you answered yes, what additional responsibilities do you have on the call?

CHAPTER 52 ANSWERS

REVIEW QUESTIONS

1. Scene size-up for danger should begin during response and be based on dispatch information, knowledge of the area, and physical assessment of the scene during the approach.
(Objective 1)

2. a. Past history of problems or violence
   b. Known drug or gang area
   c. Loud noises indicating violent activity
   d. Presence of alcohol or drug use
   e. Presence of dangerous pets
   f. Unusual silence or darkened residence
(Objective 2)

3. a. Avoid use of lights and sirens as you get close; use unconventional pathways to approach the house; avoid positioning yourself between the ambulance lights and the residence; listen for signs of danger before entry; and stand on the doorknob side of the entry door.
(Objective 2)

   b. One crew member should approach the car while the other remains in the ambulance; ambulance lights should be used to light the vehicle; the approach should be made from the passenger side; and the paramedic should not walk between the ambulance and the other vehicle. Observe for unusual activity in the rear seat and do not move forward from post C if a threat is suspected. If any warning signs of danger are noted, retreat until law enforcement secures the scene.
(Objective 3)

4. a. Avoidance should be used. The EMS crew should stage their ambulance at a safe distance until law enforcement officers indicate that the scene is safe enough to proceed.
   b. Tactical retreat should be used and cover should be sought. The paramedics should immediately retreat to a safe area of cover for protection against the projectiles and the possibility of further crowd violence.
   c. Cover and concealment should immediately be sought. Seek cover behind a solid object that will not allow penetration of a bullet and conceal yourself from the perpetrator until the scene is safe or retreat can be done safely.
   d. Distraction and evasive maneuvers may be attempted during retreat. Try to move something between you and the patient to slow an attack as you quickly retreat.
(Objective 6)

5. a. Fingerprints
   b. Footprints
   c. Blood or other body fluids
   d. Hair
   e. Carpet fibers
   f. Clothing fibers
(Objective 8)

STUDENT SELF-ASSESSMENT

6. d. Locations of unsafe scenes may be known, as may the presence of crowds, intoxicated people on the scene, violence on the scene, or weapons.
(Objective 1)

7. a. Other indications of a potentially dangerous residence are a history of violence, known drug or gang area, loud noises, witnessing acts of violence, alcohol or drug use, or dangerous pets.
(Objective 2)

8. a. Lights should be left on, and only one crew member should approach, leaving the second crew member to call for help if needed.
(Objective 3)

9. c. Police may lose control of the scene, which would put you, your partner, and the patient in danger. Leave the scene as quickly as possible. Angry people may direct violence at uniformed paramedics.
(Objective 4)

10. d. Gang-related activity varies by region. All these agencies may provide you with information that can alert you to danger related to gang activities.
(Objective 5)

11. c. This process can produce hazardous gases, explosive forces, or fires.
(Objective 5)

12. d. Injuries that aren't consistent with the history or mechanism of injury should be viewed with suspicion. An inaccurate medical history may reflect poor patient knowledge. Excessive nervous talking may be related to many factors.
(Objective 5)

13. a. Avoidance requires alertness to detect and avoid dangerous situations.
(Objective 6)

14. c. The other choices provide concealment but can easily be penetrated by a bullet and therefore should not be used for cover.
(Objective 6)

15. d. The boxer stance and clenched fists are also signs of increasing aggression.
(Objective 6)

16. c. High-velocity rifle bullets or thin- or dual-edged weapons, such as ice picks, may penetrate body armor.
(Objective 7)

17. a. Other areas of training include hostage survival, care under fire, weapons and ballistics, medical threat assessment, forensic medicine, assessment under special situations, safe searches, dental injury management, medical issues related to drug lab raids, and rescue and extraction.
(Objective 7)

18. b. Document only objective findings; try not to disturb any evidence; save patient items in a paper bag.
(Objective 8)

WRAP IT UP

1. If the patient is violent, he may come after the EMS crew, injuring or killing crew members or taking a hostage.
(Objectives 1, 2)

2. The house is dark, the patient has numerous visible weapons, and a dangerous pet is on the premises.
(Objective 2)

3. a (staging); b (behind ambulance); d (running from house)
(Objective 6)

4. d. It would temporarily hide you from the perpetrator, but it does not afford complete protection from gunfire.
(Objective 6)

5. Yes. Objective observations should be carefully worded. Any significant statements from the patient should be recorded in quotes.
(Objective 8)

Hazardous Materials Incidents

READING ASSIGNMENT
Chapter 53, pages 1286-1305, in *Mosby's Paramedic Textbook*, ed. 3

OBJECTIVES
Upon completion of this chapter, the paramedic student will be able to:
1. Define hazardous materials terminology.
2. Identify legislation about hazardous materials that influences emergency health care workers.
3. Describe resources to assist in identification and management of hazardous materials incidents.
4. Identify the protective clothing and equipment needed to respond to selected hazardous materials incidents.
5. Describe the pathophysiology, signs, and symptoms of internal damage caused by exposure to selected hazardous materials.
6. Identify the pathophysiology, signs and symptoms, and prehospital management of selected hazardous materials that produce external damage.
7. Outline the prehospital response to a hazardous materials emergency.
8. Describe medical monitoring and rehabilitation of rescue workers who respond to a hazardous materials emergency.
9. Describe emergency decontamination and management of patients who have been contaminated by hazardous materials.
10. Outline the eight steps to decontaminate rescue personnel and equipment at a hazardous materials incident.

SUMMARY
- A hazardous material is any substance or material that is capable of posing an unreasonable risk to health, safety, and property.
- The Superfund Amendments and Reauthorization Act of 1986 established requirements for federal, state, and local governments and industry regarding emergency planning and the reporting of hazardous materials-related incidents. In 1989 OSHA and the EPA published rules to govern training requirements, emergency plans, medical checkups, and other safety precautions for workers at uncontrolled hazardous waste sites and those responding to hazardous chemical spills. In addition, the NFPA has published standards that address competencies for EMS workers at hazmat scenes.
- There are two methods used to identify hazardous materials. One is informal product identification. (This includes visual, olfactory, and verbal clues.) The other is formal product identification. (This includes, for

example, placards and shipping papers.) Resources for hazardous materials reference include the North American Emergency Response Guidebook, regional poison control centers, CHEMTREC, CHEMTEL, and CAMEO.

- It is crucial that anyone dealing with hazardous materials use proper protection. This includes using the proper respiratory devices. It also includes wearing protective clothing. This clothing is made of a variety of materials. The clothing is designed for certain chemical exposures. Thus, the manufacturer's guidelines must be followed.
- Hazardous materials may enter the body through inhalation, ingestion, injection, and absorption. Internal damage to the human body from hazardous materials exposure may involve the respiratory tract, CNS, or other internal organs. Chemicals producing internal damage include irritants, asphyxiants, nerve poisons, anesthetics, narcotics, hepatotoxins, cardiotoxins, nephrotoxins, neurotoxins, and carcinogens.
- Exposure to hazardous materials may result in burns. It also may result in severe tissue damage.
- The first agency to arrive at the scene of a hazardous materials incident must detect and identify the materials involved, assess the risk of exposure to rescue personnel and others, consider the potential risk of fire or explosion, gather information from on-site personnel or other sources, and confine and control the incident.
- A hazmat medical monitoring program may include medical examination for members of hazmat response teams, providing medical care, record-keeping, and periodic evaluation of the surveillance program.
- The primary goals of decontamination are to reduce the patient's dosage of material, decrease the threat of secondary contamination, and reduce the risk of rescuer injury.
- Rescuers should follow strict protocols for proper decontamination of themselves, their clothing, and any contaminated equipment.

REVIEW QUESTIONS

Match the HAZMAT terms in column II with the appropriate definition in column I. Use each term *only* once.

Column I		Column II
1. _____ Weight of pure vapor compared with the weight of an equal volume of dry air		**a.** Flammable/exposure limits
2. _____ Dose of chemical that will kill 50% of animals		**b.** Flash point
3. _____ Exposure limit of 15 minutes		**c.** IDLH
4. _____ Gas or vapor concentration that will burn or explode with ignition source		**d.** Ignition temperature
5. _____ Safe exposure for a 40-hour work week		**e.** LD50
6. _____ Minimum temperature to ignite gas without spark or flame		**f.** PEL
7. _____ Atmosphere that causes immediate harm		**g.** TLV-C
8. _____ Vapor's ability to mix with water		**h.** TLV-STEL
9. _____ Maximum concentration not to be exceeded even for a moment		**i.** Vapor density
10. _____ Temperature at which liquid produces enough vapor to ignite and flash over but not continue to burn without more heat		**j.** Vapor pressure
		k. Vapor solubility

Match each of the hazardous chemicals in column I with *all* the terms in column II that describe the chemical's associated health hazards. Answers may be used *more* than once.

Column I	Column II
11. _____ Arsenic	a. Asphyxiant
12. _____ Halogenated hydrocarbons	b. Anesthetic
13. _____ Hydrochloric acid	c. Carcinogen
14. _____ Hydrogen cyanide	d. Cardiotoxin
15. _____ Lead	e. Hemotoxin
16. _____ Malathion	f. Hepatotoxin
17. _____ Mercury	g. Irritant
	h. Nephrotoxin
	i. Nerve poison
	j. Neurotoxin

18. Briefly describe each of the five categories of emergency response personnel who may respond to a hazardous materials situation:

   a. First responder–awareness:

   _____

   _____

   b. First responder–operations:

   _____

   _____

   c. Hazardous materials technician:

   _____

   _____

   d. Hazardous materials specialist:

   _____

   _____

   e. On-scene incident commander:

   _____

   _____

19. You arrive on the scene of a motor vehicle collision involving an overturned tanker truck. You note a cloud of white vapor escaping from a relief valve on top of the truck. Describe the formal and informal means of identifying hazardous materials that may be involved in this situation.

   a. Formal:

   _____

   _____

b. Informal:

_____

20. After a hazardous material has been identified, what other resources can help the emergency response crew to determine the dangers and management of the scene?

_____

_____

21. Describe the protective clothing needed in the following hazardous materials response situations:

a. The hazardous materials crew provides emergency care to a seriously injured worker who is lying in an area contaminated with a liquid acidic chemical. No contaminated gas is present from the spill.

_____

_____

b. Your fire rescue team must enter a burning building to extricate trapped victims. No known hazardous materials are reported on the scene.

_____

_____

c. An equipment malfunction inside a chemical manufacturing plant has resulted in the release of toxic gases. Hazardous materials specialists must enter to attempt to locate a victim known to be just inside the hot zone.

_____

_____

22. Describe the health problems that can be encountered when an individual is exposed to the following agents:

a. Irritants:

_____

b. Asphyxiants:

_____

c. Nerve poisons, anesthetics, and narcotics:

_____

d. Hepatotoxins:

_____

e. Cardiotoxins:

_____

f. Neurotoxins:

_____

g. Hemotoxins:

_____

h. Carcinogens:

_____

23. You respond to the scene of a fire in which hazardous materials of unknown origin are involved. Describe signs and symptoms shown by scene workers that may cause you to suspect exposure to hazardous materials.

_____

24. Your crew arrives at an industrial chemical manufacturing plant where a worker has sustained a splash exposure of a corrosive chemical to the eyes. Describe patient management in this situation.

_____

25. Label Fig. 53-1 and briefly describe each of the three safety zones for a hazardous materials situation that have been established by hazardous materials specialists.

A. _____

B. _____

C. _____

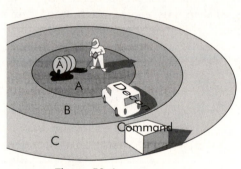

Figure 53-1

Questions 26 to 28 refer to the following case study:

> You are the first team dispatched to the scene of a train derailment where three victims remain trapped. The bystanders who called in the incident report that several of the involved train cars have placards indicating the presence of hazardous materials.

26. Describe any actions you should take during your initial response to this situation.

_____

_____

_____

_____

_____

_____

27. Describe special considerations in the prehospital management of contaminated patients.

_____

_____

_____

_____

_____

_____

28. The incident commander at this scene delegates your EMS crew to establish a medical monitoring station. Describe the responsibilities of this role.

_____

_____

_____

29. What measures should rescuers follow as they leave the hot zone of a HAZMAT scene?

_____

_____

STUDENT SELF-ASSESSMENT

30. What term is used for substances and materials that can pose an unreasonable risk to health, safety, and property?
  a. External hazards
  b. Hazardous materials
  c. Immediately dangerous to life and health
  d. Internal hazards

31. What term describes the legislation, enacted in 1986, that established requirements for federal, state, and local governments and industry regarding emergency planning and the reporting of hazardous materials?
  a. Hazardous Materials Control Act
  b. Occupational Health and Safety Law
  c. Ryan White Law
  d. Superfund Amendments and Reauthorization Act

32. According to the HAZWOPER rules, the five categories of individuals who may respond to an emergency involving hazardous materials include all of the following _except_
  a. First responder–operations   **c.** Hazardous material specialist
  b. Hazardous material technician   **d.** Rescue operation technician

33. Which of the following is a formal means of identifying hazardous products?
  a. Container characteristics   **c.** Patient signs and symptoms
  b. Incident location   **d.** United Nations labeling system

34. Which agency requires Material Safety Data Sheets when chemicals are stored, handled, or used in the workplace?
  a. International Air Transport Association
  b. National Fire Protection Association
  c. Occupational Safety and Health Administration
  d. U.S. Department of Transportation

35. General signs or symptoms of inhalation exposure to a hazardous material may include which of the following?
    a. Hemiplegia
    c. Seizure
    b. Hematemesis
    d. Urticaria
36. External exposure to corrosive chemicals generally causes which of the following?
    a. Acidosis
    c. Coughing
    b. Burns
    d. Systemic effects
37. Which of the following signs or symptoms should prompt a rescuer to seek immediate medical attention at the site of a hazardous materials incident?
    a. Confusion and lightheadedness
    b. Shortness of breath and coughing
    c. Tingling of the extremities
    d. Nausea and vomiting
    e. Any of the above
38. When responding to the scene of a hazardous materials incident, the EMS crew should approach from which direction?
    a. Downhill and downwind
    c. Uphill and downwind
    b. Downhill and upwind
    d. Uphill and upwind
39. The "pre-suit" medical monitoring of an individual who will be entering a hazardous materials situation should include all of the following *except* which one?
    a. Heart rate
    c. Temperature
    b. Reflexes
    d. Weight
40. General recommendations for emergency management of contaminated patients include all of the following *except* which one?
    a. Emergency patient care overrides all safety considerations.
    b. All patients in the hot zone are considered contaminated.
    c. Intravenous therapy should be initiated only with a physician's order.
    d. The patient's clothing should be completely cut off.
41. Which of the following is an appropriate step in the decontamination of a rescuer leaving a HAZMAT site?
    a. Shave all body hair.
    b. Shake clothing vigorously before reapplying.
    c. Take HAZMAT suit to the ambulance to be used later.
    d. Shower and wash with soap.

WRAP IT UP

The crash isn't too impressive; a car struck the rear of a delivery truck, causing it to topple over onto its side. All the occupants of both vehicles are out and moving around, but as approach, you note tears streaming down their faces, and a man is standing next to the truck coughing vigorously. "Stop," you tell your driver, "let's park upwind aways." You pick up the microphone for the loud speaker. "Move away from the truck," you command, instructing the group to follow your ambulance to a higher location, several hundred feet away from the truck. You contact dispatch to ask for fire department and HAZMAT team response. You notice a faint ammonia smell that is becoming weaker as you move away from the scene, and you pull out your binoculars to get a better look at the scene. No placards are visible, nor do you see any liquid pools around either vehicle.

When the truck driver and the two occupants of the car get to the ambulance, they report a very strong smell of ammonia and severe burning of their eyes, noses, and throats, as well as difficulty breathing. They say that they didn't see anything spilled, or any gas cloud. You immediately administer oxygen, and when you listen to their lungs, you hear diffuse wheezes. The patients are tachycardic and tachypneic but have normal blood pressure. Fire department crews douse the three with water to grossly decontaminate any affected skin and remove the patients' clothing. In the ambulance you begin treatment with a bronchodilator and place a nasal cannula over their eyes to begin continuous irrigation with normal saline. You ask the truck driver about his cargo and request his shipping papers, but he is evasive; he gets up and tries to run from the scene, but the police tackle and subdue him, confiscating a handgun from his pocket. HAZMAT teams arrive, establish zones around the contaminated area, and find a variety of hazardous chemicals in the back of the truck, which turns out to be a mobile methamphetamine lab. Apparently an ammonia tank ruptured in the collision, releasing the irritant gas and exposing your patients.

1. What methods of identification of the hazardous materials did the first rescuers attempt to use in this situation?
   a. Informal:

   _____

   _____

   b. Formal:

   _____

   _____

2. What additional resources were contacted immediately to assist with the incident?

3. Put a ✓ beside the signs or symptoms of hazardous materials exposure that were observed in these patients.
   a. _____ Confusion, dizziness   g. _____ Numbness
   b. _____ Chest tightness   h. _____ Loss of coordination
   c. _____ Double vision   i. _____ Nausea, vomiting
   d. _____ Changes in skin color   j. _____ Drooling, rhinorrhea
   e. _____ Coughing   k. _____ Tearing
   f. _____ Difficulty breathing   l. _____ Unconsciousness

4. Why was gross water decontamination done even though the situation involved a gas exposure?

   _____

   _____

5. Could the ambulance crew be charged with abandonment for pulling past the scene of an emergency? Explain your answer.

   _____

   _____

6. Describe the zones that the HAZMAT team established around the scene.

   _____

   _____

CHAPTER 53 ANSWERS

REVIEW QUESTIONS

1. i
2. e
3. h
4. a
5. f
6. d
7. c
8. k
9. g
10. b
    (Questions 1-10: Objective 1)

11. j, e
12. f, d
13. g
14. a
15. j, e
16. i
17. h, j, e
    (Questions 11-17: Objective 5)

18.

Category	Description
a. First responder–awareness	May witness or discover hazardous materials release but job does not include emergency response duties pertaining to hazardous materials
b. First responder–operations	Responds to hazardous materials release to protect nearby people, property, or the environment without trying to stop the release
c. Hazardous material technician	Responds to hazardous materials situations to stop the release
d. Hazardous materials specialist	Has direct or specific knowledge of various hazardous substances and provides support to hazardous materials technicians
e. On-scene incident commander	Trained to assume control of a hazardous materials event

(Objective 2)

19. a. Placards on trucks, shipping papers, and material safety data sheets
    b. Visual indicators (vapor), container characteristics, company name on truck, and smell
    (Objective 3)

20. Hazardous materials texts, poison control centers, CHEMTREC, federal agencies, commercial agencies, subject experts, site coordinators, and regional, state, and local agencies
    (Objective 3)

21. a. Chemical splash protective clothing to protect the skin and eyes from direct chemical contact.
    b. Structural firefighting clothing, including helmet, positive-pressure self-contained breathing apparatus, turnout coat and pants, gloves and boots, and a protective hood of fire-resistant material.
    c. Vapor-protective clothing (suit with a self-contained breathing apparatus worn inside or outside the suit or a supplied-air breathing apparatus with emergency escape capabilities).
    (Objective 4)

22. a. Irritants damage the upper and lower respiratory tracts and irritate the eyes.

b. Asphyxiants deprive the body tissues of oxygen.

c. Nerve gases, anesthetics, and narcotics act on the nervous system, causing disruption of cardiorespiratory function.

d. Hepatotoxins destroy the liver's ability to function in a normal capacity.

e. Cardiotoxins may induce myocardial ischemia and cardiac dysrhythmias.

f. Neurotoxins may cause cerebral hypoxia or neurological or behavioral disruption.

g. Hemotoxins cause destruction of red blood cells, resulting in hemolytic anemia.

h. Carcinogens are cancer-causing agents.

(Objective 5)

23. Confusion, anxiety, dizziness, visual disturbances, changes in skin color, shortness of breath or burning of the upper airway, tingling or numbness of extremities, loss of coordination, seizures, nausea and vomiting, abdominal cramps, diarrhea, unconsciousness.

(Objective 5)

24. Don protective gear, remove contact lenses, and flush with copious amounts of water, normal saline, or lactated Ringer solution.

(Objective 6)

25. A. The *hot zone* is the area that includes the hazardous material and any associated wastes. Only specially trained and clothed personnel may enter this area.

B. The *warm zone* is the area that can become contaminated if the hot zone is unstable. Decontamination and patient care activities take place here.

C. The *cold zone* is the area around the warm zone. Minimal protective clothing is required. The command post and other support agencies are located here.

(Objective 7)

26. En route to the emergency scene, the EMS crew should attempt to identify the hazardous material and obtain preliminary information about the potential hazards and recommended safety equipment, initial first aid, and a safe distance factor for response to the area. Medical control should be notified so that appropriate measures can be taken at the hospital for potential victims. If the involved substance is identified, the dispatching agency should contact the appropriate authorities and other experts (e.g., CHEMTREC) to get additional information and support. The scene should be approached from uphill and upwind, and the EMS crew should call for additional help as needed. The arriving crew should be alert to any fire hazards and leakage of gas or liquid from the involved cars and remain clear of all vapors and spills.

(Objective 7)

27. Nonambulatory patients should be removed from the hot zone by trained personnel who have adequate protective clothing. All patients in the hot zone should be considered contaminated. Patient care in the hot zone should consist only of airway and breathing management, spinal immobilization, and control of hemorrhage. Intravenous lines should be avoided unless absolutely necessary to prevent internal introduction of contaminants. Decontamination should be attempted only with adequate protection of the rescue workers; often, removal of the victim's clothing removes most of the contaminant, with the remainder being washed with copious amounts of water and mild detergent soap. All contaminated clothing from the patient and rescuers should be left in the decontamination area. Further patient care should be provided in the support area before transport. The patient should be wrapped tightly in blankets.

(Objective 9)

28. Pre-suit examination: Assess baseline vital signs and instruct rescuers about possible symptoms to anticipate if contamination or exposure occurs. Postentry examination: Assess vital signs and monitor rescuer for signs or symptoms of exposure or heat-related illness.

(Objective 8)

29. Outer gloves and boots should be removed and placed in a receptacle. Remove contaminated breathing apparatus. Remove protective clothing and assess the need to remove outer clothing (based on type of chemical). Shower and wash twice. Put on clean clothing. Obtain medical evaluation.
(Objective 8)

STUDENT SELF-ASSESSMENT

30. b. The term *external hazards* refers to materials that produce external damage, whereas *internal hazards* cause internal damage. Not all HAZMAT substances are IDLH.
(Objective 1)

31. d. The Ryan White law pertains to exposure to infectious diseases.
(Objective 2)

32. d. The categories are first responder–awareness, first responder–operations, hazardous materials technician, hazardous materials specialist, and on-scene incident commander.
(Objective 2)

33. d. All other responses are informal means of recognizing and identifying hazardous materials.
(Objective 3)

34. c. The U.S. Department of Transportation regulates hazardous materials in transit.
(Objective 3)

35. c. The others would not usually be associated with this type of exposure.
(Objective 5)

36. b. The other signs described are systemic effects, which are not the most common findings in external exposure to corrosive chemicals.
(Objective 6)

37. e. A high index of suspicion for rescuer exposure should always be maintained.
(Objective 5)

38. d. This ensures that hazardous gases and liquids are moving away from the ambulance.
(Objective 7)

39. b
(Objective 8)

40. a. Safety overrides all considerations.

41. d. Shaving may permit internal entry of chemicals. Clothing should be left at the exit point and appropriately cleaned or discarded.
(Objective 9)

WRAP IT UP

1. a. Observation of the patient's signs and symptoms; smell
   b. Checking for placards, shipping papers
   (Objective 3)

2. Fire department, HAZMAT team
   (Objective 7)

3. e, f, k
   (Objectives 5, 6)

4. To remove any chemical irritant present on the skin or clothes and to prevent subsequent off-gassing of chemicals.
   (Objective 9)

5. The first priority in an incident, especially a HAZMAT incident, is scene safety. Pulling onto the scene would have been dangerous, therefore no abandonment claim could be made.
   (Objective 7)

6. Hot (contamination) zone: Area where actual contaminant is located; only personnel in appropriate PPE are allowed entry.
   Warm (control) zone: Surrounds hot zone and is location of decontamination
   Cold (safe) zone: Normal operations
   (Objective 7)

Bioterrorism and Weapons of Mass Destruction

READING ASSIGNMENT
Chapter 54, pages 1306-1319, in *Mosby's Paramedic Textbook*, ed. 3

OBJECTIVES
Upon completion of this chapter, the paramedic student will be able to do the following:
1. List five types of weapons of mass destruction.
2. Identify actions, signs and symptoms, methods of distribution, and management of biological weapons of mass destruction.
3. Identify actions, signs and symptoms, methods of distribution, and management of chemical weapons of mass destruction.
4. Identify actions, signs and symptoms, methods of distribution, and management of nuclear weapons of mass destruction.
5. Describe security threat levels as defined by the Department of Homeland Security.
6. Identify measures to be taken by paramedics who respond to incidents with suspected weapons of mass destruction involvement.

SUMMARY
- There are five categories of weapons of mass destruction. These include biological, nuclear, incendiary, chemical, and explosive.
- Biological agents include anthrax, botulism, plague, ricin, tularemia, and smallpox.
- Person-to-person spread is possible in patients who are infected with plague or smallpox.
- Nerve agents include Sarin, Soman, Tabun, and VX. Exposure causes a cholinergic overdrive. The antidote for nerve agent exposure is atropine and pralidoxime chloride.
- Poisonous gases such as chlorine and phosgene cause severe respiratory problems. They also can cause skin and eye injury. Move exposed patients to safety, remove their clothing, and treat their symptoms.
- Dirty bombs could cause heat damage and radiation sickness, severe burns, and cancer.
- The Department of Homeland Security has identified five terrorist threat levels. Each level has specific community-wide emergency preparedness activities to be taken.

- Emergency responders at a WMD incident should recognize hazmat incidents, know protocols to detect WMD, use PPE, know crime-scene procedures, know how to activate more resources, and implement incident operations.

REVIEW QUESTIONS

Match the terms in column II with the description in column I. A term may be used more than once.

Column I	Column II
1. _____ Illness caused by bacteria found in rodents	a. Anthrax
2. _____ Nerve agent that has a camphorlike odor	b. Chlorine
3. _____ Thick, odorless liquid used as a nerve agent	c. Phosgene
4. _____ Gray, poisonous gas that smells like mown hay	d. Plague
5. _____ Odorless nerve agent	e. Ricin
6. _____ Bacterial disease spread by rodent fleas	f. Sarin
7. _____ Poisonous cytotoxin from a plant	g. Soman
8. _____ Nerve agent that has a fruity odor	h. Tabun
	i. Tularemia
	j. VX

9. Supply the words that form the following acronym for weapons of mass destruction.

B—

N—

I—

C—

E—

Match the categories in column II with the characteristics of biological agents in column I. Each category may be used *more* than once.

Column I	Column II
10. _____ Emerging pathogen	a. Category A
11. _____ Q fever	b. Category B
12. _____ Second highest priority agents	c. Category C
13. _____ Nipah virus	
14. _____ National security risk	
15. _____ Anthrax	

16. Provide the missing information for each of the following biological weapons of mass destruction.

Agent	Signs/Symptoms	Outcomes	Treatment
a. Anthrax			
b.	Fever, fainting, shortness of breath, cough, bloody sputum, GI symptoms		
c.		35% mortality from septicemia	
d. Botulism			
e.			Antibiotics, supportive treatment; vaccine under study
f. Ricin			
g.		DIC, respiratory failure, death (5%)	

17. You are called to investigate multiple reports of difficulty breathing at the airport. When you arrive, approximately 30 people rush toward the ambulance with tears streaming down their faces. They report a sudden onset of difficulty breathing, blurred vision, headache, and weakness. Most were in the baggage pickup area when their symptoms began. You note that they are sweating profusely, some are faint, and they have fasciculations.

    a. List four agents that can cause this clinical presentation.

    b. What precautions should you take prior to transport of these patients?

    c. List three drugs that may be indicated in the management of these patients.

18. Your patients were working at an immigration center when they smelled an odor they described as "like fresh cut hay." They then developed severe dyspnea, a burning sensation in the chest, and a nonproductive cough.

    a. What WMD agent do you suspect?

b. What interventions would you perform?

_____

_____

_____

19. List three factors that would affect the degree of contamination from a dirty bomb.

a.

b.

c.

20. Describe three special considerations for a paramedic responding to a WMD incident.

a.

b.

c.

STUDENT SELF-ASSESSMENT

21. People in your community are becoming very ill with a rash and severe respiratory symptoms. Many have died, and new cases are spreading among people who appear to have had contact with the first group. What WMD infectious agent may be involved?
a. Anthrax   **c.** Smallpox
b. Plague   **d.** Tularemia

22. According to the CDC categorization of biological agents, which category includes agents that cause moderate morbidity and low mortality and includes Q fever?
a. Category A   **c.** Category C
b. Category B   **d.** Category D

23. Which WMD exposure route has the potential for the greatest number of casualties?
a. Aerosol   **c.** Liquid ingestion
b. Direct contact   **d.** Solid ingestion

24. Which of the following is _true_ about anthrax infection?
a. All those who come in contact with the infected patient should be quarantined.
b. It can cause severe respiratory distress and sepsis in later stages.
c. Treatment with antibiotics is not indicated and is ineffective.
d. Vaccination is routinely recommended for health care workers.

25. A large number of patients who ate at the salad bar of a local restaurant are complaining of nausea, blurred vision, and dry mouth. Several have difficulty swallowing and complain that they are having trouble breathing. Which of the following may be associated with this presentation?
a. Botulism   **c.** Soman
b. Ricin   **d.** Tularemia

26. Which of the following WMD agents can be spread from person to person?
a. Botulism   **c.** Ricin
b. Plague   **d.** Tularemia

27. You are caring for a patient who has just been exposed to a WMD agent. You know that you must remove the patient's clothing to protect yourself from illness or injury caused by which of the following?
a. Chlorine
b. Smallpox
c. VX
d. All of the above

28. You are called to a government building where a large number of patients have excessive tearing, salivation, severe dyspnea with wheezing, weakness, drooling, and hypotension. After HAZMAT teams have decontaminated the patients and while oxygen is administered, which treatments should you give next to improve their condition?
    a. Albuterol, fluid bolus
    b. Albuterol, atropine
    d. Atropine, fluid bolus
    d. Atropine, pralidoxime chloride
29. A tanker transporting chlorine has collided with a van carrying six occupants. A slow gas leak is streaming from the side of the truck. All those involved in the accident are ambulatory but complaining of severe burning of the eyes, coughing, and difficulty breathing. You have staged away from the incident. After calling for appropriate additional resources, what should your immediate priorities be for these patients?
    a. Administer oxygen and an antidote.
    b. Have them remain in place until the HAZMAT team arrives.
    c. Instruct them to move upwind to higher ground.
    d. Take oxygen and albuterol to the patients to begin care.
30. When a yellow Homeland Security threat level is activated, what special measures should be taken?
    a. Consider canceling or alternative venues for special events.
    b. Implement appropriate contingency and emergency response plans.
    c. Monitor, redirect, or constrain transportation systems.
    d. Refine and exercise preplanned protective measures.
31. According to the Office for Domestic Preparedness, what are the responsibilities of EMS providers in preparing for and responding to incidents of terrorism involving WMD agents?
    a. Contain hazardous materials.
    b. Detect and identify agents used as a WMD.
    c. Implement incident operations.
    d. Protect the crime scene perimeter.

WRAP IT UP

As you pull up on the scene, you see more than 100 people streaming from a church where your dispatcher tells you there have been multiple calls for difficulty breathing. People report noticing a faint "fruity" odor when the minister lit the incense oil pots, and watering eyes, drooling, sweating, and coughing quickly developed. You call for an MCI response and a HAZMAT team. Several people have fallen to the ground, and you note a child having a grand mal seizure on the grass. Other people are running from the scene to their cars. The incident commander and HAZMAT team arrive, and a decision is quickly made that a vaporized nerve agent has been used. Therefore the patients' clothing should be removed and gross decontamination should be performed before treatment and transport to eliminate any possibility of off-gassing. You and your partner are in charge of the triage division and direct next-arriving crews to initiate START triage. The supply branch is in charge of locating and procuring MARK-I kits deployed in the city and having them sent to the treatment division and appropriate receiving hospitals. After disrobing and undergoing gross decontamination, patients are moved to the treatment division, where antidote administration and supportive care begin until appropriate transport can be arranged. It is 2 hours before the ninety-seventh patient is transported to the hospital, leaving only seven who were tagged unsalvageable to be transported to the county medical examiner's office and the police and HAZMAT teams to finish up their work.

1. Which nerve agent has the characteristics described in this scenario?

2. Put a ✔ beside the signs or symptoms that a patient exposed to a nerve agent may experience (even if not described in the above scenario).

a. _____ Blurred vision   h. _____ Hypotension
b. _____ Bradycardia   i. _____ Renal failure
c. _____ Cardiac arrest   j. _____ Seizures
d. _____ Drooling   k. _____ Sweating
e. _____ Dry skin   l. _____ Watery eyes
f. _____ Headache   m. _____ Wheezing
g. _____ Hypertension   n. _____ Loss of consciousness

3. What drugs does the MARK-I kit contain?

4. What additional interventions are needed for patients poisoned by a nerve agent?

REVIEW QUESTIONS

1. d, i
   (Objective 2)

2. b
   (Objective 3)

3. j
   (Objective 3)

4. c
   (Objective 3)

5. f
   (Objective 3)

6. d
   (Objective 2)

7. e
   (Objective 2)

8. h
   (Objective 3)

9. B—biological; N—nuclear; I—incendiary; C—chemical; E—explosives
   (Objective 1)

10. c
11. b
12. b
13. c
14. a
15. a
   (Questions 10-15: Objective 2)

16.

Agent	Signs/Symptoms	Outcomes	Treatment
a. Anthrax	Itching, papular lesion that becomes vesicular, black eschar; signs and symptoms resembling those of a cold, followed by respiratory distress, sepsis	High mortality if untreated	Antibiotics, vaccines (controversial)
b. Plague (*Yersinia pestis*)	Fever, fainting, short of breath, cough, bloody sputum, GI symptoms	Septic shock; high mortality	Antibiotics, post-exposure drug therapy, isolation
c. Smallpox (variola virus)	High fever, fatigue, headache and backache; within 2 to 3 days, rash and skin lesions that crust and scar; joint deformities; blindness	35% mortality from septicemia	Vaccine, antivirals (experimental), supportive care, isolation
d. Botulism	Nausea, dry mouth, blurred vision, dysphagia, fatigue, dyspnea	Recovery may occur with weeks of supportive care	Antitoxin, mechanical ventilation
e. Tularemia	Fever, HA, chills, malaise, GI illness, DIC, ARF; death possible	Severe incapacitation; low death rate	Antibiotics, supportive treatment; vaccine under study
f. Ricin	Severe respiratory symptoms within 8 hours; respiratory failure in 36 to 72 hours; severe GI symptoms; vascular collapse; seizures	Respiratory failure, shock, death	No antidote; only supportive care possible; avoid exposure, eliminate toxin, and decontaminate
g. Tularemia	Fever, chills, general malaise, GI illness	DIC, respiratory failure, death (5%)	Antibiotics, supportive care; vaccine under review

(Objective 2)

17. a. Sarin, soman, tabun, VX
b. Secondary exposure is possible from off-gassing of clothes; clothing should be removed before transport.
c. Atropine, pralidoxime chloride, and diazepam or lorazepam are indicated for the management of nerve agent poisoning.
(Objective 3)

18. a. Phosgene gas; b. decontamination if needed, supportive care with oxygen and management of symptoms.
(Objective 3)

19. The size of the explosive, the amount and type of radioactive material used, and the weather (Objective 4)
20. Danger to EMS crews from secondary devices or armed resistance; crowd control and public panic situations; the need to preserve the crime scene.
(Objective 6)

STUDENT SELF-ASSESSMENT

21. c. Smallpox is spread easily from person to person, causes a progressive rash, and has a high mortality rate in unvaccinated individuals.
(Objective 2)

22. b. Category A agents (which include anthrax) have a high morbidity and mortality; category C agents (which include Nipah virus) are emerging pathogens. There is no category D.
(Objective 2)

23. a. Aerosolized agents can be distributed easily over a wide area, exposing large numbers of victims in a short time.
(Objective 2)

24. b. Person-to-person contact does not transmit the infection. Antibiotics should be given as soon as possible to minimize the risk of death. Vaccination is recommended only for military personnel and for researchers who work with anthrax.
(Objective 2)

25. a. Ricin produces pulmonary symptoms; soman is a nerve agent; and tularemia does not typically cause blurred vision or dysphagia.
(Objective 2)

26. b. Botulism and tularemia are not known to spread from person to person. Ricin is not an infectious agent.
(Objective 2)

27. d. Direct skin contamination or secondary contamination from off-gassing is possible with many WMD agents. As a precaution, if full decontamination is not indicated, clothing should be removed before transport to prevent secondary exposure.
(Objective 3)

28. d. Atropine and pralidoxime chloride (PAM) are direct antidotes to nerve agents and should be given immediately to reverse the effect of the nerve poisons.
(Objective 3)

29. c. Any attempt to move to the contaminated area without appropriate PPE would be dangerous. Supportive care can begin after patients are in a safe area and their clothing has been removed.
(Objective 3)

30. b. In an orange level activation, public event modifications would be considered. In a red condition situation, transportation modifications may need to be made. Preplanning should be done at the green level and modified as needed at each level of activation.
(Objective 4)

31. c. HAZMAT teams are typically responsible for containing the hazardous material and identifying specific agents using special monitoring devices. Police should control the perimeter of the crime scene.
(Objective 5)

WRAP IT UP

1. Tabun; it has a fruity odor, vaporizes when heated, causes symptoms within seconds of exposure to the vapor, and produces the signs and symptoms described.
(Objective 3)

2. a, b, c, d, f, h, i, j, k, l, m
(Objective 3)

3. Atropine and pralidoxime chloride
(Objective 3)

4. IV fluids, oxygen, and diazepam or lorazepam for seizures
(Objective 3)

Emergency Drug Index

1. List the actions, indications, and side effects of steroids.

   _____

   _____

2. For each of the following two drugs, list the time of onset, duration, and dose:
   a. Methylprednisolone:

   _____

   b. Dexamethasone:

   _____

   For each of the scenarios in questions 3 to 28, complete the corresponding flashcard (after the electrocardiogram flashcards at the end of this workbook) with the appropriate drug information, including trade name, class, description, indications, contraindications, adverse reactions, onset, duration, dose (adult and pediatric, if appropriate), and special considerations. Verify your drug choice before completing the flashcard by looking at the generic drug name on the back.

3. Your patient is experiencing urticaria and severe itching resulting from an allergic reaction. His vital signs are

   stable, and no wheezes are audible on auscultation of his lungs. You administer _____.
   (Complete Flashcard 23.)

4. After delivering a defibrillation to your patient who is in ventricular fibrillation cardiac arrest and continuing CPR, you wish to give a potent vasoconstrictor with a long duration of action. What do you administer? _____. (Complete Flashcard 24.)

5. Your crew is unable to initiate an intravenous line on an unconscious diabetic patient who is known to be hypoglycemic. Transport time is 45 minutes. The drug of choice to increase the blood glucose level is

   _____. (Complete Flashcard 25.)

6. Your patient is in stable ventricular tachycardia. List two specific antidysrhythmic drugs you may administer. _____. Both drugs can also be used to treat some narrow QRS tachycardias (Complete Flashcards 26 and 27.)

7. A 65-year-old woman calls you and complains of shortness of breath and chest pain radiating down her left arm.

Her blood pressure is 110/70 mm Hg. The initial drug of choice to relieve her pain is _____. (Complete Flashcard 28.)

8. You place a 42-year-old patient with a pounding sensation in her chest on a monitor and discover ventricular tachycardia. The patient's blood pressure is normal, she has no chest pain, and the rest of the history and physical examination is unremarkable. If amiodarone is not available, the appropriate drug to use to suppress ventricular dysrhythmia in this situation is _____. (Complete Flashcard 29.)

9. Your 30-year-old patient fell while in-line skating and has obvious deformity of the right wrist with significant pain.

What nonnarcotic analgesic can you give him intramuscularly or intravenously? _____ (Complete Flashcard 30.)

10. You are called to an outpatient surgery center to evaluate a nurse who is unconscious. Co-workers confide that they have suspected drug abuse for some time, and an empty meperidine (Demerol) tubex is found in her pocket. All other available medical history is negative. Pupils are pinpoint, and respirations are 12 and shallow.

What drug do you administer first if an overdose is suspected? _____ (Complete Flashcard 31.)

11. You perform transcutaneous pacing on a conscious patient. He complains of severe discomfort related to the procedure. BP is 110/70 mm Hg. What short-acting IV medicine can you administer to reduce anxiety, relax skeletal muscles, and provide amnesia? _____ (Complete Flashcard 32.)

12. You are called to a nursing home to care for an 88-year-old woman who has fainted. The patient is extremely bradycardic (pulse 40) and has a blood pressure of 80 mm Hg systolic by palpation. Her only history is hypertension. What emergency care drug is indicated initially to correct her sinus bradycardia?

_____ (Complete Flashcard 33.)

13. An initial electrical countershock and good CPR do not successfully convert your cardiac arrest patient from ventricular fibrillation. An adrenergic drug that should be repeated every 3 to 5 minutes is _____. (Complete Flashcard 34.)

14. A 32-year-old patient fell while playing softball and has an apparent dislocation of the left shoulder, which is very painful. Medical direction wishes to administer a short-acting analgesic so that accurate emergency department evaluation will be possible. What is an appropriate, self-administered analgesic in this situation?

_____ (Complete Flashcard 35.)

15. You have been trying without success to resuscitate a 73-year-old woman who is in cardiac arrest. Tricyclic antidepressant overdose is suspected. What electrolyte may be considered at this point? _____ (Complete Flashcard 36.)

16. The police call you to evaluate an unconscious person. The patient is a known alcoholic, and friends say that he has not eaten for several days. He has a blood glucose level of 40 mg/dL (normal range 80 to 120 mg/dL). No drug use is suspected. The two drugs indicated for this patient are _____ and _____. (Complete Flashcards 37 and 38.)

17. A frantic husband calls you to evaluate his wife, who has been having seizures for 10 minutes. She is experiencing repetitive grand mal seizures. She is a known epileptic who has not taken any phenytoin (Dilantin) for 2 days. What is your drug of choice under these circumstances (you do not have lorazepam or midazolam)?

_____ (Complete Flashcard 39.)

18. Your 24-year-old patient is a known asthmatic who is experiencing an acute attack. Inspiratory and expiratory wheezes are audible throughout the chest, and the patient's HR is 100/min. What drug would you initially administer by inhalation? _____ (Complete Flashcard 40.)

19. A 56-year-old woman has severe crushing substernal chest pain and diaphoresis. You administer vasodilators and a narcotic analgesic to relieve pain. What antiplatelet drug should you also administer?

_____ (Complete Flashcard 41.)

20. You are called to treat a 32-year-old woman with a sudden onset of palpitations. The electrocardiogram reveals a rapid supraventricular tachycardia. What is the safest drug to use to convert this rhythm to sinus rhythm? _____ (Complete Flashcard 42.)

21. Airport authorities call you to care for a mechanic whose arm is trapped in the landing gear of a small aircraft. Extrication time is lengthy, and the patient is in extreme distress because of pain. Vital signs are stable, and no other injuries are noted. List two narcotic analgesics that may be administered to this patient. _____ and _____ (Complete Flashcards 43 ands 44.)

22. Your 67-year-old patient is experiencing a headache resulting from his elevated blood pressure, which is now 230/160 mm Hg. He is awake and cooperative. After you consult with medical direction, which alpha- and beta-adrenegic blocker drug may improve this situation by lowering the blood pressure? _____ (Complete Flashcard 45.)

23. A 21-year-old took an SSRI overdose of an antidepressant 10 minutes ago and is awake and alert. What drug may be used to prevent absorption of the antidepressant in the gastrointestinal tract? _____ (Complete Flashcard 46.)

24. Your patient is 8 months pregnant and has been diagnosed with preeclampsia. Co-workers found her experiencing a grand mal seizure in the restroom. The patient appears to be in a postictal state. Blood pressure is 160/116 mm Hg.

    What drug may be given for her seizure activity? _____ (Complete Flashcard 47.)

25. You have a 30-minute estimated time of arrival to the hospital with an 86-year-old patient from a nursing home whose vital signs are blood pressure, 80/50 mm Hg; pulse, 124; and respirations, 24. The urine in her Foley catheter bag is milky green and foul smelling. Cardiac history is negative, and no reason exists to suspect blood or fluid volume loss. What is the drug of choice to treat her hypotension quickly after fluid resuscitation in this

    situation? _____ (Complete Flashcard 48.)

26. The 65-year-old patient you are called to evaluate has the following vital signs: blood pressure, 130/90 mm Hg; pulse, 160; and respirations, 24. The electrocardiogram monitor shows atrial fibrillation with a rapid ventricular response. She has mild signs of congestive heart failure, but all other physical findings are negative. What Class

    IV antidysrhythmic drug is indicated for this patient? _____ (Complete Flashcard 49.)

27. Your 72-year-old patient is experiencing severe dyspnea that began suddenly during the night. She is in obvious distress, with cyanosis of the nail beds and lips. Lung sounds reveal rales and wheezes throughout, and she has a cough that produces frothy, pink sputum. History reveals two previous myocardial infarctions. Vital signs are blood pressure, 170/108 mm Hg; pulse, 132; and respirations, 32. Identify the diuretic to administer in an

    attempt to improve this patient's condition. _____ (Complete Flashcard 50.)

28. You have just delivered a healthy baby boy, followed minutes later by a complete placenta. Despite vigorous massage, the patient's uterus is very soft, and she is experiencing profuse vaginal bleeding. What pharmaco

    logical agent can you administer to help control this bleeding? _____ (Complete Flashcard 51.)

    Complete the remaining flashcards with drugs not included in the previous questions that are administered within your emergency medical services system.

STUDENT SELF-ASSESSMENT

29. When is the use of dopamine most clearly indicated?
    a. Cardiac arrest
    b. Cardiogenic shock
    c. Head injury
    d. Internal bleeding

30. Which of the following is the appropriate drug to administer to a patient with multiple injuries who was in a motor vehicle collision and is complaining of severe abdominal pain?
    a. Meperidine
    b. Morphine
    c. Nitrous oxide
    d. None of the above

31. Which of the following is an indication for administration of epinephrine 1:1000 subcutaneously?
    a. Anaphylaxis
    c. Electromechanical dissociation
    b. Asystole
    d. Ventricular fibrillation
32. Which drug is recommended to control atrial fibrillation with a rate of 170 beats/min when the patient has Wolff-Parkinson-White syndrome?
    a. Adenosine
    c. Atenolol
    b. Amiodarone
    d. Diltiazem
33. Which of the following is *not* true regarding use of atropine?
    a. It is indicated for management of bradycardia.
    b. The initial dose in bradycardia is 0.5 mg intravenously.
    c. It should be given in asystole.
    d. It is an antidote for verapamil.
34. What is dopamine used to treat?
    a. Hypovolemic shock
    b. Postresuscitation hypotension
    c. Cerebral edema
    d. Ventricular dysrhythmias
35. Your patient has severe chest pain and is nauseated and diaphoretic. His 12-lead electrocardiogram shows ST segment elevation in leads II, III, and aV_F. His breath sounds are clear and his blood pressure is 86/50 mm Hg, pulse is 64 per minute, and respirations are 20 per minute. Which of the following drugs would be indicated during your 10-minute transport to the emergency department?
    a. Aspirin
    c. Nitroglycerin
    b. Morphine
    d. Verapamil
36. Your patient is in ventricular fibrillation and has been shocked twice. An intravenous infusion has been started. Your first choice for drug therapy is which of the following?
    a. Epinephrine
    c. Magnesium sulfate
    b. Calcium chloride
    d. Sodium bicarbonate
37. Which of the following drugs does *not* cause bronchodilation?
    a. Albuterol
    c. Diphenhydramine
    b. Epinephrine
    d. Isoproterenol
38. Verapamil is contraindicated if the patient can be described as which of the following?
    a. Complaining of palpitations
    c. Tachycardic
    b. Hypotensive
    d. Under age 45
39. Which of the following drugs is self-administered by mask for relief of pain?
    a. Albuterol
    c. Nitroglycerin
    b. Morphine sulfate
    d. Nitrous oxide:oxygen
40. Which of the following is a drug indicated to treat stable narrow QRS complex atrial fibrillation at a rate of 152/min?
    a. Adenosine
    c. Lidocaine
    b. Diltiazem
    d. Magnesium
41. Which of the following drugs affects blood clotting by inhibition of platelets?
    a. Aspirin
    c. Streptokinase
    b. Reteplase
    d. Tissue plasminogen activator
42. Which treatment is appropriate for the patient suffering from coma of unknown origin?
    a. Naloxone, glucagon, and $D_{50}W$
    b. Butorphanol (Stadol), glucagon, and thiamine
    c. Naloxone, thiamine, and $D_{50}W$
    d. Dexamethasone, glucagon, and $D_{50}W$
43. In which of the following situations is mannitol indicated?
    a. Myocardial infarction
    c. Digoxin toxicity
    b. Acute cerebral edema
    d. Shock
44. Which of the following pharmacological agents is useful in status epilepticus, as an antianxiety agent, and as a skeletal muscle relaxant?
    a. Diazepam
    c. Naloxone
    b. Morphine
    d. Phenytoin

45. Which of the following drugs is indicated for management of postpartum bleeding?
    a. Dopamine
    b. Insulin
    c. Magnesium sulfate
    d. Oxytocin
46. Diphenhydramine is contraindicated in which of the following situations?
    a. Anaphylactic shock
    b. An acute asthma attack
    c. Allergic reactions
    d. Patients over 35 years of age
47. Charcoal should be administered for toxic ingestion if the patient has ingested?
    a. Cyanide
    b. Ethanol
    c. Lithium
    d. Strattera
48. Naloxone is an antagonist to all of the following, except which?
    a. Propoxyphene
    b. Heroin
    c. Oxycontin
    d. Phenobarbital
49. Which of the following medications may cause respiratory depression?
    a. Atropine
    b. Dexamethasone
    c. Magnesium sulfate
    d. Thiamine
50. A patient has monomorphic ventricular tachycardia at 160 beats/min (normal Q-T interval). Her blood pressure is 100 mm Hg, and the patient has crackles in both lung bases. Which drug is preferred to manage this rhythm?
    a. Amiodarone
    b. Magnesium sulfate
    c. Metoprolol
    d. Lidocaine
51. Which of the following side effects may occur after nitroglycerin ingestion?
    a. Headache
    b. Hypotension
    c. Burning under the tongue
    d. All of the above
52. Which of the following drugs exerts a positive chronotropic effect?
    a. Adenosine
    b. Epinephrine
    c. Labetolol
    d. Propranolol
53. Furosemide is indicated in the management of which of the following?
    a. Angina
    b. Dysrhythmias
    c. Hypotension
    d. Pulmonary edema
54. Which of the following is a calcium channel blocker that slows conduction and is useful to slow the heart rate in atrial flutter?
    a. Adenosine
    b. Albuterol
    c. Dobutamine
    d. Diltiazem
55. All of the following drugs are indicated to manage pulmonary edema that develops from left ventricular failure, except which?
    a. Atropine
    b. Furosemide
    c. Morphine
    d. Nitroglycerin
56. When meperidine is given alone, which of the following side effects should be anticipated?
    a. Increased heart rate
    b. Nausea and vomiting
    c. Vasoconstriction
    d. Hyperactivity
57. Your patient is a 35-year-old man who is psychotic and violent. Which of the following is the drug of choice for his care?
    a. Haloperidol
    b. Hydroxyzine
    c. Meperidine
    d. Midazolam
58. Dexamethasone and methylprednisolone belong to which of the following classes of drugs?
    a. Analgesics
    b. Inotropics
    c. Sympathomimetics
    d. Steroids

EMERGENCY DRUG INDEX ANSWERS

1. Actions: suppress acute or chronic inflammation and potentiate relaxation of vascular smooth muscle by beta-adrenergic agonist. Indications: anaphylaxis, asthma, shock, and spinal cord injury. Adverse reactions: hypertension, sodium and water retention, hypokalemia, hypocalcemia, alkalosis, and headache

2. a. Onset: 1 to 2 hours. Duration: 8 to 24 hours. Dose: 40 to 125 mg IV (in spinal cord injury, initial dose of 30 mg/kg, followed by IV infusion of 5.4 mg/kg/hr)

   b. Onset: 4 to 8 hours. Duration: 24 to 72 hours. Dose: 4 to 24 mg IV

3. Diphenhydramine (Benadryl). *Class:* antihistamine. *Description:* drug that prevents histamine from reaching H_1 and H_2 receptor sites. *Indications:* allergic reactions, anaphylaxis, and acute extrapyramidal reactions. *Contraindications:* asthma attacks, patients taking monoamine oxidase inhibitors, hypersensitivity, narrow-angle glaucoma, newborns, and nursing mothers. *Adverse reactions:* drowsiness, sedation, disturbed coordination, hypotension, palpitations, tachycardia or bradycardia, thickening of bronchial secretions, and dry mouth and throat. *Onset:* maximal effects in 1 to 3 hours. *Duration:* 6 to 12 hours. *Dose:* adult—25 to 50 mg deep IM or slow IV injection; pediatric—5 mg/kg/day in divided doses IV or IM. *Special considerations:* pregnancy category C.

4. Vasopressin (Pitressin). *Class:* antidiuretic hormone. *Description:* stimulation of smooth muscles; in high doses acts as a nonadrenergic peripheral vasoconstrictor. *Indications:* adult ventricular fibrillation asystole or PEA to replace the first or second dose of epinephrine; vasodilatory shock. *Contraindications:* responsive patients with coronary artery disease. *Adverse reactions:* ischemic chest pain, abdominal distress, sweating, nausea, vomiting, tremors. *Onset:* immediate. *Duration:* variable. *Dose:* adult cardiac arrest—40 U IV push 1 time; pediatric—not recommended. *Special considerations:* Drug may cause cardiac ischemia and angina. Drug may be given IO.

5. Glucagon. *Class:* pancreatic hormone and insulin antagonist. *Description:* used to elevate blood glucose level if sufficient stores of glycogen are available; has a positive inotropic effect on the heart. *Indications:* altered level of consciousness resulting from hypoglycemia if glucose administration not possible; calcium channel blocker or beta-blocker toxicity. *Contraindications:* hypersensitivity to proteins. *Adverse reactions:* tachycardia, hypotension, nausea, vomiting, and urticaria; may potentiate the effects of oral anticoagulants. *Onset:* within 1 minute. *Duration:* 60 to 90 minutes. *Dose:* adult—0.5 to 1.0 mg IM; pediatric—0.025 to 1.0 mg IM (may repeat in 7 to 10 minutes). Calcium channel blocker or beta-blocker toxicity, adult 1 to 5 mg over 2 to 5 minutes. *Special considerations:* not first-line choice for hypoglycemia.

6. a. Procainamide (Pronestyl). *Class:* antidysrhythmic (Class Ia). *Description:* reduces automaticity of ectopic pacemakers and suppresses reentry dysrhythmias by slowing IV conduction. *Indications:* suppression of monomorphic ventricular tachycardia (with a pulse) and paroxysmal supraventricular tachycardia with wide-complex tachycardia of unknown origin; atrial fibrillation with a rapid rate if Wolff-Parkinson-White syndrome is present. *Contraindications:* second- and third-degree AV block, complete heart block, tricyclic antidepressant toxicity, digitalis toxicity, and torsades de pointes. *Adverse reactions:* hypotension, bradycardia, reflex tachycardia, AV block, widened QRS complex, prolonged P-R or Q-T interval, premature ventricular contractions, ventricular tachycardia, ventricular fibrillation, asystole, central nervous system depression, confusion, and seizure. *Onset:* 10 to 30 minutes. *Duration:* 3 to 6 hours. *Dose:* adult—20 mg/min slow IV infusion (100 mg IV push in refractory ventricular fibrillation) to maximum dose 17 mg/kg, maintenance infusion after resuscitation or after initial bolus; 1 g mixed in 250 mL of solution infuse at (1 to 4 mg/min). *Special considerations:* Administration should be discontinued if dysrhythmia is suppressed, hypotension develops, the QRS complex widens by 50% of its original width, or a total of 17 mg/kg has been given; use caution with patients with asthma, digitalis-induced dysrhythmias, acute myocardial infarction, or cardiac, renal, or hepatic insufficiency. Do not use in combination with other drugs that prolong the Q-T interval or if pre-existing prolonged QT interval.

   b. Amiodarone (Cordarone). *Class:* Class III antidysrhythmic. *Description:* multiple mechanisms of action; prolongs action potential and refractory period; alpha adrenoreceptor and calcium channel blocker. *Indications:* treatment and prophylaxis of frequently recurring ventricular fibrillation and unstable ventricular tachycardia. *Contraindications:* pulmonary congestion, cardiogenic shock, hypotension, sensitivity to amiodarone. *Adverse reactions:* hypotension, bradycardia, headache, dizziness, atrioventricular conduction abnormalities, flushing, abnormal salivation. *Onset:* within minutes. *Duration:* variable. *Dose:* adult cardiac arrest—300 mg IV push; supplemental bolus for cardiac arrest—150 mg IV push in 3 to 5 minutes; loading infusion after reestablishment of spontaneous circulation—360 mg (diluted) over 6 hours. Wide complex tachycardias—150 mg IV over 10 min; may repeat in 10 min if needed. Follow with 1 mg/min infusion for 6 hours, then 0.5 mg/min infusion for 18 hr.

7. Nitroglycerin (Nitrostat). *Class:* vasodilator. *Description:* drug that dilates peripheral venous and arteriolar blood vessels and reduces cardiac workload and oxygen demand. *Indications:* ischemic chest pain, pulmonary hypertension, hypertensive emergencies, and congestive heart failure. *Contraindications:* hypersensitivity, hypotension, head injury, and cerebral hemorrhage. Do not give if patient has taken a phosphodiesterase inhibitor for erectile dysfunction within 24 hours (longer for some drugs); or SBP <90 mm Hg or >30 mm Hg below baseline; if HR <50 bpm or >100 bpm. *Adverse reactions:* headache, postural syncope, reflex tachycardia, hypotension, nausea, vomiting, and diaphoresis. *Onset:* 1 to 3 minutes. *Duration:* 30 to 60 minutes. *Dose:* tablet—0.3 to 0.4 mg sublingually that may be repeated in 5 minutes, twice; metered spray—0.4 mg/spray, one sublingual spray that may be repeated in 5 minutes, twice; infusion at a rate of 10 to 20 mcg/min, increased by 5 to 10 mcg/min every 5 to 10 minutes to desired effect. *Special considerations:* keep in an airtight container protected from light; older adults have an increased risk of hypotension. Administer with caution if at all to patients with inferior wall MI and suspected to have RV infarct.

8. Lidocaine (Xylocaine). *Class:* antidysrhythmic, local anesthetic (Class Ib). *Description:* Suppresses premature ventricular contractions and raises ventricular fibrillation threshold. *Indications:* ventricular fibrillation, ventricular tachycardia, significant ventricular ectopy in the presence of myocardial ischemia or infarction; wide-complex tachycardia of unknown origin. *Contraindications:* hypersensitivity, Stokes-Adams syndrome, and second- or third-degree heart block in the absence of an artificial pacemaker. *Adverse reactions:* light-headedness, confusion, blurred vision, hypotension, cardiovascular collapse, bradycardia, and central nervous system depression (including seizures) with high doses. *Onset:* 30 to 90 seconds. *Duration:* 10 to 20 minutes. *Dose:* adult—administration IV or via endotracheal bolus (at 2 to 2 1/2 times IV dose) followed by a continuous infusion; for ventricular fibrillation, 1.0 to 1.5 mg/kg IV repeated at 0.5–0.75 mg/kg in 3 to 5 minutes to a total loading dose of 3 mg/kg; for ventricular ectopy or stable ventricular tachycardia, 1 to 1.5 mg/kg IV repeated in 5 to 10 minutes at 0.5 to 0.75 mg/kg to a total dose of 3 mg/kg; given via infusion—maintenance infusion at 1 to 4 mg/min; pediatric—1 mg/kg/dose IV or IO; infusion—20 to 50 mcg/kg/min. *Special considerations:* The drug has a short half-life; if bradycardia is present with premature ventricular contractions, the bradycardia is treated first with atropine; high doses can result in coma or death; decrease dose in elderly. Avoid lidocaine in reperfusion dysrhythmias after thrombolytic therapy; use extreme caution in patients with hepatic disease, heart failure, marked hypoxia, severe respiratory depression, hypovolemia, or shock.

9. Ketorolac tromethamine (Toradol). *Class:* nonsteroidal antiinflammatory. *Description:* an antiinflammatory drug that also exhibits peripherally acting nonnarcotic analgesic activity by inhibiting prostaglandin synthesis. *Indications:* Short-term management of moderate to severe pain. *Contraindications:* hypersensitivity, allergies to aspirin or other nonsteroidal antiinflammatory drugs, bleeding disorders, renal failure, active peptic ulcer disease. *Adverse reactions:* anaphylaxis from hypersensitivity, edema, sedation, bleeding disorders, rash, nausea, and headache. *Onset:* within 10 minutes. *Duration:* 6 to 8 hours. *Dose:* adult— 30 to 60 mg IM, followed by 15 to 30 mg q6h prn up to 5 days; or 30 mg IM over 1 minute (patients >65 years); one half dose (15 mg) for patients more than 65 years old and those with renal impairment. *Special considerations:* pregnancy category B safety; clear, slightly yellow solution; use with caution and reduce dose in elderly.

10. Naloxone (Narcan). *Class:* synthetic opioid antagonist. *Description:* a competitive narcotic antagonist used to manage and reverse overdoses caused by narcotics and synthetic narcotic agents. *Indications:* complete or partial reversal of narcotic depression and ventilatory depression resulting from opioids, including narcotic agonists, narcotic agonist/antagonists, and others; decreased level of consciousness, coma of unknown origin, and circulatory support in refractory shock (investigational), phencyclidine, and ethanol ingestion (investigational). *Contraindications:* hypersensitivity and caution with narcotic-dependent patients, who may experience withdrawal syndrome. *Adverse reactions:* tachycardia, hypertension, dysrhythmias, nausea, vomiting, blurred vision, withdrawal, and diaphoresis. *Onset:* within 2 minutes. *Duration:* 30 to 60 minutes. *Dose:* adult—0.4 to 2.0 mg IV or 0.4-0.8 mg lm or SQ. May be repeated in 5-minute intervals to a maximum of 10 mg; children —0.1 mg/kg/dose IV, IM, or SQ or via endotracheal administration (diluted). *Special considerations:* Seizures have been reported; drug may not reverse hypotension and may cause withdrawal syndrome; use caution if patient is a suspected narcotic addict. Naloxone has shorter duration than some narcotics; monitor patient carefully after administration.

11. Midazolam hydrochloride (Versed). *Class:* short-acting benzodiazepine. *Description:* benzodiazepine that may be administered for conscious sedation to relieve apprehension or impair memory before tracheal intubation or cardioversion. *Indications:* premedication for trachea intubation or cardioversion. *Contraindications:* hypersensitivity to midazolam; glaucoma; shock; coma; alcohol intoxication (relative); depressed vital signs; concomitant use of barbiturates, alcohol, narcotics, or other central nervous system depressants. *Adverse reactions:* respiratory depression, hiccups, cough, oversedation, pain at injection site, nausea and vomiting, headache, blurred vision, fluctuations in

vital signs, hypotension, and respiratory arrest. *Onset:* 1 to 3 minutes. *Duration:* 2 to 6 hours, dose dependent. *Dose:* adult—1 to 2.5 mg slow intravenously (over 2 to 3 minutes); repeat as needed in small increments (total maximum dose not to exceed 0.1 mg/kg); elderly—0.5 mg slow intravenously (maximum of 1.5 mg in a 2-minute period); pediatric—loading dose 0.05 to 0.2 mg/kg, followed by continued infusion at 1 to 2 mcg/kg/min. *Special considerations:* pregnancy category D; continuously monitor respiratory and cardiac function; have resuscitation equipment and medication readily at hand; never administer medication as an intravenous bolus.

12. Atropine sulfate (atropine and others). *Class:* anticholinergic agent. *Description:* drug that inhibits the action of acetylcholine at postganglionic parasympathetic receptor sites; blocks vagus nerve and causes increased heart rate and enhanced atrioventricular conduction. *Indications:* hemodynamically significant bradycardia, asystole, pulseless electrical activity, organophosphate or nerve-gas poisoning. *Contraindications:* tachycardia, hypersensitivity, unstable cardiovascular status in acute hemorrhage and myocardial ischemia, and narrow-angle glaucoma, obstructive disease of the gastrointestinal tract, obstructive uropathy, and thyrotoxicosis. *Adverse reactions:* tachycardia; paradoxical bradycardia when pushed slowly or when used at doses less than 0.5 mg; palpitations; dysrhythmias; headache; dizziness; anticholinergic effects (dry mouth, nose, skin, photophobia, blurred vision, urine retention); nausea; vomiting; flushed, hot, dry skin; and allergic reactions. *Onset:* rapid. *Duration:* 2 to 6 hours. *Dose:* Bradydysrhythmias: adult—0.5 mg intravenously every 3 to 5 minutes as needed (maximum total dose 3 mg); pediatric—0.02 mg/kg/dose intravenously or intraosseous (minimum total dose dose 0.1 mg; maximum single dose 0.5 mg for a child and 1.0 mg for an adolescent; may repeat in 5 minutes for maximum total dose of 1.0 mg child and 2.0 mg adolescent). Asystole: adult—1.0 mg intravenously or endotracheally; repeat to total dose 0.03 to 0.04 mg/kg; pediatric—same dose as bradycardia. Pulseless electrical activity: if absolute or relative bradycardia, same dose as asystole. Anticholinesterase poisoning: adult—2-4 mg intravenously every 5 to 15 minutes to dry secretions, repeated as needed; pediatric—0.05 mg/kg/dose (usual dose 1 to 5 mg) intravenously, repeated as needed every 20 minutes until atropine effect is observed. *Special considerations:* potential adverse effects when given with digitalis, cholinergics, and neostigmine; effects of atropine may be enhanced by antihistamines, procainamide, quinidine, antipsychotics, antidepressants, and benzodiazepines.

13. Epinephrine (Adrenalin). *Class:* sympathomimetic. *Description:* drug that stimulates alpha- and beta-receptors; causes bronchodilation and, when administered via rapid intravenous injection, causes rapid increases in systolic pressure, ventricular contractility, and heart rate; causes vasoconstriction of the arterioles of the skin, mucosa, and splanchnic areas; and antagonizes the effects of histamine. *Indications:* bronchial asthma, acute allergic reactions, asystole, pulseless electrical activity, ventricular fibrillation, and pulseless ventricular tachycardia. *Contraindications:* hypersensitivity, hypovolemic shock, coronary insufficiency (should be used with caution). *Adverse reactions:* headache, restlessness, weakness, dysrhythmias, hypertension, and precipitation of angina pectoris and tachycardia. *Onset:* 5 to 10 minutes (subcutaneously), 1 to 2 minutes (intravenously). *Duration:* 5 to 10 minutes. *Dose:* Asystole, pulseless electrical activity, pulseless ventricular tachycardia, or ventricular fibrillation: adult—1 mg intravenous push repeated every 3 to 5 minutes; pediatric—(0.1 ml/kg 1:10,000) intravenously or intraosseously, high (0.1 mL/kg 1:1000) via endotracheal administration (diluted to 3 to 5 mL). Bradycardia refractory to other interventions: adult—2 to 10 mcg/min (1 mg 1:1000 in 500 mL of normal saline or D_5W); pediatric—dilute 0.6 mg/kg to create 100 mL solution; begin infusion at 1 mL/hr (0.1 mcg/kg/min) and adjust every 5 minutes for desired effect (0.1 to 1.0 mcg/kg/min). Anaphylactic reaction or bronchoconstriction: adult—mild to moderate: 0.3 to 0.5 mL (1:1000) subcutaneously IM for anaphylaxis; severe: 0.1 mg (1 ml of 1:10,000) slow intravenous injection; pediatric—0.01 mL/kg subcutaneously (1:1000), maximum of 0.3 mL. *Special considerations:* Syncope has been reported after administration in children; it may increase myocardial oxygen demand.

14. Nitrous oxide:oxygen (50:50; Nitronox). *Class:* gaseous analgesic and anesthetic. *Description:* drug that depresses the central nervous system and causes anesthesia. *Indications:* moderate to severe pain. *Contraindications:* impaired level of consciousness, head injury, chest trauma, inability to comply with instructions, decompression sickness, undiagnosed abdominal pain, bowel obstruction, hypotension, shock, and chronic obstructive pulmonary disease. *Adverse reactions:* dizziness, apnea, cyanosis, nausea, vomiting, and malignant hyperthermia. *Onset:* 2 to 5 minutes. *Duration:* 2 to 5 minutes. *Dose:* adult—invert cylinder several times before use and instruct the patient to inhale deeply through the mask or mouthpiece, which the patient must hold; pediatric—same. *Special considerations:* The drug increases the incidence of spontaneous abortion; it diffuses into gas-filled pockets trapped in the patient (for example, pneumothorax, intestinal obstruction) and may cause rupture; nitrous oxide is a nonexplosive gas.

15. Sodium bicarbonate. *Class:* buffer, alkalinizing agent, electrolyte supplement. *Description:* drug that reacts with hydrogen ions to form water and carbon dioxide to buffer metabolic acidosis. *Indications:* known preexisting

metabolic acidosis, tricyclic antidepressant overdose, and alkalinization for treatment of specific intoxications. *Contraindications:* patients with chloride loss from vomiting or gastrointestinal suction, metabolic and respiratory alkalosis, hypernatremia, hypokalemia, hypocalcemia, and abdominal pain of unknown origin. *Adverse reactions:* metabolic alkalosis, hypoxia, rise in intracellular PCO_2 and increased tissue acidosis, hypernatremia, seizures, and tissue sloughing at injection site. *Onset:* 2 to 10 minutes. *Duration:* 30 to 60 minutes. *Dose:* urgent forms of metabolic acidosis: adult—1 mEq/kg intravenously repeated in 5 minutes with 0.5 mEq/kg every 10 minutes; pediatric—same. *Special considerations:* If possible, arterial blood gas analysis should guide administration of this drug; it may increase edematous or sodium-retaining states; it initially may worsen cellular acidosis; it may worsen congestive heart failure.

16. a. Thiamine (Betaxin). *Class:* vitamin (B_1). *Description:* vitamin necessary for carbohydrate metabolism. *Indications:* coma of unknown origin (with administration of dextrose 50% or naloxone), delirium tremens, beriberi, and Wernicke's encephalopathy. *Contraindications:* none significant. *Adverse reactions:* hypotension (from rapid injection or a large dose), anxiety, diaphoresis, nausea, vomiting, and allergic reaction (rare). *Onset:* rapid. *Duration:* depends on degree of deficiency. *Dose:* adult—100 mg slow intravenous or intramuscular injection. *Special considerations:* Anaphylactic reactions have been reported.

    b. Dextrose 50%. *Class:* carbohydrate and hypertonic solution. *Description:* the principal carbohydrate used in the body. *Indications:* hypoglycemia, altered level of consciousness, coma of unknown cause, seizure of unknown cause. *Contraindications:* intracranial hemorrhage, increased intracranial pressure, or suspected cerebral vascular accident in the absence of hypoglycemia. *Adverse reactions:* warmth, pain, burning from medication infusion, thrombophlebitis. *Onset:* less than 1 minute. *Duration:* depends on degree of hypoglycemia. *Dose:* adult—12.5 to 25 g slow intravenous injection (may repeat once); pediatric—0.5 to 1 g/kg/dose intravenously or intraosseously; 1 to 2 mL/kg 50%; 2 to 4 mL/kg 25%; 5 to 10 mL/kg 10%. *Special considerations:* Blood glucose analysis should be performed before administration, if possible; extravasation may cause tissue necrosis; it may sometimes precipitate severe neurological symptoms (Wernicke's encephalopathy) in patients with thiamine depletion, such as alcoholics; high-risk groups should receive thiamine before dextrose 50%.

17. Diazepam (Valium and others). *Class:* benzodiazepine. *Description:* drug that raises the seizure threshold in the cerebral cortex and acts on the limbic, thalamic, and hypothalamic regions of the brain to potentiate the effects of inhibitory neurotransmitters. *Indications:* acute anxiety states, acute alcohol withdrawal, muscle relaxation, seizure activity, and premedication to countershock or transcutaneous pacing. *Contraindications:* hypersensitivity, substance abuse, coma, shock, central nervous system depression following head injury, respiratory depression. *Adverse reactions:* hypotension, reflex tachycardia, respiratory depression, ataxia, psychomotor impairment, confusion, and nausea. *Onset:* 1 to 5 minutes (intravenously); 15 to 30 minutes (intramuscularly). *Duration:* 15 minutes to 1 hour (intravenously), 15 minutes to 1 hour (intramuscularly). *Dose:* Seizure activity: adult—5 mg intravenously over 2 minutes (may give up to 10 mg for most adults); pediatric—infants more than 30 days to 5 years: 0.2 to 0.5 mg slow intravenously or intraosseously every 2 to 5 minutes as necessary (maximum total dose 5 mg); children greater than 5 years: 1 mg every 2 to 5 minutes to maximum 10 mg slow intravenously. Premedication for cardioversion: adult—5 to 15 mg intravenously 5 to 10 minutes before procedure. *Special considerations:* Diazepam may cause local venous irritation; dose should be reduced by 50% in older adults; resuscitation equipment should be readily available; anticonvulsant effect has a short duration.

18. Albuterol (Proventil, Ventolin). *Class:* sympathomimetic bronchodilator. *Description:* a beta$_2$-specific sympathomimetic stimulant that relaxes bronchiolar smooth muscle and peripheral vasculature. *Indications:* relief of bronchospasm in patients with reversible obstructive airway disease and prevention of exercise-induced bronchospasm. *Contraindications:* hypersensitivity, cardiac dysrhythmias associated with tachycardia. *Adverse reactions:* restlessness, apprehension, dizziness, palpitations, increased blood pressure, and dysrhythmias. *Onset:* 5 to 15 minutes via inhalation. *Duration:* 3 to 4 hours via inhalation. *Dose:* bronchial asthma: adults—via metered-dose inhaler, 1 to 2 inhalations (90 to 180 mcg) every 4 to 6 hours (5 minutes between inhalations); via inhalation, 2.5 mg (0.5 mL of 0.5% solution) diluted to 3 mL with 0.9% NaCl administered over 5 to 15 minutes; pediatric—via solution, 0.01 to 0.03 mL (0.05 to 0.15 mg) per kilogram per dose to a maximum of 0.5 mL/dose diluted in 2 mL of 0.9% normal saline (may be repeated every 20 minutes, 3 times). *Special considerations:* Sympathomimetics may exacerbate adverse cardiac effects; drug may potentiate hypokalemia; it may precipitate angina pectoris and dysrhythmias; it should be used with caution with patients with diabetes mellitus, hyperthyroidism, prostatic hypertrophy, cardiovascular disorder or seizure disorder; it should be administered only by inhalation in prehospital care.

19. Aspirin (ASA, Bayer, Ecotrin, St. Joseph, others). *Class:* analgesic, antiinflammatory, antiplatelet, antipyretic. *Description:* drug that blocks pain impulses in the central nervous system, dilates peripheral vessels, and decreases platelet aggregation. *Indications:* mild to moderate pain or fever; prevention of platelet aggregation in

ischemia and thromboembolism; unstable angina; prevention of myocardial infarction or reinfarction. *Contraindications:* hypersensitivity to salicylates; gastrointestinal bleeding; active ulcer disease; hemorrhagic stroke; bleeding disorders; children. *Adverse reactions:* stomach irritation, heartburn or indigestion, nausea or vomiting, allergic reaction. *Onset:* 15 to 30 minutes. *Duration:* 4 to 6 hours. *Dose:* adult—mild pain or fever: 325 to 650 mg PO q4h; myocardial infarction—160 to 325 mg PO (chew).

20. Adenosine (Adenocard). *Class:* endogenous nucleotide, miscellaneous antidysrhythmic agent. *Description:* drug that slows tachycardia associated with the atrioventricular node via modulation of the autonomic nervous system without causing negative inotropic effects and acts directly on sinus pacemaker cells and vagal nerve terminals to decrease chronotropic and dromotropic activity. *Indications:* treatment of supraventricular tachycardia. *Contraindications:* second- or third-degree atrioventricular block, sick sinus syndrome, and hypersensitivity to adenosine; adenosine will not convert atrial flutter, atrial fibrillation, and ventricular tachycardia. *Adverse reactions:* light-headedness, paresthesia, headache, diaphoresis, palpitations, chest pain, hypotension, dyspnea, nausea, and metallic taste. Transient sinus bradycardia, sinus pause, bradyasystole ventricular ectopy. *Onset:* immediate. *Duration:* 10 seconds. *Dose:* adult—initial, 6 mg over 1 to 3 seconds, if no response in 1 to 2 minutes, administration of 12 mg over 1 to 3 seconds, 12-mg dose repeated once as necessary; pediatric—0.1 mg/kg rapid intravenous injection; may be doubled once (maximum single dose 12 mg). *Special considerations:* Methylxanthines antagonize the action of adenosine; dipyridamole potentiates the effect of adenosine; carbamazepine may potentiate the atrioventricular-nodal blocking effect of adenosine; adenosine may produce bronchoconstriction in patients with asthma or bronchopulmonary disease; asystole (up to 15 seconds) followed by normal sinus rhythm is common after administration.

21. a. Morphine sulfate (Astramorph/PF and others). *Class:* opioid analgesic. *Description:* drug that increases peripheral venous capacitance and decreases venous return; promotes analgesia, euphoria, and respiratory and physical depression; decreases myocardial oxygen demand; a Schedule II drug. *Indications:* chest pain associated with myocardial infarction, moderate to severe acute or chronic pain, and pulmonary edema with or without pain. *Contraindications:* hypersensitivity to narcotics, hypovolemia, hypotension, head injury or undiagnosed abdominal pain, and patients who have taken monoamine oxidase inhibitors within 14 days; increased intracranial pressure; and severe respiratory depression. *Adverse reactions:* hypotension, tachycardia, bradycardia, palpitations, syncope, facial flushing, respiratory depression, euphoria, bronchospasm, dry mouth, and allergic reaction. *Onset:* 1 to 2 minutes. *Duration:* 2 to 7 hours. *Dose:* adult—2 to 4 mg intravenously every 5 to 15 minutes titrated to relief of pain; pediatric—0.1 to 0.2 mg/kg/dose intravenously (maximum 15-mg total dose). *Special considerations:* Narcotics rapidly cross the placenta; drug should be used with caution with older adults, patients with asthma, and patients susceptible to central nervous system depression; naloxone should be readily available; drug may worsen bradycardia or heart block in inferior myocardial infarction (vagotonic effect).

    b. Meperidine (Demerol). *Class:* opioid analgesic. *Description:* an opioid agonist that produces analgesia, euphoria, and respiratory and central nervous system depression. *Indications:* moderate to severe pain, preoperative medication, obstetrical analgesia. *Contraindications:* hypersensitivity to narcotics, concurrent use of monoamine oxidase inhibitors or selective serotonin reuptake inhibitors, labor or delivery of a premature infant, and head injury. *Adverse reactions:* respiratory depression, euphoria, delirium, agitation, hallucination, seizures, headache, visual disturbances, coma, facial flushing, hypotension, circulatory collapse, dysrhythmias, allergic reaction, nausea, and vomiting. *Onset:* 10 to 45 minutes (intramuscularly), within 5 minutes (intravenously). *Duration:* 2 to 4 hours. *Dose:* adult—50 to 100 mg every 3 to 4 hours (intramuscularly), 15 to 35 mg (intravenously); pediatric—1 to 2 mg/kg/dose (intramuscularly) every 3 to 4 hours. *Special considerations:* Drug should be used with caution in patients with asthma and chronic obstructive pulmonary disease and may aggravate seizures in patients with convulsive disorders; nalaxone should be readily available.

22. Labetalol (Normodyne, Trandate). *Class:* alpha- and beta-adrenergic blocker. *Description:* competitive alpha$_1$-receptor blocker and a nonselective beta-receptor blocker used to lower blood pressure in hypertensive crisis. *Indications:* hypertensive emergencies. *Contraindications:* bronchial asthma (relative), uncompensated congestive heart failure, second- and third-degree heart block, bradycardia, cardiogenic shock, pulmonary edema, BP <100 mm Hg. *Adverse reactions:* dose-related orthostatic hypotension, headache, dizziness, edema, fatigue, vertigo, ventricular dysrhythmias, dyspnea, allergic reaction, facial flushing, diaphoresis. *Onset:* within 5 minutes. *Duration:* 3 to 6 hours. *Dose:* adult—10 mg slow intravenous bolus over 2 minutes; additional injections at 10-minute intervals as needed (maximum 150 mg); infusion—mix 200 mg in 250 mL D$_5$W (0.8 mg/mL) and infuse at a rate of 2 to 8 mg/min, titrated to supine blood pressure (maximum 300 mg). *Special considerations:* pregnancy safety category C; monitor blood pressure, pulse, electrocardiogram continuously; observe for signs of congestive heart failure, bradycardia, bronchospasm; administer with patient in supine position.

23. Activated charcoal (Actidose-Aqua, Liqui-Char). *Class:* adsorbent, antidote. *Description:* drug that binds and adsorbs ingested toxins. *Indications:* many oral poisonings and medication overdoses. *Contraindications:* corrosives, gastrointestinal bleeding, caustics, and petroleum distillates. *Adverse reactions:* nausea (indirectly), vomiting, and constipation. *Onset:* immediate. *Duration:* continual in gastrointestinal tract. *Dose:* prepared in a slurry and administered by mouth or slowly by gastric tube; adult—30 to 100 g; pediatric—15 to 30 g; infant less than 1 year—1 g/kg. *Special considerations:* Drug does not adsorb all drugs and toxic substances (for example, phenobarbital, aspirin, cyanide, lithium, iron, lead, and arsenic).

24. Magnesium sulfate. *Class:* electrolyte, anticonvulsant. *Description:* drug that reduces striated muscle contractions and blocks peripheral neuromuscular transmission by reducing acetylcholine release at the myoneural junction. *Indications:* seizures resulting from eclampsia, torsades de pointes, refractory ventricular fibrillation, with suspected hypomagnesemia. *Contraindications:* heart block or myocardial damage. *Adverse reactions:* diaphoresis, facial flushing, hypotension, depressed reflexes, hypothermia, reduced heart rate, circulatory collapse, diarrhea, and respiratory depression. *Onset:* (intravenously) immediate. *Duration:* 30 minutes. *Dose:* seizures associated with pregnancy: 1 to 4 g (8 to 32 mEq) intravenously; maximum dose of 1.5 mL/min. Pulseless arrest (torsades de pointes, or hypomagnesemic state): adult—1 to 2 g in 10 mL of D_5W intravenously over 5-20 minutes; pediatric—25 to 50 mg/kg over 10 to 20 minutes. *Special considerations:* Other central nervous system depressants may enhance central nervous system depressant effects; drug should not be administered in the 2 hours before delivery; calcium gluconate or calcium chloride should be available as antagonist; drug may be needed for up to 48 hours after delivery; use with caution in patients with renal failure.

25. Dopamine (Intropin). *Class:* sympathomimetic. *Description:* drug that acts on alpha$_1$- and beta-adrenergic receptors, increasing systemic vascular resistance and exerting a positive inotropic effect on the heart. *Indications:* hemodynamically significant hypotension in the absence of hypovolemia. *Contraindications:* tachydysrhythmias, ventricular fibrillation, and patients with pheochromocytoma. *Adverse reactions:* dose-related tachycardias, hypertension, and increased myocardial oxygen demand. *Onset:* 2 to 4 minutes. *Duration:* 10 to 15 minutes. *Dose:* adult—dosage range of 2 to 20 mcg/kg/min recommended; pediatric—2 to 20 mcg/kg/min; intravenously or intraosseously titrated to patient response (not to exceed 20 mcg/kg/min). *Special considerations:* Drug should be infused through a large, stable vein to avoid extravasation injury; patient should be monitored for signs of compromised circulation; infusion pump is recommended.

26. Verapamil (Isoptin). *Class:* calcium channel blocker (Class IV antidysrhythmic). *Description:* antidysrhythmic, antianginal, antihypertensive; inhibits the movement of calcium ions across cell membranes, decreases atrial automaticity, reduces atrioventricular conduction velocity, prolongs the atrioventricular nodal refractory period, decreases myocardial contractility, reduces vascular smooth muscle tone, and dilates coronary arteries and arterioles. *Indications:* paroxysmal supraventricular tachycardia (unresponsive to vagal maneuvers or adenosine), atrial flutter with rapid ventricular response, and atrial fibrillation with a rapid ventricular response; chronic stable angina. *Contraindications:* hypersensitivity, sick sinus syndrome (unless the patient has a pacemaker), second- or third-degree heart block, hypotension, cardiogenic shock, severe congestive heart failure, Wolff-Parkinson-White syndrome with atrial fibrillation or flutter, patients receiving intravenously administered beta-blockers, wide-complex tachycardias. *Adverse reactions:* dizziness, headache, nausea, vomiting, hypotension, bradycardia, complete atrioventricular block, and peripheral edema. *Onset:* 2 to 5 minutes. *Duration:* 30 to 60 minutes. *Dose:* adult—2.5 to 5.0 mg intravenous bolus over 2 minutes; repeat with 5 to 10 mg in 15 to 30 minutes, as necessary (maximum of 30 mg). Alternative dosing: 5mg IV over 2 min every 15 min to maximum dose of 30 mg. *Special considerations:* Vital signs should be monitored closely; be prepared to resuscitate the patient; atrioventricular block or asystole may occur because of slowed atrioventricular conduction; decrease dose when administering to elderly or borderline hypotensive patients.

27. Furosemide (Lasix). *Class:* loop diuretic. *Description:* drug that inhibits reabsorption of sodium and chloride in the proximal tubule and loop of Henle; intravenous doses can increase venous capacitance and decrease preload. *Indications:* pulmonary edema associated with congestive heart failure, and hepatic or renal disease. *Contraindications:* anuria, hypersensitivity; states of severe electrolyte depletion; dehydration; known allergy to sulfonamides. *Adverse reactions:* hypotension, electrocardiogram changes, dry mouth, hypercalcemia, hypochloremia, hypokalemia, hyponatremia, and hyperglycemia; may cause hearing loss if infusion of large doses is too rapid. *Onset:* vascular effects within 5 minutes intravenously; diuresis, 15 to 20 minutes. *Duration:* 2 hours. *Dose:* adult—0.5 to 1.0 mg/kg slow intravenous injection (not to exceed 20 mg/min); if no response, double dose to 2 mg/kg slow over 2 minutes; pediatric—1 mg/kg/dose. *Special considerations:* Drug has been known to cause fetal abnormalities; it should be protected from light.

28. Oxytocin (Pitocin). *Class:* pituitary hormone. *Description:* drug that indirectly stimulates uterine smooth muscle contractions, which transiently reduce uterine blood flow, and stimulates the mammary gland to increase lactation. *Indications:* postpartum hemorrhage after infant and placental delivery; induces labor at term (not a prehospital indication). *Contraindications:* presence of a second fetus; hypertonic or hyperactive uterus. *Adverse reactions:* tachycardia, hypertension, dysrhythmias, angina pectoris, anxiety, seizure, nausea, vomiting, allergic reaction, and uterine rupture (excessive dose). *Onset:* intravenous—immediate; intramuscular—3 to 5 minutes. *Duration:* intravenous—20 minutes; intramuscular—30 to 60 minutes. *Dose:* intramuscular—3 to 10 units after delivery of the placenta; intravenous—mix 10 units in 1000 mL normal saline or lactated Ringer's solution and infuse at 20 to 30 drops/min, titrated to the severity of bleeding and uterine response. *Special considerations:* Vasopressors may potentiate hypertension; vital signs and uterine tone should be monitored closely.

29. b. Dopamine is used to increase stroke volume.

30. d. Narcotic analgesics and nitrous oxide are contraindicated in undiagnosed abdominal pain because they may mask symptoms.

31. a. Epinephrine 1:10,000 intravenously is indicated for all other conditions listed.

32. b. Adenosine, beta-blockers (atenolol), and calcium blockers (diltiazem) are Class III recommendations to control rate in atrial fibrillation/flutter in the presence of Wolff-Parkinson-White syndrome.

33. d. Calcium and pacemaker are used to treat calcium channel blocker overdose.

34. b. Treat hypovolemia with IV fluids. Dopamine can cause ventricular arrhythmias.

35. a. Aspirin and oxygen should be administered. The patient's legs should be elevated, and a fluid bolus should be administered in an attempt to increase the blood pressure. His electrocardiogram and clinical presentation suggest inferior STEM 1, the probability of right ventricular infarction, so nitroglycerin would not be given. Morphine would not be given until the blood pressure increases. Verapamil is not indicated in this setting.

36. a. All other drugs may be used later to treat specific causes of cardiac arrest.

37. c. All others are beta-agonists.

38. b. Verapamil vasodilates and further decreases blood pressure.

39. d. Albuterol is a bronchodilator. Morphine is given IV or IM. Nitro is given by infusion, SL tablet, or spray for chest pain.

40. b.

41. a. The other drugs listed increase the plasmin in the blood, which causes degradation of fibrin threads and fibrinogen.

42. c. Naloxone is administered to reverse potential narcotic intoxication. Thiamine promotes uptake of glucose in the brain and prevents the development of Wernicke's encephalopathy when glucose is administered. Dextrose 50% in water corrects underlying hypoglycemia.

43. b. It is an osmotic diuretic and pulls excess fluid from the brain, temporarily decreasing intracranial pressure.

44. a.

45. d. Oxytocin should be administered only after delivery of all the babies.

46. b. Benadryl causes thickening of the bronchial secretions and exacerbates an asthma attack.

47. d. It is contraindicated with the other ingestions listed.

48. d. It is not effective against barbiturates.

49. c. It also may cause hypotension.

50. a. Magnesium would be given if the Q-T interval were prolonged. Beta-blockers would be an option for polymorphic ventricular tachycardia. Lidocaine can be used if amiodarone is not available.

51. d.

52. b.

53. d. Furosemide decreases intravascular volume and causes vasodilation, which causes decreased preload and therefore less fluid to back up in the lungs.

54. d. Adenosine is not a calcium channel blocker and is not used to treat atrial flutter.

55. a. Atropine would increase the heart rate and the work of the heart and make the patient's condition worse.

56. b. Vistaril or phenergen often is ordered concurrently to prevent this side effect.

57. a. Haloperidol (Haldol) is a major tranquilizer.

58. d.

National Registry of Emergency Medical Technicians
Advanced Level Practical Examination

PATIENT ASSESSMENT - TRAUMA

Candidate: _____   Examiner: _____

Date: _____   Signature: _____

Scenario # _____

Time Start: _____

NOTE: Areas denoted by "**" may be integrated within sequence of Initial Assessment	Possible Points	Points Awarded
Takes or verbalizes body substance isolation precautions	1	
SCENE SIZE-UP		
Determines the scene/situation is safe	1	
Determines the mechanism of injury/nature of illness	1	
Determines the number of patients	1	
Requests additional help if necessary	1	
Considers stabilization of spine	1	
INITIAL ASSESSMENT/RESUSCITATION		
Verbalizes general impression of the patient	1	
Determines responsiveness/level of consciousness	1	
Determines chief complaint/apparent life-threats	1	
Airway -Opens and assesses airway (1 point) -Inserts adjunct as indicated (1 point)	2	
Breathing -Assess breathing (1 point) -Assures adequate ventilation (1 point) -Initiates appropriate oxygen therapy (1 point) -Manages any injury which may compromise breathing/ventilation (1 point)	4	
Circulation -Checks pulse (1point) -Assess skin [either skin color, temperature, or condition] (1 point) -Assesses for and controls major bleeding if present (1 point) -Initiates shock management (1 point)	4	
Identifies priority patients/makes transport decision	1	
FOCUSED HISTORY AND PHYSICAL EXAMINATION/RAPID TRAUMA ASSESSMENT		
Selects appropriate assessment	1	
Obtains, or directs assistant to obtain, baseline vital signs	1	
Obtains SAMPLE history	1	
DETAILED PHYSICAL EXAMINATION		
Head -Inspects mouth**, nose**, and assesses facial area (1 point) -Inspects and palpates scalp and ears (1 point) -Assesses eyes for PERRL** (1 point)	3	
Neck** -Checks position of trachea (1 point) -Checks jugular veins (1 point) -Palpates cervical spine (1 point)	3	
Chest** -Inspects chest (1 point) -Palpates chest (1 point) -Auscultates chest (1 point)	3	
Abdomen/pelvis** -Inspects and palpates abdomen (1 point) -Assesses pelvis (1 point) -Verbalizes assessment of genitalia/perineum as needed (1 point)	3	
Lower extremities** -Inspects, palpates, and assesses motor, sensory, and distal circulatory functions (1 point/leg)	2	
Upper extremities -Inspects, palpates, and assesses motor, sensory, and distal circulatory functions (1 point/arm)	2	
Posterior thorax, lumbar, and buttocks** -Inspects and palpates posterior thorax (1 point) -Inspects and palpates lumbar and buttocks area (1 point)	2	
Manages secondary injuries and wounds appropriately	1	
Performs ongoing assessment	1	
TOTAL	43	

Time End: _____

CRITICAL CRITERIA

____ Failure to initiate or call for transport of the patient within 10 minute time limit
____ Failure to take or verbalize body substance isolation precautions
____ Failure to determine scene safety
____ Failure to assess for and provide spinal protection when indicated
____ Failure to voice and ultimately provide high concentration of oxygen
____ Failure to assess/provide adequate ventilation
____ Failure to find or appropriately manage problems associated with airway, breathing, hemorrhage or shock [hypoperfusion]
____ Failure to differentiate patient's need for immediate transportation versus continued assessment/treatment at the scene
____ Does other detailed/focused history or physical exam before assessing/treating threats to airway, breathing, and circulation
____ Orders a dangerous or inappropriate intervention

You must factually document your rationale for checking any of the above critical items on the reverse side of this form.

p301/8-003k

PATIENT ASSESSMENT - MEDICAL

Candidate: _____ Examiner: _____

Date: _____ Signature: _____

Scenario:_____

Time Start: _____

	Possible Points	Points Awarded
Takes or verbalizes body substance isolation precautions	1	
SCENE SIZE-UP		
Determines the scene/situation is safe	1	
Determines the mechanism of injury/nature of illness	1	
Determines the number of patients	1	
Requests additional help if necessary	1	
Considers stabilization of spine	1	
INITIAL ASSESSMENT		
Verbalizes general impression of the patient	1	
Determines responsiveness/level of consciousness	1	
Determines chief complaint/apparent life-threats	1	
Assesses airway and breathing -Assessment (1 point) -Assures adequate ventilation (1 point) -Initiates appropriate oxygen therapy (1 point)	3	
Assesses circulation -Assesses/controls major bleeding (1 point) -Assesses skin [either skin color, temperature, or condition] (1 point) -Assesses pulse (1 point)	3	
Identifies priority patients/makes transport decision	1	
FOCUSED HISTORY AND PHYSICAL EXAMINATION/RAPID ASSESSMENT		
History of present illness -Onset (1 point) -Severity (1 point) -Provocation (1 point) -Time (1 point) -Quality (1 point) -Clarifying questions of associated signs and symptoms as related to OPQRST (2 points) -Radiation (1 point)	8	
Past medical history -Allergies (1 point) -Past pertinent history (1 point) -Events leading to present illness (1 point) -Medications (1 point) -Last oral intake (1 point)	5	
Performs focused physical examination [assess affected body part/system or, if indicated, completes rapid assessment] -Cardiovascular -Neurological -Integumentary -Reproductive -Pulmonary -Musculoskeletal -GI/GU -Psychological/Social	5	
Vital signs -Pulse (1 point) -Respiratory rate and quality (1 point each) -Blood pressure (1 point) -AVPU (1 point)	5	
Diagnostics [must include application of ECG monitor for dyspnea and chest pain]	2	
States field impression of patient	1	
Verbalizes treatment plan for patient and calls for appropriate intervention(s)	1	
Transport decision re-evaluated	1	
ON-GOING ASSESSMENT		
Repeats initial assessment	1	
Repeats vital signs	1	
Evaluates response to treatments	1	
Repeats focused assessment regarding patient complaint or injuries	1	

Time End: _____

CRITICAL CRITERIA   **TOTAL** 48

_____ Failure to initiate or call for transport of the patient within 15 minute time limit

_____ Failure to take or verbalize body substance isolation precautions

_____ Failure to determine scene safety before approaching patient

_____ Failure to voice and ultimately provide appropriate oxygen therapy

_____ Failure to assess/provide adequate ventilation

_____ Failure to find or appropriately manage problems associated with airway, breathing, hemorrhage or shock [hypoperfusion]

_____ Failure to differentiate patient's need for immediate transportation versus continued assessment and treatment at the scene

_____ Does other detailed or focused history or physical examination before assessing and treating threats to airway, breathing, and circulation

_____ Failure to determine the patient's primary problem

_____ Orders a dangerous or inappropriate intervention

_____ Failure to provide for spinal protection when indicated

You must factually document your rationale for checking any of the above critical items on the reverse side of this form.

p302/8-003k

VENTILATORY MANAGEMENT - ADULT

Candidate:_____ Examiner:_____

Date: _____ Signature: _____

NOTE: If candidate elects to ventilate initially with BVM attached to reservoir and oxygen, full credit must be awarded for steps denoted by "**" so long as first ventilation is delivered within 30 seconds.

	Possible Points	Points Awarded
Takes or verbalizes body substance isolation precautions	1	
Opens the airway manually	1	
Elevates tongue, inserts simple adjunct [oropharyngeal or nasopharyngeal airway]	1	
NOTE: Examiner now informs candidate no gag reflex is present and patient accepts adjunct		
**Ventilates patient immediately with bag-valve-mask device unattached to oxygen	1	
**Hyperventilates patient with room air	1	
NOTE: Examiner now informs candidate that ventilation is being performed without difficulty and that pulse oximetry indicates the patient's blood oxygen saturation is 85%		
Attaches oxygen reservoir to bag-valve-mask device and connects to high flow oxygen regulator [12-15 L/minute]	1	
Ventilates patient at a rate of 10-20/minute with appropriate volumes	1	
NOTE: After 30 seconds, examiner auscultates and reports breath sounds are present, equal bilaterally and medical direction has ordered intubation. The examiner must now take over ventilation.		
Directs assistant to pre-oxygenate patient	1	
Identifies/selects proper equipment for intubation	1	
Checks equipment for: -Cuff leaks (1 point) -Laryngoscope operational with bulb tight (1 point)	2	
NOTE: Examiner to remove OPA and move out of the way when candidate is prepared to intubate		
Positions head properly	1	
Inserts blade while displacing tongue	1	
Elevates mandible with laryngoscope	1	
Introduces ET tube and advances to proper depth	1	
Inflates cuff to proper pressure and disconnects syringe	1	
Directs ventilation of patient	1	
Confirms proper placement by auscultation bilaterally over each lung and over epigastrium	1	
NOTE: Examiner to ask, "If you had proper placement, what should you expect to hear?"		
Secures ET tube [may be verbalized]	1	
NOTE: Examiner now asks candidate, "Please demonstrate one additional method of verifying proper tube placement in this patient."		
Identifies/selects proper equipment	1	
Verbalizes findings and interpretations [compares indicator color to the colorimetric scale and states reading to examiner]	1	
NOTE: Examiner now states, "You see secretions in the tube and hear gurgling sounds with the patient's exhalation."		
Identifies/selects a flexible suction catheter	1	
Pre-oxygenates patient	1	
Marks maximum insertion length with thumb and forefinger	1	
Inserts catheter into the ET tube leaving catheter port open	1	
At proper insertion depth, covers catheter port and applies suction while withdrawing catheter	1	
Ventilates/directs ventilation of patient as catheter is flushed with sterile water	1	
TOTAL	27	

CRITICAL CRITERIA

_____ Failure to initiate ventilations within 30 seconds after applying gloves or interrupts ventilations for greater than 30 seconds at any time
_____ Failure to take or verbalize body substance isolation precautions
_____ Failure to voice and ultimately provide high oxygen concentrations [at least 85%]
_____ Failure to ventilate patient at a rate of at least 10/minute
_____ Failure to provide adequate volumes per breath [maximum 2 errors/minute permissible]
_____ Failure to pre-oxygenate patient prior to intubation and suctioning
_____ Failure to successfully intubate within 3 attempts
_____ Failure to disconnect syringe **immediately** after inflating cuff of ET tube
_____ Uses teeth as a fulcrum
_____ Failure to assure proper tube placement by auscultation bilaterally **and** over the epigastrium
_____ If used, stylette extends beyond end of ET tube
_____ Inserts any adjunct in a manner dangerous to the patient
_____ Suctions the patient for more than 15 seconds
_____ Does not suction the patient

You must factually document your rationale for checking any of the above critical items on the reverse side of this form.

p303/8-003k

DUAL LUMEN AIRWAY DEVICE (COMBITUBE® OR PTL®)

Candidate: _____ Examiner: _____

Date: _____ Signature: _____

NOTE: If candidate elects to initially ventilate with BVM attached to reservoir and oxygen, full credit must be awarded for steps denoted by "**" so long as first ventilation is delivered within 30 seconds.

	Possible Points	Points Awarded
Takes or verbalizes body substance isolation precautions	1	
Opens the airway manually	1	
Elevates tongue, inserts simple adjunct [oropharyngeal or nasopharyngeal airway]	1	
NOTE: *Examiner now informs candidate no gag reflex is present and patient accepts adjunct*		
**Ventilates patient immediately with bag-valve-mask device unattached to oxygen	1	
**Hyperventilates patient with room air	1	
NOTE: *Examiner now informs candidate that ventilation is being performed without difficulty*		
Attaches oxygen reservoir to bag-valve-mask device and connects to high flow oxygen regulator [12-15 L/minute]	1	
Ventilates patient at a rate of 10-20/minute with appropriate volumes	1	
NOTE: *After 30 seconds, examiner auscultates and reports breath sounds are present and equal bilaterally and medical control has ordered insertion of a dual lumen airway. The examiner must now take over ventilation.*		
Directs assistant to pre-oxygenate patient	1	
Checks/prepares airway device	1	
Lubricates distal tip of the device [may be verbalized]	1	
NOTE: *Examiner to remove OPA and move out of the way when candidate is prepared to insert device*		
Positions head properly	1	
Performs a tongue-jaw lift	1	

☐ USES COMBITUBE®	☐ USES PTL®	Possible Points	Points Awarded
Inserts device in mid-line and to depth so printed ring is at level of teeth	Inserts device in mid-line until bite block flange is at level of teeth	1	
Inflates pharyngeal cuff with proper volume and removes syringe	Secures strap	1	
Inflates distal cuff with proper volume and removes syringe	Blows into tube #1 to adequately inflate both cuffs	1	
Attaches/directs attachment of BVM to the first [esophageal placement] lumen and ventilates		1	
Confirms placement and ventilation through correct lumen by observing chest rise, auscultation over the epigastrium, and bilaterally over each lung		1	
NOTE: *The examiner states, "You do not see rise and fall of the chest and you only hear sounds over the epigastrium."*			
Attaches/directs attachment of BVM to the second [endotracheal placement] lumen and ventilates		1	
Confirms placement and ventilation through correct lumen by observing chest rise, auscultation over the epigastrium, and bilaterally over each lung		1	
NOTE: *The examiner confirms adequate chest rise, absent sounds over the epigastrium, and equal bilateral breath sounds.*			
Secures device or confirms that the device remains properly secured		1	
TOTAL		**20**	

CRITICAL CRITERIA

_____ Failure to initiate ventilations within 30 seconds after taking body substance isolation precautions or interrupts ventilations for greater than 30 seconds at any time

_____ Failure to take or verbalize body substance isolation precautions

_____ Failure to voice and ultimately provide high oxygen concentrations [at least 85%]

_____ Failure to ventilate patient at a rate of at least 10/minute

_____ Failure to provide adequate volumes per breath [maximum 2 errors/minute permissible]

_____ Failure to pre-oxygenate patient prior to insertion of the dual lumen airway device

_____ Failure to insert the dual lumen airway device at a proper depth or at either proper place within 3 attempts

_____ Failure to inflate both cuffs properly

_____ **Combitube** - failure to remove the syringe immediately after inflation of each cuff
   PTL - failure to secure the strap prior to cuff inflation

_____ Failure to confirm that the proper lumen of the device is being ventilated by observing chest rise, auscultation over the epigastrium, and bilaterally over each lung

_____ Inserts any adjunct in a manner dangerous to patient

You must factually document your rationale for checking any of the above critical items on the reverse side of this form.

p304/8-003k

PEDIATRIC (<2 yrs.) VENTILATORY MANAGEMENT

Candidate: _____ Examiner _____

Date: _____ Signature: _____

NOTE: If candidate elects to ventilate initially with BVM attached to reservoir and oxygen, full credit must be awarded for steps denoted by "**" so long as first ventilation is delivered within 30 seconds.

	Possible Points	Points Awarded
Takes or verbalizes body substance isolation precautions	1	
Opens the airway manually	1	
Elevates tongue, inserts simple adjunct [oropharyngeal or nasopharyngeal airway]	1	
NOTE: Examiner now informs candidate no gag reflex is present and patient accepts adjunct		
**Ventilates patient immediately with bag-valve-mask device unattached to oxygen	1	
**Hyperventilates patient with room air	1	
NOTE: Examiner now informs candidate that ventilation is being performed without difficulty and that pulse oximetry indicates the patient's blood oxygen saturation is 85%		
Attaches oxygen reservoir to bag-valve-mask device and connects to high flow oxygen regulator [12-15 L/minute]	1	
Ventilates patient at a rate of 20-30/minute and assures adequate chest expansion	1	
NOTE: After 30 seconds, examiner auscultates and reports breath sounds are present, equal bilaterally and medical direction has ordered intubation. The examiner must now take over ventilation.		
Directs assistant to pre-oxygenate patient	1	
Identifies/selects proper equipment for intubation	1	
Checks laryngoscope to assure operational with bulb tight	1	
NOTE: Examiner to remove OPA and move out of the way when candidate is prepared to intubate		
Places patient in neutral or sniffing position	1	
Inserts blade while displacing tongue	1	
Elevates mandible with laryngoscope	1	
Introduces ET tube and advances to proper depth	1	
Directs ventilation of patient	1	
Confirms proper placement by auscultation bilaterally over each lung and over epigastrium	1	
NOTE: Examiner to ask, "If you had proper placement, what should you expect to hear?"		
Secures ET tube [may be verbalized]	1	

TOTAL 17

CRITICAL CRITERIA

_____ Failure to initiate ventilations within 30 seconds after applying gloves or interrupts ventilations for greater than 30 seconds at any time
_____ Failure to take or verbalize body substance isolation precautions
_____ Failure to pad under the torso to allow neutral head position or sniffing position
_____ Failure to voice and ultimately provide high oxygen concentrations [at least 85%]
_____ Failure to ventilate patient at a rate of at least 20/minute
_____ Failure to provide adequate volumes per breath [maximum 2 errors/minute permissible]
_____ Failure to pre-oxygenate patient prior to intubation
_____ Failure to successfully intubate within 3 attempts
_____ Uses gums as a fulcrum
_____ Failure to assure proper tube placement by auscultation bilaterally **and** over the epigastrium
_____ Inserts any adjunct in a manner dangerous to the patient
_____ Attempts to use any equipment not appropriate for the pediatric patient

You must factually document your rationale for checking any of the above critical items on the reverse side of this form.

National Registry of Emergency Medical Technicians
Advanced Level Practical Examination

DYNAMIC CARDIOLOGY

Candidate: _____ Examiner: _____

Date: _____ Signature: _____

SET #_____

Level of Testing:　　　□ NREMT-Intermediate/99　　　　□ NREMT-Paramedic

Time Start:_____	Possible Points	Points Awarded
Takes or verbalizes infection control precautions	1	
Checks level of responsiveness	1	
Checks ABCs	1	
Initiates CPR if appropriate [verbally]	1	
Attaches ECG monitor in a timely fashion or applies paddles for "Quick Look"	1	
Correctly interprets initial rhythm	1	
Appropriately manages initial rhythm	2	
Notes change in rhythm	1	
Checks patient condition to include pulse and, if appropriate, BP	1	
Correctly interprets second rhythm	1	
Appropriately manages second rhythm	2	
Notes change in rhythm	1	
Checks patient condition to include pulse and, if appropriate, BP	1	
Correctly interprets third rhythm	1	
Appropriately manages third rhythm	2	
Notes change in rhythm	1	
Checks patient condition to include pulse and, if appropriate, BP	1	
Correctly interprets fourth rhythm	1	
Appropriately manages fourth rhythm	2	
Orders high percentages of supplemental oxygen at proper times	1	
Time End: _____ 　　　　　　　　　　　　　　　　**TOTAL**	24	

CRITICAL CRITERIA

_____ Failure to deliver first shock in a timely manner due to operator delay in machine use or providing treatments other than CPR with simple adjuncts

_____ Failure to deliver second or third shocks without delay other than the time required to reassess rhythm and recharge paddles

_____ Failure to verify rhythm before delivering each shock

_____ Failure to ensure the safety of self and others [verbalizes "All clear" and observes]

_____ Inability to deliver DC shock [does not use machine properly]

_____ Failure to demonstrate acceptable shock sequence

_____ Failure to order initiation or resumption of CPR when appropriate

_____ Failure to order correct management of airway [ET when appropriate]

_____ Failure to order administration of appropriate oxygen at proper time

_____ Failure to diagnose or treat 2 or more rhythms correctly

_____ Orders administration of an inappropriate drug or lethal dosage

_____ Failure to correctly diagnose or adequately treat v-fib, v-tach, or asystole

You must factually document your rationale for checking any of the above critical items on the reverse side of this form.

p306/8-003k

National Registry of Emergency Medical Technicians
Advanced Level Practical Examination

STATIC CARDIOLOGY

Candidate: _____ Examiner: _____

Date: _____ Signature: _____

SET #_____

Level of Testing: □ NREMT-Intermediate/99 □ NREMT-Paramedic

Note: No points for treatment may be awarded if the diagnosis is incorrect.
Only document incorrect responses in spaces provided.

Time Start:_____

	Possible Points	Points Awarded
STRIP #1		
Diagnosis:	1	
Treatment:	2	
STRIP #2		
Diagnosis:	1	
Treatment:	2	
STRIP #3		
Diagnosis:	1	
Treatment:	2	
STRIP #4		
Diagnosis:	1	
Treatment:	2	
Time End: _____ **TOTAL**	12	

p307/8-003k

INTRAVENOUS THERAPY

Candidate: _____ Examiner: _____

Date: _____ Signature: _____

Level of Testing: ❏ NREMT-Intermediate/85   ❏ NREMT-Intermediate/99   ❏ NREMT-Paramedic

Time Start: _____

	Possible Points	Points Awarded

Checks selected IV fluid for:
    -Proper fluid (1 point)
    -Clarity (1 point)
	2	

Selects appropriate catheter	1	
Selects proper administration set	1	
Connects IV tubing to the IV bag	1	
Prepares administration set [fills drip chamber and flushes tubing]	1	
Cuts or tears tape [at any time before venipuncture]	1	
Takes/verbalizes body substance isolation precautions [prior to venipuncture]	1	
Applies tourniquet	1	
Palpates suitable vein	1	
Cleanses site appropriately	1	

Performs venipuncture
    -Inserts stylette (1 point)
    -Notes or verbalizes flashback (1 point)
    -Occludes vein proximal to catheter (1 point)
    -Removes stylette (1 point)
    -Connects IV tubing to catheter (1 point)
	5	

Disposes/verbalizes disposal of needle in proper container	1	
Releases tourniquet	1	
Runs IV for a brief period to assure patent line	1	
Secures catheter [tapes securely or verbalizes]	1	
Adjusts flow rate as appropriate	1	

Time End: _____   **TOTAL**   21

CRITICAL CRITERIA

_____ Failure to establish a patent and properly adjusted IV within 6 minute time limit
_____ Failure to take or verbalize body substance isolation precautions prior to performing venipuncture
_____ Contaminates equipment or site without appropriately correcting situation
_____ Performs any improper technique resulting in the potential for uncontrolled hemorrhage, catheter shear, or air embolism
_____ Failure to successfully establish IV within 3 attempts during 6 minute time limit
_____ Failure to dispose/verbalize disposal of needle in proper container

NOTE: Check here (_____) if candidate did not establish a patent IV and do not evaluate IV Bolus Medications.

INTRAVENOUS BOLUS MEDICATIONS

Time Start: _____

Asks patient for known allergies	1	
Selects correct medication	1	
Assures correct concentration of drug	1	
Assembles prefilled syringe correctly and dispels air	1	
Continues body substance isolation precautions	1	
Cleanses injection site [Y-port or hub]	1	
Reaffirms medication	1	
Stops IV flow [pinches tubing or shuts off]	1	
Administers correct dose at proper push rate	1	
Disposes/verbalizes proper disposal of syringe and needle in proper container	1	
Flushes tubing [runs wide open for a brief period]	1	
Adjusts drip rate to TKO/KVO	1	
Verbalizes need to observe patient for desired effect/adverse side effects	1	

Time End: _____   **TOTAL**   13

CRITICAL CRITERIA

_____ Failure to begin administration of medication within 3 minute time limit
_____ Contaminates equipment or site without appropriately correcting situation
_____ Failure to adequately dispel air resulting in potential for air embolism
_____ Injects improper drug or dosage [wrong drug, incorrect amount, or pushes at inappropriate rate]
_____ Failure to flush IV tubing after injecting medication
_____ Recaps needle or failure to dispose/verbalize disposal of syringe and needle in proper container

You must factually document your rationale for checking any of the above critical items on the reverse side of this form.

p309/8-003k

PEDIATRIC INTRAOSSEOUS INFUSION

Candidate: _____ Examiner: _____

Date: _____ Signature: _____

Time Start:_____	Possible Points	Points Awarded
Checks selected IV fluid for: -Proper fluid (1 point) -Clarity (1 point)	2	
Selects appropriate equipment to include: -IO needle (1 point) -Syringe (1 point) -Saline (1 point) -Extension set (1 point)	4	
Selects proper administration set	1	
Connects administration set to bag	1	
Prepares administration set [fills drip chamber and flushes tubing]	1	
Prepares syringe and extension tubing	1	
Cuts or tears tape [at any time before IO puncture]	1	
Takes or verbalizes body substance isolation precautions [prior to IO puncture]	1	
Identifies proper anatomical site for IO puncture	1	
Cleanses site appropriately	1	
Performs IO puncture: -Stabilizes tibia (1 point) -Inserts needle at proper angle (1 point) -Advances needle with twisting motion until "pop" is felt (1 point) -Unscrews cap and removes stylette from needle (1 point)	4	
Disposes of needle in proper container	1	
Attaches syringe and extension set to IO needle and aspirates	1	
Slowly injects saline to assure proper placement of needle	1	
Connects administration set and adjusts flow rate as appropriate	1	
Secures needle with tape and supports with bulky dressing	1	
Time End: _____ **TOTAL**	23	

CRITICAL CRITERIA

_____ Failure to establish a patent and properly adjusted IO line within the 6 minute time limit
_____ Failure to take or verbalize body substance isolation precautions prior to performing IO puncture
_____ Contaminates equipment or site without appropriately correcting situation
_____ Performs any improper technique resulting in the potential for air embolism
_____ Failure to assure correct needle placement before attaching administration set
_____ Failure to successfully establish IO infusion within 2 attempts during 6 minute time limit
_____ Performing IO puncture in an unacceptable manner [improper site, incorrect needle angle, etc.]
_____ Failure to dispose of needle in proper container
_____ Orders or performs any dangerous or potentially harmful procedure

You must factually document your rationale for checking any of the above critical items on the reverse side of this form.

National Registry of Emergency Medical Technicians
Advanced Level Practical Examination

SPINAL IMMOBILIZATION (SEATED PATIENT)

Candidate:_____ Examiner:_____

Date: _____ Signature:_____

Time Start: _____	Possible Points	Points Awarded
Takes or verbalizes body substance isolation precautions	1	
Directs assistant to place/maintain head in the neutral, in-line position	1	
Directs assistant to maintain manual immobilization of the head	1	
Reassesses motor, sensory, and circulatory function in each extremity	1	
Applies appropriately sized extrication collar	1	
Positions the immobilization device behind the patient	1	
Secures the device to the patient's torso	1	
Evaluates torso fixation and adjusts as necessary	1	
Evaluates and pads behind the patient's head as necessary	1	
Secures the patient's head to the device	1	
Verbalizes moving the patient to a long backboard	1	
Reassesses motor, sensory, and circulatory function in each extremity	1	

Time End: _____   **TOTAL**   12

CRITICAL CRITERIA

_____ Did not immediately direct or take manual immobilization of the head
_____ Did not properly apply appropriately sized cervical collar before ordering release of manual immobilization
_____ Released or ordered release of manual immobilization before it was maintained mechanically
_____ Manipulated or moved patient excessively causing potential spinal compromise
_____ Head immobilized to the device **before** device sufficiently secured to torso
_____ Device moves excessively up, down, left, or right on the patient's torso
_____ Head immobilization allows for excessive movement
_____ Torso fixation inhibits chest rise, resulting in respiratory compromise
_____ Upon completion of immobilization, head is not in a neutral, in-line position
_____ Did not reassess motor, sensory, and circulatory functions in each extremity after voicing immobilization to the long backboard

You must factually document your rationale for checking any of the above critical items on the reverse side of this form.

SPINAL IMMOBILIZATION (SUPINE PATIENT)

Candidate:_____Examiner:_____

Date: _____Signature:_____

	Possible Points	Points Awarded
Time Start: _____		
Takes or verbalizes body substance isolation precautions	1	
Directs assistant to place/maintain head in the neutral, in-line position	1	
Directs assistant to maintain manual immobilization of the head	1	
Reassesses motor, sensory, and circulatory function in each extremity	1	
Applies appropriately sized extrication collar	1	
Positions the immobilization device appropriately	1	
Directs movement of the patient onto the device without compromising the integrity of the spine	1	
Applies padding to voids between the torso and the device as necessary	1	
Immobilizes the patient's torso to the device	1	
Evaluates and pads behind the patient's head as necessary	1	
Immobilizes the patient's head to the device	1	
Secures the patient's legs to the device	1	
Secures the patient's arms to the device	1	
Reassesses motor, sensory, and circulatory function in each extremity	1	
Time End: _____ **TOTAL**	14	

CRITICAL CRITERIA

_____ Did not immediately direct or take manual immobilization of the head

_____ Did not properly apply appropriately sized cervical collar before ordering release of manual immobilization

_____ Released or ordered release of manual immobilization before it was maintained mechanically

_____ Manipulated or moved patient excessively causing potential spinal compromise

_____ Head immobilized to the device **before** device sufficiently secured to torso

_____ Patient moves excessively up, down, left, or right on the device

_____ Head immobilization allows for excessive movement

_____ Upon completion of immobilization, head is not in a neutral, in-line position

_____ Did not reassess motor, sensory, and circulatory functions in each extremity after voicing immobilization to the device

You must factually document your rationale for checking any of the above critical items on the reverse side of this form.

p312/8-003k

BLEEDING CONTROL/SHOCK MANAGEMENT

Candidate: _____ Examiner: _____

Date: _____ Signature: _____

Time Start:_____	Possible Points	Points Awarded
Takes or verbalizes body substance isolation precautions	1	
Applies direct pressure to the wound	1	
Elevates the extremity	1	
NOTE: The examiner must now inform the candidate that the wound continues to bleed.		
Applies an additional dressing to the wound	1	
NOTE: The examiner must now inform the candidate that the wound still continues to bleed. The second dressing does not control the bleeding.		
Locates and applies pressure to appropriate arterial pressure point	1	
NOTE: The examiner must now inform the candidate that the bleeding is controlled.		
Bandages the wound	1	
NOTE: The examiner must now inform the candidate that the patient is exhibiting signs and symptoms of hypoperfusion.		
Properly positions the patient	1	
Administers high concentration oxygen	1	
Initiates steps to prevent heat loss from the patient	1	
Indicates the need for immediate transportation	1	
Time End: _____ **TOTAL**	10	

CRITICAL CRITERIA

_____ Did not take or verbalize body substance isolation precautions

_____ Did not apply high concentration of oxygen

_____ Applied a tourniquet before attempting other methods of bleeding control

_____ Did not control hemorrhage in a timely manner

_____ Did not indicate the need for immediate transportation

You must factually document your rationale for checking any of the above critical items on the reverse side of this form.

ILLUSTRATION CREDITS AND ACKNOWLEDGMENTS

Fig. 6-1 Thibodeau GA: *Structure & function of the body,* ed 9, St Louis, 1992, Mosby.

Figs. 6-4, 6-5, 6-13, 6-14 Thibodeau GA: *Structure & function of the body,* ed 9, St Louis, 1992, Mosby (Illustrator E.W. Beck).

Figs. 6-6, 6-8 Seeley R, Stephens T, Tate P: *Anatomy & physiology,* ed 2, St Louis, 1992, Mosby (Illustrator David J. Mascaro & Associates).

Fig. 6-18 Thibodeau GA: *Structure & function of the body,* ed 9, St Louis, 1992, Mosby (Illustrator Branislav Vidic).

Figs. 6-10, 6-11 Thibodeau GA: *Structure & function of the body,* ed 9, St Louis, 1992, Mosby (Illustrator Christine Oleksyk).

Fig. 6-15 Seeley R: *Anatomy & physiology,* ed 2, St Louis, 1992, Mosby (Sims/Illustrator Jody L. Fulks).

Fig. 6-16 Thibodeau GA: *Structure & function of the body,* ed 9, St Louis, 1992, Mosby (Illustrator Barbara Cousins).

Fig. 6-17 Thibodeau GA: *Structure & function of the body,* ed. 9, St Louis, 1992, Mosby (Illustrator William Ober).

Figs. 29-1, 29-3 Cotton S: *Mosby's paramedic study guide,* St Louis, 1989, Mosby.

Figs. 29-4, 29-12 Huszar R: *Basic dysrhythmias,* ed 2, St Louis, 1994, Mosby.